Natural Brain Support

Your Guide to Preventing and Treating Alzheimer's, Dementia and Other Related Diseases Naturally

Michael Edson, MS, L.Ac.

Copyright 2021 by Michael Edson, L.Ac.

All Rights Reserved

No part of this book may be reproduced in any form

without the written consent of the authors.

ISBN 978-15136-6311-1

Library of Congress Control Number:2020946315

Printed in the United States of America

Published by Safe Goods

561 Shunpike Rd., Sheffield, MA 01257

SafeGoodsPublishing.com

Natural Brain Support is not intended as medical advice. No claims are made for the ability of products mentioned to treat, cure, or prevent any disease. No promise is made for health, and no diagnostic or health claims are stated. This literature is for informational purposes only and is not meant to diagnose, or prescribe for, any health condition. Always see a doctor for matters relating to your health. The FDA has not evaluated this information.

Table of Contents

Introduction

My interest in dementia and Alzheimer's disease began in my 20s when my grandmother suffered a stroke which resulted in memory dysfunction and dementia. I was impressed by my father's initiative in playing simply games with her to try to stimulate her brain. Unfortunately, all the appropriate games were designed and labeled for children. I was inspired to create an activity called "Remember With Me" that used a dozen 6" x 10" photographs of common daily life occurrences such as a picture of a plane, monkey, train, etc. These photos corresponded to related sounds on a tape (converted CD format) with questions on the back of each picture; they start in the 1920s and continue to the present. The idea was to try and stimulate long-term memory (the most enduring) and then work forward into short-term memory. Short-term memory loss is an early symptom of Alzheimer's; long-term memories remain the longest before advanced Alzheimer's sets in.

Recreational therapists in long-term care Alzheimer's facilities used this kit in test form and helped me refine it. I bought it to market and sold thousands to (mostly) recreational therapists and social workers. There was one incident in which a resident suffering from serious dementia (had not spoken a word in a year) saw the picture of the plane, heard the sound of the plane flying overhead, then opened her pocketbook and took out pictures from a trip she had taken many years earlier.

My interest over the years in this field has continued as I have seen my great aunt and uncle suffer from AD, as well as my parents developing late-stage dementia. My business partner and I recently wrote a 799-page book called *Natural Eye Care: Your Guide to Healthy Vision and Healing*. While writing this book, I found it fascinating that the many of the nutrients that help the eyes also directly support brain health, even to the effect of reducing beta amyloid and tau protein build-up found in AD patients. The body actually allows many of these nutrients to cross the blood-brain barrier, while blocking out unwanted substances and pathogens. Writing a book on brain health had been in the back of my mind for many years, and I finally decided to embark on this mission.

In the process, I have read some great books (see the Appendix for recommended readings), and determined that as excellent as these books were, there was much more I could add to the conversation. This includes analyzing the research on over seventy nutrients that benefit brain health and summarizing them in a more compact way in a nutrient chart. Some nutrients provide multiple benefits from helping prevent and even reducing amyloid beta and build-up of neurofibrillary fibers (from excess tao protein) to supporting neurogenesis (production of new neurons), reducing brain inflammation, preventing premature brain cell death, supporting mitochondria, and much more.

As a licensed acupuncturist, I also wanted to introduce "alternative approaches" to supporting brain health. For example, Chinese medicine and Ayurvedic medicine has been practiced for thousands of years and offers great wisdom in ways to keep the brain (and overall body) healthy. It approaches health from a whole-body perspective, where all parts of the body are interconnected and when we are "out of balance" in one part of the body, this can eventually cause other health problems over time.

These approaches focus on looking at each person as a unique individual, so treatment strategies will vary depending on each person's imbalances despite similar symptoms. Western medicine tends to offer the same medications (and often same dosages regardless of weight, size, and individual sensitivities), without really looking at people in this manner, with the medications often addressing only single factors. In the case of AD for example, one of the main medications used is Memantine (Namenda), which focuses on by regulating the activity of glutamate, a messenger chemical widely involved in brain functions. This approach doesn't look at the multiple contributing causative factors to AD so ultimately has limited benefit. Functional medicine is an exception as an evolving Western medicine approach, often focusing on the underlying (root) cause of disease, particularly related to gut health and nutrition.

The brain is connected to the health of the whole body, so when one looks at brain health, we also have to look at many other variables that contribute both to its healthy function as well as its decline. Medications may help in the short-term, but single solutions are not going to bring overall positive results without evaluating the complex relationship of the whole body to the brain at which this book attempts to look.

I hope my book brings more light to the discussion of how to keep our brain healthy for a lifetime, and address the serious growing crisis surrounding dementia and AD.

Michael Edson, MS, L.Ac.
President, Natural Eye Care, Inc.
Co-Author, *Natural Eye Care: Your Guide to Vision Health and Healing (2019),*
Natural Eye Care: A Comprehensive Guide for Practitioners of Oriental Medicine (2003),
Author, *Natural Parkinson's Support: Ways to Keep Your Brain Healthy Naturally (2020).*

A note on sources

Not all research is equal, and sometimes it is difficult to identify poorly done research. Some studies may be poorly designed, not be placebo-controlled, not be randomized, not have a large enough sample size, be of too short period, not be free of conflict-of-interest, and so forth. We have attempted to rely on research that avoids those weaknesses, but we are not statisticians. The best studies are probably those that are reviews of the literature, or meta-analysis where the researcher is looking at a number of studies that meet certain standards. Other studies that we favor are those where the same results are corroborated by different teams of researchers. In short, we've done our best to rely on good results.

The abstracts (summaries) and sometimes the entire text of almost all of the research in our endnotes may be found at PubMed – the research database of the National Institutes of Health. that is located at https://www.ncbi.nlm.nih.gov/pubmed. The website has an excellent search feature, so you can input your search query (e.g. the name of an herb and a condition) to look for newer or additional corroborating research.

Author

Michael Edson, MS, L.Ac is a co-founder and President of Natural Eye Care, Inc. He is a New York State licensed acupuncturist and teaches workshops on vision care with co-founder Dr. Marc Grossman, specializing in Qi Gong for vision. He is co-author of *Natural Eye Care: A Comprehensive Manual for Practitioners of Oriental Medicine* and *Natural Eye Care: Your Guide to Healthy Vision and Healing*, 2019. Recent titles are *Natural Parkinson's Support: Your Guide to Preventing and Managing Parkinson's* (2020). His upcoming book, *Natural Brain Support Your Guide to Preventing and Treating Alzheimer's, Dementia and Other Related Diseases Naturally* (2021) and is co-author with Dr. Marc Grossman of the *Natural Eye Care Series*.

Chapter 1. How the Brain Works

The amazing brain is composed of over one hundred billion neurons with over one trillion supporting cells. It is the primary center that drives our responses to our environment. The healthy brain is resilient and neural circuitry adapts to a new situation along with underlying changes in gene expression.[1] Each neuron can have up to ten thousand connections to other neurons, and it is these interconnections that are critical to one's ability to think, feel, analyze, remember and process new information. The neurons communicate with each other by releasing chemical signals called "neurotransmitters" into the spaces between each of the neurons. These are known as "synapses."

Parts of the Brain

Physiologists have divided the brain into sections depending on the apparent function of that part of the brain.

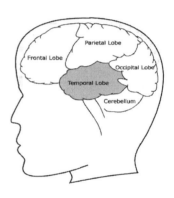

The frontal lobe, containing the **prefrontal cortex** which controls higher-order cognitive functions including planning and decision-making, problem solving, abstract rule learning, cognitive flexibility, and spatial working memory. The **parietal lobe** is associated with perceiving tactile sensory information such as pressure, touch, and pain. The **occipital lobe** interprets visual information, and the **temporal lobe** interprets sounds and language. The temporal lobe is linked to memory since it includes the hippocampus. The **cerebellum** is located at the rear of the brain and is critical for fine motor control.

Memory is one of the important functional aspects of the central nervous system (CNS) and is categorized as sensory, short term, and long-term. **Sensory memory** is dependent upon the parietal and temporal lobes. **Short-term memory** is dependent on the function of the prefrontal and parietal lobes, while **long-term memory** depends on the function of larger areas of the brain.[2]

Prefrontal Cortex

The prefrontal cortex (PFC) is located at the front of the frontal lobe. It is implicated in a variety of complex behaviors, including planning, and greatly contributes to personality development. Studied under stress, it has provided important clues to age-related loss of resilience and impaired memory as well as effects of circadian disruption and extinction of fear memory.[3] Within the prefrontal cortex chronic stress causes some neurons (medial PFC neurons) to lose branches and shrink dendrites. However, some types of neurons (orbitofrontal cortical neurons) experience expanding dendrites which may be related to increased vigilance.[4][5][6]

The Temporal Lobe

The temporal lobe is involved in primary auditory perception, such as hearing, and holds the primary auditory cortex. It is home to a number of glands and clusters of neurons with specific functions. The **amygdala** is linked to emotions. The **striatum**, in addition to its role in control of motivated movement, is also involved in working memory, abstract rule learning, and attention control. The **hippocampus** is responsible for memory storage and is critical for the formation and consolidation of declarative (factual) memories.

Cognition means reception and perception of perceived stimuli and its interpretation, which includes learning, decision making, attention, and judgment,[7] which is mainly formed in the hippocampus, amygdala, and temporal lobe.[8]

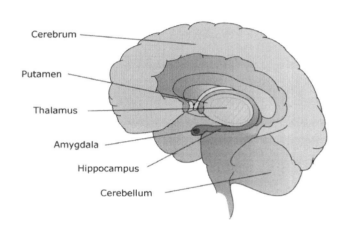

Hippocampus

Total function of memory and the conversion of short-term memory to long-term memory are dependent on the hippocampus,[9] an area of the brain with the highest density of glucocorticosteroid receptors and also represents the highest level of response to stress.

Glucocorticosteroids are a class of corticosteroid hormones more commonly known as glucocorticoids. They bind to glucocorticoid receptors in the hippocampus[10] and are necessary to improve learning and memory. Studies have shown that stress can cause functional and structural changes in the hippocampus[11] including atrophy and neurogenesis disorders.[12]

Chronic stress and, consequently, an increase in plasma cortisol, leads to a reduction in the number of dendritic branches,[13] and neurons,[14] structural changes in synaptic terminals,[15] and decreased neurogenesis in hippocampus tissue.[16] Glucocorticosteroids induce these changes by effecting the cellular metabolism of neurons,[17] increasing the sensitivity of hippocampus cells to stimulatory amino acids,[18] and/or increasing the level of extracellular glutamate.[19] Excitatory amino acids, particularly glutamate, play a key role in structural as well as functional changes in the brain since glutamate is the major excitatory transmitter. At the same time, excess causes damage and inflammation.[20]

Amygdala

The amygdala, thought to be part of the limbic system, produces the emotional experiences of memory.[21] Within the amygdala are two hormones involved in the memory process that responds to daily stress. There is a mutual balance between them for creating a response in the memory process.[22] First, noradrenaline, a hormone and neurotransmitter, creates emotional aspects of memories stored in the basolateral amygdala area.[23] Second, corticosteroids facilitate the memory process. However, if high levels of chronic stress cause excessive release of corticosteroids, noradrenaline effectiveness is suppressed. This can cause a negative effect on memory formation in the amygdala.[24]

Basal Ganglia

The basal ganglia are involved in a wide range of processes such as emotion, reward processing, habit formation, movement, and learning. This part of the brain is particularly involved in coordinating sequences of motor activity, as would be needed when playing a musical instrument, dancing, or playing basketball. It is the section of the brain along with the substantia nigra pars compacta and locus coeruleus are most effected by Parkinson's disease.

Parietal Lobe

The parietal lobes have two roles: sensation and perception, and integrating sensory input, primarily with the visual system.

Cerebellum

The cerebellum is a separate structure located at the rear of the brain and it is critical for fine motor control.

Brain Cells

The neuron is the brain cell at the core of our ability to process information. The adult brain contains an estimated 100 billion neurons which communicate with each other through junction points called synapses in order for us to think and to send messages to other cells in the body. Neurons have dendrites that branch out like tree branches into secondary and tertiary dendrites. Each of these dendrites creates thousands of synapse connections with other neurons. Neurons fire impulses at a rate of approximately 10-100 times per second, depending on the type of neuron. Each neuron is connected to an average of 7,000 – 10,000 other neurons (and some more).

The human brain is capable of forming new connections between neurons. When we take in new information, an electro-chemical signal is sent across the space between neurons (called the synaptic space). This ability of the brain to form new connections or neural pathways to communicate with each other is often referred to as brain plasticity. Brain plasticity is now understood to be the very foundation of learning and memory. Through the mid-1990's, it was thought that the brain was not capable of generating new neurons and neural passages. This theory has been now totally debunked. Neurogenesis, and the growth of nerve cells is now part of our understanding of how the brain regenerates parts of itself and maintains its plasticity.

Microglia

Microglia are the resident macrophages (large cells) and primary immune cells of the brain, and they have a multitude of functions, including attacking and consuming bacteria (phagocytosis), removing waste, providing neuroprotection, and contributing to the growth of new neurons. They interact with a number of cell types, including astrocytes, neurons, and endothelial cells.

Glial Cells

Glial cells maintain homeostasis, form the myelin sheath that protects nerve cells, and provide support and protection for neurons. In addition, they support synaptic contacts and the signaling abilities of neurons. Glia are more numerous than nerve cells in the brain, outnumbering them by a ratio of perhaps 3 to 1.

- Star-shaped **astrocytes** are the largest and most numerous types of glial cell in the CNS. Their broad role is to maintain brain homeostasis and neuronal metabolism. They support brain plasticity and synaptogenesis, provide neurons with mechanical support, control neuronal cell development, release nutritional and energy substrates like glucose and lactate that regulate neurotransmission, vaso-modulation, and repair, and protect neurons from oxidative damage, and control the blood brain barrier and blood flow.[25] [26]
- **Oligodendroglia cells** are found in the central nervous system. Their main function of along with Schwann cells (found in the peripheral nervous system) is the formation of myelin, the protective covering of nerve cells.
- **Satellite cells** are glial cells that cover the surface of nerve cell bodies in sensory, sympathetic, and parasympathetic ganglia, and help regulate the external chemical environment. Like astrocytes, they are interconnected by gap junctions and respond to ATP (a neurotransmitter) by elevating intracellular concentration of calcium ions.

The Effects of Aging

With aging, we lose brain plasticity, which results in a loss of cognitive function. That's why a young person with an active, flexible brain, easily latches on to new ideas and simply thinks faster than an older person whose brain has lost plasticity and is more fixed in its patterns.[27] Loss of resilience can, for example, can be counteracted by regular physical activity.[28] The pliability of the brain is reliant on its ability to branch out and connect to new neural circuitry through:

- the ongoing elimination of old neural cells and natural waste,
- the ability to utilize glucose and essential nutrients, and
- the production of new neurons.

Protecting Plasticity

Synaptic Plasticity

Synaptic plasticity is a term that arises frequently in brain research. It refers to the process through which patterns of synaptic activity stimulate changes at synapses. Patterns of synaptic activity or inactivity regulates the amount of communication at the synapse. Synapses can change and the degree of change depends on how much they are used.[29]

Neurotropic Factors

The ability to utilize and put into action essential proteins in the brain is possible through the action of neurotrophic factors. These are molecules produced by the body (biomolecules), mostly peptides and proteins. The three known neurotrophins are brain-derived: neurotrophic factor (BDNF), vascular endothelial growth factor (VEGF), and nerve growth factor (NGF).

Neurotrophic factors keep the brain nourished. When they are working well our ability to think and process information stays healthy. When their action is impaired, learning and remembering becomes more difficult, and the brain actually withers and shrinks over time. Neurotrophic factors are positively affected by a having a healthy diet, being emotional balanced, managing stress and exercising regularly. Negative influences include an unhealthy diet, sedentary lifestyle, tobacco and alcohol use, mood disorders, oxidative stress, emotional imbalances such as excessive fear or anger, chronic pain, deficiencies in certain essential vitamins and in some cases, medications.

Glucocorticoids

In response to signals from the hypothalamus, the adrenal glands secrete glucocorticoids, hormones that produce an array of effects in response to stress. Natural glucocorticoids (also called glucocorticosteroids, corticosteroids or steroids) are present in almost all organs and tissues, including brain, and effect homeostasis, the body's ability to adapt to stress, and mediate hormonal activity through the stimulation or suppression of target gene transcription.[30]

Glucocorticoids can diffuse through the blood-brain barrier and exert long-term effects on processing and cognition.[31] Excess chronic stress causes the increased release of glucocorticoids, which in turn causes changes seen in AD patients in glutamate neurotransmission in the prefrontal cortex and the hippocampus, thereby influencing some aspects of cognitive processing.[32] A decrease in the secretion of glucocorticosteroids causes preservation of spatial memory in adults and has also been shown to have neuroprotective effects. Lifelong corticosterone levels determine age-related decline in neurogenesis and memory.[33]

Stress and Brain Function

The term "stress" covers a wide range of experience.

- **Good stress** makes us more adaptive and resilient in the face of daily challenges. Sometimes good stress can actually improve memory or enable us to take quick action.[34]
- **Tolerable stress** occurs when things go wrong but we are able to cope, re-evaluate, and grow.
- **Toxic stress** happens when things go wrong and we don't have good support to get through it. It can often be managed by good impulse control and judgment and adequate self-esteem. "With toxic stress, the inability to cope is likely to have adverse effects on behavior and physiology, and this will result in a higher degree of allostatic overload."[35] This refers to maintaining stability through altering physiologic parameters to counteract challenges within the body that work together to achieve a healthy balance. This is also referred to as "homeostasis" which includes: the sympathetic and parasympathetic systems, hypothalamic–pituitary– adrenal (HPA) axis, immune system and metabolic hormones and molecular processes within all organs including the brain, which all operate non-linearly.

Chronic Stress

Negative or toxic stress leaves us chronically in the "fight and flight" mode where we are not able to relax after we deal with the daily life challenges. This form of stress overtime affects one's health and even changes the brain architecture.

- Chronic stress results in immune suppression,[36] [37] as well as many other health conditions including high blood pressure and digestive disorders.
- Chronic stress can result in reduced brain plasticity. With persistence of this condition, involving excessive activation of excitatory amino acids, potentiated by glucocorticoids, irreversible damage occurs; this is postulated to be a key step in the irreversible activation of the cascade leading to Alzheimer's disease involving inactivation of the adaptive insulin receptor mechanism.[38]
- Chronic stress effects on the brain varies on different parts of the brain. For example, the medial amygdala shows a chronic stress-induced loss of spines[39] and shrinkage of dendrites.[40]
- These alterations are implicated in increased anxiety, posttraumatic stress disorder (PTSD)-like behaviors,[41] [42] as well as social avoidance as in social defeat.[43] [44]

In contrast, normal brain aging involves potentially reversible loss of resilience, which, for example, can often be counteracted by regular physical activity,[45] as well as regular forms of meditation, stress management, a healthy diet, and targeted supplementation, particularly related to deficiencies in certain nutrients.

Recreational Drugs

Basically, all illegal substances abused accelerate aging. For example, methamphetamine damages the blood-brain barrier, the tight junctions in the vasculature that prevent damaging molecules from entering the brain. Structural and functional differences in the brain have been linked to early and heavy cannabis use.[46] Cocaine induces alterations in neurotransmitters, neurotrophins, glucocorticoids, and promote inflammatory agents that affect neurogenesis in the hippocampus.[47]

Smoking and Brain Cell Loss

Nicotine can kill brain cells, stop new neurons forming in the hippocampus, and significantly impact the ability to promote new neurons.[48] Nicotine may also lead to higher levels of dependence by exerting neurotoxic effects in the prefrontal cortex (PFC) interfering with cognitive development, executive functioning, and inhibitory control. These effects are particularly evident under stressful or emotionally intense states and are most pronounced when smoking begins during early adolescence.[49] Once nicotine has entered the body, it is distributed quickly through the bloodstream and crosses the blood–brain barrier reaching the brain within ten to twenty seconds after inhalation.[50] Smoking may affect plasticity and refinement of cortical connections,[51] and may it may have functional implications for maturation and function of the prefrontal network.[52]

Chapter 2. Epigenetics

Genes, DNA and RNA

Our genes are what make us unique, what we look like and how our body functions. Genes carry the blueprint of essential proteins that regulate our functioning. Genes are built of DNA molecules formed in the shape of a double helix. The helix strands are sugar and phosphate molecules and the rungs of the double helix are pairs of four types of "nitrogenous bases". These are adenine (A), always paired with thymine (T), and guanine (G), always paired with cytosine (C).[53]

DNA can make copies of itself. Separated strands are able to build new second strands; these are new DNA molecules. DNA carries information. The arrangement of bases along the DNA molecule double helix is a blueprint for making proteins. DNA molecules are arranged around histone proteins (nucleosomes) to make chromosomes, which may contain from about 300 to 8000 genes.[54]

In addition, DNA can build smaller segments of itself, called RNA. RNA strands are single strands, not double, and act as signaling messengers within the body. Their roles include coding and decoding genes and expressing and regulating genetic information.[55]

Genes Turn On and Off

Genes continually turn on and off through a process, stimulated by enzymes, involving spooling and unspooling around the histone proteins. The enzymes are activated by diverse factors such as physical activity, mood, bacterial invasion, hormonal changes, or the environment. They can get 'stuck' in the on or off position with serious consequences in learning and long and short-term memory capacity.[56]

Epigenetics

Epigenetics is the study of the effect of the environment on gene expression, that is, how genetic inheritances change, not the DNA sequence itself, but how the gene is expressed.[57] Prior to the study of epigenetics, it was thought that our genes and how they express themselves were present at birth. With the onset of epigenetics, it has been found the genes turn on and off all during life. Epigenetic mechanisms are implicated in gene regulation and the development of different diseases.[58] The epigenome, the biochemicals that tell each human's set of genes, instructs the unique gene expression program of each cell type to define its functional identity during development or disease.[59] The epigenome represents, in a way, how we are able to adapt to our ever-changing environment.[60] Cytokines, growth factors, alterations in hormonal levels as well as release of stress-response and neurotropic factors are some examples of molecules that can be affected and go through changes due to one's exposure to a range of environmental factors.

Genetics versus Epigenetics

Genetics (DNA) is the foundation that drives our growth, development and even our personality types. It controls the myelination of the nerves in our body and brains and is the blueprint of the "brain" in each cell in our body. It was always thought that genes and related instructions were permanent and unchangeable. Then came the study of epigenetics, which showed that gene expression could change throughout one's lifetime, determined by many environmental factors including diet, emotional nurturing, social interactions, exercise, smoking, alcohol consumption, air pollution and other exposure to toxins, working habits (particularly those who have shift work), chronic stress, and even how one sleeps. All of these influences affect the healthy determination of gene activity. In diseases such as cancer, congenital diseases, neurodegenerative diseases, and neuropsychiatric disorders,[61][62][63][64] various genes are switched into an opposite state, away from the normal/healthy state. With over 200,000 genes, epigenetics can play a significant role in disease onset and prevention.

Factors that Influence Epigenetics

DNA Methylation

Methylation of DNA is a signaling tool that the body uses to lock genes in the "off" position. It is an important factor in many cellular processes, including prenatal development, inactivation of X chromosomes, and how and whether parental genes are expressed in children.[65] Hypermethylation refers to increases in the rate of DNA methylation, present for example, in cancer.

One researcher describes DNA methylation as an archetypal example of epigenetic modification.[66] DNA can be modified by the addition of a methyl group to the 5-position of the cytosine-guanine pair. DNA methylation changes the activity of DNA segment without changing its structure by repressing gene transcription. Gene transcription is the first step in copying segments of DNA into RNA before they are expressed in the body.

Histone Methylation

Histone methylation involves adding a methyl group to the amino acids making up the histone proteins (nucleosomes). Histone methylation can repress or enhance gene transcription.[67]

There is a complex interplay between DNA methylation and histone methylation.[68] Unlike DNA methylation which causes lasting changes to the expression of genes, histone methylation causes more rapid changes in cellular life cycles. For example: histone lysine methylation may help to target prenatal DNA methylation and vice versa. Histone lysine methylation affects changes in chromatin histones, which sends more changes back to DNA methylation. "The timing and placement of DNA methylation in the genome is essential for normal development and cellular function"[69] so this inter-related dance has critical consequence.

Transcription Factors

Transcription factors are proteins (at least 2600 of them) that control rates of gene transcription rates from DNA to RNA messengers through specific binding sequences. These factors turn on and turn off certain gene segments. They function by themselves or in combination with other biochemicals to enhance or repress enzymes that perform gene transcription.[70]

Permanent Epigenetic Modification

What is important to understand about epigenetic modification is that it heavily influences neurotrophic factor (BDNF), vascular endothelial growth factor (VEGF), and nerve growth factor (NGF), and consequently loss of brain plasticity which results in loss of cognitive capacity expressed in conditions like Alzheimer's disease. These growth factors are responsible for the ability to utilize and put into action essential proteins in the brain and the promotion of health and re-growth of neurons.

Processes like DNA methylation control intracellular signaling that can cause lasting changes in DNA function in the brain and cognitive capacity. Such processes can be triggered by a broad range of factors ranging from harmful drugs to mental well-being. Diet, exercise, and other aspects of our daily interaction with the environment have the potential to alter our brain health and mental function. Even our thoughts can impact how our DNA expresses itself and instructs how genes turn on and off.

The remarkable thing is that how one's lifestyle effects gene expression which then affects future generations. Numerous historical studies show that patterns of famine, smoking, or breast feeding, affect future generations related to potential impact on development and health,[71] especially during critical developmental periods.[72]

Drugs can have a direct effect on normal histone methylation controls, resulting in aberrant gene expression.[73] Histone modification can also make people more vulnerable to developing addictions.[74] Indirect negative effects include alterations in transcription factors, essential for healthy gene expression.[75] Screening protocols have been developed to distinguish between therapeutic drugs positive therapeutic capacity and those with a potential negative epigenetic impact.[76]

Exposure to therapeutic drugs may cause persistent epigenetic changes, possibly manifesting as permanent adverse side-effects[77] Recreational drugs like cocaine, opiates, amphetamines, alcohol, and nicotine modify the epigenome by altering methylation patterns in areas such as the nucleus accumbens (located in the midbrain), the major pleasure reward center.[78]

Smoking causes DNA methylation changes. For example, cigarette smoke causes abnormal expression of a lung cancer oncogene (a gene that can transform a cell into a cancer cell) through NDA hypermethylation.[79] It can result in tumor suppressor genes being inactivated, and methylation of the tumor suppressor gene p16 has frequently been associated with the development of cancer. Of particular interest is the finding that not only maternal smoking but also grandmaternal smoking is linked to pediatric disease as a result of epigenetic changes to DNA and histones.[80][81]

Alcohol also causes epigenetic changes. The epigenetic effects of alcohol on liver and neuronal tissue are well documented.[82] Chronic alcohol consumption can lead to a deficiency in the growth process of new cells (S-adenosylmethionine (SAM) levels) and alter carbohydrate metabolism, cell death, and mitochondrial well-being – all contributing to epigenetic modification.[83]

Obesity. In obesity studies, it has been shown that obese mothers tend to have obese children.[84] It has also been shown that weight-loss surgery before pregnancy not only results in fewer obesity-related problems during pregnancy, but has a positive effect on reducing risk of obesity (and related problems) in the offspring continuing into adolescence. [85]

Diet. Prenatal dietary deficiencies in essential nutrients that are required for correct DNA methylation are known as "methyl donors" gives rise to fetal development issues. Methyl donors include essential nutrients such as the choline, methionine, methyltetrahydrofolate (methyl-THF) and vitamins B-6 and B-12.[86] [87]

Maternal mental health. Domestic violence causes permanent epigenetic changes in the DNA of the cortisol receptor in offspring observed during adolescence.[88] In rats, prenatal stress during late gestation has been shown to modify epigenetic signatures that are linked to neurological disease during the critical period of fetal brain development.[89]

Birth. Babies born by caesarean delivery have different gut microbiota in the first hours and days of life to those born vaginally, [90] and there is mounting evidence that the development of IgE-mediated sensitization to food allergens is higher in children born by caesarean delivery.[91] Studies also indicate the risk of marked increase in children's susceptibility to a range of immune related disorders if they are born by caesarean delivery, and particularly when it is performed electively without concurrent labor.[92]

Childhood mental health. Under stress conditions the hypothalamus signals the adrenal glands to secrete the glucocorticoids which produce stress responses such as fight or flight. Childhood abuse causes epigenetic modifications affecting glucocorticoid receptors and related gene transcription and results in poor hypothalamic-pituitary-adrenal functioning and increased risk of suicide.[93]

Maternal behavior. Poverty and neglect have direct negative impacts upon future development. The quality of family life including maternal care influences the physiology and psychology of the child such that persistent neglect, emotional abuse, or sexual abuse hampers growth and intellectual development and increases risk of disorders like obesity[94] or mood disorders[95] and increased stress response[96] in both childhood and adulthood. Maternal behavior such as maternal bonding, maternal grooming, and related behaviors in lab animals[97] has the ability to cause epigenetic modification[98] ranging from physical and cognitive functioning to mental well-being and decrease in stress and anxiety through adulthood.[99] Early life experiences like maternal care, stress adaptation, and early life adversities contribute to a biological memory. Epigenetic modifications of DNA are responsible for imprinting such influences into the neuronal circuits of the developing brain which can have life-long impacts.[100]

Lifestyle Changes Can Help

Exercise has been shown to induce positive changes in DNA methylation within adipose (fat) tissue and regulate metabolism in both healthy and diseased individuals.[101] The health benefits of physical exercise, especially on a long-term and strenuous basis, has a positive effect on epigenetic mechanisms and ultimately may reduce incidence and severity of disease.[102]

Two new studies published in 2019 lend more clarity to how to exercise. In a ten-year review of the aerobic fitness of over thirty-thousand people, three groups were identified: those who remained in the lowest twenty percent of fitness measures over the entire ten-year period, those who moved in and out of that lowest percentile, and those who never were in the lowest twenty percent group. They found that people who remained fit throughout the ten years were fifty percent less likely to develop dementia. Moreover, and even more encouraging, they found that people who didn't get in shape until middle age or later still enjoyed the benefits of markedly lowered risk of dementia.[103]

The second study looked more to the *type* of exercise. The researchers started with sixty-four sedentary men and women sixty or older and measured their fitness and cognitive capacity, especially memory, often an indicator of mild cognitive impairment. The subjects were divided into three groups. One was to meet together and stretch, one to spend fifty minutes three times a week walking moderately on a treadmill, and the third to do *interval walking*.

In interval walking, the incline of the treadmill was increased more steeply for four-minute periods, so that the people had three minutes of easy walking and three minutes of walking in which heart rates were about ninety percent of maximum for each person's condition. After twelve weeks, the results were striking.

Compared to continuous moderate walking the interval walkers showed marked improvements in both physical endurance and memory performance. The more fit they became, the more their memory improved.[104] [105]

A 2020 study reported that exercise causes the liver to increase the amount of a special protein in blood plasma, GPLD1, (glycosylphosphatidylinositol (GPI)-specific phospholipase D1). GPLD1 enhances messaging and related enzyme cascades that support the aged brain by improving cognitive function and impaired neurogenesis capacity.[106]

Diet. Although the molecular mechanisms for the influence of diet on epigenetics are unknown, it is also known that the brain-derived neurotrophic factor (BDNF) system is particularly susceptible to epigenetic modifications that influence cognitive function.[107] Nutrients extracted from the diet enter metabolic pathways and are transformed into useful molecules. These nutrients are known to have epigenetic targets in cells such that they can be used to modify the epigenome in order to correct abnormally activated or silenced genes and can be combined into an "epigenetic diet" useful as a therapeutic or chemo-preventive measure.[108] Studies in genomic imprinting have revealed how DNA methylation patterns are influenced by diet, and how epigenomic sensitivity to environmental cues and specifically diet can be used to influence (both positively and negatively) disease susceptibility.[109] [110] [111]

Summary

The study of epigenetics has demonstrated that health is not just determined by our genes (even those prone to certain genetic diseases), but that genes can be turned on and off throughout our life, and that the nurturing we receive in early childhood, diet and lifestyle all effect disease onset and prevention later in life. Even positive health and emotional factors from prior generations affect future generations.

Chapter 3. Neurogenesis

Neurogenesis reflects the process by which new neurons are created, the way in which the brain renews and upgrades itself. Up to the 1990's, it was thought that the brain stopped growing and that brain cells could not regenerate. But in 1998 researchers determined that neurogenesis occurs within the brain throughout life.[112] Neurogenesis and hippocampal plasticity can be stimulated (and even negatively regulated) by extrinsic factors including environment, exercise, and diet.[113]

The ability to utilize and put into action essential proteins (neurotrophins) is possible through the action of growth factors produced by the body. Examples are basic fibroblast growth factor (bFGF), brain-derived neurotrophic factor (BDNF), ciliary neurotrophic factor (CNTF), and glial cell line-derived neurotrophic factor (GDNF). Neurotrophic factors act dynamically to prevent or lessen dysfunction and neuron cell death due to neurologic disorders.[114] Neurotrophic factors also play a role in angiogenesis, the production of new blood vessels.[115]

The rate of neurogenesis is tied to the quality of your life and has everything to do with: healthy cognitive function, better memory and faster learning, an effective immune system, depression, and anxiety (or not being depressed or anxious), and overall brain function. Neuroplasticity, or neural plasticity, allows neurons to regenerate both anatomically as well as functionally, and to form new synaptic connections, and enables the brain to recover and restructure itself from oxidative stress, free radicals, injury, and basic aging. The neural pathways in our brain interconnect. The communication is called "synapsis", and basically enables us to think and create communication to the rest of our cells in our body.

How the Brain Regulates Neurogenesis

Researchers noted in the 90s that neurogenesis decreases with aging.[116] But the number and type of stem cells in the neurogenic region of the hippocampus apparently does not decrease with aging, rather they become inactive or dormant.[117]

Stem Cells

Neurogenesis occurs through stem cells that can differentiate into many other types of cells, including nerve cells. Long-lived stem cells that allow for neurogenesis originate in underside of the fetal hippocampus late in pregnancy and then later relocate into the dorsal hippocampus.[118] Researchers have found that neurogenesis takes place not only in the hippocampus, but also in the amygdala, hypothalamus, olfactory tubercle (a multi-sensory processing center), and piriform cortex (related to sense of smell).[119] Epigenetic processes involving both DNA and RNA have important roles in different aspects of neurogenesis.[120]

Neurotropic Factors

Neurotrophic factors are molecules called polypeptides which have neuroprotective functions. They regulate the growth, health, movement, and differentiation of nerve cells in the nervous system.[121] A neurotrophic factor is synthesized by and released from target cells of the neurons.

Neurotrophic factors are sometimes referred to as neurotrophins (NTs) and there are a number of groups of NTs.[122] The family of growth factors also includes NGF, brain-derived neurotrophic factor (BDNF), NT-3, NT-4 (NT-4/5 or NT-5),[123] and NT-6.[124]

The glial cell-derived neurotrophic factors (GDNF) family and neuropoietic cytokines, such as ciliary neurotrophic factor (CNTF) and leukemia inhibitory factor, are also considered members of the neurotrophic factor family.[125] [126] [127]

Brain Derived Neurotropic Factor

Brain derived neurotropic factor (BDNF) regulates hippocampal neurogenesis.[128] [129] It is required for the development of the nervous system, proper cognitive function, and memory formation, and is known to be critical for the development of the brain, neurons survival,[130] neuronal regeneration and synaptic plasticity.[131] [132] [133] [134] [135] It regulates the survival of immature neurons.[136] [137] BDNF decreases with age and is associated with reduced hippocampal volume and corresponding impaired spatial memory in aged humans (59–80 years old).[138] [139]

When BDNF levels are irregular or declining, neurological diseases such as Alzheimer's, Parkinson's, Huntington's disease, and amyotrophic lateral sclerosis can develop.[140] BDNF also participates in learning and memory,[141] modulates synaptic transmission,[142] and affects long-term potentiation (LTP).[143] [144] [145] LTP is the long-lasting signal strength in a synapse after stimulation. Signal pathway activation by BDNF, can lead to the transcription of genes needed for synaptic plasticity[146] and neurogenesis.[147] [148]

BDNF supports cell differentiation,[149] maturation,[150] and shows a neuroprotective effect under adverse conditions such as glutamatergic stimulation, cerebral ischemia, hypoglycemia, and neurotoxicity.[151] Endothelial cells secrete soluble factors that increase stem cell proliferation, neurogenesis,[152] maturation, and migration, in part, by secreting BDNF.

Nerve Growth Factors

Nerve growth factors (NGF) have been shown to improve neural regeneration in neurodegenerative diseases, such as Alzheimer's,[153] Parkinson's[154] and Huntington's disease.[155] Neurotrophins have also been found to be located in adult stem cells niches and therefore may promote tissue regeneration outside of the nervous system.

Microglia

The process of neurogenesis and the function of the immune system are closely related.[156] Through phagocytosis (attacking bacteria) microglia regulate neurogenesis and shape neurogenesis in the adult hippocampus.[157] They dynamically interact with a number of cell types, including astrocytes, neurons, and endothelial cells. Even when apparently inactive microglial cells are highly dynamic surveillants of brain parenchyma (neurons and glial cells) in vivo.[158]

Glial Cells

Glial cells help create a microenvironment that permits neurogenesis and are themselves generated alongside the new neurons in an associated but independently regulated process.[159]

Astroglia (astrocytes) induce differentiation of stem cell progeny [160] [161] (neural progenitor cells, NPCs) and identification of astrocyte-expressed factors that modulate neural stem/progenitor cell differentiation.[162]

- Astrocytes are also known to release molecules important for neuronal survival and neurite formation. 57 percent of synapses in the mature hippocampus are in direct contact with astrocytes.[163] Other proteins in hippocampal astrocytes, such as ephrins (specifically ephrin-B2), have also been identified to play a role in regulating neurogenesis through cell
- To cell contact.[164]
- Interleukin-6 is an example of a neurotrophic factor that is derived from astrocytes. It supports differentiation of neural progenitor cells in the adult hippocampus.[165]

Endothelial cells (blood vessels) represent an abundant source of extrinsic factors that can modulate adult neurogenesis.[166] [167] Astrocytes are tightly linked physically with endothelial cells, wrapping their end feet around blood vessels.

Brain Plasticity

Brain plasticity refers to the capacity of the nervous system to change its structure and its function over a lifetime, in reaction to environmental diversity. Plasticity in the adult brain enables lifelong learning. Current evidence indicates that lifelong addition of new hippocampal neurons may extend from early developmental plasticity to adulthood, which continuously rejuvenates in the adult brain. [168]

"Plasticity, or neuroplasticity, refers to the ways that neural pathways are able to re-form in the brain. It's true that these pathways such as the one between the hippocampus and the amygdala can get severely damaged due to constant exposure to stress, but such changes are not necessarily permanent. While stress can negatively affect the brain, the brain and body is able to recover."[169]

How Lifestyle and Daily Experience Affect Neurogenesis

There is a great variation in people's rate of nerve cell regeneration, which is affected by the quality of your lifestyle which includes diet, quality of relationships, mental health, stress, exposure to toxins and amount and type of exercise. Providing an enriched environment for the brain increases BDNF levels, stimulating neurogenesis and neural growth.

Chronic Inflammation

Inflammation in the brain causes shrinkage, decreased neurogenesis, and neurodegeneration in pathologically vulnerable regions of the brain, as in AD.[170][171][172] Chronic intestinal inflammation is associated with decreased neurogenesis in the subgranular region of the hippocampus which is responsible for learning, memory, and mood control.[173]

Oxidative Stress

The brain is particularly susceptible to free radical damage due to its high polyunsaturated fatty acid and DHA content and high rate of metabolic activity.[174][175] Oxidative stress has many causes, including lack of antioxidants from food, antioxidant deterioration, reactive oxygen species (free radicals) formation, free radical accumulation, and lipid oxidation.

Chronic Stress

Good stress helps keep our body strong and increases neurogenesis, but chronic tolerable or toxic stress can lead to atrophy of the brain, shriveled neurons, decreased neurogenesis and BDNF, and decreased brain weight.[176] The hippocampus has higher levels of glucocorticoid receptors than any other part of the brain and therefore is most affected by high levels of chronic stress.[177] Studies of people with some forms of PTSD show that the hippocampus is one quarter smaller than normal, affecting cognition, memory, and the ability to handle emotions.[178][179]

Chronic stress withers the dendrite neurons, reducing synapsis. Neurogenesis is reduced as the body is less able to produce new brains cells needed, resulting in the lessened ability of the hippocampus to make new memories.[180][181]

Trauma

Traumatic brain injury (TBI) is the leading cause of death and disability of persons under forty-five years old in the United States. It had been thought that recovery from such injuries is severely limited due to the inability of the adult brain to replace damaged neurons. Heightened levels of cell proliferation and neurogenesis have been observed in response to brain trauma or insults suggesting that the brain has the inherent potential to restore populations of damaged or destroyed neurons. [182][183]

Exercise

Although the production of new neurons declines with age, neurogenesis can be promoted later in life by regular exercise[184][185] as demonstrated in research with adult rodents[186][187] and humans.[188] Similarly, aerobic exercise has shown to suppress dopaminergic nerve loss in Parkinsonian rodents.[189]

Regular exercise promotes increases in brain-derived neurotrophic factor in blood serum,[190] neurotrophic factors,[191][192] improvements in learning, memory (in healthy young adults),[193][194][195][196] and cognitive function.[197][198] Although much of the research connecting aerobic exercise with neurogenesis is with healthy young adults, researchers do feel that exercise supports neurogenesis throughout the lifespan.[199]

Exercise, along with a flavonoid-enriched diet increases the ability of genes to have a positive effect on neuronal plasticity and decreases the expression of genes involved in harmful processes, such as inflammation and cell death.[200] Exercise also counteracts the effects of a high fat diet and supports neurogenesis.[201][202]

Molecules that could explain the synergistic effects of diet and exercise include BDNF, which has emerged as an important factor for translating the effects of exercise on synaptic plasticity and cognitive function.[203][204] As discussed in the previous chapter, interval walking, alternating moderate and intense (especially hills if possible) are most beneficial.

Learning

The process of learning new knowledge, skills, and information also stimulates hippocampal neurogenesis.[205] Learning tasks that are related to the hippocampus are linked to new cell generation there, while learning tasks that do not require the hippocampus do not alter the number of new cells.[206] Learning, spaced over time, induces more enduring memory, which is linked to the number of new cells in the hippocampus.[207]

Diet

Scientists agree that nutritional factors have a role in protecting and enhancing neurogenesis.[208][209] Diets that include lots of sugars and high fats reduce neurotrophic factors in the hippocampus, nerve plasticity and learning capacity.[210] Many plant foods help to reduce the ill-effects of a high-fat, high-sugar diet on neurogenesis and brain health. Examples are lion's mane mushrooms[211] and zinc.[212] Periodic fasting (as opposed to prolonged fasting, which does promote stress resistance) alternated with a nutrient-rich diet improves hippocampal neurogenesis as well as reducing body fat, cancer, bone loss, and biomarkers for aging, diabetes, and heart disease.[213] Some carotenoids, such as astaxanthin, are as helpful for memory, hippocampus-based neural plasticity, and neurogenesis as exercise, and even more effective when combined.[214]

These top four nutrients or foods are the most important for supporting neurogenesis and/or BDNF. They are discussed in detail in the diet and nutrition chapters.

- **Blueberries.** The polyphenols contained in blueberries support neurogenesis,[215][216] and protect cognitive capacity.[217][218]
- **Curcumin** induces neurogenesis,[219][220] protects against fat oxidation, and reduces neuron deterioration due to free radicals in neurodegenerative conditions.[221][222]
- **Goji Berries** (lycium barbarum). Goji berry supports neurogenesis,[223] and protects against chemical-caused neurogenesis suppression.[224] Goji contains high amounts of antioxidants, and other vitamins and flavonoids.
- **Omega-3 Fatty Acids.** Not only do omega-3s induce neurogenesis via synapse support and neurite growth,[225][226][227] but they reduce inflammation, are neuroprotective,[228] and enhance BDNF synthesis. They are essential for learning and memory.[229][230]

Other important nutrients and foods to support brain health and neurogenesis include: acetyl-l-carnitine, apigenin, ashwagandha, choline, curcumin, ginkgo, ginseng, goji berry, grapeseed extract, green tea, gut microbia, hesperidin, huperzine A, iron, lecithin, lotus root extract, lutein, magnesium, magnolol, melatonin, milk thistle extract, mulberry, mushrooms (lion's mane, shiitake, reishi), olive leaf extract, omega-3s, pantethine, piperine, phosphatidylserine, pinocembrin, PQQ, quercetin, red sage (salvia), resveratrol, rhodiola, selenium, shankhpushpi, taurine, theanine, trytophan, vinpocetine, and vitamins A, B6, B12, E, and D.

Chapter 4. About Memory and Dementia

As we age, we become more prone to health issues for many reasons. Some people can remain healthy and sharp through their natural life, while others suffer from some form of dementia even as early as in their fifties.

As people are living longer, the onset of dementia in our aging population is becoming a major health challenge, both for individuals suffering from dementia, and also for the family and caregivers, notwithstanding the cost of caring for an aging population. In 2019, an estimated 5.6 million Americans have Alzheimer's Disease (AD); and fourteen percent of those over seventy have some form of dementia.[231] AD and dementia cost 19-times more to society when compared with age-matched people without dementia, estimated to be around $290 billion in 2019.[232]

At present trends, fifty percent of the adults eight-five plus-years-old can expect to receive a diagnosis of AD. As the population is living longer, this is creating a tremendous cost to each individual and to society.

An Integrated Perspective of the Brain

Looking at the brain from a holistic, integrated perspective gives us the best opportunity to maintain our whole body and brain health. Whole body means the relationship between the mind, body, emotions, and spirit. This perspective has been the good health foundation for thousands of years in Chinese and ayurvedic medicine, as well as more recent holistic practices such as homeopathy and functional medicine.

The onset of dementia is often connected to the health of the whole body. For example, studies have shown that illnesses such as anemia,[233] diabetes mellitus,[234] and cardiovascular disease all increase the risk of onset of dementia as well as those with fewer teeth (often related to poor health habits).

The brain is the most active organ in our body and requires a significant and ongoing supply of blood and essential nutrients. Fortunately, the brain has its own circulatory system with multiple power back-up systems to maintain integrity. The system is called the "circle of Willis," a circular cross-connection of blood circulation supported by the carotid artery. The sides of the neck provide most of the blood flow to the front and top of the brain and the vertebral arteries which climb up through the spinal column along with parts of the carotids.

The foods we eat and the health of our gastrointestinal system play a major role in our brain health because although the brain is only one to two percent of our body weight, it utilizes twenty percent of our body's energy. We absorb nutrients through our digestive system, and the liver processes the blood and filters out toxins before they reach the brain. Intake of excessive alcohol, and from a Chinese medical perspective, anger (or excessive anger) being held, both affect the health of the liver. Epidemiological and experimental studies have demonstrated that a diet rich in fruit and vegetables has a beneficial effect on cognitive function.[235] Essential food groups are rich in antioxidants that act as free radical scavengers that protect the brain from neuronal damage.[236] Specific micronutrients in specific vitamins, herbs and mushrooms, may ease these debilitating pathologies.[237] [238]

Correspondingly, our exercise strongly affects the health of the brain. Multiple studies demonstrate that exercise, both intensive (such as running) and more moderate (such as dancing or walking) also support brain health because they induce neurogenesis. [239] [240] Moreover exercise even helps to mitigate the ill-effects of a high-fat or high-sucrose diet. [241] [242] [243]

Types of Dementia

Alzheimer's Disease

The best-known form of dementia is Alzheimer's disease (AD), a fatal neurodegenerative disease characterized clinically by progressive memory loss as well as aberrant behavior.[244] [245]

Patients with AD display:

- Loss of synapses and neurons
- Extracellular senile plaques consisting of aggregations (clump) of amyloid beta peptide
- Intracellular neurofibrillary tangles (NFTs) consisting primarily of tau protein, which normally is important as it forms part of a structure called microtubules. In Alzheimer's disease, however, the tau protein is abnormal and the microtubule structures collapse.

Development of AD

- The hippocampus and its connected structures which are related to forming new memories, learning, and retrieving memories.
- Amygdala is typically affected later than the hippocampus. This part of the brain is responsible for emotions, survival instincts, and memory, and plays a role in the libido and sex drive.
- The cortex overall becomes thinner (so memories from longer ago are lost) and the brain gradually shrinks.
- Damage to the left hemisphere is linked to problems with semantic memory and language, causing a struggle to find the right word.
- Damage to the visual system in the temporal lobes makes recognizing familiar faces and objects harder. The person may seem to forget who a familiar person is.
- As the damage spreads to the frontal lobes, someone with Alzheimer's may struggle with decision-making, planning or organizing (such as family finances). A more complex task with a sequence of steps, such as following a new recipe, might also become much harder.
- There are rarer atypical forms of AD where the hippocampus is not affected, but instead the damage is done to the occipital lobes and parts of the parietal lobes, which help to process visual information and deal with spatial awareness. Someone with this type of AD may also struggle to judge distances walking down stairs or parking the car. Or they may seem uncoordinated, such as when dressing.

Vascular Dementia

Vascular dementia (multi-infarct dementia), second only to Alzheimer's, is a general term referring to difficulty in thought processes like reasoning and memory. It is caused by brain damage from poor circulation to the brain due to multiple conditions like a stroke, mini-stroke, or atherosclerosis. In addition, the person may be left with weakness down one side of the body or problems with vision or speech. If related to mini-strokes, each stroke can result in small patches of dead tissue in the cortex of the brain.

Subcortical vascular dementia. Another version of vascular dementia is called subcortical vascular dementia resulting from deterioration of the small blood vessels deep in the brain. This often causes widespread damage to white matter beneath the cortex, affecting nerve fibers that carry signals between different parts of the cortex, including the frontal lobes. A person with subcortical vascular dementia will therefore often have slowed thinking and problems with executive function.

The commonality of vascular dementia suggests that dyslipidemia is in the blood (containing an abnormal amount of lipids such as triglycerides, cholesterol, and/or fat phospholipids). Also, the results of having high cholesterol related to AD are mixed, and a number of studies reported that high total cholesterol levels increased risk of AD significantly.[246][247]

Dementia with Lewy Bodies

Lewy body dementia (DLB) is a progressive dementia third after Alzheimer's in which protein deposits (Lewy bodies) accumulate within nerve cells in parts of the brain involving thinking, memory and movement, the cerebral cortex, limbic system, and brain stem.

The brain of a person with DLB often shows less overall shrinkage than the brain of someone with Alzheimer's or frontotemporal dementia. In DLB, early damage is seen in the visual pathways and possibly also in the frontal lobes, which may explain why problems with vision and attention are commonly found as early symptoms of DLB. Similarly, Lewy bodies in the brain stem may be linked to the problems with movement, as also seen in Parkinson's disease which is why Robin Williams was diagnosed with Parkinson's when he suffered from DLB (discovered in his autopsy).

Post Traumatic Stress Disorder

Post-traumatic stress disorder (PTSD) was once thought to be a mental health-only condition triggered by a terrifying event, involving flashbacks, anxiety, nightmares and erratic thoughts and behavior. However, the triggering event causes changes in the amygdala, medial prefrontal cortex, and hippocampus. The amygdala displays heightened responsivity, the prefrontal cortex shrinks and is hyporesponsive, and the hippocampus is smaller, exhibits nerve damage, and also is dysfunctional.[248]

Frontotemporal Dementia

In all forms of frontotemporal dementia (FTD), the frontal and/or temporal lobes shrink, affecting the persons' ability to speak and their behavior. The person tends to repeat the same word, phrase, or action over and over again. Changes in the cortex also can result in the person becoming withdrawn and losing motivation. In the early stages, the person may have fluent speech but struggle to find the right word for something, or they may ask what a familiar word (example: 'knife') means. Damage to the right temporal lobe leads to problems recognizing faces and also objects.

Parkinson's Disease

Parkinson's is the second-most common neurological condition in the world. It is characterized by cognitive impairment, physical tremors, slowness of movement (brandykinesia), instability, muscular rigidity, and other non-motor symptoms. Lewy bodies made of protein accumulate within specific nerve cells in the brain stem resulting in their death.

Other Forms of Dementia

Other forms of dementia include Creutzfeldt-Jakob disease (an infectious brain disease), HIV-associated dementia, chronic traumatic encephalopathy (caused by repeated head injuries), and Picks disease (involving localized atrophy in the brain).

Brain Pathology in Later Life

Although some form of dementia may not be specifically diagnosed or identified, many seniors still experience a decline in brain health in later life. For example, researchers now identify vascular risk during early to late adulthood with late-life brain structure decline. By vascular risk, we mean systolic blood pressure, antihypertensive medication need, smoking, presence of diabetes, and body mass index. In a large, long-term British study of participants free of dementia who had high vascular risk in early life were strongly linked with smaller whole-brain size and greater amounts of brain lesions which appear in MRI, and referred to as white-matter hyperintensities. These often show up in CTs or MRI's of elderly patients, even though there may be no evidence of amyloid beta accumulation.[249] The researchers' conclusion was that **"reducing vascular risk with appropriate interventions should be considered from early adulthood to maximize late-life brain health."**[250]

Symptoms

Dementia isn't a specific disease. Instead, dementia describes a group of symptoms affecting memory, thinking and social abilities severely enough to interfere with daily functioning.

Word-object problems. People experience difficulty in finding the right words or even recognizing common words as the relate to objects

Difficulty in daily life. Patients experience difficulty with common tasks, organizing and planning, recognizing people they know, reasoning and problem-solving.

Motor functions. People have trouble with coordination and motor functions, being confused and disoriented.

Brain "fog" is a constellation of symptoms that include reduced mental acuity and cognition, inability to concentrate and multitask, as well as loss of short and long-term memory. It is considered the early clinical presentation of AD,[251] though there may be other reasons this occurs (see Brain Fog chapter).

Psychological symptoms such as depression, anxiety, difficulty sleeping, agitation, paranoia, personality changes, hallucinations.

Causes of Dementia

In addition to aging, a general lifestyle pattern appears to be a major risk factor for development of dementia. Risks include long-term consumption of high-fat, high-sucrose, refined-grains diet, poor nutrition and/or nutrient absorption, sedentary lifestyle, chronic insomnia, social isolation, chronic stress, cognitive inactivity, and epigenetic (environmental) factors.

More specifically, research points to genetic inheritance, cardiovascular and cerebrovascular problems, excessive alcohol consumption, traumatic brain injury, chronic inflammation, compromised blood-brain barrier, biochemical imbalances, oxidative stress, and having one or two copies of the APOE∈4 genetic variant.

General Causes

- **Aging**. Neurodegeneration increases with age and is characterized by progressive deterioration of the structure and function of neurons, crucially accompanied by severe cognitive deficits. Aging is the major risk factor for neurodegenerative disorders in Alzheimer's disease (AD), as co-equal risk factors Parkinson's disease (PD), and Huntington's disease (HD).
- **Genetics**. Family history of some forms of dementia is a strong factor.
- **Medications** including anticholinergic drugs (drugs that block the neurotransmitter acetylcholine in the central and the peripheral nervous system).[252] These drugs are typically used to treat a variety of conditions such as including urinary incontinence, overactive bladder (OAB), chronic obstructive pulmonary disorder (COPD), and certain types of poisoning. Examples of these medications include: atropine (Atropen), belladonna alkaloids, benztropine mesylate (Cogentin), clidinium, cyclopentolate (Cyclogyl), darifenacin (Enablex), dicylomine, fesoterodine (Toviaz), flavoxate (Urispas), glycopyrrolate, homatropine hydrobromide, hyoscyamine (Levsinex), ipratropium (Atrovent), orphenadrine, oxybutynin (Ditropan XL), propantheline (Pro-banthine), scopolamine, methscopolamine, solifenacin (VESIcare), tiotropium (Spiriva), tolterodine (Detrol), trihexyphenidyl, and trospium. Sleeping pills, anti-anxiety drugs, antidepressants, and some cold remedies can worsen dementia.
- **Diet and nutrition**. Poor diet and/or poor absorption of essential nutrients is a factor. Deficiency or low levels in specific vitamins such as vitamin D3, and B vitamins can result in cognitive difficulty, mood swing, and depression. These deficiencies can mimic symptoms

of dementia and AD. In contrast to the healthful effects of diets that are rich in omega-3 fatty acids and antioxidants, epidemiological studies indicate that diets with high contents of trans and saturated fats adversely affect cognition.[253] A diet high in "junk food" and saturated fats elevates the neurological burden that is associated with brain injury, as evidenced by a worse performance in learning tasks and a reduction of BDNF-mediated synaptic plasticity.[254] [255] [256] This type of diet increases the vulnerability of cells to damage[257] by causing free-radical formation that surpasses cellular buffering capacity.

Specific nutrient deficiencies such as zinc, vitamins B1, B2, B6, B12 and magnesium contribute to brain dysfunction. Zinc deficiency may induce learning and memory impairment. B12 deficiency has been linked to mental decline (which can often be mistaken for dementia). Magnesium is essential for learning and memory, and has been shown to support brain plasticity for optimal learning, memory, and cognitive function. It also suppresses amyloid beta build-up in the brain.

- **Lack of exercise**. As one ages, we become more sedentary. Exercise helps maintain healthy circulation, supports ongoing detoxification, improves overall mood (reducing onset of depression), and helps keep us more mobile. It reduces inflammation, stimulates the brain to create new neural connections and helps improve insulin sensitivity. Daily running, fast walking, gym workouts, swimming, tennis, dancing are all good examples of good daily exercises.

- **Lack of social support.** Mood may influence social behavior, and social support is one of the most studied psychosocial factors in relation to health and disease, possibly resulting in mimicking symptoms of dementia.

- **Sleep**. Not getting enough sleep at night and chronic insomnia cause many cognitive and related problems.

- **Circadian Rhythm**. Related to sleep is the circadian rhythm which runs twenty-four hours and is often referred to as your "sleep/wake cycle." Part of your hypothalamus controls your circadian rhythm which works best with regular sleep schedule habits. Circadian rhythms have regulatory effects on cell proliferation, cell metabolism, cell senescence, and cell death. Circadian dysfunction also impacts negatively on immune, metabolic, and cardiovascular systems.[258] [259] Increasing evidence indicates that circadian rhythms play an important role in the pathogenesis of many ailments. These include including neurodegenerative diseases.[260] [261] [262]

Chronotherapeutic approaches refers to the best time of the day to take medication related to the circadian rhythm, optimizing the benefits of the drug(s) while minimizing the dosage. With circadian rhythms significantly disturbed in AD, they may have a direct link to the pathogenesis of AD, and accumulating evidence shows that chronotherapeutic approaches may generate benefits in the treatment of AD.[263]

- **Chronic stress.** Studies have shown that stress has many effects on the human nervous system and can cause structural changes in different parts of the brain (especially in the hippocampus), including the response to stress, cognition, behavior, and memory.[264][265][266] During extended periods of high stress, neuron growth decreases[267][268] and the hippocampus can shrink in size.[269] Both psychological and emotional stress, experienced over time causes the body to stay in a "flight and fight" mode, which can result in autoimmune disease, chronic inflammation, high blood pressure, high cholesterol, cardiovascular disease, stroke, digestive issues, fertility difficulties, depression, anxiety, memory (especially spatial memory),[270] and cognitive problems, as well as behavioral, cognitive, and also mood disorders.[271]

When someone experiences tolerable or toxic stress, signals go to the command center of the brain, the hypothalamus, resulting in an increased cortisol level which causes the fight-or-flight response. Heart rate increases, senses heighten, more oxygen is taken in, and adrenaline level surges. Next, cortisol is released, which helps to restore the energy lost in the response. When the stressful event is over, cortisol levels fall, and the body returns to stasis. When chronic stress is experienced, the body makes more cortisol than it has a chance to release, which can overtime wear down the brain, disrupt synapse regulation,[272] kill brain cells,[273] and actually shrink the size of the brain.[274]

One study looked at neural stem cells in the hippocampus of the brains of adult rats under acute or chronic stress. These stem cells which were thought to mature only into astrocytes, can also mature in the hippocampus, to an oligodendrocyte.[275] which produces the myelin that sheaths nerve cells. Due to the increase in cortisol the brain generates more myelin-producing cells and fewer neurons.[276] In adult humans, oligodendrocytes are not typically produced from neural stem cells. They are like vines that spread out, wrapping around, supporting, and insulating axons. Overproduction of oligodendrocytes due to chronic stress may also account for brain damage and affect cognitive function.[277]

Chronic mild stress can cause complications such as "increased IL-6 and plasma cortisol, as well as decreased amounts of cAMP responsive element binding protein and brain-derived neurotrophic factor (BDNF). This is very similar to what is observed in people with depression and mood disorders that exhibit a wide range of cognitive problems."[278]

- **Oxidative stress**. Free radical damage contributes to all types of disease. Cognitive decline observed during aging and in AD and is associated with increased oxidative stress, which may be partially responsible for the time-dependent accumulation of cellular damage,[279] ultimately leading to neuronal death and neurodegenerative disorders.

  o **Antioxidants from food**. The body produces some of its own antioxidants that neutralize free radicals before they destroy healthy cells, but it also needs antioxidants from food. If antioxidants are missing in the diet, then higher levels of oxidative stress exist within the brain.[280]

  o **Antioxidant deterioration.** The antioxidant system deteriorates as a function of age, bringing about disruption of the delicate balance between radical oxygen species (ROS) production and elimination. This leads to oxidative cellular damage, resulting in oxidative damage to the body such as to the brain, heart and skeleton muscles which are more susceptible to aging, compared with other organs.[281]

- o **Free radical accumulation**. Free radicals are considered a key factor in the aging of brain cells (as well as overall aging). In the central nervous system (CNS), cellular damage due to free radicals may be responsible for neurodegeneration.[282]

- o **Reactive oxygen species.** The majority of free radicals contain an atom of oxygen and, therefore, are called reactive oxygen species (ROS). The accumulation of free radicals and attenuation of respiratory chain enzyme complex activity causes damage to cerebral mitochondria,[283] leading to the onset of neurodegenerative diseases, such as Parkinson's, Alzheimer's, and Huntington's disease.

- o **Lipid oxidation.** Lipid peroxidation may be a major factor in the aging process resulting in the quantity and integrity of white matter.[284] Blood cell membranes lose flexibility under the influence of free radicals that oxidize some of their component lipids. Elevated DHA oxidation has been observed in the brains of Alzheimer's disease and cognitively impaired patients.[285] Inhibition of DHA oxidation (helped by essential antioxidants such as lutein and other carotenoids) not only helps to maintain membrane structure and fluidity but also preserves DHA. Therefore, it remains available for cleavage and for conversion into anti-inflammatory molecules.[286]

- **Environmental toxins**. In people, there is evidence that lead (Pb), a neurotoxin, raises the risk of age-related cognitive decline. A small percentage of circulating Pb is highly toxic because it is free and bioavailable in the plasma.[287] Exposure in children affects IQ and behavior[288][289] and is a significant risk factor for accelerated declines in cognition in adults.[290][291] High levels of blood Pb is associated with reduced ability to recall and define words, identify line-drawn objects, difficulty in a perceptual comparison test,[292] as well as fatigue, decreased processing speed, fine and gross motor deficits, and generally decreased cognitive functioning.[293] These declines are greater than changes observed with normal aging alone.[294]

  Cumulative lead exposure is associated with an increased risk of amyotrophic lateral sclerosis[295][296] and Parkinson's disease.[297] In regions with high levels of air pollution even children exhibit the hallmarks of Alzheimer's: twisted protein fibers, deteriorating neurons, and amyloid plaque deposits.[298][299][300] The same is true of industrial-, combustion- and friction-derived nanoparticles.[301]

- **Chronic Inflammation**. Over time chronic inflammation can cause the immune system to go into overdrive, resulting in it attacking its own healthy cells.
  - o Microglial cells in the brain, which are needed to break down redundant or dead nerve tissue,[302][303] are part of the immune system. In conditions such as AD they fail to clear away waste, including beta-amyloid deposits.[304] Chronic inflammatory conditions associated with autoimmune diseases show high microglial activity. Such activity also includes high sugar levels (as in uncontrolled diabetes) and oxidative stress which produces high amounts of free radicals.[305]

- o The TREM2 gene directs microglia cells called astrocytes to fight inflammation and remove plaque from the brain. A TREM2 mutation hinders this function; astrocytes (and other microglia cells) accumulate around neurons but are dysfunctional and also release neurotoxins. [306]
- o Chronic inflammation can also be caused by emotional stress; there is a physiological link between stress and mood-based cognitive disorders.[307][308][309]

Contributory Conditions

- **Circulation** – People with dementia seldom have just changes in their brains. One major condition often seen is vascular/cardiovascular problems which interfere with the free flow of oxygen and essential nutrients to the brain. In a person with dementia, a faulty blood-brain barrier prevents glucose from reaching the brain, allows pathogens and toxins to get to the brain, and prevents the clearing away of toxic beta-amyloid and tau proteins.
  - o **Strokes** are the second most common cause of dementia,[310] known medically as multi-infarct dementia, demonstrating the case that AD is a vascular disease.[311] Studies have also found that baseline high density lipoprotein levels were lower and triglyceride levels were higher in elderly men who developed dementia with vascular components.[312] An ischemic stroke occurs when not enough oxygen reaches the brain. Even in mild cases of stroke, some apoptosis (cell death) occurs. Free radicals are also generated that damage brain cell membranes.
  - o **Carotid atherosclerosis.** There is compelling evidence that carotid atherosclerosis is associated with brain atrophy. As we age, atherosclerosis occurs where accumulation of fat-laden, calcified plaque builds up in the blood vessels.[313]
  - o **Chronic high blood pressure** in which blood vessels lose their elasticity cause the muscular layer of the vessels to enlarge, making it more difficult for the body to get the blood effectively to the brain.[314]
  - o **Hypertension** may contribute to cognitive decline by causing cerebral small vessel pathology and increasing neurofibrillary tangles and amyloid plaques.[315]
  - o **Elevated plasma homocysteine** is an independent risk factor for cardiovascular disease, stroke and dementia including AD.[316]
- **Metabolic deficiencies or dysfunction.**
  - o **Cholinergic circuit dysfunction.** Problems of the cholinergic circuit, such as with the neurotransmitter acetylcholine, are important factors. Cholinergic circuit dysfunction has been associated with neurodegenerative diseases such as Alzheimer's, Parkinson's, and Huntington's as well as in psychiatric disorders such as schizophrenia.[317]
  - o **Seratonin** is a chemical produced in the brain by nerve cells that is essential for nerve cell signaling. It is found mostly in the digestive system, although it's also in blood platelets and throughout the central nervous system. Low levels of serotonin in the brain may cause depression, anxiety, and sleep trouble. In a series of recent studies, negative emotions [318] were associated with increased disability due to mental and physical disorders. increased incidence of depression, increased suicide, and increased mortality (even up to two decades later).

o **Removal of ovaries**. A Mayo Clinic study concluded that women whose ovaries are removed by the age of forty without having hormone replacement therapy, have double the risk of AD onset.[319]

o **Insulin imbalances.** Messaging by insulin is essential for neuron survival and is compromised by chronically high levels of insulin. Insulin-degrading enzyme (IDE) is an enzyme responsible for the breakdown of insulin once insulin has done its job. IDE also degrades amyloid beta. If the IDE is tied up resolving excess insulin, there is less available to manage the levels of amyloid beta.[320]

o **High blood sugar** levels, even in people without diabetes, are strongly linked to increased risk of dementia, and most specifically, AD (which is sometimes called type 3 diabetes).[321] Excess sugar also results in an increase of advanced glycation end products (AGEs). These cause increases in free radicals and promote inflammation, damage blood vessels which can result in nutritional deficiencies in the brain.

Tests for Dementia

At this point, most diagnosis for dementia and AD is based on ability to perform common tasks, remember recent events, evaluating behavioral changes, etc. Common tests take only about five to fifteen minutes to complete and can serve as a baseline for comparison should further testing be necessary.

- Mini-Mental State Examination, the Montreal Cognitive Assessment test (MOCA), the Short Test of Mental Status or the Cognitive Capacity Screening Examination, are given to check for any general cognitive impairment.
- The Clock-drawing Test and the Time and Change Test: two other simple tests
- Other tests may include: Orientation Test, Word Repetition (Registration and Memory), Language (for example naming animals or supermarket items), Test of Attention and Working Memory (WM) for example, who is the current President or recent events, and Executive Function (ability to complete complex tasks).

The American Academy of Neurology recommends the following tests in the routine evaluation of a patient with suspected dementia:

- Complete blood cell count
- Electrolyte levels in the blood (potassium, sodium, and chloride)
- Blood levels of glucose, urea nitrogen and creatinine
- Blood levels of vitamin B12
- Liver function tests and thyroid function tests
- Depression screening
- Non-contrast computed tomography (CT) or magnetic resonance imaging (MRI)

A routine evaluation would not include an amyloid PET (photon emission tomography) scanning, genetic screening, or testing for a variant form of the apolipoprotein E (APOE) gene that significantly increases the risk of developing Alzheimer's disease. Testing for syphilis, HIV disease or performing a lumbar puncture to check the spinal fluid for infection or biochemical "red flags" (markers) of Alzheimer's disease would only be done in special circumstances. Some lab tests may be ordered including blood tests that can identify anemia, liver disorders, thyroid problems, nutritional deficiencies, and infections such as syphilis.

Misdiagnosis. Current use of PET scans reveals that many patients being treated for Alzheimer's do not actually have accumulations of amyloid beta.[322]

Conventional Treatment

There are many drugs that have been approved for use with Alzheimer's patients which may slow progression of the condition. Some of them may be appropriate for other forms of dementia.

- Given the connection of cardiovascular health, neuroprotective effects of drugs used in patients with CVD have great potential and these would add benefits to patients' overall outcome.
- Drugs used for the treatment of AD include tacrine and donepezil. Deonepezil inhibits acetylcholinesterase (AChE); by increasing levels of available acetylcholine, and may compensate for the loss of functioning cholinergic brain cells
- Ibuprofen and other anti-inflammatory drugs may slow its progression.
- Dementia caused by small strokes cannot be treated medically; however, treating co-existing conditions, such as hypertension and diabetes, can slow or stop the progression of symptoms.
- If depression is the cause, antidepressants and counseling may help.
- If dementia is caused by hydrocephalus, removing excess fluid by shunting may help.
- Antipsychotic drugs such as thorazine or haloperidol may be prescribed if the patient has paranoia or hallucinations.
- For those with cardiovascular risk factors, studies indicate early intervention could reduce the risk of several cognitive deficits.[323]

Note: As discussed in further detail in the above section "Causes of Dementia" under Circadian Rhythm, applying the practice of Chronotherapy when determining medication for AD can optimize the benefits of medication while minimizing the dosage.

Complementary Approach

Diet and Nutrition

See the Alzheimer's and Parkinson's chapters for more specific information and studies about the nutrients listed below (plus more related nutrients) and the Nutrient Spreadsheet, the Diet, and Alzheimer's chapters.

Top brain nutrients that have the widest range of brain benefits include: acetyl-L-carnitine, ashwagandha, apigenin, curcumin, DHA (or fish oil), gingko biloba, ginseng, grapeseed extract, green tea extract, lutein, N-acetyl-cysteine, resveratrol, olive leaf extract, phosphatidylserine, PQQ (pyrroloquinoline quinone), vinpocetine, vitamin E, and zeaxanthin.

Top brain foods include avocado, blueberries (and other dark berries) dark chocolate, eggs, fish, fruits and vegetables, goji berry, green and black teas, mulberry, nuts. mushrooms (reiki, shitake, and lion's mane for example), pomegranate juice, prunes, pumpkin seeds, yogurt (organic plain), and walnuts.

Nutrient deficiencies that can mimic dementia include vitamins B1, B6, B12, D3, iron, magnesium, selenium, zinc, as well as low levels of serotonin (essential neurotransmitter in the central nervous system and acts as a hormone in the periphery) and dopamine (a hormone).

Essential and aromatic oils. Essential and aromatic oils are great for helping support memory and cognition, improving circulation, reducing inflammation, reducing anxiety and depression, improving digestion and sleep, and much more. Top essential oils include bergamot, ginger, lavender, lemon balm, frankincense, peppermint, rosemary, sage, and ylang ylang.

Juicing recipe. Green, leafy vegetables, broccoli, avocado, apples, berries (especially blueberries), strawberry, bilberry, black currant, blackberry, mulberry, lemon, goji berries, chia seeds, kale, citrus fruits, apple, curcumin, garlic, parsley, pomegranate juice, prunes, walnuts, yogurt.

Exercise

Many researchers have noted that exercise enhances and protects cognition[324] and sensorimotor functions. Regular exercise might delay a rare form of early-onset Alzheimer's disease. Researchers found that two and one-half hours of walking or other physical activity a week thwarts mental decline tied to autosomal dominant Alzheimer's disease (ADAD), a genetic form of Alzheimer's. Participants of the study did at least 150 minutes a week of walking, running, swimming or other exercise. The result was lowered levels of key biological markers of Alzheimer's disease in their cerebrospinal fluid, including tau (a protein that builds up in the brains of people who are diagnosed with Alzheimer's).[325]

Another study showed that people with a history of exercise that have the ApoE4 gene (that increases the risk of AD onset 10-30%) did not develop dementia and has less *b*-amyloid in their brains.[326]

Meditation

Studies show that meditation reduces stress and changes brain structure. In one meta-analysis, the study compared those that meditated with non-meditators. The result was that the meditators showed better interoceptive and exteroceptive awareness, memory, emotional regulation, intra and interhemispheric communication between brain regions.[327]

There is evidence that even a short-term meditation practice may alter large-scale brain networks. In beginners after two weeks of training, an increase in functional connections were detected, involving the neural circuitry related to attention, cognitive and affective processing among others.[328]

Several studies have documented the positive impact of mindfulness-based programs on symptoms of anxiety and depression [329] [330] and improvements in sleep patterns,[331] [332] and attention. [333]

In one mindful breath group of seniors who completed an eight-week session, the group showed significant behavioral and electrophysiological responses related to Stroop task performance. Stroop tasks refer to testing person's selective attention capacity and skills, as well as their processing speed ability.[334]

Mental Health

- Manage stress levels. Preventing and managing long-term stress can lower your risk for other conditions like heart disease, obesity, high blood pressure, and depression.[335]
- Socialize with positive people.

Chapter 5. Alzheimer's Disease

Alzheimer's disease (AD) is a multi-neurological/multifaceted disease characterized clinically by a progressive and gradual decline in cognitive function associated with the build-up of amyloid beta, neurofibrillary tangles, and tau protein in the brain. This build-up results in specific neuron loss, and synapse loss in addition to the hallmarks of memory loss, cognitive problems, and other symptoms of dementia.[336] Increase in age is a major risk factor. It affects ten percent of individuals over the age of sixty-five, rising to over forty percent in those aged over eight-five[337] and is the most common cause of dementia, accounting for sixty to eighty percent of dementia cases. AD is the third leading cause of death in the United States, following only cardiovascular disease and cancer.[338]

An estimated 5.7 million Americans of all ages were living with Alzheimer's in 2018, and this figure is projected to triple to 14 million people by 2060.[339] The number includes almost forty percent of those aged sixty-five and over, and five percent of people under age sixty-five with early-onset Alzheimer's. Between the years 2000 and 2015, deaths from heart disease decreased eleven percent while those from AD increased 123 percent(primarily due to living longer).[340] [341]

Common symptoms can include difficulty with daily activities, decreased and poor judgment, changes in mood and behavior, and often onset of depression. Delaying the onset of the AD clinical phase by just one year can reduce disease prevalence by twenty-five percent,[342] with enormous positive economic and social impacts for society.

Alzheimer's Onset

Symptom onset usually follows a period of great stress, sleep loss, or menopause; presentation is not predominantly amnestic but is instead cortical, with dyscalculia (difficulty in remembering the day and doing math calculations), aphasia (difficulty in understanding expressing speech), executive dysfunction, or other cortical (related to the outer layer of the cerebrum) deficits; and the neurological presentation is often preceded or accompanied by depression.

Alzheimer's is categorized as either early-onset or late-onset.

- **Early-onset AD**, appearing as early as age thirty, is strongly linked to genetic inheritance (see Genetic Factors: Early-Onset AD below). It is strongly linked to genetic inheritance.
- The more common **late-onset AD** may start as early as late forties or fifties (see Genetic Factors: Late-Onset AD below). This variant is linked to genetic inheritance and/or other epigenetic and related health factors.

The accumulation of amyloid beta plaque, a hallmark of Alzheimer's is gradual. Imaging can detect the presence of amyloid beta plaque in cognitively normal adults. This is known as being "amyloid positive" and it may be many years before enough accumulation is present to cause dementia.

Types of Alzheimer's

Metabolic profiling has allowed for identifying three sub-types of Alzheimer's: biochemically, genetically, and symptomatically.[343]

Type 1 (Inflammatory)

Inflammatory AD is reflected in such laboratory results as a high-sensitivity C-reactive protein (high hs-CRP), low albumin:globulin ratio, and high cytokine levels such as interleukin-1 and interleukin-6.

Type 2 (Non-inflammatory or Atrophic)

Atrophic AD is characterized by an atrophic profile (breakdown of organs and cells), with reduced support from molecules such as estradiol, progesterone, testosterone, insulin, and vitamin D, often accompanied by increased homocysteine and insulin resistance.

Type 3 (Cortical)

Cortical AD is very dissimilar to the other two types and may be mediated by a fundamentally different pathophysiological process (although, by definition, still amyloid positive and phospho-tau positive): the onset is typically younger (late forties to early sixties). Type 3 Alzheimer's disease is the result of exposure to specific toxins and is most commonly inhalational (IAD) which would be due to biotoxins such as mycotoxins. However, type 3 may be genetically driven as well.

It is possible that type 3 represents on the order of ten percent of patients with Alzheimer's disease, thus potentially affecting hundreds of thousands of Americans. This percentage would be much higher for the subgroup of patients who are ApoE4-negative and whose symptoms begin prior to the age of sixty-five.[344]

Pathology

Over Production of Amyloid Beta (Aβ or b-amyloid)

The problem arises in the over production of Aβ, which is toxic to the brain causing apoptosis (neuron death). This occurs when three things take place:

1. It goes through a structural change whereupon it folds back on itself called *cross-sheets*, resulting in it forming insoluble fibrils (referred to as fibrillation). Aβ is normally easily soluble and reabsorbed into one's body through the lymph system;
2. excess copper binds with iron;
3. the presence of the amino acid methionine [345]

When methionine binds to Aβ, the clumps of the b-amyloid begin generating oxidizing molecules that damage surrounding neurons (think of rusting of metal as the effect of oxidation).

Amyloid Precursor Protein

There are two compounds at work: amyloid beta protein and amyloid beta peptide. The latter is derived from the former. According to Dr. Dale Bredeson in his book, *The End of Alzheimer's*, the build-up of beta-amyloid plaque, neurofibillary fibers, and tau protein is actually the attempt by the body to deal with a variety of metabolic imbalances such as inflammation, a decline and shortage of essential nutrients, hormones, and/or exposure to toxins such as metals or biotoxins including metals toxicity and poisons produced by microbes such as molds.[346]

Amyloid precursor protein (APP) is found in many tissues and concentrated in the synapses of neurons. It is thought to be a regulator of the synapse formation, and essential in supporting neural plasticity and iron export. It is found in abundance in Aβ. APP is produced by the neurons and consists of 695 amino acids (Aβ is 40-42 amino acids). In an analysis by Dr. Bredeson, APP is split by molecular scissors called "proteases". If APP splits into two sections (peptides), healthy synaptic connections and neurogenesis are supported. But if APP divides into four sections, synaptic connections are damaged, and neurogenesis is inhibited. Such a division creates an excess of beta amyloid which comes from the cleavage of APP, binding it to APP and causing a cascade of creating excess beta-amyloid. The cascade is referred to as the "prionic loop," producing more and more synapse and neuron destroying amyloid beta.[347]

The theory as to the reason for this on one level is a molecule called netrin-1, floating around in the molecular fluid. When APP grabs hold of netrin-1, APP functions in a healthy manner in the brain. When APP fails to grab hold of netrin-1, and lacks other trophic support, the signal it emits causes the neurons to commit suicide. The second effect is that it ends up grabbing the beta-amyloid molecule, unleashing a cascade of biochemical reactions that cause the APP to be cut in a manner the produces more amyloid beta.

Amyloid Cascade Hypothesis

The amyloid cascade hypothesis outlines probable steps in development of AD.[348]
- Beta-amyloid deposits are the initial pathological event,
- This leads to the formation of senile plaques (SPs) neuronal cell death,
- ultimately and finally, dementia.
- In addition is the formation of neurofibrillary tangles and tau protein build-up

There are limitations to this hypothesis:[349]
1. SPs and NFTs may develop independently, and
2. SPs and NFTs may be the products, rather than causes, of neurodegeneration.
3. In addition, studies targeting the amyloid pathway via drugs, etc. are not conclusive.

1. Beta-amyloid deposits are the initial event.

Amyloid beta (Aβ) plaque accumulation caused by amyloid beta precursor protein (APP) and apolipoprotein E (APOE) genetic mutations and increased inflammation and oxidative damage have been shown to be associated with AD.[350]

2. This leads to the formation of senile plaques (SPs).

The aggregation and fibrillization of amyloid beta protein (Aß), leading to the deposit of amyloid plaques in the brain, is one of the major pathological features in AD. Although AD brains typically harbor senile plaques that consist of insoluble aggregates of Aβ, different assemblies of Aβ, including fibrils as well as soluble dimers, trimers and dodecamers (biomolecular complexes of proteins with nucleic acids and other cofactors), may differentially contribute to AD pathogenesis.[351][352]

3. And then to neurofibrillary tangles (NFTs).

Tau proteins hold together microtubules, which in turn protect axons (neurons that provide outgoing information in the brain) as well as dendrites. Microtubules are made of tubulin and tau interacts with tubulin to protect the stability of microtubules.

When tau has an excessive amount of phosphate attached to it (known as hyperphosphorylated tau), the microtubules diminish in number and density and this loss of microtubule mass negatively impacts the capacity of the neuron to maintain axonal transport and synaptic connections.

Neurofibrillary tangles are clumps of hyperphosphorylated tau. [353][354][355] Increasing numbers of these malformed proteins compromise the ability of microtubules to provide structure and stability inside and around the cells, as well as acting as highways transporting nutrients around and inside the cells. This structure is found in the axons that provide outgoing information, not the dendrites that handle incoming signals in the brain. Think of telephone wires sending data and bringing calls in. Axons and dendrites are extension neurons.

There is an additional degree of complexity. "Tau is normally less enriched in dendrites than axons. In AD, tau invades dendrites abnormally through deregulation of its normal sorting mechanism, and this somehow leads to microtubule loss from dendrites."[356]

4. Neuronal cell death.

When the microtubule structure breaks down, the axons (and dendrites) lose their integrity resulting in various ions flowing into the cells, causing neurons to die.

5. Dementia develops.

Causes of Alzheimer's

AB May be a Trigger, Not a Cause

Tough amyloid plaques are a major indicator of possible onset of AD, it may be more complex than that. While potential floor or ceiling effects in the amount of Aβ deposition could contribute, there is also the possibility that Aβ exerts its major effects early by triggering a cascade of processes that, once begun, proceed independently of Aβ. For example, in spite of this markedly lower amount of Aβ, presumably caused by the immunotherapy, the subjects continued to decline cognitively to an end stage dementia that was clinically indistinguishable from untreated

AD.[357] It is tempting to speculate that the implication of these results is that Aβ acts as a trigger for a degenerative process that continues even if it is removed.[358] Two major enzymes, neprilysin (NEP) and insulin degrading enzyme (also known as insulysin; IDE), are believed responsible for most Aβ degradation.[359] [360]

Genetic Factors: Late-Onset AD

Many general risk factors, discussed in Chapter 4, *About Memory and Dementia,* are also risk factors for Alzheimer's. Genetics accounts for one-third of AD onset causes. Both genetic inheritance and influence of genetic expression have an influence.

APOE Gene

There are three types (alleles) of the apolipoprotein E (APOE) gene: APOE2, APOE3, and APOE4. Everyone has two copies (one from each parent) of the APOE gene which can be different types. The APOE4 allele is the gene which most puts you at risk for AD, although some researchers now feel that the APOE3 gene also carries some risk. Which pair you have, determines your risk for AD development: E2/E2, E2/E3, E2/E4, E3/E3, E3/E4, or E4/E4.[361]

- **APOE2** is rare; having even one copy of this gene variant may reduce AD risk by up to forty percent.[362]
- **APOE3** is the most common APOE polymorphism in the general population and considered risk-neutral.[363]
- **APOE4** is present in present is fifty percent of the AD population and approximately 10-15 percent of general people. Having this gene increases AD risk and lowers the age of onset. [364] [365] [366] The APOE4 gene binds amyloid beta and regulates clumping or clearing of amyloid beta.[367]
  - *a.* Twenty-five percent (or 75 million Americans) carry a single ApoE4 gene which increases their risk of AD to thirty percent (two to three times).[368] Symptoms of onset typically start in the late fifties or sixties.

Those that carry two copies are at a higher risk of getting AD. About 7 million people carry two copies which increases the risk of AD to well above 50 percent [369] (10-30 times higher). This gene along with other factors which include Amyloid precursor protein (APP), Presenilin 1 (PSEN1) and Presenilin 2 (PSEN2) may be related to "Early Onset Dementia" which can start as early as people in their thirties, forties, or fifties.[370]
  - *b.* Poorer outcomes associated with ApoE4 might relate to its reduced ability to repair and remodel synapses and protect neurons upon injury compared with ApoE3.[371]

However not everyone who has the APOE4 develops Alzheimer's, and some people develop AD who do not have APOE3 or 4. Other genetic or environmental factors may trigger development of AD

Other Genes

Researchers are finding other genetic links for late-onset Alzheimer's, including the following:[372]

ABCA7. This gene may be linked to a higher risk of Alzheimer's involving how the body processes cholesterol.[373]

CLU. The clusterin gene helps regulate the removal of amyloid beta; it is a biomarker for the ability of the body to remove cholesterol and reduce inflammation.[374]

CR1. A deficiency of the protein produced by CR1 (complement receptor type 1) contributes to chronic inflammation in the brain.[375]

PICALM. The "phosphatidylinositol binding clathrin assembly" gene is involved in the ability of brain neurons to communicate with each other.[376]

PLD3. The "phospholipase D family member 3" gene is linked to processing of amyloid beta precursor protein, and consequently, with AD development.[377]

TREM2. Mutations of this gene, which with another gene, TYROBP regulates development of dendritic immune cells, and is therefore linked the behavior of micrologia, the immune cells found in the brain. It is involved in the regulation of the brain's response to inflammation.[378]

SORL1. (Also known as LR11) variations of this gene are linked to accumulation of amyloid beta by way of its role in regulating the amyloid precursor protein, destruction of amyloid beta, and interaction with the APOE gene and tau protein.[379]

Epigenetic Factors

Epigenetics is the study of how environmental factors affect genes getting turned on and off through life. Epigenetics plays an important regulatory role in gene expression. Epigenetic dysregulation of important AD tau and amyloid processing pathway genes may point to a potential mechanism for AD disease progression. Evidence for the role of epigenetics in AD pathogenesis is found in human studies of various tissues, animal models, and cell culture.[380] [381] Factors that affect epigenetics include: "lifestyle" habits such as nutrition, behavior, stress, physical activity, working habits, smoking and alcohol consumption, as well as environmental pollutants, psychological stress, and working on night shifts (see Epigenetics chapter for details).

- **Epigenetic alterations** have been reported in AD at different levels. Bulk histone acetylation (ac), phosphorylation (ph), and methylation (me) changes, as well as DNA methylation (5mC) and hydroxymethylation (5hmC) alterations. Alterations in epigenetic marks have also been associated with a variety of human diseases, including cancer, cardiovascular, respiratory, and neurodegenerative diseases.[382]

- **Environmental pollution**. As discussed earlier, children and young adults who live in   areas with significant air pollution are much more likely to have the hallmarks of Alzheimer's. These include twisted protein fibers, deteriorating neurons and amyloid beta plaque deposits.[383] [384] [385] The same risk is true of industrial-, combustion-, and friction-derived nanoparticles.[386]

Circulatory Factors

- **Aging** is associated with a reduction of blood flow to the brain, which contributes to adverse changes in cognitive function.[387] A significant body of evidence points to diminished cerebral circulation as a precursor to both vascular and Alzheimer's dementia.
- Growing evidence supports a strong and likely causal association between **cardiovascular disease** (CVD) and its risk factors with incidence of cognitive decline and AD.[388] Individuals with subclinical CVD are at higher risk for dementia and AD.[389] [390]

Metabolic Factors

- **Blood sugar imbalances.** A strong school of thought is that insulin resistance[391] with chronic blood sugar elevations are involved in depression and neurodegenerative disorders such as Alzheimer's disease.[392] [393] [394] The brain, as well as the pancreas, produces insulin. Insulin regulates glucose (sugar) and directs the body to store energy, primarily in the form of fat. In the brain, insulin not only breaks down glucose, but also regulates the clearance of b-amyloid protein and tau phosphorylation (essential for avoiding AD). Insulin supports healthy blood flow and the removal of fats from the brain, inhibits apoptosis (cell death), manages the response to inflammation, supports the ability for the formation of new synapsis, and supports new memory formation. It can also facilitate neurotransmitter receptor trafficking.[395]

  Therefore, any change in insulin balance can have serious consequences. There is a great similarity between AD and type 2 diabetes as both ultimately result in one's body becoming resistant to insulin, thereby reducing its effectiveness. In both conditions, inflammation with increased levels of oxidative stress occurs. The b-amyloid levels increase in both the brain and pancreas, as well as hyperphosphorylated tau protein and cognitive decline. Fifty percent of Americans between the ages of forty-five to sixty four and seventy-six percent of those over sixty-five have an insulin imbalance which becomes a critical health issue for Americans. Factors that contribute to insulin resistance over time include: having a sedentary lifestyle (lack of consistent exercise), poor diet that includes high amounts of refined carbohydrates, poor quality oils, high levels of stress, health conditions that cause chronic inflammation, emotional imbalances that may result in being easily angered, having chronic, excess worry and/or fear for example.

- **Hormonal deficiencies**. Imbalances in estrogen, testosterone, and thyroid hormone.
- **Hyperhomocysteinemia**. Elevated plasma homocysteine is an independent risk factor for cardiovascular disease, stroke and dementia including AD.[396] [397]
- **Cholesterol/lipid metabolism**. Researchers note that it has become obvious that AD is closely linked to lipid metabolism. [398] "Aβ is derived from sequential proteolytic processing of the amyloid precursor protein (APP). Interestingly, both, the APP and all APP secretases are transmembrane proteins that cleave APP close to and in the lipid bilayer. Moreover, apoE4 has been identified as the most prevalent genetic risk factor for AD. ApoE is the main lipoprotein in the brain, which has an abundant role in the transport of lipids and brain lipid metabolism."[399]

Aβ affects and alters cholesterol levels in neurons, which leads to neurodegeneration with abnormally phosphorylated tau.[400] In one study, high levels of LDL or total cholesterol were reported to correlate with lower Modified Mini Mental State Exam scores in clinically nondemented patients.[401] In another study, high total cholesterol levels at midlife have been associated with a nearly threefold increase in the likelihood of developing AD, even after controlling for ApoE genotype.[402]

It has been further suggested that cholesterol levels exert some influence over the well-established correlation of the ApoE4 allele with risk of AD.[403] Researchers note that although cholesterol itself cannot cross the blood-brain barrier; oxidized cholesterol metabolites known as oxysterols are able to do so. Two main oxysterols, 24S-hydroxycholesterol and 27-hydrosycholesterol are found to be altered in the brains of AD patients and they appear to play a role in AD's progression.[404]

Note. Statin drugs are the most common treatment for lowering cholesterol. Though they tend to work well, they can have significant side effects including muscle wasting over time. There are ways you can discuss with your doctor to naturally lower cholesterol that may enable you to avoid taking statin drugs including: regular exercise, weight management, a healthy, high fiber diet (rich in beans, oats, fruits and raw or lightly steamed vegetables), avoiding high levels of saturated fats and trans fatty acids, not smoking, drinking in moderation (a glass of red wine at night is typically fine), and supplements including red rice yeast, fish oil, CoQ10, psyllium, garlic, green tea.

- **Acetylcholine deficiency.** In the brain, the acetylcholine receptor is a membrane-based protein that can be activated by the neurotransmitter molecule, acetylcholine. The acetylcholine receptor is responsible for cognitive function and it consists of two members, muscarinic[405] and nicotinic receptors.[406] Muscarinic receptors are one of two major receptors being targeted in Alzheimer's research. They mediate acetylcholine-induced neurotransmission. Five muscarinic receptors have been identified so far and some of them are implicated in many forms of brain dysfunction. Investigating these members is one of the recent research targets because dysfunctional acetylcholine reception triggers a series of problems.

  Alzheimer's disease sufferers have been found to have a lack of the enzyme responsible for converting **choline** into acetylcholine.[407] [408] [409] Choline is a water-soluble nutrient essential for synthesis of phospholipids needed for cell membrane integrity. It is needed to reduce homocysteine levels. High homocysteine levels double the risk of Alzheimer's.[410] Choline also reduces excess microglia action causing brain inflammation and nerve cell death.

  Acetylcholine (ACh) is one of the most important neurotransmitters, promoting cell proliferation as well as neuron and glial cell survival and differentiation. It is used both in the central and peripheral nervous system. In advanced AD, loss of cholinergic innervation in the cerebral cortex is widespread, with the most severe losses in the temporal lobes.[411] [412] These cortical cholinergic losses in AD have primarily been associated with cognitive impairment and dementia.[413]

- **Glutathione (GSH) deficiency**. Researchers have observed that AD patients have significantly depleted levels of glutathione, a powerful antioxidant that protects the brain from oxidative stress. By implementing non-invasive imaging techniques in the hippocampus, it was discovered that when GSH is depleted in the hippocampus regions of an elderly person the healthy brain suffers mild cognitive impairment, which is known to be present in the earlier stages of AD.[414]

- **Methylation.** Cell studies suggest that AD is associated with lower levels of DNA methylation.[415] Higher Aβ levels induce a general DNA hypomethylation as measured by DNA methylation-sensitive antibodies.[416 417]

- **Mitochondrial function.** Mitochondria are the energy batteries of our cells, producing APT which powers metabolic processes. Mitochondrial dysfunction appears to be a critical factor in the pathogenesis of AD.[418 419] Hypometabolism (low metabolism) develops as a function of aging in the brain[420] and is evident in affected brain regions,[421 422] where mitochondrial structure is altered.[423 424]

  AD brain mitochondria abnormalities reduce membrane potential, increase permeability, and produce excess free radicals which damage proteins, lipids, and nucleic acids. Growing evidence suggests that elevated amyloid beta levels contribute to these mitochondrial abnormalities and although the mechanism is not clearly established, both amyloid precursor protein (APP) and Aβ are found in mitochondrial membranes and interact with mitochondrial proteins. Overproduction of the APP and Aβ may affect dynamics of mitochondrial fusion/fission,[425 426 427] impair mitochondrial transport, disrupt the electron transfer chain, increase ROS production,[428 429] and impair mitochondrial function.[430 431] These findings build a strong case for mitochondrial dysfunction in AD and effective treatment will likely include targets that address mitochondrial function.[432 433]

- **Mitochondrial biogenesis** plays an essential role in maintaining an adequate functional neuronal mitochondrial mass by compensating for damaged mitochondria that have been eliminated. It is highly regulated and requires coordination and crosstalk between the nuclear and mitochondrial genomes.[434] While mitochondrial biogenesis occurs on a regular basis in healthy cells where mitochondria constantly divide and fuse with each other,[435 436] it also occurs in response to oxidative stress, increased energy demand, exercise training and certain diseases.

- **Mitophagy** is the process of removal of damaged mitochondria through autophagy (the body's natural regeneration process) and is delivered to lysosomes to be degraded and recycled by the cell.[437 438] Lysosomes are more than mere cellular "trash cans". They are an important part of the signaling process through which autophagy occurs. High levels of ROS may trigger autophagy; dysfunctional mitochondria are selectively targeted for mitophagy.[439] In sum, autophagy is critical for neuronal homeostasis and survival[440 441 442] and mutations in several key autophagy proteins have been linked to the progression of neurodegenerative disease in humans.[443 444 445]

  Note. Nutrients that support mitochondrial function (and against mitochondrial dysfunction) include: Vitamins B1, B2, B6, C, D and E, l-carnosine, l-taurine, CoQ10, benfotiamine, alpha-R-lipoic acid, PQQ (pyrroloquinoline quinone), luteolin [from orange extract fruit), l-carnitine, trans-resveratrol, curcumin, magnesium, and schisandra.

- **Transglutaminases** are a large family of related and ubiquitous enzymes capable of catalyzing other reactions important for the cell viability. "Tissue" transglutaminase (TG2) has been shown to be involved in very in a number of health conditions including celiac disease, neurodegenerative diseases, Alzheimer's, Parkinson's, supranuclear palsy, and Huntington's disease.[446]

Chronic Inflammation and Oxidative Stress

Increases in chronic inflammation results in increases in oxidative molecules, chemokines, cytokines, and immune cells, (such as bradykinin, serotonin, and histamine) which in turn result in insulin resistance in the brain, causing a cascade of events that end up affecting healthy neurons. They increase both endothelial permeability and vessel diameter, together contributing to significant leak across the blood-brain barrier and cerebral edema. Chronic inflammation[447][448][449][450] and oxidative stress[451][452] are prominent issues related to contributing nerve damage and the onset of AD, and may play a role in other forms of dementia.[453]

Exaggerated oxidative stress in AD,[454][455][456][457][458][459] leads to overproduction of amyloid beta protein associated free radical production and cell death,[460][461] causing yet more oxidative stress,[462] a dangerous cycle. Inflammation is recognized as a risk factor for degenerative diseases of the brain, including Alzheimer's disease and dementia[463][464] The pathophysiology of CIRS (chronic inflammatory response system) includes effects are relevant to all three types of Alzheimer's disease.

Neuroinflammation has been tied to disease progression and severity in AD, where misfolded and aggregated proteins trigger an immune response resulting in neuronal death and progressive cognitive decline.[465][466][467][468]

Astrocyte destruction. Astrocyte destruction is associated with BBB (blood-brain-barrier) disruption.[469] Astrocytes induce and maintain the BBB, and in particular form the glia limitans.[470][471] This abundant form of glial cells is closely associated with neuronal synapses. They regulate the transmission of electrical impulses within the brain, provide metabolic support and essential nutrients to the neurons.

Exposure to Toxins

Toxic exposure has been shown to be connected to onset of AD, including exposure to various heavy metals, chemical compounds, molds, as well as herbicides and pesticides.

- **Aluminum.** A possible relationship between Al and the pathogenesis of AD has been discussed for several decades,[472][473] with considerable number of studies have provided evidence to support an association between AD and Al in drinking water. [474][475] Accumulation of excess aluminum due to leakage from cookware, unpurified municipal drinking water (aluminum is frequently used to filter municipal water and often not removed completely) and baking powder used in cooking and antacid tablets for example.

  A 2016 meta-analysis reviewing eight studies of over 10,000 people found that chronic exposure to aluminum caused a seventy-one percent increased risk of developing

AD.[476] Even so, other studies still find the linkage controversial.[477]

- **Heavy metals** including mercury, arsenic, lead, and cadmium can all affect healthy brain function. Mercury can induce the buildup of amyloid beta and neurofibrillary tangles in the brain. It also destroys parts of glutathione essential for neutralizing and eliminating free radicals.[478] [479] Zinc, copper and iron are also implicated influencing oligomerization and conformational changes of AβP as cross-linkers. This increasing evidence suggests the implication of these metals in the pathogenesis of AD.[480] [481]

  Elevated levels of metals may induce various detrimental intracellular events, including oxidative stress, mitochondrial dysfunction, DNA fragmentation, protein misfolding, endoplasmic reticulum (a network of tubules in cells) stress, unregulated cell cleansing/removal, and premature cell death.[482] [483]

- **Arsenic.** High levels of exposure to arsenic has been associated with impaired executive function, reduced mental acuity, deterioration in verbal skills, as well as depression.[484]

  Note: If you going to have a blood test for arsenic levels, it is best to avoid eating seafood for at least a few days. Seafood may contain some non-toxic organic arsenic, so the test could result in a false positive reading.

- **Excess lead exposure** has been shown in a rat study to increase amyloid formation (lead can be found in old paint and dust particles in cities).[485] The presence of lead in the human body causes damage to the nervous system through several mechanisms. One way affects babies in the prenatal thru childhood stage. Such effects include disruption of key molecules during neuronal migration and differentiation,[486] interfering with synapse formation, mediated by a reduction in neuronal sialic acid production,[487] and causing and premature differentiation of glial cells.[488] In addition, it disrupts the function dopaminergic, and cholinergic systems as well as inhibiting NMDA-ion channels during the neonatal period.[489] [490] Other conditions that exposure to lead can lead to include: adverse effects on nervous system function, hypertension, impaired renal function, impaired thyroid function, vitamin D deficiency, and preterm birth.[491]

  The most severe neurological effect of lead exposure is lead encephalopathy,[492] with symptoms that include irritability, headache, mental dullness and attention difficulty, memory loss, tremor, and hallucinations within weeks of exposure. Even low dosages of exposure to lead can lead to effects on nervous system function. Some research also. has demonstrated lowered learning and memory scores in occupational lead-exposed adults. [493] [494]

- **Cadmium** is more known as a carcinogenic substance but rat studies indicate that excess cadmium acts with lead and arsenic induce Alzheimer-like changes in the brain.[495]

- **Pesticides and environmental chemicals**. Recent studies, including a 2019 meta-analysis reported that exposure to pesticides and herbicides increases the risk of developing neurodegenerative conditions such as ALS, Parkinson's[496] [497] and Alzheimer's[498] by fifty percent.[499] Poisoning by organophosphorus pesticides affects the neurophysiology by causing oxidative stress, inflammation, through acting on enzymes crucial to neurotransmission, as well as genetic mutations.[500]

These toxins may alter neurotransmission and lead to neurodegeneration, which can manifest as cognitive problems, movement disorders, learning/memory dysfunction. To date, metal-induced neurotoxicity has been associated with multiple neurological diseases in humans, including AD, amyotrophic lateral sclerosis (ALS), autism spectrum disorders (ASDs), Guillain–Barré disease (GBD), Gulf War syndrome (GWS), Huntington's disease (HD), multiple sclerosis, Parkinson's disease (PD), and also Wilson's disease (WD).[501 502 503]

- **Mycotoxins.** Type 3 AD may be more indicative of mycotoxin exposure.[504] There is an estimated twenty-five percent of the population with mycotoxin exposure where the mold is not readily identified by the body that can cause chronic inflammation, along with a variety of illnesses including: chronic fatigue, fibromyalgia, asthma, shortness of breath, rashes, nosebleeds, headaches and cognitive decline. This is well described in a 2010 book by Dr. Ritchie Shoemaker called *Surviving Mold: Life in the Era of Dangerous Building.*

  The resulting syndrome has been designated chronic inflammatory response syndrome (CIRS). The most common cause of CIRS is exposure to mycotoxins, typically associated with molds such as stachybotrys, penicillium, or aspergillus, present in water-damaged buildings. However, other biotoxins, from herpes simplex virus, which can migrate to the brain, the borrelia burgdorferi of Lyme disease, or other tick-borne pathogens, or aquatoxins such as those from dinoflagellates, may also cause CIRS. A good genetic blood test is the HLA-DR/DQ test, which tests for the twenty-five percent of the population exposed to mycotoxins, where the body does not readily identify them but still results in a chronic inflammatory response.

- **Blood-brain barrier (BBB) permeability.** The blood-brain barrier is essential in preventing toxins, bacteria, viruses, mold, fungi, and other unwanted substances from reaching the brain. Unfortunately, a list of disease-causing bacteria, viruses, fungi, and other microbes have been identified in the brains of AD patients. For example, a bacterium called porphromonas gingivitis has turned up repeatedly in patients' brains with AD, as has some of the proteins made by this microbe.[505]

- **Excessive alcohol consumption** can result in BBB permeability.[506] Bacterial overgrowth has been observed with alcohol consumption, whereas antibiotics may be able to decrease the bacterial load and attenuate ALD (alcoholic liver disease).[507 508 509 510] Probiotic lactobacillus is significantly suppressed during alcohol consumption (so supplementing with this probiotic is highly recommended to help restore proper flora balance).[511 512]

Lymphatic System Factors

The lymphatic system maintains the body's fluid balance, blood circulation, and immune mechanisms. Although a direct correlation between compromised lymphatic drainage and amyloid beta build-up has not been proven, and the brain lacks lymphatic channels, there is a possible connection found in that Aβ is present in the "interstitial cerebral fluid" (ICF) and that it might be drained into lymph nodes.[513 514] The route by which lymphatic drainage of Aβ may occur was suggested to be along basement membranes of cerebral capillaries and arteries.[515 516]

Glymphatic System Factors

The function of the glymphatic system (also known as "astroglial-mediated interstitial fluid (ISF) bulk flow") is to clear waste through tunnels around blood vessels on the macroscopic level. Formed by astroglial cells, it may contribute to clearance of amyloid beta. The glymphatic system is most active during sleep, when it supports distribution of glucose, fats, amino acids, growth factors, and neuromodulators throughout the brain.[517][518]

Emerging evidence suggests that Aβ clearance is impaired in both early-onset and late-onset forms of AD.[519][520]

Diet and Nutrition

Deficiencies in certain vitamins such as Vitamin D and the B vitamins may cause dementia. High calorie diets could lead to onset of AD. Caloric restriction has been shown to prevent onset of neurological disorders.[521]

Aβ in its healthy state supports brain health as follows: 1) binds and removes trace minerals. When trace minerals such as copper, iron, mercury, and zinc become excessive, the body sends additional b-amyloid with the goal removing these minerals.[522][523] A diet that increases inflammation, such as a diet high in red meat, processed meat, peas and legumes, and low in whole grains show increased cognitive decline over a ten-year period.[524] Other foods that increase inflammation include sugar, processed food, fast food, and trans-fatty acids often found in chips, fast food and margarine (see the Diet chapter for more information).

"Leaky gut" results from an unhealthy gut lining that has large cracks or holes, allowing partially digested food, toxins, and bacteria to penetrate and pass through the tissues. In pathologic conditions, the permeability of the epithelial lining may be compromised allowing the passage of toxins, antigens, and bacteria in the lumen to enter the blood stream. Growing evidence shows that the gut microbiota is important in supporting the epithelial barrier and therefore plays a key role in the regulation of environmental factors that enter the body.

Many things can affect gut permeability, such as various diet-derived compounds, alcohol consumption, a diet high in sugar (particularly corn syrup), gluten sensitivity, medications such as aspirin and acetaminophen, processed foods, preservatives, excessive use of antibiotics, chemicals in food, and chronic stress or anger. Excess use of antibiotics can kill off both unhealthy bacteria as well as the healthy flora needed for proper digestion and effective mucosal lining to prevent permeability. People taking antibiotics should be on a good probiotic formula to replenish the healthy flora which keeps the "bad" bacteria and yeast in check. Nutrients and food ingredients have been reported to contribute to the maintenance or alterations of gut microbiota and the intestinal barrier function.[525]

Besides the effect of poor absorption due to flora imbalances, the worst aspect increasing the risk of AD is the chronic, low level inflammation caused by "leaky gut", which is due to larger particles escaping into the bloodstream and tissues, resulting in the body mistakenly attacking them as pathogens

Note. To correct leaky gut syndrome, eat a diet high in vegetables and fruits (particularly berries), avoid fried foods and trans fatty acids, keep away from sugary foods, add high grade olive oil, maintain a diet low in carbohydrates, avoid any foods with gluten (if gluten sensitive). To facilitate digestion and repair leaky gut, take probiotics and digestive enzymes, and even a good GI Repair formula, detoxify if necessary (such as mild fasting starting with a two-week elimination diet or cleanse), avoid NSAIDs (non-steroidal anti-inflammatories) if possible. Add foods high in the amino acid L-glutamine such as bone broth, grass-fed beef, asparagus, and broccoli, or it can be taken as a supplement. In addition, manage stress (do some form of meditation daily), and exercise regularly.

Trans fatty acids. Studies have found that when people consume higher amounts of trans fats, they tend to have an increased risk of Alzheimer's disease, poorer memory, lower brain volume and cognitive decline.[526][527][528][529] Trans fatty acids are found commonly in many foods including: most margarines and many fast foods, frosting, crackers, and chips

Lifestyle Factors

As lifestyle factors are associated with Alzheimer's and other neurodegenerative conditions including cardiovascular disease and diabetes, consideration of lifestyle, exercise, (and diet) become important.[530] Similarly, obesity and metabolic dysfunction, both affected by lifestyle, are known to contribute to cognition decline.[531]

Sleep

It is estimated that one out of three adults get less than 7 hours of sleep during a twenty-four-hour period. Proper amount of sleep is essential for:

- flushing out excess waste including amyloid beta cells,
- helping prevent excess formation of amyloid,
- maintaining insulin sensitivity, and
- activating autophagy.

Autophagy is the process of "cellular housekeeping". This process enables the brain to recycle waste products including damaged mitochondria or large protein aggregates such as misfolded proteins.[532][533][534]

Because lack of sleep reduces autophagy, the production of ATP (cellular energy), which is needed for metabolic processes, is reduced. In cognitively normal adults, poor sleep is also associated with increased CSF biomarkers of amyloid pathology. Worse subjective sleep quality, more sleep problems, and daytime somnolence are linked to greater AD pathology.[535] Those who sleep walk and/or talk in their sleep are fifty percent more likely of developing Parkinson's or dementia.[536] In rodent models of AD, sleep restriction alters amyloid metabolism and tau phosphorylation,[537][538] and tau-deficient mice show disturbed sleep architecture.[539] Maintenance of axons and synapses occurs during sleep,[540] and sleep loss elevates inflammation and microglial activation.[541] Specifically, carriers of EOAD-associated presenilin mutations show both increased

Aβ production,[542] [543] and decreased Aβ clearance.[544] It has also been shown in mice that clearance of exogenous amyloid is greater during sleep, as a result of increased glymphatic flow.[545] PBP is associated with neurofibrillary tangles in Alzheimer's disease brain, and the expression of PBP increases the phosphorylation of tau in cultured cells. Therefore, PBP may have a regulatory role in tau phosphorylation and in the genesis of neurofibrillary tangles.[546]

Exercise

The causes of diseases like Parkinson's and Alzheimer's are complex; because it is difficult to isolate causal behavior most research has focused on genetic and environmental factors.[547] A sedentary lifestyle does not significantly increase Parkinson's risk, but exercise does help to decrease PD symptoms.[548] However, sedentary behavior increases the risk of Alzheimer's as much as genetic factors because "inactivity may negate the protective effects of healthy genes."[549] [550]

Immune Dysfunction

A weak immune system has been identified in T- and B-cells, macrophages, and microglia activation.[551] AD is associated with increased T cell infiltration, changes in immune populations are associated with disease progression, reduction in T- and B-cell numbers and reductions in CD4+CD25+ Tregs (regulatory T cells).[552]

Conventional Treatment

Cholinesterase inhibitors

Cholinesterase inhibitors are a class of drugs now being offered to try to slow down the effects of AD. These drugs work by slowing the breakdown of acetylcholine, a chemical that is linked to the formation of new memories. By delaying the breakdown of acetylcholine, these drugs effectively increase their concentration in the synapses that connect cells. People taking cholinesterase inhibitors, however, experienced increased risk of falls and slow heartbeat.[553]

Donepezil (Aricept). Second-generation cholinesterase inhibitors produce fewer and less severe side effects. Donepezil appears to be at least as effective as other treatments of cognitive function, such as rivastigmine, galantamine, tacrine, and vitamin E.

One UK study of 486 patients with mild-to-moderate Alzheimer's, "Patients taking donepezil had significantly higher cognition and functionality scores at two years than those taking placebo, and some differences in institutionalization were seen at one year (nine percent donepezil versus fourteen percent placebo). But this latter difference was not statistically significant (P=0.15) and not sustained at three years (forty-two percent donepezil versus forty-four percent placebo, respectively, P=0.4). Results for the other primary outcome (progression of disability) showed little difference at one year and no benefit at three years."[554] The most common adverse effects caused by Donepezil recorded in clinical trials include nausea (sickness), diarrhea, insomnia (trouble sleeping), vomiting, muscle cramps, fatigue, and anorexia (loss of appetite).

Rivastigmine (Exelon) is another cholinesterase inhibitor for mild to moderate AD, with markedly better scores in standard cognitive function tests in four placebo-controlled trials. (24 percent in one trial showed markedly better scores).[555]

Galantamine (Razadyne). Also, for mild to moderate AD, galantamine showed cognitive improvements and better daily functioning in four placebo-controlled trials.[556]

Receptor Antagonist

Memantine (Namenda, Ebixa) is approved for treatment of moderate to advanced AD. It helps block the neurotransmitter glutamate by binding to N-methyl D-aspartate receptors on brain cell surfaces. Glutamate normally plays an important role in learning and memory but if levels are too high, it overstimulates nerve cells, leading to cell death. It is less effective than the cholinesterase inhibitors.[557]

Note. Most people who take the drugs, however, have limited benefit and may not be able to tell the difference between the prescription drug and a placebo. In addition, they are very expensive and have potential side effects. There are important considerations as to whether to start medications or not, so this should be discussed with your doctor.

Metabolic Enhancement

A programmatic approach involving metabolic enhancement (MEND) offers promising anecdotal results.[558]

Diagnosis

Imaging technologies, including new amyloid imaging agents based on the chemical structure of histologic dyes, are now making it possible to track amyloid pathology along with disease progression in the living patient. The two hallmark pathologies required for a diagnosis of Alzheimer's disease (AD) are the extracellular plaque deposits of the amyloid beta peptide (Aβ) and the flame-shaped neurofibrillary tangles of the microtubule binding protein tau. Familial early-onset forms of AD are associated with mutations either in the precursor protein for Aβ (APP).

The main issue becomes insulin resistance. This is very similar to what occurs in Type 2 Diabetes, where the insulin cannot break down the glucose efficiently nor perform its necessary functions. One of the strategies to optimize treatment development is to identify specific subtypes of Alzheimer's disease that may respond to different optimal programs.

Testing

Two laboratory tests, called the ADmark Assays, can aid in the diagnosis of Alzheimer's disease. One of these assays measures beta-amyloid and tau protein in the cerebrospinal fluid (and therefore requires a spinal tap, in which a thin needle is inserted into the lower back to withdraw the cerebral spinal fluid that bathes the spinal cord and brain). Its use is currently discouraged because its accuracy is equivalent to that of a careful clinical evaluation, which should be conducted anyway.

The second test identifies which variation of APOE the person carries. The test assesses the probability that a person's dementia stems from Alzheimer's on the basis of whether the APOE4 variation is present. The test is not definitive because some individuals with this allele will never develop Alzheimer's. As a result, this test is not part of a routine evaluation of people with dementia and is not recommended at this time.

Certain markers indicative of AD that can be tested are:

- increase of c-reactive protein,
- change in ratio of albumin (needed for elimination of waste in the brain),
- increase in interleukin-6 often associated with chronic inflammation,
- increase in TNF (tumor necrosis factor) related to inflammation,
- metabolic and hormonal imbalances with related insulin resistance,
- high levels of toxins such as mercury,[559] and lead as well as mycotoxins and mold,
- infections such as herpes simplex-1, borrelia (Lyme disease), p. gingivitis (oral bacterium), various fungi and others,
- diabetes (including high insulin and glucose levels), and/or
- high levels of homocysteine.

Complementary Approach

In a complementary approach we look for those factors which are readily available and which can play a supportive or even a preventative role in reducing neurodegeneration risk and/or managing the symptoms. In examining the research, we looked for the following neuroprotective qualities in the lifestyle, diet, or nutrient:

- can cross the blood brain barrier,
- supports neurogenesis,
- supports brain plasticity
- reduce development of amyloid plaque or its precursors,
- provides antioxidant support to reduce free radical toxicity,
- reduces or inhibits neuroinflammation,
- protects against cell death (apoptosis),
- supports mitochondrial function,
- supports cognitive capacity and learning, and
- improves side effects such as anxiety, sleep disruptions and depression.

Mediterranean Diet

Much research suggests that the Mediterranean diet reduces the incidence of dementia (including a meta-analysis of 32 studies)[560] [561] and Alzheimer's disease.[562] [563] [564] [565] The benefit appears to reduce amyloid beta accumulation[566] [567] (there is some contradictory research[568]) and improve neuroimaging biomarker profiles.[569] [570]

Researchers also note that the anti-inflammatory and antioxidant polyphenols in the diet reduce the risk of microglia-mediated neuroinflammation.[571]

Caloric Restriction (CR)

Caloric restriction involves consuming twenty to forty percent lower calories than normal. This has been suggested as a promising intervention to increase both median and maximal lifespan in humans.[572] It may prevent or delay several diseases including cancer, cardiovascular diseases, neurodegenerative disorders, diabetes, and autoimmune diseases, can extend one's lifespan,[573] and has been reported to protect against age-related mitochondrial dysfunction[574] and to reduce mtDNA damage.[575]

In animal models of neurodegenerative diseases, CR promotes neurogenesis and enhances synaptic plasticity,[576] improves cognitive capability, has anti-inflammatory mechanisms, reduces neural oxidative stress, induces various stress and neurotrophic/neuroprotective factors, and prevents Aβ neuropathology in AD transgenic models.[577]

Removing Heavy Metals

Heavy metal build-up that can cause ill health and disease include, lead, mercury, arsenic, aluminum, cadmium, nickel, uranium, and cadmium. Certain essential nutrients found in excess can also be toxic including: manganese, iron, lithium, zinc, and calcium.[578]

When they become severe, heavy metal poisoning symptoms can even mimic symptoms associated with Alzheimer's disease, Parkinson's disease and multiple sclerosis, including those considered just "aging issues" such as fatigue and loss of memory, brain fog, poor recovery from exercise and weakness, insomnia, depression, poor motor control and balance, and digestive issues.

Foods for detoxifying include: water, cruciferous vegetables, blueberries, cranberries, garlic, coffee, apples, grapefruit, green, leafy vegetables.

Note that Chelation therapy may be helpful for those found to have metal toxicity. There are various fasting methods as well that can be explored. This should be managed with a healthcare provider who is familiar with fasting methods as fasting too quickly or intensively can exacerbate symptoms.

Exercise Training

Exercise, alone or in combination with caloric restriction may also represent an efficient strategy to delay mitochondrial aging and age-related as it improves oxidative capacity, protein quality control, and has been shown in aging men to promote mitochondrial biogenesis,[579] [580] and may have important implications, not only with regard to fatigue, but also with respect to various central nervous system diseases and age-related dementia that are often characterized by mitochondrial dysfunction.[581]

ReCODE: Reversing Cognitive Decline

Functional medicine is a growing field, and approaches disease such as AD from a much broader perspective than single of multiple medication approaches. Chinese and ayurvedic medicine was founded on the principal that we are all unique individuals, and that treatment strategies should be based on the fact that each individuals' condition(s) may be due to a different pattern of energy imbalances (meridians in the case of Chinese medicine). So, for example, ten patients may come in with the same symptoms and even same medical diagnosis, but each treatment may vary based on the practitioner intake and evaluation.

Functional medicine views each person as a unique individual, evaluating diet, exercise, stress, hormonal imbalances, nutrient deficiencies, genetics, inflammation, and other lifestyle considerations to determine the underlying cause of the "disease" to determine an optimal treatment strategy.

ReCODE is well described in Dr. Bredesen's book, *The End of Alzheimer's: The First Programmed to Prevent and Reverse the Cognitive Decline of Dementia*[582] which views and treats AD and dementia from a multifaceted (whole body) perspective. Bredesen identifies thirty-six factors that determine whether the brain follows a synapse-destroying pathway that ends in Alzheimer's. A few of those factors are addressed by drugs with minimal benefit.

The good news that by addressing what combination of the thirty-six factors described in Dr Bredesen's book that can cause this negative spiral from happening, it has been shown that it is possible that dementia and AD can sometimes be stopped and even reversed.

According to Dr. Bredeson the build-up of beta-amyloid plaque, neurofibillary fibers, and tau protein is actually the attempt by the body to deal with variety of metabolic imbalances such as inflammation, a decline and shortage of essential nutrients, hormones and/or exposure to toxins such as metals or biotoxins including metals toxicity and poisons produced by microbes such as molds.

Reduce Oxidative Stress

Oxidative stress is generated by the accumulation of oxygen free radicals and is the result of the natural aging process. Cumulative oxidative damage has been associated in cell death and over time systemic functional breakdown.[583] [584] [585]

Antioxidants are essential for neutralizing free radicals. The body can produce some on its own, but most are derived from healthy food as well as targeted supplements.

One study of centenarians looked at contributing factors that could be attributed to their living such a long life and found that there was a drop in oxidative stress compared to those younger due to their adherence to a high antioxidant dietary regimen.[586]

Nutrients, Foods, and Medicinal Herbs

These nutrients, foods, and medicinal herbs may be beneficial for patients or those at risk for Alzheimer's according to studies with human AD patients or animal models of AD. Read about them in more detail in the Nutrients chapter. Herbal therapies such as traditional herbal combinations, have received attention as alternative and complementary interventions for neurodegenerative diseases, especially AD.[587] [588] [589]

Acetyl-L-Carnitine HCI (500mg, along with alpha lipoic acid (ALA) (150mg – 300mg). In pretreatment the amino acid acetyl-l-carnitine has been shown to increase mitochondrial biogenesis and decrease production of free radicals. In the body, acetyl-L-carnitine is made from L-carnitine that the body produces naturally. Since the late 1990s, it has been demonstrated that it slows the development of AD.[590] [591] It reduces the ill effects of high levels of homocysteine,[592] lessens physical and mental fatigue, and improves cognitive functioning.[593] It may raise the levels of nerve growth factor and increase the activity of acetylcholine, a neurotransmitter that is critical to healthy brain function.[594] ALA supports neurogenesis (production of new neurons) in the brain. This results in improvements in memory and learning as well as mental status and cognitive function.[595] [596] [597]

A small double-blind placebo-controlled twelve-week trial, using 2250 to 3000mg daily found that neuropsychological tests (MMSE, CGI, etc.) was markedly better than placebo, and did not depend on the baseline cognitive impairment. The researchers recommend it for early stages of Alzheimer's and vascular dementia.[598]

Ashwagandha root extract (Indian winter cherry or Indian ginseng/withania somnifera) (500mg twice per day with meals). Ashwagandha reverses behavioral deficits and plaque load in AD models[599] and inhibiting amyloid beta fibrillation.[600] Its withanamides reduce accumulation of beta-amyloid peptides in AD models and is neuroprotective.[601] [602] [603] [604] [605] Extracts increase acetylcholine content and choline acetyl transferase activity in rats which might partly explain the cognition-enhancing and memory-improving effects.[606] [607] The leaves also have nootropic potential with multiple benefits including reversing Alzheimer pathologies, protecting against environmental neurotoxins, and enhancing memory.[608]

Astaxanthin (6mg – 12 mg per day). A combination of **astaxanthin and DHA** are more effective in reducing oxidative stress,[609] enhancing learning, memory, and reducing tau hyperphosphorylation, and neuroinflammation than either alone.[610]

Bacopa monnieri extract (Brahmi, 150mg – 300mg). Bacopa monnieri is known to have neuroprotective[611] and cognition enhancing effects and has traditionally been a therapy for Alzheimer's disease.[612] It improves circulation to the brain, improves mood, cognitive function, and general neurological function.[613] Bacopa extract protects neurons from beta-amyloid-induced cell death by suppressing cellular acetylcholinesterase activity, and reduces oxidative stress[614] by inhibiting release of proinflammatory cytokines from microglial cells (in vitro).[615] It protects cells from oxidative damage from free radicals and DNA damage in the hippocampus, reduces lipid oxidation, and is comparable to donepezil (and other drugs) in reducing anticholinesterase activity.[616]

Baicalein (200mg-800 mg in multiple doses, once in the morning and once again at night) has been of great interest to investigators due to its versatility as a therapeutic agent for neurological diseases.[617][618] It shows therapeutic potential for Alzheimer's disease[619] and significantly improves the biochemical and histopathological condition of AD in lab animals.[620] It protects synaptic functions and memory, by preventing amyloid beta impairment in the hippocampus of animal models of AD.[621][622] It may be that indirect action on impaired insulin signaling and glucose metabolism accounts for the protective effect.[623]

Berries. In general, blueberries, bilberries, mulberries, raspberries, blackberries, black currant, and strawberries exert a neuroprotective effect[624] because they contain natural plant antioxidants and anti-inflammatory compounds. Much of current research suggests that inflammation plays a central role in the cause and development of Alzheimer's.[625]

Blueberries (1 cup a day). Blueberries contain anthocyanins that give blueberries their color and are able to cross the blood-brain barrier. In this way they support brain antioxidant capacity,[626] neurogenesis, BDNF levels,[627] reduce inflammation,[628] and increase cognitive memory, as well as modulate hippocampal plasticity.[629] Other berries that are believed to have similar effects include black currents, blackberries, and bilberries. Studies have demonstrated that patients with mild cognitive decline showed improvement when eating blueberries daily.[630]

Citicoline (250mg per day) is a choline precursor and as such has been proposed for use in traumatic brain injury, stroke, vascular dementia, and brain aging.[631] Due to its effects on cognitive disturbance some researchers recommend it as long-term preventive treatment for patients at high risk of Alzheimer's.[632]

Coffee (1-3 cups per day, recommended dosages can vary depending in certain body types). Quercetin, not caffeine, is the major neuroprotective element in coffee, consumption of which reduces the risk of Alzheimer's.[633] Although study results are not consistent, three out of five reviewed supported coffee's favorable effects against cognitive decline, dementia, or AD. A 2007 review of observational studies suggested that coffee consumption was associated with a reduced risk of AD by approximately by thirty percent as compared to non-coffee consumer.[634]

Coffee combined with melatonin has been shown to have a range of benefits including antioxidative, antiapoptotic and neuroprotective effects.[635]

Curcumin (500mg – 1200mg per day) is the key component responsible for the major therapeutic properties attributed to turmeric that affect AD pathology and age-related mental decline. It is found to inhibit amyloid beta plaque, inhibit formation of amyloid beta oligomers and fibrils, inhibit acetylcholinesterase, mediate insulin signaling, reduce tau hyperphosphorylation, and binding to copper.[636] It decreases the low-density lipoprotein oxidation[637] and the free radicals that cause the deterioration of neurons.[638][639] Curcumin also has strong anti-inflammatory activity. This is attributed to its unique molecular structure. It increases neurogenesis, regulates enzymes essential for enzyme disbursement, mitochondrial regulation, gene expression oxidative stress and is also anti-mutagenic, and anti-microbial.[640] One of the unique properties of curcumin is its ability protect[641] and cross the blood-brain barrier offering an unusual opportunity to support brain health through its neuroprotective, anti-inflammatory and antioxidant properties around neurons and glial cells that is significantly associated with brain aging and injury.[642]

Other studies show that curcumin boosts brain-derived neurotrophic factor, a type of growth hormone that helps brain cells grow. It may help delay age-related mental decline.[643] Reports have suggested lower dementia prevalence in South Asia may be directly attributable to the amount of turmeric (an excellent source of curcumin) used in daily cooking.[644] Studies suggest that curcumin should be considered as part of a treatment strategy as well to treat or prevent age-related neurodegenerative diseases such as AD, PD, and cerebrovascular disease.[645] [646]

Food sources are primarily the turmeric spice often used in Indian and Indonesian food. The limitations of curcumin are primarily in its lack of ready absorption when taken orally and researchers are exploring ways to improve bioavailability.[647] An older study showed that adding 20mg of piperine to 2g of curcumin improved its bioavailability markedly.[648] About 5% of turmeric is curcumin and about 5 percent of black pepper (by weight) is piperine. Even 1/20th of piperine improves bioavailability. Curcumin is also fat soluble, so cook your turmeric and black pepper (freshly ground) briefly in oil before adding.

Note. Curcumin taken in high dosages may be toxic, so higher doses than what is recommended above should only be done under a health professional's care. For some people, higher dosages in the amount suggested above may result in some numbness, so start with a lower amount first then work your way up to the higher dosage depending on how you feel. It may also have slight blood thinning properties so should not be taken without your doctors' supervision if on blood thinners.

Caution: Curcumin is not recommended for persons with biliary tract obstruction because it stimulates bile secretion or those with gallstones, obstructive jaundice, or acute biliary colic.

DHA (docosahexaenoic acid) (1,000mg – 4,000mg per day for prevention and maintenance/4,000mg-6,000mg per day for depression). Because of the close link between AD and lipid metabolism, DHA[649] (and EPA) are important.[650] [651] Modulation of lipid composition in the brain by DHA improves behavior motor function and survival.[652] It promotes brain-derived nerve factor,[653] supports cognition,[654] and enhances neurogenesis. It supports cell differentiation, maturation, neuron survival, reducing inflammation, as well as reduced amyloid beta (A-β) build-up.[655]

Note. DHA is also found in fish and omega-3 fatty acid supplements, as well as algae for vegetarians. See comment above regarding synergy with **astaxanthin**.

Flavonoids. Many epidemiological studies have shown that regular flavonoid-rich fruit intake is associated with delayed Alzheimer's and aging effects.[656] [657] [658] Flavonoids are plant compounds that are potent antioxidants, and are found in almost all fruits and vegetables, giving them the rich variety of colors. Examples of flavonoids that help protect against or slow Alzheimer's development include nobiletin and tangeretin in citrus fruits.[659] Other examples are resveratrol (red wine, berries, dark chocolate), anthocyanins (berries, currants, grapes, cherries), and tea. One study combined grape seed extract with resveratrol and grape juice extract, which had different polyphenolic compositions and saw that total amyloid content in the brain was greatly reduced.[660] The point of view of these researchers was to combine different flavonoids to address multiple pathological mechanisms.

Aged Garlic, (600mg per day). Compared to regular garlic, aged garlic extract stands out as having superior beneficial effects with respect to inhibiting platelet aggregation in cardiovascular disease,[661] strengthening the immune system and boosting levels of natural glutathione,[662 663 664 665] supporting working memory and cognitive capacity, slowing cholinergic cell death due to amyloid beta accumulation,[666 667] being neuroprotective,[668] and protecting neuronal PC12 cells against amyloid beta.[669] Aged garlic extract restricts several of the cascades related to synapse deterioration and neuroinflammation,[670] improves cognitive impairment, and reduces neurodegeneration caused by amyloid beta accumulation,[671 672] regulates cholinergic function,[673] improves short-term recognition memory in lab animals, and slows inflammatory response.[674]

Ginger root (500mg – 700mg per day). Ginger root stimulates anti-Alzheimer activity, and researchers are now investigating the mechanics of why.[675] Fermented with Schizosaccharomyces pombe, it reduces memory impairment by protecting neurons in the hippocampus.[676] Combined with peony root it inhibits amyloid beta accumulation and pathology in AD mice.[677]

In AD rat models of ginger root extract reverses behavioral dysfunction and reduces AD-like symptoms.[678] In an in vitro study ginger extract increases cell survival in AD rat hippocampus and prevents formation of destructive oligomers.[679] In biochemistry, an oligomer usually refers to a macromolecular complex. They give rise to Alzheimer's disease, and are small enough to spread easily around the brain, killing neurons and interacting harmfully with other molecules. How oligomers are formed and why is still not known.

Theoretical simulations of the mechanical process suggest that ginger acts as an inhibitor of acetylcholinesterase and is as effective as donepezil.[680] It increases neurogenesis, raises BDNF levels, enhances cognitive function, and helps in reducing amyloid beta plaque for those with Alzheimer's.[681 682 683 684] The role of ApoE4 in amyloid pathology is supported by evidence that it binds Aβ and modulates the aggregation and clearance of Aβ.[685] Ginger extract inhibits beta-amyloid peptide-induced cytokine and chemokine expression in cultured THP-1 monocytes.[686]

One of the many health claims attributed to ginger is its purported ability to decrease inflammation, swelling, and pain. A dried ginger extract, [6]-gingerol,[687] and a dried gingerol-enriched extract[688] were each reported to exhibit analgesic and anti-inflammatory effects.[689]

Gingko biloba (120mg – 240mg per day). Though research is inconsistent regarding memory for those with Alzheimer's, research does support that gingko may increase neurogenesis, raise BDNF levels, enhance cognitive function and help in reducing amyloid beta plaque for those with Alzheimer's.[690 691]

Ginseng (500mg – 1,000mg per day of Asian ginseng (panax ginseng) root extract). Ginseng root has been widely used in the far eastern countries such as China, Japan, and Korea for thousands of years as a traditional tonic for longevity. It is known for energizing the body or increasing vital energy and mood elevation with few if any side effects. Ginseng may reduce amyloid and neurofibrillary fiber build-up related to Alzheimer's.[692]

A number of studies have shown that the long-term administration of Korean red ginseng extract to patients with AD, combined with conventional AD drugs, gradually improved cognitive function. This was assessed using the mini-mental state examination (MMSE) and Alzheimer's Disease Assessment Scale–Cognitive Subscale (ADAS-Cog) tests, with minor adverse effects,[693] [694] [695] and with positive indication of frontal cortical activity, such as right temporal, parietal, and occipital areas, in elderly patients with AD. Gintonin found in ginseng when applied to neuroblastoma cells decreased Aβ formation and attenuated Aβ-induced neurotoxicity, indicating that gintonin could affect the brain's APP processing[696]

Glutathione (best taken sublingually or intravenously) (reduced) (700mg – 900mg per day if taken in capsule or tablet form). Glutathione is the most abundant antioxidant found in the brain. Glutathione levels are becoming an important therapeutic target both to reduce the impacts of aging[697] as well as in the treatment of age-associated neurological diseases such as AD.[698] Glutathione levels are of interest to AD researchers because glutathione levels are depleted in AD patients[699] [700] [701] and AD-caused increases in oxidative stress are attributed to reduced levels of glutathione[702] (in fact, glutathione levels in the brain are relevant AD biomarkers).[703] Scientists are currently examining the methods for increasing these levels as an AD therapy.[704]

Food sources: sulfur rich foods including cruciferous vegetables such as broccoli, cauliflower, cabbage, as well as bok choy, kale, mustard and collard greens, radish, turnip, arugula.

Grapeseed Extract (GSE) (300mg – 600mg per day). GSE has potent antioxidant and neurogenesis properties, protects the central nervous system from reactive oxygen species. GSE potently inhibits the aggregation of amyloid beta peptides into amyloid fibrils (through its component, gallic acid).[705] GSE's antioxidant and anti-inflammatory flavonoids inhibit aggregation[706] [707] [708] of amyloid beta peptides into neurotoxic soluble amyloid beta.[709] [710] [711]

Hesperidin (100mg – 500mg per day) promotes nerve cell differentiation and survival,[712] and enhances the neuroprotective capacity of astrocytes, by inducing them to secrete soluble factors involved in neuronal survival in vitro and increasing the number of neural progenitors.[713] It reduces cognitive impairment, oxidative stress, and cell death in animal models of Alzheimer's[714] and inhibits amyloid fibril formation.[715]

Food sources: citrus fruits including grapefruit, as well as apricots, plums, and bilberry. Vegetables containing hesperidin include green and yellow peppers, peas, green leafy vegetables, and broccoli. Whole grains, such as buckwheat, also contain hesperidin.

Huperzia A. While some small studies indicate that HupA may be valuable in an AD treatment strategy, the Alzheimer's Association recommends not taking huperzine A, especially if you're taking a prescribed cholinesterase inhibitor, such as donepezil (Aricept), rivastigmine (Exelon) or galantamine (Razadyne). Taking both could increase your risk of serious side effects.[716] See the full description in the nutrients chapter for more information.

Lycopene (3mg per day). Lycopene, a carotenoid, has demonstrated greater singlet oxygen quenching abilities compared with the other carotenoids, such as β-carotene, lutein, and zeaxanthin.[717] Lycopene has been shown to exhibit neuroprotective effects by reducing oxidative stress, suppressing production of inflammatory cytokines, and reducing accumulation of amyloid plaques.[718][719]

Lycopene has also been shown to attenuate cognitive deficits by improving inflammation in the gut–liver–brain axis as well improving glycolipid metabolism,[720] mechanisms by which lycopene provides neurocognitive protection as well as inhibition of neuronal apoptosis and restoration of mitochondrial function. [721]

Food sources. Several fruits including tomatoes and watermelon

Magnesium (3,000mg – 6,000mg per day). Although blood levels of magnesium do not vary between AD patients and controls, levels of magnesium in cerebrospinal fluid and hair are much lower in AD patients.[722] Magnesium can reduce the BBB permeability and promote clearance of amyloid beta from the brain.[723]

Food sources: nuts, seed, unprocessed cereals, green vegetables, as well as (in lower quantities) legumes, fruit, fish, and meat.

Melatonin (1mg – 3 mg at bedtime). Melatonin is a hormone produced by the pineal gland and its production runs parallel to AD progression. Quality of sleep is dependent upon melatonin, and it appears to be a safe and effective treatment for AD patients with sleep dysfunction.[724] Melatonin stimulates non amyloidogenic processing and inhibits beta amyloid precursor protein processing which culminates in amyloid aggregates – a neuroprotective function in AD pathology.[725] It decreases AD-like tau hyperphosphorylation, protects the cholinergic system and is anti-inflammatory. It may be a useful agent in preventing and treating AD.[726] Weak melatonin signaling (melatonin receptor type 1A gene) appears to contribute to the cascade of AD pathology.[727]

Mushrooms have long been used not only as food but also for the treatment of various ailments. Studies have shown both within in vitro and mammal studies to have potential roles in the prevention of many age-associated neurological diseases including Alzheimer's,[728] including the following mushrooms:[729] lion's mane (Hericium erinaceus),[730] reishi (Ganoderma lucidum),[731] Sarcodon scabrosus, Antrodia camphorata, Pleurotus giganteus, maitake (Grifola frondosa), and many more. Reishi mushrooms help reduce inflammation. For example, the inhibition of COX-2 could relieve cerebral ischemic injury and slow down the progress of Alzheimer's disease or Parkinson's disease, has antioxidant effects, anti-neurodegenerative and anti-tumor benefits.[732][733]

Nattokinase (100mg – 200mg per day) and **serrapeptase** (30mg – 120mg 1-2 times per day away from food). In animal models of AD either nattokinase or serrapeptase, improves brain metabolism, increases BDNF and IGF-1 levels, increases the expression of relevant genes (ADAM9 and ADAM10), has neuroprotective value,[734] reduces neuroinflammation,[735] and therefore may have a therapeutic value in AD therapy.[736] Tests of nanoencapsulation delivery find that nattokinase is able to reduce amyloid aggregation and reduce fibril formation.[737][738][739] It is also associated with improved learning and memory.[740]

Nuts. A 2014 review showed that nuts can improve cognition and even help prevent neurodegenerative diseases such as Alzheimer's.[741][742] In animal models, walnuts are found to reduce amyloid beta fibrillization, reduce amyloid beta-caused oxidative stress and apoptosis.[743]

Olive Leaf Extract (500mg per day with or without food). Olive leaf extract is a potential nutraceutical against Alzheimer's. A key polyphenol of olives, oleuropein, binds amyloid beta 1–40 peptide molecules counteracting amyloid plaque generation and deposition. Furthermore, oleuropein inhibits tau, which aberrantly forms the amyloid-positive aggregates characteristic of AD.[744] Thus, olive helps treat and prevent build-up of Aβ, decreased fibril formation risk, and as well is antioxidant, anti-inflammatory, anti-cancer, antimicrobial, antiviral, anti-atherogenic, hypoglycemic, hepatic-, cardiac, and neuro-protective.

Phosphatidylserine (100mg – 400mg per day) is key to proper brain function. Combined with phosphatidic acid (from soy lecithin) it improves memory, mood, and cognition in the elderly, and has a general stabilizing effect in AD patients.[745] In other studies, it improves mood, brain function, learning memory, and vocabulary in people with Alzheimer's.[746] Additionally, cholinesterase and hippocampal inflammation injury decreases.[747]

Polygalae radix (35mg – 45mg per day) is found typically as part of the Chinese herbal formulas Kai-xin-san or Bushen Tiansui. An extract of polygalae radix prevents cognitive deficit and neuron axon degeneration associated with amyloid plaque accumulation in a mouse model of AD. But. it does not influence the formation of plaque. It protects the area of growth at the tips of axons.[748] Other extracts of kai-xin-san have been tested and some are found to increase both NGF and BDNF expression.[749]

Pomegranate juice is higher in polyphenols, with anti-inflammatory and antioxidant action, than most other juices. A specific polyphenol called punicalagin is believed to be the source of pomegranate's anti-inflammatory properties. An animal study showed mice fed pomegranate juice experienced lower levels of amyloid plaque.[750][751] Pomegranate has been shown to be neuroprotective against Alzheimer's, possibly due to gut microbiota called urolithins which contribute to pomegranate's anti-AD effects by inhibiting amyloid beta fibrillation.[752]

Pycnogenol reduces neuroinflammation and neurodegeneration in animal models,[753] and has been found to improve cognitive functioning in animal and human studies.[754]

Pyrroloquinoline quinone (PQQ) (10mg - 20mg per day). In Alzheimer's models PQQ has been found to prevent mitochondrial dysfunction. In a mouse model of AD, a nutraceutical containing PQQ clearly improved motor dysfunction and cognitive impairment, protected mitochondrial function, reduced free radicals, and reduced membrane hyperpolarization. It slightly reduced soluble amyloid beta-42 levels which resulted in reduced tau levels.[755]

Food sources: Good non-meat food sources include parsley, papaya, green peppers, and oolong and green teas. Animal sources include eggs and dairy.

Quercetin (250mg-500mg 1-2 times per day). Studies show that quercetin protects brain cells against excitotoxicity, the damage done by repeated excitatory electrical impulses observed in AD and other neurodegenerative diseases.[756][757][758][759] Quercetin is the component in coffee responsible for coffee's beneficial effects.

Resveratrol (125mg per day). Because resveratrol has strong anti-inflammatory and anti-oxidative effects, researchers have hypothesized that it could be useful for neurological disorders. Resveratrol crosses[760][761] and restores the integrity[762] of the blood-brain barrier. It helps to prevent neurodegeneration caused by amyloid beta peptides[763] by enhancing glutathione and consequently, antioxidant status[764] in AD. It reduces inflammation,[765] and alters AD biomarker trajectories.[766] It is helpful against a number of AD mechanisms and metabolic pathologies.[767][768][769]

Food sources: Resveratrol is a naturally occurring polyphenolic phytoalexin which occurs in plants such as grapes, peanuts, berries, pines and in red wine.

Red sage (salvia). Sage appears to halt the breakdown of the chemical messenger acetylcholine (ACH),[770] which levels appear to fall in Alzheimer's disease. It may enhance cognition and protect against neurodegenerative disease[771] well as having a strong effect in increasing neurogenesis. Salvia miltiorrhiza (red sage, Chinese sage, or danshen) constituents have multiple neuroprotective effects including anti-amyloid beta, antioxidant, and anti-inflammation that are potentially useful in development of drugs to combat AD.[772]

Rutin has a potential protective role in neurogenerative disorders, such as AD,[773][774][775] due to its capacity as a potent antioxidant.[776][777][778] It includes a strong effect on processing and clumping of amyloid beta, and changes to the oxidant-antioxidant balance linked to nerve cell death.[779]

Saffron (30mg – 80mg per day) was found to be as effective as donepezil but with fewer side effects.[780] It is considered promising due to its anti-oxidant and neuroprotective properties.[781]

Taurine (750mg – 1,000mg per day) is of interest to researchers because of its link to cognitive function.[782] In Alzheimer mice, taurine improved cognitive impairment.[783]

Theanine (100mg – 200mg per day). L-theanine is theanine's chemical mirror image, and is most often tested. Long-term L-theanine administration has demonstrated facilitating long-term potentiation and an increase in brain-derived neurotrophic factor (BDNF) expression in the hippocampus over three to four weeks.[784][785] There is mounting evidence supporting its neuroprotective effect.[786][787][788] In a recent study l-theanine treated AD patients experienced reduced stress-related symptoms, such as sleep disturbances as well as cognitive improvements in verbal fluency and executive function.[789]

     The combination of theanine and luteolin improved AD-like symptoms by increasing hippocampal insulin signaling power and decreasing neuroinflammation and norepinephrine degradation in animal models of AD.[790][791]

Vinpocetine. (30mg – 60mg per day). Vinpocetine's antioxidant and anti-inflammatory properties have been central to its role in AD treatments. It clearly improved deterioration in the cerebral cortex and hippocampus of AD isolated rats.[792] Physical and mental activities enhance the neuroprotective capacity of vinpocetine and CoQ10 which markedly reduce neurodegeneration as evidenced by improvement in AD, oxidant, and inflammatory biomarkers in brain tissue.[793] Vinpocetine acts as a phosphodiesterase inhibitor (PDE1-1) against reduced plasticity and neurogenesis in AD patients. PDE1-1 has a possible positive effect on memory impairment.[794]

Vitamin B deficiencies, linked to nerve damage and dementia, are found in Alzheimer's patients but the mechanisms and direct causal relationships are still under investigation. See the Nutrients chapter for more information.

Vitamin D (2,000IU - 5,000IU per day) As with the B vitamins, vitamin D is linked to neurological development and is being investigated as a therapeutic tool for cognitive impairment and dementia. While it offers some protection and support, clinical interventional studies don't link increased D with improved cognition.[795] See the Nutrients chapter for more information.

Zeaxanthin (2-12mg per day). Zeaxanthin inhibits amyloid beta aggregation,[796] and, combined with lutein, reduces AD mortality.[797] Supplementation with lutein and zeaxanthin improved cognitive function in community-dwelling, older, men and women.[798] With the addition of mesozeaxanthin it was clinically shown to improve vision in AD patients.[799]

Summary

Below is a summary of nutrients that support brain health. Some we have explained in this chapter. The others you can read about them in the Nutrients chapter.

Neurogenesis support: Acetyl-l-carnitine, astaxanthin, and phosphatidylserine.

Improve Cognition: Astaxanthin, ashwagandha, curcumin, lycopene, ginseng, green tea, n-acetylcysteine, omega-3s, phosphatidylserine, PQQ, vinpocetine, and vitamin E.

Reduce Brain Inflammation: Alpha lipoic acid, Apigenin, ashwagandha, astaxanthin, baicalein, CoQ10, curcumin, garlic, ginseng, green tea, omega-3, 6, 7 essential fatty acids, pycnogenol, reishi mushrooms, resveratrol, sage, SAM-e, vinpocetine, and zeaxanthin.

Reduce Depression: 5-HTP, baicalein, ginger, ginseng, goji berry, n-acetylcysteine, olive leaf extract, omega-3 fatty acids, phosphatidylserine, sage, SAM-e, tryptophan, and vitamin B12.

Support Brain Plasticity: Blueberries, DHA, fisetin, ginseng, goji berry, magnesium, omega-3 fatty acids, and resveratrol.

Physiological Causes

Major variables that can result in Alzheimer's include chronic inflammation, high oxidative stress, insulin resistance, mitochondrial dysfunction.

Lifestyle Causes

Lifestyle considerations that contribute to onset of AD include poor diet (including high caloric, low nutrient diets, and regular intake of trans-fatty acids), lack of regular exercise, poor sleeping habits, toxic build-up due to exposure, for example to mold, poor oral hygiene, poor sleep habits, and contracting Lyme disease.

Eat a healthy diet, get moderate exercise regularly, manage chronic stress, get enough sleep, and take targeted supplements based on the recommendations above. Some of the best foods include avocado, green, leafy vegetables, colored fruits and vegetables, blueberries (and other dark berries), mushrooms (reishi, shiitake, lion's mane) pomegranate juice, and walnuts.

Chapter 6. Parkinson's Disease

Parkinson's disease (PD) is the second most common neurodegenerative disease in the world, with a prevalence rate of one percent in the population over age of sixty,[800] and is the second most common neurodegenerative disease involving movement disorder.[801] [802] Males are most likely to develop PD (50 percent more men than women) and its incidence in Caucasians seems higher than in other races.[803] [804]

The condition is characterized by cognitive impairment, physical tremors, slowness of movement (brandykinesia), instability, muscular rigidity, and other non-motor symptoms. Clumps of protein accumulate within specific nerve cells resulting in their death (apoptosis). These neurons are known as "dominergetic neurons" because they are responsible for the production of dopamine (DA).[805] DA is a neurotransmitter produced from the dietary amino acid tyrosine and plays significant roles in a variety of motor, cognitive, motivational, and neuroendocrine functions. As these neurons die, dopamine production is lost and message transmission between brain cells and the body breaks down. Parkinson's is linked to among other issues antioxidant loss, free radical increases[806] and mitochondrial dysfunction.

Pathology

The protein associated with Parkinson's development is known as protein alpha synuclein. Its function in the brain is relatively unknown. But, has become of great interest to Parkinson's researchers because it is a major constituent of the hallmark protein clumps, which are called Lewy bodies[807] (cytoplasmic inclusion bodies).

Although Parkinson's has been viewed as a neurodegenerative condition resulting from reduced dopamine production, along with Lewy body inclusions in the nerve cells, it is now acknowledged to be caused by multisystem neurodegeneration affecting multiple neurotransmission systems (much like Alzheimer's disease). [808] [809]

- Accelerated oligomerization of two different alpha-synuclein mutations is a hallmark of early-onset Parkinson's. This is the process of changing single molecules (monomers) into chains of similar molecules (oligomers).[810]
- Parkinson's pathology has a special emphasis on the degeneration of the cholinergic system in which is often more severe than in AD.[811] The cholinergic system has a role in both large-scale and local brain messaging circuits, with impacts that go well beyond cognition.[812]

PD patients have a build-up in plaque primarily in the **substantia nigra pars compacta** and **locus coeruleus** regions in the midbrain. These cells produce the neurotransmitters or biochemicals that help regulate the nervous system and body functions.

The substantia nigra pars compacta region of the brain is involved in a wide range of processes such as emotion, reward processing, habit formation, movement, and learning. This part of the brain is particularly involved in coordinating sequences of motor activity, as would be needed when playing a musical instrument, dancing, or playing sports, as it is the section of the brain most effected by Parkinson's disease.

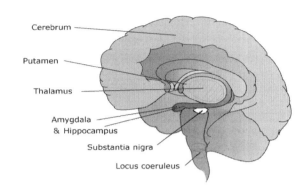

Causes and Contributing Factors

Genetic and Epigenetic Factors

Genetic factors. Genetic mutations can cause Parkinson's, including mutations to α-synuclein or the PRKN (parkin) gene (which is involved in mitochondria maintenance)[813] or the LRRK2 gene (linked to late-onset Parkinson's),[814] which are associated with the most common inherited form of the condition.

Environmental factors. Epigenetics is the study of the effect of the environment on gene expression. Environmental factors such as how we are nurtured as infants and children, our parents' diet and ours, levels of stress and many other factors affect how one's brain develops. Neurotrophic factors, which are growth factors that can promote the survival and regeneration of neurons, can be impacted by environmental factors.

Environmental pollution. Researchers first noted in 2002, and have since validated that children and young adults who live in areas with significant air pollution are much more likely to have the hallmarks of Parkinson's: twisted protein fibers, deteriorating neurons and amyloid plaque deposits.[815][816][817] The same is true of industrial-, combustion-, and friction-derived nanoparticles.[818]

Metabolic Factors

α-synuclein aggregation. Clumping of this protein, forming Lewy bodies within dopaminergetic nerve cells resulting in nerve cell death.

Dopamine loss. Researchers believe a loss of the neurotransmitter dopamine, neurological damage, inflammation, and brain cell deterioration are among the primary factors that trigger Parkinson's development.

Cholinergic circuit dysfunction has been associated with neurodegenerative diseases such as Alzheimer's, Parkinson's, Huntington's diseases, and in psychiatric disorders such as schizophrenia.[819] Central cholinergic circuits participate in aspects of memory formation, motivational and volitional behaviors.

High sugar levels. Many researchers feel that chronic blood sugar elevations are involved in depression and neurodegenerative disorders such as Alzheimer's disease.[820][821][822]

Hormonal imbalances and other medical conditions[823] that affect cognitive health and increase inflammation.

Mitochondrial dysfunction plays a role in contributing to neurodegeneration.[824][825]

Excitotoxicity and signals mediating an apoptosis cascade.[826] This is the process through which cells die.

Misfolded protein. Autography, the process of "cellular housekeeping" enabling the brain to recycle waste products, including damaged mitochondria, large protein aggregates, is critical for neuronal homeostasis and survival.[827][828][829] The accumulation of misfolded protein is a defining hallmark for the progression of various neurodegenerative diseases including amyotrophic lateral sclerosis (ALS), Huntington's, Parkinson's, and Alzheimer's diseases.[830]

Neurotoxins are directly implicated in Parkinson's. L-methyl-4-phenyl-1,2,3,6-tetra-hydropyridine (MPTP) was discovered to produce acutely PD-like symptoms. Two groups of natural MPTP-like and amine-related neurotoxins may cause oxidative stress, mitochondrial dysfunction, cell death, and PD symptoms.[831]

Enzyme imbalance. Transglutaminases are a large family of related and ubiquitous enzymes which catalyze the cross-linking of a glutaminyl residue of a protein/peptide substrate to a lysyl residue of a protein/peptide co-substrate. These enzymes are also capable of catalyzing other reactions important for the cell viability. "Tissue" transglutaminase (TG2) has been shown to be involved in the molecular mechanisms responsible for a very widespread human pathology including celiac disease. Transglutaminase activity has also been hypothesized to be directly involved in the pathogenetic mechanisms responsible for several human neurodegenerative diseases, which are characterized in part by aberrant cerebral transglutaminase activity and by increased cross-linked proteins in affected brains, such as AD, PD, supranuclear palsy, and Huntington's disease.[832]

High magnesium levels are also noted in PD patients' blood and cerebrospinal fluid and are considered a risk factor according to a meta-analysis of seventeen published studies.[833]

Oxidative Stress and Inflammation

Free radical increase and nigral cell loss.[834] Oxidative stress is a factor.[835][836][837] The excessive production of reactive oxygen species (ROS), such as superoxide anion, hydroxyl radical and hydrogen peroxide, may either directly damage the cellular macromolecule to cause cell necrosis or affect normal cellular signaling pathways and gene regulation to induce apoptosis.[838] Excess iron is a source of oxidative damage and iron neurochemistry has been linked to several neurodegenerative conditions, including PD.[839]

Inflammation. Parkinson's[840] (and Alzheimer's) is characterized by neuroinflammation, appearing in old age when chronic inflammation in the body compromises the immune system.[841] [842]

Exposure to Toxins

Heavy metal build-up may alter neurotransmission and lead to neurodegeneration, which can manifest as cognitive problems, movement disorders, and learning and memory dysfunction. To date, metal-induced neurotoxicity has been associated with multiple neurological diseases in humans, including AD, amyotrophic lateral sclerosis, autism spectrum disorders, Guillain–Barré disease, Gulf War syndrome, Huntington's disease (HD), multiple sclerosis, PD, and Wilson's disease.[843] [844] [845] Molecular epidemiology studies show cumulative lead exposure is associated with an increased risk of amyotrophic lateral sclerosis[846] [847] and Parkinson's,[848] suggesting that lead exerts a significant neurodegenerative effect.

Drugs. Drugs with an ACB (anticholinergic burden) score of 3 that have been prescribed for depression, Parkinson's disease, and loss of bladder control are linked to higher risk of dementia up to twenty years after exposure. These include many antidepressant, urological, and anti-Parkinson drugs. The following drugs may cause symptoms to Parkinson's but do not cause Parkinson's: these include medications such as Haldol (Haloperidol) and Thorazine (Chlorpromazine) used to treat psychiatric disorders, as well as drugs used to treat nausea such as Reglan (Metoclopramide). The anti-seizure drug, Depakene (Valproic Acid), also may cause some of the features of parkinsonism, notably severe tremor.

Diet and Digestion

Increased PD symptoms are found in a diet with canned fruits and vegetables, diet and non-diet soda, fried foods, beef, ice cream, and cheese.[849]

Dairy product consumption and drinking milk may increase one's risk of PD independently of calcium intake,[850] [851] particularly in men.[852] In addition, the possible presence of dopaminergic neurotoxins, including pesticides and polychlorinated biphenyls in dairy products may increase the risk of PD.[853] Consumption of dairy (not yogurt) such as milk, ice cream, and cream (butter is questionable but not fully researched) worsened PD symptoms.[854] [855]

Canned foods. Consumption of canned fruits and vegetables is a strong predictor of PD progression, most likely due to the leakage of Bisphenol A (BPA) used in the inner coating of the cans. It is a well-established endocrine conductor associated with obesity, and more recent evidence suggests that it is an energy balance disruptor.[856] The aluminum content of the cans may be contributing to the association as aluminum is a neurotoxicant.[857]

Dysfunction in the brain-gut microbiota axis which has a role in irritable bowel syndrome, inflammatory bowel disease, depression, and anxiety, also may be important in neurodevelopmental disorders such as autism, Parkinson's disease, and AD.[858] [859] [860] [861]

Low uric acid levels. Preliminary research shows that individuals who consume large amounts of dairy products may often have low serum uric acid levels.[862] Serum urate and uric acid is inversely correlated with the risk of PD and disease duration.[863 864 865 866] The neuroprotective effects of serum urate may be limited to men [867 868] since the same is not observed in women.[869]

Alcohol consumption. Low to moderate alcohol consumption may exert neuroprotective effects in PD. One case-controlled study found an inverse association between total alcohol consumption and PD.[870] More recent studies suggest that low to moderate alcohol or beer consumption may be associated with a lower PD risk, whereas greater liquor consumption increases the risk of PD [871] and earlier onset.[872] Specific components found in red wine including resveratrol and quercetin, may elicit neuroprotection against PD.

Sugary drinks such as soda has a strong association with obesity,[873] which is also associated with PD progression. Diet soda is associated with a faster rate of PD progression possibly due to the consumption of aspartame, which metabolizes into phenylalanine, aspartic acid, and methanol. The increase in phenylalanine and aspartic acid interferes with the transport of serotonin and dopamine to the brain, increases neuronal hyperexcitability, and leads to degeneration in astrocytes and neurons.[874 875]

Fried goods should be avoided as they produce reactive ROS observed in PD. ROS destroys healthy cells, and produces aldehydes such as acrolein that bind covalently with thiol groups of proteins, leading to protein aggregation and dysfunction in the brain.[876] In PD they accumulate in the substantia nigra, and in the dopaminergic neurons. This modifies alpha-synuclein, and inhibits proteasome activity which is needed to degrade unneeded or damaged proteins by proteolysis.[877]

Beef consumption may lead to PD progression, due to its high iron content (along with added pesticides and hormones). Beef contains alpha-synuclein in the enteric nervous system which is associated with immune cell activation.[878] Iron supplementation as well has been implicated in PD and PD progression.

Daily Life Factors

Sleep disturbances. Research finds that those who sleepwalk or/and talk in their sleep have a fifty percent chance of developing Parkinson's or dementia within the decade.[879] A variety of sleep disturbances are common in PD patients including insomnia and REM sleep disorders.[880]

Traumatic brain injury (TBI). Trauma to the head, as evidenced by boxers, football players, people who've been in an accident, may slightly increase risk, or may trigger or hasten PD onset. One study looked at more than 350,000 vets, half of whom had some level of TBI. (TBI is identified by loss of consciousness and/or memory loss.) They concluded that mild TBI increases risk fifty-six percent and moderate to severe increases risk by eighty-three percent.[881]

Diagnosis

There are no specific tests that indicate Parkinson's, but a neurologist looks to analyze physical manifestations.

"Four motor symptoms are considered cardinal in PD: slowness of movement (bradykinesia), tremor, rigidity, and postural instability. Typical for PD is an initial asymmetric distribution of these symptoms, where in the course of the disease, a gradual progression to bilateral symptoms develops, although some asymmetry usually persists. Other motor symptoms include gait and posture disturbances such as decreased arm swing, a forward-flexed posture, and the use of small steps when walking; speech and swallowing disturbances; and other symptoms such as a mask-like facial expression or small handwriting are examples of the range of common motor problems that can appear."[882]

Conventional Treatment

There is no cure for PD, but there are drugs available that can help reduce some symptoms.

Drug treatments include the following:

- **Drugs that increase dopamine in the brain**, or mimic dopamine or prevent or slow its breakdown. The most common drug used in Levodopa (L-Dopa) which crosses the blood brain barrier. It is commonly used with Carbidopa which prevents the dopamine from being produced in the body, limiting it to production in the brain. This drug allows the majority of people with PD to extend the period of time in which they can lead active, productive lives, reducing bradykinesia and rigidity.

   But these drugs can elicit a number of possible side effects including: abnormal thinking or hallucination with agitation or anxiety, confusion or mood change, teeth grinding, problems swallowing or mouth-watering, unsteadiness or clumsiness, clenching or grinding of teeth, clumsiness or unsteadiness, dizziness, feeling faint, general discomfort feeling, hand tremors or other involuntary movements, nausea or vomiting, numbness, and unusual tiredness or weakness.

   Dyskinesias, or involuntary movements such twisting and writhing commonly develop in people who take levodopa over an extended period. There are also a number of less common side effects as well. Motor complications have been found to occur in forty percent and as well, seventy percent of patients after five years and fifteen years of levodopa treatment, respectively.[883] [884]

   Dopamine dysregulation syndrome is the result of addictive use, over-medication, or extended uses of dopamine agonists such as levodopa. It occurs in about four percent of PD patients (mostly early onset). This is a complication of long-term therapy for Parkinson's.[885] [886]

- **Caffeine-based compounds**. In a 2016 study, caffeine-based chemical compounds which contained certain nutrients including nicotine, metformin and aminoindan prevented the misfolding of alpha-synuclein, which is the protein that has been shown to be necessary for dopamine regulation.[887]

Other drugs in this category include dopamine agonists, MAO-B inhibitors, OMT inhibitors, amantadine, anticholinergics.

- These drugs **affect other neurotransmitters** in the body in order to ease some of the symptoms of the disease. These can help reduce tremors
- Other drugs include medications that help **control the non-motor symptoms** of the disease such as antidepressants.

Additional Side Effects of Conventional Treatments

Side effects from conventional treatment can include mouth dryness, constipation, nausea, insomnia, palpitation, and mental problems.

Surgery May Sometimes be Recommended:

1. Pallidotomy and thalamotomy selectively destroy specific parts of the brain that contribute to PD symptoms.

2. Deep brain stimulation (DBS) uses an electrode surgically implanted into part of the brain (typically the subthalamic nucleus or the globus pallidus) to gently stimulate the brain in a way that helps to block signals that cause many of the motor symptoms of PD.

Note: Herbs such as bacopa monnieri (also supports motor behavior), baicalein and alpha lipoic acid have been shown to help breakdown alpha synuclein in the brain. Others include ginseng, melatonin and olives (helps prevent a-syn build-up) the macuna plant that contains high amounts of natural l-dopa, and a broad range of the herbs promote neurogenesis, synapsis, help prevent apoptosis, breakdown excess amyloid beta, neurofibrillary fibers and tau protein build-up and more as described below. See below for more details.

Complementary Support

There are no current therapies that, by themselves, stop nerve cell death, or cure Parkinson's. It is becoming increasingly clear that neurological diseases such as PD are multi-factorial involving disruptions in multiple cellular systems.[888]

The following recommendations are based on the concept that PD must be addressed from the point of view of all of its constituent symptoms: neurodegeneration, mitochondrial dysfunction, motor dysfunction, inflammation, oxidative stress, apoptosis (cell death), weak blood-brain barrier, gut-brain axis imbalances, poor dopamine production, and also alpha-synuclein build-up.

Diet

A poor diet will have a negative impact on an individual's health. Nutrition affects multiple aspects of neurodevelopment, neurogenesis and the functions of neurons and neural networks.[889] Nutrition-gene interactions play a critical role in dysfunction and disease.[890]

Epidemiological studies found that high intake of fruits, vegetables and fish was inversely associated with PD risk,[891][892][893] and the risk of many other health conditions. Epidemiological studies have found a decrease in PD risk in individuals who consume foods containing carotenoids and β-carotene,[894] as well as cruciferous vegetables such as cauliflower, cabbage, and broccoli (rich in antioxidants with neuroprotective capacity).

Food choices: Reduced Parkinson's symptoms are found in a diet high in fresh vegetables, fresh fruit, nuts, and seeds, nonfried fish, olive oil, wine, coconut oil, fresh herbs, and spices. Consumption of green tea, coffee, and blueberries as well as avoiding dairy are associated with reduced risk of being diagnosed with PD.[895][896]

Mediterranean Diet

Studies have shown that the dietary patterns characteristic of a Mediterranean diet significantly reduce the risk of Parkinson's. These results are emerging as a potential neuroprotective alternative for PD,[897] and are linked to later age of diagnosis.[898] Some of these foods include fresh fish, olive oil, nuts and seeds, fresh fruit, and vegetables.

Keto Diet

Limited studies indicate that a Keto diet improve symptoms related to PD.[899][900] Although the mechanisms are not yet well defined, it is plausible that neuroprotection results from enhanced neuronal energy reserves, which improve the ability of neurons to resist metabolic challenges, and possibly through other actions including antioxidant and anti-inflammatory effects. It may as well have beneficial disease-modifying activity applicable to a broad range of brain disorders characterized by the death of neurons.

Note: Having protein at the dinner meal only (along with vegetables, particularly green, leafy vegetables) can keep inflammation down. Keeping protein levels moderate throughout the day has been shown to help reduce the symptoms of Parkinson's.[901]

Juicing Recipe for Brain Health

Below are recommended foods for juicing for brain health. Choose some combination of these foods and add your favorite fruits and vegetables as well.
- Green, leafy vegetables, avocado, broccoli, avocado, kale, and red beets
- Apples, berries (especially blueberry), bilberry, black currant, blackberry, mulberry, goji berry citrus fruits (especially lemon), kiwi, grapes, pomegranate juice, and prunes
- Garlic, ginger, chia seeds, parsley, ginseng, walnuts, yogurt, and honey
- Coconut oil

Limit the Following

- Limit the amount of protein. Consuming lots of beef, fish, or cheese may affect the effectiveness of certain Parkinson's medications.
- Limit sodium, trans fats, cholesterol, and saturated fats.

Nutrients, Food, and Medicinal Herbs

> These nutrients, food, and medicinal herbs may be beneficial for patients or those at risk for Parkinson's according to studies with human PD patients or animal models of PD. Read about them in more detail in the Nutrients chapter.

We discussed a number of essential brain nutrients in the Alzheimer's chapter related to a broad spectrum of benefits including promoting neurogenesis, reducing apoptosis, supporting synapsis and mitochondria, helping strengthen the blood-brain barrier and eliminate waste (and much more), but targeted herbs in particular for PD include bacopa monnieri and baicalein which have been shown to help breakdown alpha-synuclein, and the macuna plant that contains high amounts of natural l-dopa.

Acetyl-L-Carnitine HCI (500mg, along with alpha lipoic acid (ALA) (150mg – 300mg). In pretreatment acetyl-l-carnitine has been shown to increase mitochondrial biogenesis and decrease production of free radicals. When combined with ALA (specifically the r-lipoic acid version), l-carnitine improved its benefits for PD 100-1000-fold compared to these nutrients taken individually.[902] The combination of alpha lipoic acid, acetyl-l-carnitine, CoQ10, and melatonin supports energy metabolism via carbohydrate and fatty acid utilization, assists electron transport and adenosine triphosphate synthesis, counters oxidative and nitrosative stress.[903] Acetyl-l-carnitine is a precursor to glutathione, increases dopamine transporter density, and in PD patients has shown corresponding improvements in clinical outcomes.[904] [905]

Alpha lipoic acid (300mg – 600mg per day or 150mg – 300mg in the "R" form), which boosts glutathione levels and is a potent antioxidant, protects dopaminergic neurons in a Parkinson's model and decreased alpha-synuclein aggregation in the substantia nigra.[906] The R-form, most easily utilized by the body, decreases cell death, and reverses decreased dopamine in PD models. It is neuroprotective, perhaps because of improved mitochondrial action and autophagy.[907] Alpha lipoamide, a derivative of alpha lipoic acid appears to have a stronger beneficial effect on mitochondria than alpha lipoic acid.[908]

Ashwagandha root extract (Indian winter cherry or Indian ginseng/withania somnifera) (500mg twice per day with meals) is useful as part of a treatment strategy in neurodegenerative diseases such as PD.[909] Ashwagandha withanoids may reduce inflammation, nerve cell death, and behavioral deficits.[910] It may stimulate dendrite formation,[911][912] and neurite outgrowth,[913] [914] [915] improve synaptic function, increase acetylcholine content and choline acetyl transferase activity,[916] [917] and modulate mitochondrial function.[918]

Astaxanthin (6mg – 12 mg per day) is able to cross the blood-brain barrier bringing neuroprotection to the brain.[919] It has been shown to be protective across various models of PD[920] by reducing the pathophysiology that causes neurodegeneration.[921] It accomplishes this, in part, by suppressing oxidative damage in certain signaling pathways[922] and by protecting against mitochondria dysfunction.[923] Its action as an anti-inflammatory, an antioxidative, and an anti-apoptotic may underly its effectiveness in protecting against neurodegeneration.[924]

Food sources: Natural AXT is produced from algae, yeast, and crustacean byproduct.

Bacopa monnieri extract (150mg – 300mg). Bacopa monnieri (BM) is known to have neuroprotective and cognition enhancing effects. It reduces alpha synuclein aggregation, prevents dopaminergic neurodegeneration and restores the lipid content in nematodes, thereby suggesting its potential as a possible anti-Parkinsonian agent.[925] It significantly supports motor behavior, improve normal levels of a number of Parkinson biomarkers, and enhanced levels of dopamine, DOPAC and HVA.[926] This was accomplished by inhibiting pathways for cell death of dopaminergic neurons. It reduces alpha synuclein clumping, prevents dopaminergic neurodegeneration, and normalizes lipid content in a nematode model of PD.[927]

Baicalein (200-800 mg in multiple doses, once in the morning and once again at night) is of great interest to investigators due to its versatility as a therapeutic agent for neurological diseases.[928] It shows therapeutic potential for Parkinson's disease[929] because it protects mitochondrial function and biogenesis,[930] by restoring the body's ability to get rid of waste materials (autophagy). In so doing it reduces behavioral deficits, dopaminergic neuronal cell loss, cell death and mitochondrial dysfunction.[931]

Recent studies show that its neuroprotective efficacy,[932][933] is closely related to reducing inflammation, oxidative stress, cytotoxicity,[934][935] glutamate neurotoxicity, and inhibiting alpha-synuclein protein-aggregate activities, as well as disaggregating existing α-syn fibrils.[936] Studies also show that it protects condriosome (an organelle containing enzymes responsible for producing energy) and promotes nerve growth.[937]

Blueberries and other berries, rich in anthocyanins and proanthocyanidins, may reduce PD risk because they protect mitochondrial respiration in a dopaminergic cell line.[938]

Catechins. In one study a greater intake of epicatechin (EC) and proanthocyanidin dimers was associated with a lower risk of PD. Among other benefits, the author reported that proanthocyanidins may increase brain dopamine concentrations, inhibit monoamine oxidase-A activity, and reduce the 6-OHDA-induced dopaminergic loss.[939] It was implied that catechin derivatives may be involved in tea's beneficial effect on PD.

Food sources: Apricots, blackberries, black grapes, blueberries, black grapes, brewed black tea such as Darjeeling, peaches, raspberries, strawberries, chocolate, and red wine.

Citicoline (250mg per day) is a choline precursor and as such has been proposed for use in traumatic brain injury, stroke, vascular dementia, PD, and brain aging.[940][941] It may also help improve memory,[942] and play a possible role as a retardant agent for the cognitive deterioration of the eventual subsequent dementia.[943] Combined with the drug Nacom (Levodopa and Carbidopa) it reduces muscle rigidity more effectively than either constituent alone.[944] It crosses the blood brain barrier, is well absorbed when taken orally, and experimentally increases levels of norepinephrine and dopamine.[945]

Food sources: eggs, caviar, brewer's yeast, shiitake mushrooms, poultry, fish, raw beef liver, dairy foods, pasta, rice, and egg-based dishes, spinach, beets, wheat, and shellfish.

Curcumin (500mg – 1200mg per day) decreases the low-density lipoprotein oxidation and the free radicals that cause the deterioration of neurons,[946] in neuron degenerative disorders such as Parkinson's.[947] Studies suggest that curcumin should be considered as part of a treatment strategy as well to treat or prevent age-related neurodegenerative diseases such as Parkinson's disease PD.[948] [949] For best absorption, a curcumin supplement should have either piperine (a pepper extract) added and/or phospholipids such as lecithin to improve bioavailability.

Aged garlic stands out as having superior beneficial effects. With respect to Parkinson's, it is neuroprotective, reduces neuroinflammation,[950] [951] and reduces motor dysfunction.[952]

Fisetin, a flavonoid, helps prevent oxidative stress-induced nerve cell death and may reduce the impact of PD.[953] It has been shown that fisetin can activate the Ras-ERK cascade, a signaling pathway that regulates gene expression and prevents apoptosis in nerve cells.[954] Activation of this pathway is associated with the neuroprotective, neurotrophic and cognition enhancing effects of fisetin.[955] [956] [957] [958]

Food sources: This flavonoid is found in strawberries, apples, and persimmons, and lesser amounts in kiwi fruit, peaches, grapes, tomatoes, onions, and cucumbers.

Ginger (500mg – 700mg per day) increases neurogenesis, raises BDNF levels, enhances cognitive function, and is able to cross the blood brain barrier.[959] One of the active compounds of ginger, 6-shogaol, which has neuroprotective and anti-inflammatory effects, increased neurons in the substantia nigra, reduced inflammation biomarkers, and significantly inhibited motor rigidity, and microglial activation.[960] [961]

Goji berry (wolfberry or Lycium barbarum) (500mg once or twice per day). It contains powerful antioxidants and has strong neuroprotective and neurogenesis supporting properties.[962] [963] It has great potential in the treatment of Parkinson's disease.[964]

Gingko biloba (120mg – 240 mg per day). Gingko is known for its antioxidant, neuroprotective, and anti-apoptotic activity.[965] [966] Combined with donepezil, cognitive and dementia test scores and the quality of life improved for PD patients.[967]

Note: Gingko has slight blood thinning properties so consult your doctor if on any blood thinning medications before adding as a supplement.

Ginseng (500mg – 1,000mg per day of Asian ginseng (panax ginseng) root extract). Evidence of the effectiveness of various extracts of ginseng in their potential efficacy in Parkinson's treatment is increasing.[968] These ginsenosides are promising anti-Parkinson's agents through their neuroprotective actions, accomplished through a variety of mechanisms including "inhibition of oxidative stress and neuroinflammation, decrease in toxins-induced apoptosis and nigral iron levels, and regulation of N-methyl-D-aspartate receptor channel activity".[969] Korean red ginseng suppresses dopaminergic neuronal death in a mouse model of Parkinson's.[970]

Only the Rb1 ginsenoside of ginseng inhibits alpha-synuclein fibrillation and toxicity.[971] Other ginsenosides didn't prevent cell loss, but did prevent neuronal degeneration,[972] were anti-inflammatory, neuroprotective, and exhibited other anti-Parkinson effects.[973]

Glutathione [best taken sublingually (preferred) or intravenously) (reduced)] (700mg – 900mg per day in capsule or tablet form or 250mg in a sublingual/liposomal form). Levels of GSH is becoming an important therapeutic target both to reduce the impacts of aging[974] as well as in the treatment of age-associated neurological diseases such as PD.[975] A 2016 publication demonstrated that the glutathione precursor, NAC, produced a mean thirteen percent improvement in Unified Parkinson's Disease Rating Scale (UPDRS scores), and significantly increased dopamine transporter density in the caudate and putamen in PD, suggesting that NAC and/or GSH can affect dopaminergic neurotransmission.[976]

Food sources: sulfur rich foods including cruciferous vegetables such as broccoli, cauliflower, cabbage, as well as bok choy, kale, mustard and collard greens, radish, turnip, arugula.

Grape seed extract (GSE) (300mg – 500mg per day), modulates CNS function and supports the striato-thalamo-cortical pathways in Parkinson's, which improves PD motor dysfunction.[977] GSE, containing anthocyanins and proanthocyanidins, has greater neuroprotective effect than extracts rich in other polyphenols. **Grape seed and blueberry extract** protect mitochondrial respiration in a dopaminergic cell line.[978] **Grape seed and grape skin extract** shows promise in protecting against Parkinson's in a mouse model. Rich in antioxidants, GSSE has neuroprotective effects on dopaminergic neurons both in vitro and in vivo, reduces cell death, reduces inflammation, and improves motor function.[979]

Lutein (10mg – 20mg per day). Lutein provides potent antioxidant properties in the brain. It protects dopaminergic neurons against cell death and motor dysfunction by reducing mitochondrial disruption and oxidative stress.[980] Macular pigment density also has been found to be significantly related to multiple measures of temporal processing speed,[981] an important aspect of sensory and cognitive function. Only case-control studies show a link between PD risk and lutein intake[982] and higher intake of carotenoids like lutein are linked to slower progression of PD.[983]

Melatonin (1mg – 3 mg at bedtime). Melatonin is a hormone produced by the pineal gland which regulates sleep[984] and REM sleep,[985] that are common problems for PD patients. Researchers have learned that PD is linked to impaired brain expression of melatonin and its receptors.[986] Melatonin not only improves sleep in PD patients, but has important neuroprotective, anti-inflammatory, and antioxidant effects. It has shown to regulate neurotrophin expression affecting dopaminergic neuron integrity and reduces a-synuclein aggregation. Research shows the benefits of melatonin for PD cognitive, motor and nonmotor impairments, including insomnia, anxiety.[987]

Mucuna plant (dopa bean) (250mg of mucuna prurients seed extract per day or more as prescribed by your healthcare practitioner) has long been used in Ayurvedic medicine and contains a relatively high amount of L-dopa than other plants[988] in a natural form (versus synthetic medication). It provides additional benefits as an antioxidant.[989] It has been shown in both a PD mice model and patients, to be more effective than L-Dopa without the accompanying increase in dyskinesia (uncontrolled movements).[990][991]

Mulberry (500mg per day). protects neurons from toxin-caused damage,[992] and has antioxidant and anti-inflammatory properties.[993] In a mouse model of Parkinson's black mulberry juice reduced involuntary movement.[994]

Mushrooms. Numerous studies have shown both within in vitro and mammal studies to have potential roles in the prevention of many age-associated neurological diseases including Parkinson's.[995][996] See important species of mushrooms in the Nutrients chapter, especially Hericium erinaceus (lion's mane).

Nuts and berries. The interaction of nuts and berries supports cognition, reduces oxidative stress, inflammation and other factors contributing to the development of Parkinson's.[997][998] Walnuts are especially valuable in their neuroprotective potential related to Parkinson's.[999][1000]

Olives. Of the olives, Koroneiki olives have the most effective antioxidant and aggregation activities against alpha-synuclein fibril formation and elongation, and against toxic alpha-synuclein oligomers implicated in Parkinson's.[1001]

Omega-3 fatty acids (2,000mg – 3,000mg per day). Researchers have found that omega-3s reduce inflammation, and are neuroprotective,[1002] enhance the synthesis of brain-derived neurotrophic factor (BDNF), and promote neurogenesis via enhanced synaptogenesis and neurite outgrowth.[1003][1004] One study showed that supplementation with omega-3 PUFA reduced depression in PD patients.[1005] About sixty percent of your brain is made of fat, and half of that fat are omega-3 fatty acids.[1006] Your brain uses omega-3s to build brain and nerve cells, and these fats are essential for learning and memory.[1007][1008] One trial found that omega-3s combined with vitamin E had beneficial results in PD patients.[1009]

Food sources: Krill oil, fish, and seafood. Vegetarians can get DHA from algae sources.

Phosphatidylserine (100mg – 400mg per day) is key to proper brain function, and people with Parkinson's often have low levels of phosphatidylserine, which affects sleep patterns and disturbances.[1010] In one study, taking 100 milligrams of PS three times per day improved mood and brain function in people with Parkinson's.[1011]

Polygalae radix (35mg – 45mg per day). One in vivo mouse study concluded that polygalae radix protected dopaminergic neurons and fibers from MPTP-induced toxicity. These results suggest that it has protective effects on dopaminergic neurons via its antioxidant and anti-apoptotic activity.[1012] Onjisaponin B, derived from polygalae radix, was able remove mutant A53T a-synuclean associated with PD makes it a candidate for regulating neurodegenerative disorders.[1013]

Pueraria thomsonii benth (typically part of a Chinese herbal formulation). The active compounds of Pueraria (daidzein and genistein) have neuroprotective effects on the dopaminergic neurons. Rather than showing antioxidant activity, they inhibit activation of caspase 8 and partially inhibit activation of caspase 8 (both are pro-apoptosis proteases), thereby preventing cell death.[1014] Another isoflavonoid from P. thomsonii is tectorigenin which offers neuroprotection against 1-methyl-4-phenylpyridinium in a cellular model of Parkinson's. Research suggests that it does so by improving antioxidant defenses.[1015]

Pycnogenol inhibited neuroinflammation and neurodegeneration in Parkinsonian mice.[1016]

Pyrroloquinoline quinone (PQQ) (10mg - 20mg per day). PQQ promotes mitochondrial biogenesis and regulates mitochondrial fission and fusion offering neuroprotection in Parkinsonian mice. Additionally, PQQ may offer neuroprotection through gene modulation of Ndufs1 and Ndufs4.[1017] In vitro, it prevents fibril formation of alpha-synuclein.[1018]

Food sources: good non-meat food sources include parsley, papaya, green peppers, and oolong and green teas. Animal sources include eggs and dairy.

Quercetin (250mg-500mg 1-2 times per day). Quercetin has potent antioxidant and anti-inflammatory properties[1019] and therefore may limit brain cell death due to chronic inflammation[1020] that often leads to PD.[1021] It attenuates chemical-induced behavioral impairment, reduces oxidative stress, reduces cell death, and helps remove waste material in a rat model of Parkinson's.[1022] Quercetin, not caffeine, is the major neuroprotective element in coffee, consumption of which reduces the risk of Parkinson's (and Alzheimer's).[1023]

Red sage (aka Danshen/Salvia miltiorrhiza/ Salvia officinalis/red sage) (100mg per day). Tanshione IIA is a major constituent of red sage known to have neuroprotective effects. Treatment with Tanshione IIA prevents neurodegeneration of nigrostriatal DA neurons and increases striatal dopamine levels. These findings, along with its anti-inflammatory and anti-oxidative capacity suggest that it may be helpful in PD therapy.[1024] Another salvia flavonoid, tanshione I also exerts anti-inflammatory action and prevents damage to nigrostriatal dopaminergic neurons in a mouse model of PD.[1025]

Resveratrol (125mg per day). Research suggests that resveratrol has a therapeutic effect against PD due to its ability to modulate the MALAT1/miR-129/SNCA signaling pathway.[1026] Because resveratrol has strong anti-inflammatory and antioxidative effects, researchers have hypothesized that it could be a useful treatment for neurological disorders.

Food sources: Resveratrol is a naturally occurring polyphenolic phytoalexin which occurs in plants such as grapes, peanuts, berries, pines and in red wine.

Rhodiola rosea root (artic root) (150mg - 300mg per day). Researchers report that complementary use of plants such as artic root may be more effective than use of current pharmaceutical drugs alone. These plants are neuroprotective, antioxidant, anti-proteinopathic, neural-vasodilatory, anti-inflammatory, and iron chelating and thus may treat PD at the cellular level.[1027] Current pharmacological investigation reveals that Rhodiola may have therapeutic value for PD among other diseases.[1028] A 2013 rat study showed that Rhodiola rosea reduces oxidative stress and related biochemical alteration by the neurotoxin, MPTP.[1029] Salidroside, a glycoside derived from Rhodiola rosea L. has strong antioxidant properties and may protect dopaminergic neurons through inhibition of free radicals; it modulates the ROS-NO-related mitochondrial pathway both in vitro and in vivo.[1030]

SAM-e (S-Adenosyl-L-methionine) (400mg – 1200mg per day). In one study, participants who were treated with L-methionine for periods of two weeks to six months showed improvement in akinesia and rigidity, resulting in fewer tremors than usual.[1031] Methionine may play a critical role in prevention of aging related to oxidative damage and loss of dopamine, ultimately providing a potential treatment for Parkinson's.[1032]

Saffron is considered promising due to its antioxidant and neuroprotective properties.[1033]

Taurine (750mg – 1,000mg per day). Taurine helps Parkinson's and depression.[1034][1035] Studies have showed those with PD have lower normal plasma levels of taurine. This is particularly further aggravated by the drug levodopa, which may further deplete taurine.[1036] In a mouse model of PD taurine protects noradrenergic locus coeruleus neurons.[1037]

Tea, green or black (2-3 cups per day). Several epidemiological studies have addressed the influence of drinking tea (Camellia sinensis) on the risk of PD.[1038][1039][1040][1041] In some studies, but not others, a higher consumption of green tea (as well as black and oolong) has been linked to a lower prevalence of cognitive impairment.[1042][1043] Tea flavonoids exert antioxidant, anti-inflammatory and neuroregenerative effects.[1044][1045] In vivo studies in MPTP-induced parkinsonian mice have shown that green tea extract can slow dopamine depletion and improve dopaminergic neuronal survival in the substantia nigra region of the brain.[1046][1047] It helps protect neurons from damage due to poorly regulated extracellular signaling kinases (ERK1/2) and mitogen activated protein kinases and helps protect neurons from damage due to oxidative stress.[1048][1049] Green tea can also reduce the effect of iron dyshomeostasis observed in PD patients.[1050] Iron dyshomeostasis leads to a loss of function in several enzymes requiring iron as a cofactor, the formation of toxic free radicals, and the elevated production of beta-amyloid proteins. Deleterious effects of iron accumulation are dramatically evidenced in several neurodegenerative diseases including PD.[1051]

Tyrosine (250mg per day). The rate-limiting enzyme responsible for dopamine synthesis is tyrosine hydroxylase, which catalyzes the hydroxylation of tyrosine to DA, leading to the production of different catechol monoamines such as epinephrine and norepinephrine, and acts as a chaperone for the maintenance of normal neuronal oxidative status.[1052]

Vinpocetine (30mg – 60mg per day). Certain proteins in the innate immune system ('toll-like' receptors (or TLRs) activate inflammatory or anti-inflammatory responses in Parkinson's patients. Patients were given vinpocetine, and controls had traditional levodopa therapy. The vinpocetine treatment reduced TLR2/4 mRNA levels and related proteins and consequently the expression of inflammatory cytokines. Vinpocetine increased TLR3 mRNA levels and related proteins as the expression of anti-inflammatory cytokines. Furthermore, vinpocetine treatment improved scores in a standard mental state evaluation.[1053]

In Parkinsonian rats, after fourteen days, vinpocetine attenuated MPTP-induced motor dysfunction and biochemical abnormalities, including restoring dopamine levels.[1054] In Parkinsonian mice vinpocetine prevented motor dysfunction, memory impairment, oxidative stress and neuroinflammation by the dual enhancement of antioxidants and inhibition of neuroinflammatory cytokine.[1055] Combined with piracetam, vinpocetine reversed motor dysfunction and increased dopamine in the striata.[1056]

Zeaxanthin (2mg – 4mg per day). Research studies show that along with lutein, zeaxanthin helps maintain cognitive function memory, and executive (prioritizing and decision-making) function. Higher blood levels of zeaxanthin specifically are associated with better processing speed as well as enhancing brain blood flow in the specific areas that support that cognitive function. PD patients have lower levels of carotenoids, with greater deficiencies in advanced PD.[1057]

B vitamins appear to slow cognitive and clinical decline in people with mild cognitive impairment (MCI), in particular in those with elevated homocysteine.[1058] [1059] The accelerated rate of brain atrophy in elderly with mild cognitive impairment can be slowed by treatment with homocysteine-lowering B vitamins.[1060] The class of B-vitamins includes thiamine (B1), riboflavin (B2), niacin (B3), pyridoxine (B6), folate (B9), and cobalamin (B12). Of all the B-vitamins, vitamin B12, niacin, and thiamine have the most clearly established relations with deterioration in mental state.

Vitamin B1 (50mg per day). Vitamin B1 (thiamine) is critical for memory formation.[1061] There is a significant link between low levels of B1, and B1 supplements appear to have some benefit against PD, possibly through the connection between B1 and various transcription factors, and other metabolic pathways.[1062]

Vitamin B6 (100mg per day). A low intake of vitamin B6 (pyridoxine) is associated with an increased risk of PD[1063] [1064] and intake of B6 may decrease PD risk[1065] [1066] Vitamin B6 is essential because of its participation in more than 140 enzymatic reactions, including protein metabolism, conversion of tryptophan to niacin, and neurotransmitter function, among others.[1067]

Vitamin B9 (400mcg per day). B9 (folate) is needed to support choline in the body, so a deficiency in folate may affect brain support and folate deficiency can lead to neurological disorders, such as depression and cognitive impairment.[1068] [1069] [1070] [1071] Trials and studies indicate that folic acid supplementation can help to reduce age-related decline in cognitive function.[1072] [1073]

Vitamin B12 (400IU – 800IU per day). B12 deficiency has been linked to mental decline[1074] affecting mood, cognition and depression.[1075] Vitamin B12 is essential for the production of neurotransmitters[1076] and helps reduce homocysteine levels which are a contributing cause for PD).[1077] [1078] [1079] It works synergistically with vitamin B6 and folate to regenerate (methylate) the amino acid methionine, which helps to maintain already healthy homocysteine levels within normal range, which is important for heart health.[1080]

Vitamin D3 (5,000IU per day). Vitamin D deficiency is prevalent in PD patients.[1081] Dietary regulation of vitamin D may be effective in protecting individuals from PD or slowing PD progression. In animal and cell culture models of PD, vitamin D supplementation is beneficial in slowing disease progression.[1082] [1083] [1084]

Vitamin E (400mg – 800mg per day). By itself, Vitamin E has the capacity to slow cognitive decline in patients with mild to moderate AD. ninety percent of the population does not consume the RDA of 15mg/day but average closer to half that value—around 7mg/day.[1085] Researchers find that people who consume higher vitamin E-containing foods exhibit reduced cognitive decline according to an adaptation of the standard Mini Mental State Examination (MMSE).[1086]

The most bioavailable form is the α-Tocopherol form,[1087] but a combination of the different forms may be even more effective (four tocotrienols: α (alpha), β (beta), γ (gamma) and δ (delta). In several studies, it was found that individuals who consumed higher vitamin E-containing foods exhibited reduced cognitive decline per an adaptation of the Mini Mental State Examination (MMSE).[1088]

A concrete connection between vitamin E and AD is the significant decrease of vitamin E in the cerebrospinal fluid (CSF) and plasma of AD patients.[1089] Similarly, healthy individuals who participated in the Women's Health Study were shown to have less cognitive decline when consuming higher levels of vitamin E supplementation.[1090] [1091]

Zinc (40mg-60mg per day). Changes in brain zinc status have been implicated in a wide range of neurological disorders including impaired brain development, neurodegenerative disorders, and mood disorders including depression, Parkinson's, Huntington's, amyotrophic lateral sclerosis, and prion disease.[1092] Zinc is essential for nerve signaling and synaptic function (the way neurons communicate).[1093] About ten percent of total brain zinc is found in synaptic vesicles, which may be released on excitation so that it plays a role in modulation of synaptic signaling.[1094] Synaptic vesicles store neurotransmitters at the synapse.

Note. When supplementing with zinc, copper should also be taken in a 15:1 zinc to copper ratio.

Nutrient Summary

The following nutrients support brain health (more herbs are listed in the AD chapter). You can read about them in greater detail in the Nutrients chapter.

- **Breaks down alpha synuclein/or prevents build-up:** baicalein and alpha lipoic acid have been shown to help breakdown alpha synuclein in the brain, ginseng, melatonin.
- **Neurogenesis support**: Acetyl-l-carnitine, astaxanthin, omega-3 fatty acids and phosphatidylserine.
- **Improve Cognition**: Astaxanthin, ashwagandha, curcumin, ginseng, green tea, n-acetylcysteine, omega-3s, phosphatidylserine, PQQ, vinpocetine, and vitamin E.
- **Support Brain Plasticity**: Blueberries, DHA, fisetin, ginseng, goji berry, magnesium, omega-3 fatty acids, and resveratrol.

- **Dopamine Support**: Acetyl-l-carnitine, alpha lipoic acid, choline, bacopa monnieri, baicalein, catechins, caffeine, ginseng, glutathione, green tea, lutein, n-acetyl-cysteine, polygalae radix, pueraria thomsonii benth, red sage, SAM-e, vinpocetine.
- **Reduce Brain Inflammation**: Alpha lipoic acid, Apigenin, ashwagandha, astaxanthin, baicalein, CoQ10, curcumin, garlic, ginseng, green tea, omega-3, 6, 7 essential fatty acids, pycnogenol, reishi mushrooms, resveratrol, sage, SAM-e, vinpocetine, and zeaxanthin.
- **Reduce Depression**: 5-HTP, baicalein, ginger, ginseng, goji berry, n-acetylcysteine, olive leaf extract, omega-3 fatty acids, phosphatidylserine, sage, SAM-e, tryptophan, and vitamin B12.
- **Improved Motor Performance/reduced Rigidity**: Bacopa monnieri, ginger, mulberry, SAM-e, vinpocetine

Additional benefits of herbs include those that support mitochondrial function, reduce cell death, improve synapse function, reduce neurodegeneration, improve cognitive function, strengthen the blood-brain barrier, reduce free radicals and ROS (reactive oxygen species) and oxidative stress, reduce iron levels, improve sleep and mood.

Chapter 7. Post Traumatic Stress Disorder (PTSD)

Post-traumatic stress disorder (PTSD) triggered by ongoing frightening events such those experienced in combat, or a single terrifying event such as a natural disaster, a serious accident, terrorist act, or violent personal assault, is recognized as a mental health condition. PTSD can also result from chronic high stress related to work, finances, or relationships. About 3.5 percent of American adults are affected; about one in eleven people will be diagnosed with PTSD during their lives. Women are twice as likely as men to have PTSD.

Because PTSD causes changes in the brain, supplementary nutrients can support regeneration of new nerve brain cells, and reduce causative factors such as inflammation, apoptosis (cell death), and oxidative stress as well as increase cognitive ability, improve sleep, reduce anxiety, and promote overall brain and body health.

Effect of PTSD

It is normal to have temporary difficulty adjusting to and coping with traumatic events. Some people are better able to adapt than others. With time, therapy if needed, and self-care, symptoms generally improve. Chronic stress can impair brain cells, and thereby affect the healthy functioning of key regions of the brain resulting in damaged cognitive functioning, memory, and learning ability

The chronic or extreme stresses which lead to PTSD cause "acute and chronic changes in neurochemical systems and specific brain regions which result in long-term changes in brain circuits, involved in the stress response."[1095] These give rise to symptoms that worsen and last for months or many years, and interfere with daily activities. In such cases PTSD is diagnosed. A person with PTSD may have trouble sleeping, experience nightmares and anxiety, or in severe cases may have flashbacks, panic attacks, uncontrollable thoughts, and extreme behavior that disrupt mental well-being, damage self-confidence, and impair relationships with others.

PTSD and Chronic Traumatic Encephalopathy

Chronic traumatic encephalopathy (CTE) can be caused by some of the same events that give rise to PTSD. CTE is caused by repeated brain impact such as that experienced by military personnel exposed to explosive blast force, as well as numerous hits to the head from involvement in sports such as boxing and football. Researchers used MRSI to compare the hippocampal areas of veterans with blast-related mild traumatic brain injury and PTSD, finding that those exposed to blasts had more severe cognitive and neuromotor impairment.[1096] Read the CTE chapter for more information.

How the Brain Records Traumatic Events

An important role in PTSD is played by the hippocampus, amygdala, and medial prefrontal cortex. Two key neurotransmitters, cortisol and norepinephrine are critical in the stress response. Additional key players are the hypothalamic-pituitary-adrenal (HPA) and corticotropin-releasing factor (CRF).[1097]

Cortisol triggers neurochemical responses to stress, especially via the locus coeruleus in the brainstem. This center of neurons selects and catalogs "adaptive memories," which are exciting or traumatic and which are important for survival[1098] so that we can avoid such events in the future. The locus coeruleus sends the neurotransmitter, norepinephrine,[1099] to most of the brain, including the prefrontal cortex, amygdala, hippocampus, thalamus, and anterior cingulate cortex.

Norepinephrine controls arousal, memory, attention, and cognition. During a sharply exciting or frightening event the locus coeruleus amplifies neural input so that the resources for recording memories are prioritized, making "best" use of recording resources which are available at the time.[1100]

Furthermore, in the case of PTSD, researchers are identifying impairment of the hippocampus-dependent associative learning ability, which reduces the victim's ability to recall exactly what happened. Existing smaller hippocampal volume due to previous causes is linked to increased PTSD incidence after trauma.[1101]

Brain Volume and Function

Chronic traumatic stress can actually change the shape of the brain's regions. Patients with PTSD have smaller hippocampus and anterior cingulate cortex volumes.[1102] Amygdala activity increases, and anterior prefrontal/anterior cingulate function decreases.[1103]

In adults with childhood maltreatment-related PTSD, the amygdala is shrunken in size:[1104] primarily the left amygdala, but not the hippocampus or prefrontal cortex.[1105] Amygdala size can change (and recover). In one study life stress of "relatively short duration was associated with amygdala size … while temporally distant life stress was not, suggests that amygdala size changes may occur rapidly and reversibly…"[1106]

Genetic Changes

Not only do chronic and acute stressors cause changes in volume and function in the amygdala, hippocampus, and other regions of the brain, but such stress modulates gene expression. Working with mice, researchers have learned that a history of stress can permanently alter gene expressions in the hippocampus and in the response to a new stress.[1107]

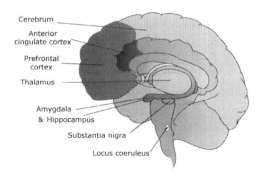

This may be the reason that severe PSTD can occur years later after an event. In terms of bio-physiology, a smaller left hippocampus volume is linked with severe PSTD occurring years after the initial experience(s).[1108]

Symptoms of PTSD

Symptoms are both mental, experienced subjectively, and physiological, reflected in the brain structure.

Symptoms and Effects
- Increased depression, emotional numbness
- Anxiety, feeling jumpy, irritable
- Flashbacks or nightmares
- Intense negative thoughts and feelings
- Poor sleep
- Diminished cognitive ability
- Increased risk of substance abuse

Neurobiological Effects
- Mast cell activation.[1109] Mast cells (mastocyte or labrocyte) are a kind of allergy-related cell derived from a stem cell that is part of the immune system. Mast cell activation refers to their releasing too many mediators and triggering allergic reactions, causing responses such as difficulty in breathing, severe diarrhea, or abnormally low blood pressure.
- Neuroinflammation and oxidative stress in the prefrontal cortex and hippocampus. Inflammation affects not only the basal ganglia and cortex, but the amygdala, insula and anterior cingulate cortex leading to changes in glutamate and monoamines.[1110]
- Reduced left amygdala and left hippocampal volumes
- Brain reserve – reduced ability to tolerate age-related change
- Changes in endocrine system: hypocortisolism in the hypothalamic-pituitary-adrenal axis causes abnormal stress encoding[1111]
- Changes in neurochemical patterns of dopamine, norepinephrine, serotonin, amino acids, and peptides.[1112]
- Anatomical changes: hippocampus volume and activity decreases, amygdala activity increases, and there is a reduced prefrontal cortex, anterior cingulate cortexes, and decreased medial prefrontal activation.[1113]

Risk Factors

Certain risk factors make one more vulnerable to PTSD. These include existing mental health conditions, genetics, previous trauma, lack of support, or chronic stress in life such as in the areas of love, work, or finances. A history of having suffered abuse or maltreatment as a child increases the risk of PTSD after a later traumatic event.[1114]

Women are more likely to develop PTSD than men (10-12 percent for women, and 4-5 percent among men).[1115] Traumatic stress affects girls and boys at different ages, and in different parts of the brain.[1116] Researchers estimate that in women about one third of the risk is due to genetic factors, much higher than for men.[1117]

There is some evidence that certain genetic structures increase vulnerability to PTSD and anxiety disorders.[1118] A gene, 5HTTLPR, with a long and a short form (5HTTLPR/short), is linked to the stress response. About forty percent of the population carries the short form and are clearly more vulnerable to all sorts of anxious behavior, including PTSD.[1119]

Treatment

According to one researcher, "PTSD may be one of the most preventable of the psychiatric disorders."[1120] Getting effective treatment after PTSD symptoms develop can be critical to reduce symptoms and improve function. Data on human PTSD support a protective role for adequate glucocorticoid levels at time of trauma. High dose hydrocortisone immediately after trauma may alter the trajectory of PTSD.[1121] [1122]

The good news is that the brain has plasticity, meaning that it has the capability of growing new neurons to regain or create new neural pathways. PTSD is usually treatable. Ways to promote healing include therapy, regular exercise, a healthy diet, doing a form of meditation or yoga daily, and seeking out support groups and healthy relationships.

Also, targeted supplementation can promote neurogenesis which promote regeneration of new nerve brain cells, and well as helping to reduce inflammation, apoptosis (cell death), increase cognitive ability, neutralize free radicals, and promote overall brain and body health.

There are nutrients and essential oils as well for helping promote a good night's sleep, reduce anxiety and depression, promote healthy circulation, and reduce blood pressure.

Some Essential Nutrients

The following have been tested in PTSD patients or animal models of PTSD.

Ashwagandha (Withania somnifera). W. somnifera root powder may protect against PTSD-induced memory impairment.[1123] In human clinical studies (with supporting preclinical evidence) it was effective for anxiety disorders.[1124]

Bacopa monnieri. In human clinical studies bacopa was found to be effective for anxiety disorders.[1125]

Bitter orange. (Citrus aurantium). Researchers found that this herb especially reduces anxiety.[1126]

Blueberries. Because PTSD is associated with increased oxidative stress and neuroinflammation in the prefrontal cortex and hippocampus powerful antioxidants are helpful against over-production of norepinephrine. In an animal model of PTSD rats on a blueberry enriched diet exhibited enzyme changes that helped restore neurotransmitter imbalances.[1127]

Curcumin. Several studies have found that curcumin, which reduces inflammation, is helpful in human and animal models of PTSD,[1128] depressive disorders,[1129][1130] and fear memories.[1131] The bioavailability of curcumin is an issue but combined with piperine (black pepper, long pepper) absorption is significantly enhanced.

DHA. Whether DHA is helpful has received strongly mixed reviews. Levels of this fatty acid are significantly lower in PTSD patients compared to healthy controls,[1132] as well as higher levels of EPA in mild PTSD.[1133] Although the American Psychiatric Association recommends omega-3s supplementation for a number of mental disorders including PTSD, 2019 research does not support this finding. This is due the likelihood of great variation in amounts and dosage of EPA and DHA.[1134] DHA, however, does improve levels of brain-derived growth factor, necessary for neurogenesis.[1135]

Ginseng. In an animal model of PTSD one of the components of ginseng, ginsenoside Rb1, reduced anxiety-like responses, suggesting that it may be helpful for patients with PTSD.[1136]

Green tea (containing epigallocatechin). In animal models of PTSD rats treated with epigallocatechin improved cognition, fear response, and reduced memory-related changes by means of inhibiting increased neuroinflammation in the face of stress. It also reversed some of the damaging hormonal changes in the brain and hypothalamic-pituitary-adrenal axis dysfunction.[1137]

Guta kola (Centella asiatica). Researchers found that this herb especially reduces anxiety.[1138]

Glycyrrhizin. Glycyrrhizin, the main constituent of licorice root, reduces PTSD-like behaviors and restores circadian rhythm of serotonin in the brain.[1139]

Lemon balm. (Melissa officianalis). Researchers find that this herb especially reduces anxiety.[1140]

N-acetyl-cysteine. PTSD carries with the high risk of substance use. Treatment with n-acetyl-cysteine during or immediately after acute stress appears to prevent stress-induced addictive drug use or a relapse.[1141]

Omega 3 fatty acids. An American panel on preparing soldiers for battle concluded that it would be unethical to not attempt to elevate the omega-3 status among military personnel.[1142] See DHA.

Passionflower (Passiflora incarnata). Researchers find that this herb especially reduces anxiety.[1143]

Resveratrol. Resveratrol[1144] and trans-resveratrol[1145] reduce anxiety in animal models of PTSD.

Sage. Researchers found that sage (salvia) species especially reduced anxiety.[1146]

Vitamin E. One study found that in a rat model of diabetes, PTSD behavior can be prevented by prolonged treatment with vitamin E.[1147]

Vinpocetine. Animal studies found the vinpocetine was effective in improving the firing rate of locus coeruleus neurons, related to its cognitive-enhancing properties.[1148]

While there is no direct PTSD research for the following supplemental nutrients, they may be helpful for specific types of support.

Neurogenesis support: Acetyl-l-carnitine, astaxanthin, curcumin, omega-e fatty acids, and phosphatidylserine.

Improve Cognition: Astaxanthin, ashwagandha, curcumin, ginseng, green tea, n-acetylcysteine, omega-3 fatty acids, phosphatidylserine, PQQ, and vitamin E.

Reduce Brain Inflammation: Apigenin, ashwagandha, astaxanthin, baicalein, CoQ10, curcumin, garlic, ginseng, green tea, omega-3, 6, 7 essential fatty acids, pycnogenol, reishi mushrooms, resveratrol, sage, SAM-e, vinpocetine, and zeaxanthin.

Reduce Depression: 5-HTP, baicalein, ginger, ginseng, goji berry, n-acetylcysteine, olive leaf extract, omega-3 fatty acids, phosphatidylserine, sage, SAM-e, tryptophan, and vitamin B12.

Support Brain Plasticity: Blueberries, DHA, fisetin, ginseng, goji berry, magnesium, omega-3 fatty acids, and resveratrol.

Essential Oils:

Improve Sleep: Lemon balm, turmeric, and ylang.

Reduce anxiety, agitation, mild depression, and stress: Bergamot, clary sage, lavender, lemon Balm, frankincense, melissa, spearmint, spike lavender (also reduces overall pain), and tea tree lemon.

Digestion Issues including a loss of appetite and constipation: Ginger, peppermint, and yarrow.

Improve Cognitive Function: Rosemary and saffron.

Chapter 8. Chronic Traumatic Encephalopathy (CTE)

Chronic traumatic encephalopathy (CTE) is a condition, first noted in boxers, and now recognized as a serious problem for athletes in collision-contact sports, such as football and related sports and occupations. It is evidenced by dementia, erratic thinking and behavior, and personality changes. It caused by repeated blows to the head, but symptoms may not appear until many years after the injuries.[1149] It appears that such trauma is necessary to the development of CTE, but is not alone the cause.[1150]

Who Gets CTE?

Although CTE is not limited to athletes, though they are the ones that experience the condition most often. Through autopsy of more than two-hundred football players who donated their brains for research, eighty-seven percent had neuropathological evidence of CTE.[1151] In general, those at risk include athletes whose careers involve repeated collision, such as in football, rugby,[1152] soccer,[1153] ice hockey,[1154] boxing,[1155] mixed martial arts,[1156] wrestling,[1157] and military personnel exposed to blast(s).[1158]

CTE has some clinical and pathological features that are similar to PTSD (and post-concussion syndrome), and may share some metabolic and neurologic causes or triggers.[1159] [1160] Additionally, brain trauma is one of the contributing causes of Parkinson's disease, although severe head injury is most often considered to be contributory.[1161]

Structural Changes

Beta-amyloid plaque. CTE is similar to Alzheimer's and Parkinson's in that tau protein becomes hyperphosphorylated leading to fibrous tangles around small blood vessels. Sometimes beta-amyloid plaque is present. Unlike Alzheimer's, the aggregates are observed more quickly than in AD. And, unlike AD, they form around blood vessels in the furrows (sulci) of the wrinkled surface of the cerebral cortex, and then spread unevenly in the cortex.[1162]

Researchers have discovered that the fibrous tangles first noted around blood vessels in the sulci also develop within the nucleus basalis neurons (an important cluster of neurons in the forebrain that are part of the cholinergic system), and contribute to disconnection of messaging.[1163] These neurons are rich in the transmitter acetylcholine with widespread connections to other parts of the brain.

Neurodegeneration. The midbrain, which regulates movement (such as eye movement), is especially vulnerable to repeated mild impact. Researchers found that the amount of neurodegeneration in the midbrain is related to the amount of rotational acceleration experienced, and it was noted that some damage occurs even after a single season of college football.[1164] In addition, researchers have found that CTE also causes increased expression of phosphorylated tau and amyloid proteins in hippocampal (important for memory) and septal neurons (that play a role in reward/reinforcement mechanisms),[1165] resulting in diminishing these capabilities.

Metabolic Changes

- **N-acetyl-aspartate levels decrease**. There is evidence (in ice hockey players) that after repetitive head impacts N-acetyl aspartate (NAA) levels decrease significantly in post-season compared to pre-season.[1166] The decrease in NAA was also noted in former NFL players.[1167] NAA, contained in neurons, is essential for neuronal mitochondrial function. Its presence indicates both density of nerve cells and nerve mitochondria integrity and reduced concentrations of NAA are common to different psychiatric disorders.[1168]

- **Choline levels decrease**. In post-season ice hockey players researchers noted a decrease in choline.[1169] Choline is essential for keeping homocysteine levels low and preventing over-activation of the microglial system which removes waste products.

- **Glutamate, glutathione, and myo-inositol levels decrease.** In the anterior of the brains of former NFL football players there was direct positive correlation between changed mood/ behavior and levels of: glutamate, thirty-two percent change; glutathione, twenty-nine percent change; myo-inositol, twenty-six percent change.[1170] Glutamate is an excitatory neurotransmitter with an important role in learning and memory. Myo-inositol is a carbohydrate that affects levels of neurotransmitters and how we experience anxiety. The antioxidant glutathione when deficiency contributes to seizures, intellectual disability, and loss of coordination.[1171]

- **Creatine levels decrease**. Early studies of NFL players that have suffered from concussions indicate that white matter signal abnormalities can occur, which as a result is associated with cognitive decline. This type of brain tissue helps you think fast, walk straight, and keeps you from falling.[1172]

Symptoms

At early stages symptoms are memory difficulties, aggression, depression, explosivity, and executive dysfunction.[1173] As the condition develops, patients experience problems with attention, mood swings, visuospatial difficulties, confusion, progressive dementia, and suicidality.[1174]

Risk Factors

The primary risk factor appears to be the number of times the head is struck, not the severity of individual blows as they can be mild.[1175] In the case of boxing, researchers found that the number of rounds fought was more indicative of CTE development rather than the number of knockouts. Researchers, however, are also beginning to think that CTE is caused by multiple factors.

Any one of the following can account for many of the symptoms.[1176]
- Repeated neurotrauma is necessary but not sufficient alone to cause CTE
- Substance abuse
- Chronic pain
- Emotional stress such as athletic career transition stress

Other researchers suggest that the following are also factors.[1177]
- Neurodevelopmental disorders
- Normal aging
- Surgeries and anesthesia
- Sleep difficulties

Diagnosis

The only positive diagnosis at this time is by autopsy after death. There are not yet any clinical guidelines for diagnosis. If CTE is suspected, often because of the patient's history, brain imaging and other tests can rule out other causes such as Alzheimer's or Parkinson's. Researchers have been investigating the possibility of fluid biomarkers to assist in diagnosis.[1178]

Treatment

There is no current treatment available for CTE other than the kind of care given to PTSD, Alzheimer's, and other patients with neurodegenerative conditions. Because CTE is caused by repetitive mild head trauma, treatments such as multidisciplinary attentive treatment (MAT) which is used for patients with severe traumatic brain injury, may not be effective for CTE.[1179] At this time the only treatment is prevention by practicing some of the following:

- **Avoidance.** Avoid participating in collision-likely contact sports such as those listed above.
- **Change the rules.** The NFL did institute a new rule outlawing using the helmet to hit an opposing player's body during a tackle.[1180] In the aftermath of this rule concussions dropped by thirty percent in the NFL.[1181] Four states, Illinois (children under twelve), New York, California, and Maryland, have introduced legislation regarding tackle football.[1182] But in every case the bills died due to parental, coaching, and organized football lobbying.[1183]
- **Nutritional support for athletes.** In 2014 a military panel recommended supplying military personnel with ample omega-3s to possible protect them from stress and increase wellness and performance.[1184] To our knowledge no research has been done as to the nutritional support athletes were offered during their lives. However, perhaps in the future guidelines will be established for the nutritional components to support neurogenesis and prevent neurodegeneration.

The following have been identified as supporting neurogenesis, memory, executive function, balance, and motor skills, and protecting against anxiety. Studies show that intake of antioxidants are applicable for both PTDS and CTE, so we included some of the related PTSD studies in this chapter.

Ashwagandha (Withania somnifera). W. somnifera root powder may protect against PTSD-induced memory impairment.[1185] In human clinical studies (with supporting preclinical evidence) it was effective for anxiety disorders.[1186]

Astaxanthin (6mg – 12 mg per day) is protective across various models of Parkinson's[1187] by reducing the pathophysiology that causes neurodegeneration.[1188] It accomplishes this, in part, by suppressing oxidative damage in certain signaling pathways[1189] and by protecting against mitochondria dysfunction.[1190] Its action as an anti-inflammatory, an antioxidative, and an anti-apoptotic may underly its effectiveness in protecting against neurodegeneration.[1191]

Baicalein (200-800 mg in multiple doses, once in the morning and once again at night). Recent studies show that its neuroprotective efficacy,[1192][1193] is closely related to reducing inflammation, oxidative stress, cytotoxicity,[1194][1195] glutamate neurotoxicity, and inhibiting alpha-synuclein protein-aggregate activities, as well as disaggregating existing α-syn fibrils.[1196] Studies also show that it protects condriosome (an organelle containing enzymes responsible for producing energy) and promotes nerve growth.[1197]

Bacopa monnieri. In human clinical studies bacopa was found to be effective for anxiety disorders,[1198] as well as having many other benefits including helping breakdown alpha synuclein and beta-alpha buildup.

Blueberries. Because PTSD is associated with increased oxidative stress and neuroinflammation in the prefrontal cortex and hippocampus powerful antioxidants are helpful against over-production of norepinephrine. In an animal model of PTSD rats on a blueberry enriched diet exhibited enzyme changes that helped restore neurotransmitter imbalances.[1199]

Curcumin. Several studies have found that curcumin, which reduces inflammation, is helpful in human and animal models of PTSD,[1200] depressive disorders,[1201][1202] and fear memories.[1203] The bioavailability of curcumin is an issue but combined with piperine (black pepper, long pepper) absorption is significantly enhanced.

DHA. Whether DHA is helpful has received strongly mixed reviews. Levels of this fatty acid are significantly lower in PTSD patients compared to healthy controls,[1204] as well as higher levels of EPA in mild PTSD.[1205] Although the American Psychiatric Association recommends omega-3s supplementation for a number of mental disorders including PTSD, 2019 research does not support this finding. This is due the likelihood of great variation in amounts and dosage of EPA and DHA.[1206] DHA, however, does improve levels of brain-derived growth factor, necessary for neurogenesis.[1207]

Ginseng. In an animal model of PTSD one of the components of ginseng, ginsenoside Rb1, reduced anxiety-like responses, suggesting that it may be helpful for patients with PTSD.[1208]

Glutathione Best taken sublingually (preferred) or intravenously) (reduced) (700mg – 900mg per day in capsule for tablet form. Levels of GSH are becoming an important therapeutic target both to reduce the impacts of aging[1209] as well as in the treatment of age-associated neurological diseases such as PD.[1210]

Guta kola (Centella asiatica). Researchers found that this herb especially reduces anxiety.[1211]

Lemon balm. (Melissa officianalis). Researchers find that this herb especially reduces anxiety.[1212]

N-acetyl-cysteine. PTSD carries with the high risk of substance use. Treatment with n-acetyl-cysteine during or immediately after acute stress appears to prevent stress-induced addictive drug use or a relapse.[1213]

Omega 3 fatty acids. An American panel on preparing soldiers for battle concluded that it would be unethical to not attempt to elevate the omega-3 status among military personnel.[1214] See the discussion on DHA above.

Pyrroloquinoline quinone, in an animal model of traumatic brain injury, improved brain electrophysiological function after trauma, decreasing lactate dehydrogenase content in primary astrocytes exposed to glutamate.[1215]

Passionflower (Passiflora incarnata). Researchers find that this herb especially reduces anxiety.[1216]

Sage. Researchers found that sage (salvia) species especially reduced anxiety.[1217]

Vitamin E. One study found that in a rat model of diabetes, PTSD behavior can be prevented by prolonged treatment with vitamin E.[1218]

The following provide support for a healthy brain. You can read more about them in the Nutrients chapter.

Neurogenesis support: Acetyl-l-carnitine, astaxanthin, and phosphatidylserine.

Improve Cognition: Astaxanthin, ashwagandha, curcumin, ginseng, green tea, n-acetylcysteine, omega-3 fatty acids, phosphatidylserine, PQQ, vinpocetine, and vitamin E.

Reduce Brain Inflammation: Alpha lipoic acid, Apigenin, ashwagandha, astaxanthin, baicalein, CoQ10, curcumin, garlic, ginseng, green tea, omega-3, 6, 7 essential fatty acids, pycnogenol, reishi mushrooms, resveratrol, sage, SAM-e, vinpocetine, and zeaxanthin.

Reduce Depression: 5-HTP, baicalein, ginger, ginseng, goji berry, n-acetylcysteine, olive leaf extract, omega-3 fatty acids, phosphatidylserine, sage, SAM-e, tryptophan, and vitamin B12.

Support Brain Plasticity: Blueberries, DHA, fisetin, ginseng, goji berry, magnesium, omega-3 fatty acids, and resveratrol.

Chapter 9. Brain Fog

One manifestation of decreased cognitive ability is the general term, "brain fog". Top descriptors of brain fog are 'forgetful,' 'cloudy,' and 'difficulty focusing, thinking, and communicating'.[1219] Symptoms of brain fog can include: slow or hazy thinking, difficulty focusing, confusion, lack of concentration, low motivation, trouble remembering things, irritability, anxiety, headaches, insomnia, and lack of incentive to exercise.

Causes of Brain Fog

Metabolic Factors

Hormonal changes. Changes to the three primary hormones dopamine, serotonin, and cortisol, determine your mood, energy, and focus. Cortisol helps keep you awake and alert and is often called the body's primary "stress hormone". Dopamine and serotonin help keep you joyful, motivated, and calm. Hormonal changes that occur with menopause can also cause brain fog as can imbalances in thyroid output.[1220]

Chronic fatigue syndrome is a clinically defined set of symptoms of unknown etiology most notable for persistent fatigue lasting greater than six months, is of new onset, not related to exertion or improved with rest, and is debilitating to a person's lifestyle.[1221]

Inflammation and Oxidative Stress

Inflammation. On a cellular level, brain fog is often caused by chronic inflammation when molecules such as adipocytokines and histamine are released from mast cells, which further stimulate microglia activation.[1222]

Fibromyalgia is a chronic inflammatory disorder characterized by widespread musculoskeletal pain, fatigue, and tenderness in localized areas.

Diet and Nutrition

Energy levels can be depleted by nutrient deficiencies, sugar, or caffeine overload, overeating of refined carbohydrates, artificial sweeteners, or other foods one may be reactive or allergic to including foods containing corn, wheat, and peanuts in particular. The brain relies on a steady stream of vitamins and minerals, amino acids, essential fatty acids, and glucose from complex carbohydrates as well as getting enough rest and relaxation.

Celiac disease results from being highly *reactive* to gluten (such as found in wheat and other grains) resulting in gut-related symptoms like abdominal pain or bloating, diarrhea, and constipation. Other symptoms can include fatigue, joint pain, or mouth sores, and brain fog. People also report feeling disoriented, unable to focus or pay attention, and claim forgetfulness.[1223] See the chapter on gluten sensitivity for more information.

Dehydration. We tend not to drink enough water each day. Recommended dosage is six to eight glasses of water per day, ideally separated in 4oz. dosages unless after exercise or other physical activity. Coffee, tea, and juice is not a replacement for water.

Food allergies includes gluten, corn, peanuts, milk, eggs, nuts, soy, and shellfish.

Iron deficiency. Brain fog is one of the early symptoms of iron deficiency.[1224]

Exposure to Toxins

Medications such as antidepressants, stimulants, sleep aids, antipsychotics, and even blood pressure medications can cause brain fog. Discuss your medications with your doctor if you have chronic brain fog.

Chemo brain is the term that refers to side effects from cancer treatments which include changes in cognitive function, memory, and attention. Such treatment can result in epigenetic changes and oxidative DNA damage.[1225]

Environmental pollutants, including indoor and outdoor air pollution, can cause brain fog.[1226] As discussed in previous chapters children and young adults who live in areas with significant air pollution are much more likely to exhibit evidence of neurodegeneration.[1227][1228][1229] The same is true of industrial-, combustion-, and friction-derived nanoparticles.[1230]

Daily Life Factors

Lack of sleep, sedentary lifestyle and high amounts of stress may impact brain functioning and cognition.

Medical Conditions

Brain fog is a symptom or side effect of many other conditions, including bacterial infections such as Lyme disease,[1231] multiple sclerosis,[1232] Sjogren's syndrome,[1233] anemia, depression, diabetes, migraine headaches, arthritis, or high levels of fats in blood plasma.[1234] As many as fifty percent of people who have the autoimmune disease lupus also have "lupus fog," with lapses in memory, difficulty concentrating, and confusion. Poor circulation can cause lack of nutrients and oxygen from reaching the brain.

Conventional Treatment

The best course of action if you experience brain fog is to get tested for the conditions listed above and get treated for them to reduce related symptoms.

Complementary Approach

Diet

Eat a healthy, alkaline-based, diet. Consuming plenty of fruit and starchy/non-starchy veggies realigns hormones and also reduces inflammation. Get enough protein in your diet through eggs, meat, fish, and dairy products. If you are a vegetarian, then use nuts, seeds, foods such as tempeh and tofu, and food-combining techniques. Avoid refined carbohydrates, artificial sweeteners, and unhealthy oils (including fried food and trans-fatty acids often found in chips and margarine). Some people may need to eliminate caffeine and alcohol, and everyone should reduce sugar, particularly refined sugar and eliminate any artificial sweeteners totally (stevia is fine).

Nutrients

Below are the most important nutrients for brain fog. Some of these are recognized as "nootropics," substances that may improve cognitive function in healthy people. Researchers call them the first "smart drugs" used for cognitive therapy.[1235] Read more about these in the Nutrients chapter, along with dosages and research.

Acetyl-l-carnitine is one of the top nutrients to stop brain fog. It increases cerebral blood flow, improves focus and concentration in healthy adults, and helps convert choline to acetylcholine.

Alpha lipoic acid crosses the blood-brain barrier to support acetylcholine synthesis. Acetylcholine is the most prominent neurotransmitter in the brain, directly linked to learning and memory.

B vitamins. Deficiencies in various B vitamins (such as B1, B2, B6 and B12) can leave you feeling sluggish and moody. B vitamins help convert nutrients from the foods you eat into usable fuel for the body. Supplementing with a high-quality B-complex supplement may possibly be recommended.

Bacopa monnieri helps cognitive function, reduces brain fog, mental fatigue, and reduces feelings of stress and anxiety.

Choline alfoscerate supplementation can be absorbed as choline and cross the blood-brain barrier. It may improve memory retention, boost brain function, and enhance mental clarity.

Ginkgo biloba is one of the most popular and well-known herbs to reduce brain fog. Ginkgo improves ocular and cerebral blood flow, as well as boosting processing speed and accuracy. Studies have shown that ginkgo biloba's effects on information recall, brain fog reduction, and mood enhancement impact all age groups.

Ginseng improves thinking, concentration, memory, and physical endurance. It can also help with depression, anxiety, chronic fatigue, and immune system health.

Huperzine A is an herbal nootropic used in traditional Chinese medicine. It is well-known for its ability to help clear the mind and improve cognitive function. It increases the amount of acetylcholine present in the brain.

Iron deficiency is often characterized by brain fog and impaired brain function being associated with oxidative stress and neurodegenerative diseases. Research suggests that iron plays an important physiological role in neuronal processes such as myelination, synaptogenesis, behavior, and synaptic plasticity.

MCTs (medium-chain triglycerides), found in coconut oil, provides ketone energy from fat, and may improve cognitive function in patients with mild cognitive impairment.[1236]

Omega-3 fish oils support brain function including enhancing cerebral blood flow, slowing cognitive decline, and helping lower inflammation. If you are a vegetarian, you can take algae supplements.

Phosphatidylserine – is another nootropic supplement that plays a vital role in enhancing cell-to-cell communication while supporting the maintenance and growth of neurons.

Rhodiola rosea helps reduce physical and mental fatigue, similar to the effects of caffeine but without the post fatigue when the caffeine wears off.

Lifestyle

Exercise regularly. Get at least twenty minutes of aerobic exercise five days a week. Your exercise can include fast walking, swimming, hiking, gym workouts, yoga, etc.

Manage stress. Do some form of meditation on a regular basis. Limit "negative" people in your life and learn how to limit your negative, anxious, or angry reaction to them.

Get plenty of sleep. Seven to eight hours a night is sufficient for most people.

Health checkup. Get tested for food allergies, hormone imbalances and vitamin deficiencies.

Essential Oils

For brain health, the most important essential oils are lavender, frankincense and vetiver. The medicinal and aromatic plants including bergamot, caraway, eucalyptus, geranium, juniper, lavender, lemon, lemongrass, mint, orange, peppermint, pine, rosemary, sage, tea tree, thyme and ylang-ylang have been used to treat a variety of physical and psychological disorders.

- Lavender essential oil is widely used for its relaxing and calming properties.
- Frankincense has been used for many years to promote healthy cellular functions. It helps balance mood by improving concentration and focus, and can help minimize irritability, impatience, hyperactivity, and restlessness.
- Vetiver is helpful for insomnia and anxiety.
- Citrus essential oils provide uplifting effects on the body and mind. For example, lemon provides uplifting effects, promotes physical energy, and reduces stress.
- Peppermint is one of the most popular essential oils used to stimulate the mind as well as support concentration, focus, memory, and overall mental performance.

Chapter 10. Brain Inflammation

Inflammation in the brain can lead to anything from brain fog to Alzheimer's Disease (AD). In AD, damaged neurons and neurites and highly insoluble amyloid beta peptide deposits and neurofibrillary tangles provide stimuli for inflammation, which then exacerbates more deposits and tangles resulting in a degenerative cycle. Many studies have proposed that inflammatory dysfunctions are associated with psychiatric disorders and neurodegeneration in both animal models and human patients.[1237] [1238]

Causes

Microglial Cells

Microglia are a collective type of neuroglia (glial cell) located throughout the brain and spinal cord. Microglia accounts for ten to fifteen percent of all cells found within the brain. In normal conditions microglia performs significant functions in maintaining healthy brain functions, including disposing of dead neurons, breaking down amyloid beta plaque (a causative factor in AD), and disposing of other brain debris. In a heightened inflammatory response, the microglia go into overtime and cause neuroinflammation. This affects neurons' ability to function at a maximum level resulting in (the short-term) brain fog, poorer recall and mental speed, and slower reflexes. It may also result in depression, and poorer endurance for daily activities for reading, driving and mental tasks. Microglial activation has also been linked with brain diseases.[1239]

A hallmark of brain damage is an increased inflammatory response capable of activating microglial cells. Neuronal damage and loss[1240] [1241] is caused by: 1) release of pro-inflammatory cytokines including interleukin (IL)-1β, IL-6 and tumor necrosis factor (TNF)-α,[1242] and 2) upregulation of nuclear factor-kappa B, mitogen-activated protein kinase, and c-Jun N-terminal kinase.[1243] The pro-inflammatory cytokines send messages through the blood-brain barrier to the brain, which results in changes in brain function and destroys brain tissue.[1244][1245][1246] In the long term, the negative effects include neuronal death, neurodegenerative disorders, and a compromised blood-brain barrier.

Medical Conditions

Rheumatoid arthritis (RA). Researchers have noted that chronic inflammation can affect the brain. MRI images taken of the brains of fifty-four people with RA showed a reduction in grey matter in an area of the brain known as the inferior parietal lobe. Researchers believe these alterations to brain tissues may have a role in converting inflammation signals to the rest of the central nervous system.[1247] RA is linked to an impaired ability to think, and may be related to the use of corticosteroids as an RA treatment.[1248]

Other medical conditions. Other conditions that can cause brain inflammation include diabetes, compromised circulation to the brain, inflammatory bowel conditions, and autoimmune diseases.

Other Causes

A poor diet with inadequate nutrition can give rise to brain fog and can mimic dementia.

Environmental Toxins

Environmental pollutants have been linked to neuro-inflammation. As discussed in previous chapters, children and young adults who live in areas with significant air pollution are at far greater risk of neuroinflammation and neurodegeneration.[1249] [1250] [1251] The same is true of industrial-, combustion-, and friction-derived nanoparticles.[1252]

Compromised Blood Brain Barrier (BBB)

The blood-brain barrier prevents unwanted material such as debris, toxins, bacteria, and viruses from reaching the brain from the body, and is essential for maintaining brain health. BBB brain homeostasis, regulation of influx and efflux transport is essential for protecting the brain. A breakdown in BBB can result in neuroinflammation, neurodegeneration, as well as cerebral small vessel disease.[1253] Read more about the blood brain barrier and ways to help repair a compromised BBB in the appendix.

Conventional Treatment

Treatment depends on diagnosis, which is based on brain imaging, blood work and sometimes analysis of spinal fluid, as well as other diagnostic tests that would indicate neurodegenerative conditions such as AD and PD. Generally, neurodegenerative treatments are through immuno-suppressive drugs such as steroids or Rituxan® (rituximab), or filtering procedures such as plasmapheresis (which filters antibodies from blood plasma) or intravenous immune globulin (**IVIG**). Nonsteroidal anti-inflammatory drugs (NSAIDs) for inflammation or arthritis may reduce neuroinflammation.[1254]

Complementary Approach

Nutrients

The Nutrients chapter includes information on research, dosage recommendations, and additional benefits of each nutrient below. These nutrients support brain health and/or reduce brain inflammation. Many of them are able to cross the blood-brain barrier.

Apigenin is a flavonoid that crosses the blood brain barrier. It has powerful anti-inflammatory benefits, promotes neurogenesis, and protects the brain neurovascular coupling against amyloid beta.

Food sources: artichokes, celery, chamomile, cloves, lemon balm, licorice, parsley, peppermint, red wine, spinach, as well as other spices such as rosemary, oregano, thyme, basil, and coriander.

Baicalein is another flavonoid that crosses the blood brain barrier. It has powerful anti-inflammatory benefits, reduces anxiety, restores blood flow, and promotes neuron development in damaged sections of the brain.

Food sources: common fruit and vegetables such as onions, parsley, as well as oranges, tea, chamomile, and wheat sprouts.

Boswellia serrata resin (frankincense) can inhibit leukotriene biosynthesis in neutrophilic granulocytes (the most common type of white blood cell) by inhibiting 5-LOX, thus affecting various inflammatory diseases that are perpetuated by leukotrienes (inflammatory mediators).

Catechin is a flavonoid that crosses the blood brain barrier. It has powerful anti-inflammatory benefits. Green tea contains a number of chemical compounds, including green tea catechins, caffeine, and theanine, which may affect brain function (see green tea below). These bioactive tea components might be useful for neuronal degeneration treatment in the future.

Food sources: apricots, blackberries, black grapes, blueberries, black grapes, brewed black tea such as Darjeeling, peaches, raspberries, strawberries, chocolate, and red wine.

Cat's claw (uncaria tomentosa) has been shown to prevent the activation of the transcriptional factor NF-kB and it directly inhibits TNF-α production by up to 65-85 percent, helping reduce inflammation.

Curcumin crosses the blood brain barrier and has powerful anti-inflammatory benefits. It is a naturally occurring yellow pigment that has long been used in both ayurvedic and Chinese medicines as an anti-inflammatory agent, a treatment for digestive disorders, and to enhance wound healing. Curcumin may be considered a viable natural alternative to nonsteroidal agents for the treatment of inflammation or used in combination with lower doses of nonsteroidal medications.

Food sources: commonly found the spice turmeric used in curry.

Ginseng (Panax) has immunomodulatory, vasodilatory, anti-inflammatory, antioxidant, anti-aging, anticancer, anti-fatigue, anti-stress, and anti-depressive effects in rodents and humans. It may also have a beneficial effect in AD by reducing tau hyperphosphorylation and neurofibrillary tangle formation.

Green tea constituents are polyphenolic compounds called catechins. Epigallocatechin-3 galate is the most abundant catechin in green tea. Green tea research now demonstrates both anti-inflammatory and chondroprotective effects.

Omega-3 polyunsaturated fatty acids are some of the most effective natural anti-inflammatory agents available. Countries that have the highest fish consumption also have a lower incidence of neurodegenerative disease and depression. Diets high in omega-3 fatty acids have been found to help protect against cognitive decline. They increase the secretion of anti-inflammatory compounds in the brain and can have a protective effect, especially in older adults.

Resveratrol is a polyphenol compound that crosses the blood-brain barrier. It is found in certain plants and in red wine that has antioxidant and anti-inflammatory properties. It has been investigated for possible anticarcinogenic effects.

Food sources: blueberries, cocoa and dark, chocolate cranberries, grapes, peanuts, pistachios, red and white wine.

Pycnogenol (maritime pine bark) is one of the most potent antioxidant compounds. It is fifty to one-hundred times more potent than vitamin E in neutralizing free radicals and it helps to recycle and prolong the activity of vitamins C and E. It inhibits matrix-degrading enzyme which is highly expressed at sites of inflammation, and it contributes to the pathogenesis of various chronic inflammatory disease.

Food sources: wine, grapes, apples, cocoa, tea, nuts, and some berries.

Rutin is a glycoside of the flavonoid quercetin, and is also known as Vitamin P. It can cross the blood brain barrier, and has powerful anti-inflammatory benefits. Rutin has been shown to have an extensive array of pharmacological applications due to its numerous properties including antioxidant, anti-inflammatory, cardiovascular, neuroprotective, antidiabetic, and anticancer activities. It also should be considered as a therapeutic approach for many health conditions in which oxidative stress is an underlying cause such as AD.

Diet

In general, it is helpful to maintain a strong alkaline diet as described in the diet chapter. The keto diet can be considered for its strong anti-inflammatory benefits, or the paleo diet,[1255] although there are potential long-term issues, also described in the diet chapter.

Your gut helps to manage levels of inflammation and therefore, keeping your gut healthy with the right foods is essential to keeping your brain healthy and reducing your risk of brain inflammation.

Top anti-Inflammatory foods. Avocados, broccoli, cocoa (dark chocolate 85 percent or higher), green, leafy vegetables, nuts (in particular hazelnuts and walnuts due to their high levels of brain-protecting, inflammation reducing vitamin E and antioxidants). Oily fish such as wild salmon, trout, tuna as well as sardines, herring, anchovies, and mackerel have strong anti-inflammatory properties.

Food Sources for vegetarians: chia seeds, flax seeds, walnuts, as well as algae.

Avoid sugar and refined carbohydrates (particularly all white, refined foods). Low carbohydrate diets how been shown to reduce inflammation. Refined carbohydrates have a high glycemic index (referring to how much a food raises your blood sugar levels, based on the serving size). Research has shown that just a single meal with a high glycemic load can impair memory in both children and adults. The effect on memory may be due to inflammation of the hippocampus, a part of the brain that affects some aspects of memory, as well as responsiveness to hunger and fullness cues.[1256] [1257] A study found that elderly people who consumed more than 58 percent of their daily calories in the form of carbohydrates had almost double the risk of mild mental impairment and dementia.[1258]

Avoid vegetable oils, sodas and other sugary drinks (including anything with artificial sweeteners such as Aspartame (NutraSweet®, Equal®), Saccharin (Sweet'N Low®, SugarTwin®), Acesulfame K (Sunett®, Sweet One®,) Sucralose (Splenda®). Also avoid trans fatty acids such as those found in most margarines and many fast foods, frosting, crackers and chips, and limit your intake of saturated fats (cheese, milk, butter and other dairy products).

Chapter 11. Leaky Gut Syndrome and Dementia

'Leaky gut' syndrome occurs when the intestinal mucosal lining of the intestine. Its impermeable status and allows molecules of microorganisms, toxins, lipopolysaccharides, antigens, and other small molecules to pass through it into the tissue of intestinal wall and then into the blood.[1259] When protection from these toxins and irritants is lost, a number of conditions may result including food allergies, infections, IBS, celiac disease, metabolic syndrome, and diabetes.[1260] Leaky gut syndrome is now of interest to investigators because some of the side effects, chronic inflammation, gastrointestinal, and blood-brain barrier integrity,[1261] are also risk factors for a number of psychological (e.g. depression) and neurodegenerative conditions.

The Gastrointestinal Tract

The gastrointestinal tract is a long tube of muscle, nerves, and intestinal digestive bacteria, with both immune system and digestive function. It receives food, extracts nutrients and energy and expels waste.[1262]

The healthy gut contains a large population of microbiota composed of ninety-nine percent anaerobic bacteria (they live without oxygen), as well as archaebacteria, protozoa, fungi, and other microorganisms.[1263] This microbiome is intimately connected to the rest of the body, and to the other microbiome constituting the microorganisms of the immune, respiratory, circulatory, endocrine, and the nervous systems. It plays a role in our health, both mental and physical.[1264] [1265] [1266] For example, over seventy percent of the immune system function lives in the gut.

Approximately sixty percent of the gut bacteria belong to the Bacteroidetes and Firmicutes phyla, and, among them, bifidobacterium, lactobacillus, bacteroides, clostridium, escherichia, streptococcus, and ruminococcus are the most commonly found in adults.[1267] Furthermore, the gut microbiota is estimated to contain 150 times more genes than the human genome. These genes have been estimated to belong to approximately 10^{13}–10^{14} microbes, with a species diversity of up to several hundred per individual.[1268]

The Gut-Brain Axis

Through two-way communication with the brain via the nervous system, endocrine system, and immune system, the gut and central nervous system form a gut-brain axis. They communicate with each other constantly, in both sickness and health.[1269] The gastrointestinal tract has a its own nervous system that includes neurotransmitters, neurons, and electrical signals. Called the enteric nervous system, it is often referred to the as the second brain. Researchers have concluded mechanisms that degenerate the neurons in the brain also degenerate neurons in the enteric nervous system.[1270] For example, exercise stimulates gut motility. If the vagus nerve is impaired, as in animal models, the gut has limited motility, and nutrient absorption is hindered.[1271]

Healthy brain function. Ninety percent of your brain's output has to do with non-voluntary functions including the digestive and elimination system, so an impaired brain often results in a compromised digestion process.

Healthy gut function is linked to healthy central nervous system. Changes in gut microbiota affect the nervous system, and dysfunction of the delicate interconnections between the two are closely associated with neurodegenerative conditions such as Parkinson's and Alzheimer's diseases.[1272] In this way intestinal microbiota are directly linked to various forms of dementia because of the action of metabolic disease and chronic low-grade inflammation.[1273]

The gut microbiota assists a number of everyday functions in the brain, including the regulation of the hypothalamic-pituitary-adrenal (HPA) axis activation state. The release of cortisol governs the activation state of brain microglia, and effects cytokine release as well as attracting monocytes from the periphery to the brain. They also can rule actions in the periphery and central nervous system by various means of communication including vagal nerve and adrenergic nerve activation as well as effecting neurotransmitters, neuropeptides, endocrine hormones and immunomodulators.

Breakdown of the Mucosal Barrier

However, the gut also contains pathogens in the form of toxins from pathogens formed as a result of candida, infection,[1274] immunosuppression,[1275] starvation,[1276] trauma,[1277] chemotherapy,[1278] intravenous feeding,[1279] radiation exposure,[1280] and emotional stress,[1281] exposure to excitotoxins such as aspartame and MSG, and exposure to pesticide chemicals such as Roundup® used pervasively in farming and home lawn management.

The mucosal lining of the intestines provides an essential barrier to preventing these pathogens and toxins from escaping through the intestines to the rest of the body. The pathogens that pass into the bloodstream due to leaky gut, activate a powerful signaling molecule called zonulin. This causes a breakdown of the close connections of cells in the gut which render the wall permeable.[1282]

Causes of Leaky Gut

Environmental pesticides. In a recent study, scientists found that the inert ingredients in Roundup® amplified the toxic effect on human cells, even at concentrations much more diluted than those used on farms and lawns.[1283] In this study, it was postulated that glyphosate, the active ingredient in the herbicide, Roundup®, is the most important causal factor in the growing epidemic of celiac disease. A 2013 paper argued that glyphosate may be a key contributor to the obesity epidemic and the autism epidemic in the United States, as well as to several other diseases and conditions, such as Alzheimer's disease, Parkinson's disease, infertility, depression, and also cancer.[1284]

Diet. A poor diet (as in excess sugar and refined carbohydrates), lack of fresh fruits and vegetables, overeating of processed and fast foods, excess intake of alcohol, exposure to environmental toxins, autoimmune disorders and certain medications can be contributing or causative factors. Diet effects the composition of the gut microbiome because it provides nutrients to microbiota as well as the individual. Long-term dietary habits form the constituents of microbiota composition.[1285]

Healthy bacteria such as *Lactobacillus* and *Bifidobacterium* species can produce short-chain fatty acids; *Escherichia*, *Bacillus* and *Saccharomyces* species can synthesize and release many neurotransmitters and neuromodulators themselves or trigger the synthesis and release of neuropeptides from enteroendocrine cells.

Vagus nerve inhibition. When poor brain health affects communication to the vagus nerve, blood flow to the intestines is inhibited, in turn compromising effective functioning of the intestinal wall and normal cell regeneration. The effects can result in low hydrochloric acid production, poor enzyme release, poor gut stretching and contraction ability, and yeast and bacteria overgrowth.[1286][1287]

Candidiasis. Normally candida exists in healthy levels along with other bacteria in the intestinal tract. However, an overgrowth can develop as the result a diet high in sugar and refined carbohydrates, high alcohol intake, weak immune system, oral contraceptives, and diabetes. People who have been on long-term antibiotics have reduced absorption as good bacteria in the gut needed to help breakdown food is killed and this can set the stage for candida overgrowth. Candida albicans overgrowth (Candidiasis) causes the intestinal wall to become permeable and allows partially digested proteins and other toxins to be released into the body.[1288]

Scientists have known for a long time that yeast overgrowth can cause a host of problems.[1289] The range of consequences is wide, including arthritis,[1290] fatigue, inflammation, auto-immune difficulties, and nutrient deficiencies (such as vitamin B6, essential fatty acids and magnesium), thrush (candidiasis that occurs in the mouth), recurring UTI, digestive issues, chronic sinus infections, skin, and nail fungal infections.[1291]

Doctors describe invasive candidiasis as an infection which has invaded other parts of the body than the genital region or mouth. Candidemia is a common infection found in patients who are hospitalized. Resulting symptoms can masquerade as other health conditions such as chronic inflammation, impaired memory, brain fog and mental illness. It can affect all parts of the body including blood, heart, brain, eyes, bones, digestive system, and immune system.[1292]

The consequences of untreated infection can be severe, even life-threatening including outcomes such as meningitis if candida invades the central nervous system.[1293] Candidemia and invasive candidiasis are major causes of mortality.[1294] Of a sample of over 300 patients with candida, sixty-two percent were elderly, and those elderly patients experienced a higher mortality rate than younger patients, particularly those who had not received any antifungal therapy.[1295]

Brain infection was found in half of patients with systemic candidiasis.[1296] In a mouse model of low-grade candidemia, cerebrum inflammation (cerebritis), was found in an area of the brain that affects functions like memory and speech. In the mouse model the cerebritis was accompanied by accumulation of activated microglial and astroglial cells around the yeast forming granulomas of white blood cells attempting to wall off the yeast. Amyloid precursor protein accumulates around the edge of these granulomas, and the mice developed mild memory impairment (which resolves when the fungus is gone).[1297] Doctors have observed a shift from C. albicans to non-albicans Candida species such as multidrug-resistant C. auris[1298] heralding a global crisis.

Consequences of Leaky Gut

Imbalanced gut flora and bacterial infections are typically a problem with leaky gut.[1299] [1300] Mucosal barrier dysfunction resulting from imbalances in the brain–gut-microbiota axis promote invasion of a variety of abnormal molecules substances, including neurotropic viruses, unconventional pathogens, or slow-acting neurotoxins.[1301]

Amyloid production. Human microorganisms can produce amyloids such as CsgA, Aβ42, and other peptides that accrue in AD brains.[1302] For example, amyloids related to fungal surface-structures and the new statement of amyloidogenic fungal proteins and diffuse mycoses in the blood of AD patients suggest that chronic fungal infection associates with high risk of AD. [1303] "Virtually every type of microbe known has been implicated in contributing to the susceptibility and pathogenesis of the AD process."[1304]

Irritable bowel syndrome may be due to a disturbed neural function along the gut-brain axis.

Increased permeability to allergens, toxins, and pathogens, leading to immunological stress response and inflammation.[1305] [1306]

GI system inflammation causes rashes, pain, food sensitivities, brain health issues and other imbalances. When the brain is affected, this can compromise the GI system, which can then cause more inflammation, creating a viscous cycle.[1307] Irritable bowel syndrome and inflammatory bowel disease are linked to gut-brain axis dysfunction.[1308]

Chronic inflammation. Many studies have shown a connection between inflammation and Alzheimer's, dementia, and cognitive decline, including circulating inflammatory markers.[1309] [1310][1311][1312] Inflammation in AD pathology is linked to activated inflammatory cells (microglia and astrocytes) and inflammatory proteins (e.g. cytokines), which surround amyloid plaque and neurofibrillary tangles.[1313]

Association with Alzheimer's. Some unique microbial patterns are seen in patients with mild cognitive impairment. One participant of the gut microbiome family, proteobacteria, positively correlated in patients with AB-42. Patients with AB-40 have a negative correlation with fecal propionate and butyrate. Several bacteria are affected in different ways in normal or impaired patients depending on their diet.[1314]

Depression and Anxiety. Microbiota dysfunction is linked to depression and anxiety.[1315]

Neurodegenerative and neurodevelopmental disorders such as autism, Parkinson's and Alzheimer's are linked to gut-brain microbiota dysfunction.[1316] [1317]

Cardiovascular disease. There is an increasing amount of proof suggesting that gut microbiota, through a variety of processes, can influence physiological processes important for the development of cardiovascular disease.[1318] The resulting restrictions in the circulatory system contribute to neurodegenerative conditions.

Blood-brain barrier. The blood-brain barrier (BBB) consists of several parallel barriers, the most studied being the vascular barrier and the choroid plexus.[1319] It is a thin lining that prevents pathogens and other unwanted particle from reaching the brain. Because leaky gut releases such pathogens across the mucosal barrier, they have a chance of also reaching the brain. Such release includes cytokines and neurotransmitters arising from inflammation in the gut.[1320][1321]

The inflammation factor is important because researchers are looking at a molecule called microRNA-155, which is elevated with inflammation. This molecule can create microscopic gaps in the blood-brain barrier that let material through, overstimulating the brains inflammatory response and triggering brain inflammation.[1322][1323]

Other conditions. Other research has identified microbiome variations which, combined with leaky gut, have an effect on a number of CNS disorders, including anxiety, depression, schizophrenia, and autism.[1324][1325][1326]

Treatment Strategies

Diet

Mediterranean/Keto diet better than heart-healthy diet. Researchers compared the Mediterranean/Keto diet (MMKD) with that American Heart Association Diet (AHAD), which indicates the MMKD diet more beneficial in supporting healthy microbial patterns. With the MMKD levels of some bacteria (Enterobacteriaceae, Akkermansia, Slackia, Christensenellaceae, and Erysipelotriaceae) increases, while other anaerobic bacteria (Bifidobacterium and Lachnobacterium) decrease. MMKD slightly reduces fecal lactate and acetate and increases propionate and butyrate. AHAD, on the other hand, increases Mullicutes (class of bacteria distinguished by the absence of a cell wall), acetate and propionate, and reduces butyrate. These AHAD microbial patterns may be typical of mild cognitive impairment. The MMKD is able to modulate gut microbiota and metabolites along with better AD biomarkers in the central nervous system.[1327]

Autoimmune Paleo Protocol (AIP) can be helpful to try for four to six weeks to start. This is a stricter version of the Paleo diet, which eliminates foods that may cause inflammation and adds nutrient rich foods.

Other diets you can investigate include:

- Autoimmune Paleo Candida Diet
- Gut and Psychology Syndrome Low Inflammatory Diet
- Low-Carbohydrate Diet Specific Carbohydrate Diet

Dietary fiber promotes the growth of beneficial Bifidobacteria which help to sustain a healthy mucus layer in the colon, and colonic barrier function, inhibiting inflammation, decreasing oxidative stress, and protecting against colon cancer.[1328]

Avoid foods that contain common allergens.

Avoid toxic foods such as sugary foods and refined carbohydrates, minimize grains which have been shown to be pro-inflammatory, and avoid artificial sweeteners, MSG, fried food, and other unhealthy oils. Remove all dietary contributing factors including sugar, refined carbohydrates and have limited complex carbohydrate foods such as grains and bread. Avoid hydrogenated oils (trans-fatty acids), preservatives, artificial colors, and flavors. Other foods that can contribute to leaky gut syndrome are: peanuts, corn seeds, chocolate, nightshades (potatoes, tomatoes, eggplants, peppers), chocolate, grains, eggs, dairy, legumes, and unfermented soy.

Add healing foods to your diet. If not vegetarian, add bone broth to your diet. It is abundant in fat-soluble vitamins and minerals to boost your overall immune health and digestion. Bone broth is also rich in gelatin, which can heal your gut from the inside out. Bones should be from grass-fed cattle or organic chickens. Other healing food sources are: grass-fed beef, wild-caught fish, grass-fed ghee (clarified butter), coconut oil, leafy greens, cruciferous veggies, aged foods as kimchi and sauerkraut, miso, kefir, kombucha, sweet potatoes, organic berries (blueberries, cranberries, raspberries, blackberries, and strawberries, for example).

Add digestive enzymes with HCL during meals (read label as to the best time to take each formula).

Cultured products including kefir, yogurt, Greek yogurt, and traditional buttermilk may be helpful.

Fermented foods in diets may confer gastrointestinal and cognitive benefits.[1329] These include kimchi, sauerkraut, kefir, fermented soy, miso and kombucha (be careful because of the alcohol-not good for everyone, especially people with eye disease) provide your gut with trillions of beneficial bacteria.

Intermittent fasting is not a full fast, but limiting your daily caloric intake to 500 or 600 a day. This restriction for a few days will allow your body to repair the gut's lining. The healing foods listed above are perfect choices to eat during intermittent fasting. Intermittent fasting works best when it is synchronized with the earth's natural circadian rhythm. Therefore, fast in the evening, after sunset.

Probiotics have been shown to have positive effects for the GI system and reducing leaky gut. They can be used to reduce intestinal permeability[1330] by strengthening the epithelial tight junctions and preserving mucosal barrier function (especially L. plantarum[1331]).

The intestinal microbiome plays an important role in normal gut function. Probiotics are the beneficial microorganisms that inhabit the gastrointestinal tract. Probiotics not only help maintain normal function of the gut mucosa, but also may protect mucosa from injurious factors such as toxins, allergens, and pathogens, and support a healthy immune system.[1332] They accomplish this by releasing bioactive factors that trigger activation of signaling pathways that in turn support strengthening of the tight junctions in the mucosal barrier.[1333]

In one animal study, mice were treated with probiotics containing Lactobacillus species and demonstrated reduced gut permeability and restored microbiome and hypothalamus-pituitary-adrenal axis functionality.[1334] This gives them the potential to diminish body's response to chronic stressors, and prevent or reverse physiologic damage[1335] with improvement in mood, anxiety, clear-mindedness and energy.[1336]

Patients given probiotics showed reduced cortisol levels and improved self-reported psychological effects to a similar degree as participants administered Diazepam, a commonly used anti-anxiety medication.[1337] Analogous studies found that probiotic therapy reduced depressive symptoms and improved HPA-axis functionality as well as Citalopram and Diazepam.[1338] [1339]

In the long run, boosting healthy bacteria is best done with ferments, as even the best supplements may contain only up to ten strains of bacteria and taking them for a long period of time can cause "monoculturing" of a few strains. This will end up with an unbalanced ecosystem. Common organisms used in the probiotic preparations include Lactobacillus, Saccharomyces, and Bifidobacterium species. Lactococcus lactis and Enterococcus species have also been used as probiotics in the treatment of different diseases.[1340] [1341] The types of probiotics used in formulas are important as they need to be able to colonize in the intestine, survival in extreme pH of gut luminal contents, ability to adhere to the intestinal epithelium.

Foods high in probiotics: fermented dairy such as yogurt, kefir, cottage cheese and probiotic cheddar cheese, sauerkraut, kimchi, miso, kombucha and Kvass tea, picked cucumber, Natto, dark chocolate, microalgae, and apple cider vinegar.

Take targeted supplements (discussed and ranked below) to help repair the GI tract including: l-glutamine, glycine, colostrum, marshmallow root, licorice, and Chinese herbs (based on the recommendation of the Chinese medical practitioner).

Check for parasite infections such as tapeworm and roundworm. Foods to help with parasites include: raw garlic, caprylic acid, wormwood extract, berberine, grapefruit seed extract, black walnut, and Chinese herbs.

Daily Life

Stress. Studies show that major effects of stress on the gut include an increase in intestinal permeability, negative effects on regeneration of gastrointestinal mucosa and negative effects on intestinal microbiota.[1342] [1343] Depression and anxiety are also linked to inflammatory responses that contribute to intestinal permeability.[1344]

Exercise. High intensity exercise, such as practiced by professional athletes, is linked to a host of gastrointestinal conditions, including leaky gut.[1345] However, moderate exercise, such as walking, hiking, dancing, or bicycling can produce a beneficial anti-inflammatory effect.[1346]

Nutrients for GI repair and Leaky Gut

Essential

DGL (deglycyrrhizinated licorice) (300mg-500mg per day) contains flavonoids that help repair and regenerate the gastric and intestinal lining, increases intestinal blood flow,[1347][1348][1349] helps secrete mucosa on the intestinal walls,[1350] and has anti-ulcer and anti-inflammatory compounds.[1351]

Note: Licorice can elevate blood pressure; removal of glycyrrhizin reduces that risk. Consult your doctor first before taking if you have any issue with high blood pressure.

Glutathione. Low glutathione levels increase the risk of leaky gut.[1352] The sublingual form is the best way to take glutathione as it is not well absorbed through the digestive system.

L-glutamine (1000mg – 1,500mg per day) is an abundant amino acid that been shown to help heal damaged gut lining[1353] closing up the tight junctions and soothing inflammation.[1354][1355][1356]

Note: Excess glutamine in the can be toxic to brain cells, so glutamine source is best recommended through food rather than supplementation.

Food sources high in L-glutamine: seafood, meat such as chicken, lamb, and beef, organ meats, bone broth, milk, yogurt, ricotta, cheese, eggs, red cabbage, nuts (such as almonds, hazelnuts, pistachios, peanuts, and walnuts (without toasting), legumes, dark, leafy greens, parsley, and asparagus.

Marshmallow extract (100mg per day) obtained from the roots and flowers of marshmallow have antibacterial, antifungal, anti-inflammatory, anti-mycobacterial and anti-cough properties,[1357] as well as antiviral, anti-yeast, anti-complement,[1358] and free radical scavenging activities. It can help heal a compromised intestinal barrier and has an enzyme that can break down hyaluronic acid in the GI tract that promotes intestinal tissue damage.[1359][1360] It helps restore integrity of the gut lining by forming a protective layer around small junctions.[1361]

MSM (methylsulfonylmethane) (2,000mg per day) reduces leaky gut by reducing inflammation,[1362][1363][1364][1365] reducing fungal[1366] and yeast growths, reducing mucosal wall gaps, and promotes detoxification and cell health.[1367]

Food sources of MSM: fruit, vegetables, grains, beer, port wine, coffee, tea, and cow's milk.

N-acetyl glucosamine (1000mg-1500mg per day) is often used to reduce joint inflammation, but also has been shown to protect your stomach and gut lining, and studies show it reduces inflammation caused by ulcerative colitis and Crohn's disease.[1368]

Food sources: shellfish and offal (meat parts high in cartilage).

Omega-3 fatty acids (2,000IU-3,000IU per day) have strong anti-inflammatory properties, and can help reduce overall inflammation regarding a number of health conditions. They influence the inflammatory status of the gut by serving as precursors to anti-inflammatory eicosanoid synthesis or enhance intestinal integrity by regulating the tight junction functions.[1369] [1370] There is emerging research that links intake of omega-3s and healthy gut microbiota.[1371]

Food sources: Overall, fatty fish is the best source of omega-3 fatty acids.

Quercetin (333mg/day) with **bromelain** (240 mcu/day) can help with leaky gut symptoms by sealing the tight junctions,[1372] enhancing barrier function[1373] and stabilizing the histamine response which can aggravate a leaky gut.[1374] It may prevent that gut-damaging histamine reaction by stabilizing the mast cells.[1375]

Food sources high in quercetin: broccoli, capers, kale, raw asparagus, raw red onion, tomatoes.

Slippery elm (100mg-200mg per day) helps coat the stomach creating a soothing barrier[1376] and has been used for centuries to treat a multitude of digestive issues, including gut inflammation, stomach ulcers, diverticulitis, colitis, and an overabundance of stomach acid.[1377] Its antioxidant effects can also be very effective for treating irritable bowel disease.[1378]

Vitamin A (5,000 IU per day or as directed by your doctor) with **zinc** (50mg per day). One study showed that supplementation with vitamin A and zinc would improve intestinal function for those deficient in these nutrients.[1379]

Zinc (30mg – 40mg per day) is important for maintaining the integrity of the intestinal lining. A small study on twelve patients with Crohn's disease in remission found that eight weeks of zinc supplementation restored normal intestinal permeability.[1380]

Note: When supplementing with zinc, there should be approximate 15:1 ratio of zinc to copper in any formula.

Food sources high in zinc: dairy, dark chocolate, eggs, legumes, meat, nuts, seeds (especially pumpkin seeds), shellfish, whole grains.

Very Important

Aloe leaf extract (300mg per day) has gastroprotective properties. The extract also possesses anti-inflammatory and anti-diabetes properties, cellular protection, restoration, and mucus-stimulating activities. It supports cholinergic intestinal motility, reduces intestinal pain, discomfort and has anti-fungal properties.[1381] [1382] [1383] [1384]

Caution: When using aloe vera long-term use is not advised as it may lower potassium levels and interferes with the liver's detoxification.

Cat's claw (500mg per day) contains nutrients and antioxidants that can enhance the immune system.[1385] It helps with leaky gut syndrome, reduce inflammation of the digestive tract (including colitis and diverticulitis). It is effective against stomach or intestinal ulcers, reducing pain associated with arthritis, fights against parasites and reduces fatigue related to chronic fatigue syndrome (as well as other benefits).[1386]

Olive leaf extract consists of olive-derived polyphenols, including oleuropein, which promotes generation of NO (nitric oxide) from nitrite in the stomach. It induces smooth muscle relaxation.[1387]

Nutrients for Candida

Essential

Aloe leaf extract. (300mg per day). Research shows that aloe vera can inhibit the growth of candida and stop the germ tubes of the yeast from forming.[1388] Additionally, aloe vera shows anti-biofilm action, destroying the protective layer around candida.[1389]

Caution: When using aloe vera long-term use is not advised as it may lower potassium levels and interferes with the liver's detoxification.

Anise seed. (330mg 4 times a day) Anise seed is known to be anti-fungal, has strong anti-candida properties,[1390] and broad anti-pathogen effects,[1391] effectively combatting harmful bacteria, viruses, and other pathogens that harm your body.

Black walnut extract (Juglans nigra) (200mg) contains a variety of phenolic compounds that exhibit antioxidant and antimicrobial properties.[1392][1393] Walnut husk extracts have demonstrated antimicrobial effects against gram-positive bacteria[1394][1395] and xanthine oxidase, an enzyme contributing to hyperuricemia, (which causes inflammation and gout).[1396] It exhibits antifungal activity against all forms of candida,[1397] and is commonly part of an anti-candida diet for intestinal yeast overgrowth management.[1398]

Coconut oil (1 tablespoon per day) Lauric, capric, and caprylic acids in coconut oil have anti-microbial, anti-fungal and antiviral properties. This is a real food medicine way to gently clean your GI system. Coconut oil should be organic, extra virgin and cold pressed. It is recommended in the treatment of Candida infections and antibiotic-resistant Candida.[1399]

Caprylic acid (400mg-800mg per day), naturally occurring in coconut oil is available as a supplement. Researchers found caprylic acid to be effective at killing candida, being superior and less expensive than the antifungal drug Diflucan.[1400] It is a medium chain fatty acid that has been used as a natural antifungal and anti-yeast product for almost fifty years. Studies indicate that caprylic acid can penetrate and dissolve yeast in the GI tract that can cause a disruption in the intestinal membrane leading to leaky gut syndrome.

Cumin. (500mg-1000mg per day). Black cumin oil attacks the membranes of candida cells, resulting in irreversible damage[1401] so that it is considered a natural inhibitor of Candida[1402] and other yeast growths.[1403]

Garlic extract (1200mg-4800mg per day) has a wealth of scientific literature that supports the proposal that garlic consumption have significant effects on lowering blood pressure, prevention of atherosclerosis, reduction of serum cholesterol and triglyceride, inhibition of platelet aggregation, and increasing fibrinolytic activity.[1404] Several studies have shown that the extract was effective against a host of protozoa including Candida albicans[1405] and other yeasts and fungi.[1406] [1407]

Marigold flower extract (calendula) is utilized for its many anti-inflammatory, antispasmodic and antifungal compounds.[1408] Among its other benefits, calendula supports digestive enzyme production, reducing inflammation and providing antibacterial activity.[1409] [1410] [1411]

Oregano oil (180mg – 360mg per day) is one of the most popular anti-candida remedies. In one study conducted carvacrol was as effective as nystatin for Candida treatment because the carvacrol (found in many plants such as wild bergamot, thyme, and pepperwort, but it is most abundant in oregano) damages the cellular envelope that surrounds the Candida yeast (once the envelope is damaged, Candida is left to die).[1412] One study found that oregano oil actually killed candida more effectively than a pharmaceutical antifungal drug, clotrimazole.[1413]

Proteases are enzymes that break down protein debris in the body, and have been proven to break down biofilms in tests. Researchers have shown that protease eats away at the sugars and proteins in biofilms, resulting in "significant eradication" of biofilms.[1414] [1415] Examples of proteases include fungal protease, pepsin, trypsin, chymotrypsin, papain, bromelain, and subtilisin.

Reishi mushroom (980mg per day) is an adaptogen that can help to positively influence your immune system, most of which is located in your gut. They help to kill dangerous cells that cause diseases (such as cancer), and can also protect healthy genes from becoming mutated.[1416] They help reduce gut inflammation,[1417] and stimulate the number and activity of a variety of immune cells and antimicrobial biochemicals,[1418] most notably, against Candida[1419]

Important

Pau d'arco tea (500mg-1,000mg per day) contains several compounds, including quinoids, benzenoids and flavonoids. This herb helps fight against infections with yeast, bacteria, viruses, or parasites, intestinal worms, stomach problems, and reduces pain related to arthritis and other health issues.[1420]

Turmeric (curcumin) (500mg -1500mg per day) used worldwide, has many health benefits including being anti-bacterial, antiviral, and strongly anti-fungal. It has been found to kill Candida albican.[1421] [1422] Best taken in a formula with Bioperine® (piper nigrum, black pepper) for improved absorption and efficacy.

Wormwood (Artemisia) has antioxidant properties, increases digestive enzymes, reduces intestinal discomfort, and is used as a treatment against parasitic worms.[1423] [1424] [1425] [1426] Wormwood has been shown to kill yeast by disrupting the function of their mitochondria,[1427] and has powerful activity against candida biofilms, the layers of slime that candida uses to protect itself.[1428]

Chinese Medical Approach

A common pattern imbalance associated with leaky gut syndrome is Spleen Qi and Yang deficiency, which means that your digestive and immune systems have become weakened. This imbalance reduces one's ability to digest and absorb nutrients and may be associated with yeast overgrowth as a result of "bad bacteria" dominating "good bacteria" in the GI tract. Related symptoms may include weight gain, muscle loss, bloating, fatigue, sinus congestion, diarrhea, and irritable bowel syndrome.

Excess use of antibiotics can be a cause of leaky gut syndrome. If this condition continues, common patterns can turn into patterns called "Spleen Insulting Liver", or "Stagnation of Liver Qi and Blood." Additional symptoms can include brain fog, anxiety, poor sleep, attention deficit, food cravings, mood swings, and hormonal dysregulation can occur.

Chapter 12. Gluten Sensitivity and Brain Function

Celiac disease (CD) is an immune-mediated affected by the intake of gluten (a protein present in wheat, rye, or barley) that occurs in about one percent of the population.[1429] [1430] It is usually characterized by gastrointestinal complaints because gluten damages the intestinal walls. More recently the understanding and knowledge of gluten sensitivity has emerged as an illness distinct from celiac disease with an estimated prevalence six times that of CD.

Also known as celiac sprue, it can manifest itself clinically at any age. At present, it is diagnosed in roughly equal measure in adults and children; it is now more commonly diagnosed in school-age children than in preschool children.

Gluten sensitivity often goes unrecognized and untreated. **Non-celiac gluten sensitivity** (NCGS) also remains undertreated and underrecognized as a contributing factor to psychiatric and neurologic manifestations. NCGS is estimated to occur six times greater in the general population than CD.[1431]

Gluten

Gluten is consumed in large quantities (10–20g per day) as part of the standard Western diet. It is a complex mixture of alcohol-soluble storage proteins found in wheat, barley, spelt, kamut, oats and rye. The main components of these proteins, called prolamins, are specific to different types of grain: wheat (gliadin), rye (secalin), and barley (hordein). They have a high proline and glutamine content which makes them water-insoluble and therefore, difficult to digest. Their partial digestion creates sequences of peptides that trigger immune responses in patients with celiac disease or who are gluten sensitive.[1432] Instead of being degraded by gastrointestinal enzymes,[1433] they pass across the epithelium of into the small-bowel mucosa.[1434]

Sources of Gluten, malt extract, dextrin, modified food starch, and clarifying

- Hidden sources of gluten include food emulsifiers, food stabilizers (agents in red wine. for example). Gluten can trigger an immune response to TG6 (transglutaminase) which is found throughout the central nervous system, leading to autoimmune destruction of brain and nervous tissue.[1435] [1436] Transglutaminase is used by the food industry to tenderize meat and hold it together. Therefore, this may be a hidden food gluten.
- Common overlooked sources of gluten are beer, soy sauce, deli meats, shampoos, imitation crab meat (often used in sushi), condiments (ketchup, mustard, and salad dressings).
- In addition, there are foods that are suspected of cross-reacting with gluten, including casein (milk protein), corn, oats, sesame, yeast, some brands of coffee.

Although going on a strict gluten diet, certain foods (as mentioned above) can continue causing similar reactions. One study showed that fifty percent of patients with gluten sensitivity had only a partial remission of symptoms when on a gluten free diet due to cross reactivity to milk.[1437]

When on a gluten free diet, many people replace the grains that contain gluten with "safe" grains such as corn, rice, or quinoa. Overtime, some people may develop a sensitivity to these grains.

Note: Most corn used in food not grown organically so is rarely GMO free. This may contribute to sensitivities from the pesticides.

Effect on the Brain

Data suggests that up to twenty-two percent of patients with CD develop neurologic or psychiatric dysfunction,[1438] and as many as fifty-seven percent of people with neurological dysfunction of unknown origin test positive for anti-gliadin antibodies.[1439] A 2006 study identified a number of patients who had cognitive impairment due to CD[1440][1441] or dementia.[1442]

Synapsins are a family of three neuron-specific genes – designated synapsins I, II and III – which encode phosphoproteins that play crucial roles in the regulation of neurotransmission and neuro-development.[1443][1444]

Researchers have learned that gliadin, the prolamin found in wheat proteins, binds with synapsin-I rendering it immunoreactive.[1445] The result is dysfunctional regulation of neurotransmitter release at synapses. Problematic synapse release affects the health of the cerebellum, which may result in balance issues, vertigo, and motor control. It may also result in anxiety as it affects an enzyme called glutamic acid decarboxylase found in the brain.[1446][1447]

Immune reactions to gluten can break down the blood-brain barrier which protects the brain by preventing unwanted particles/molecules and pathogens from reaching the brain as well as allowing essential nutrients to reach and nourish the brain. "Leaky brain" can result from this reaction to gluten by allowing pathogens and other damaging molecules to reach the brain increasing autoimmune reaction risk in the brain and nervous system.[1448][1449]

Gluten ataxia. Ataxia is a degenerative disease of the nervous system. Symptoms can include: walking balance, limb coordination, eye movements and speech.

Gluten ataxia, brought about by CD or NCGS, is characterized by changes in the cerebellum, increases in positive anti-gliadin antibodies, and lack of voluntary coordination in the limbs, gait (for example, the Parkinsonian shuffle), or slurred or slowed speech.[1450] These patients have bands of immunoglobulins (oligoclonal bands) in their cerebrospinal fluid, inflammation at the cerebellum, and anti-Purkinje cell (a type of neuron in the cerebellum) antibodies.

Other neurological manifestations. White matter lesions have also been reported, manifesting in seizures, ataxia, and loss of muscle tone (hypotonia).[1451] Peripheral neuropathy (loss of messaging between the brain and spinal cord and the rest of the body),[1452] inflammatory myopathies (muscle inflammation diseases) have been reported.[1453] With spinal cord degenerations (myelopathies) symptoms can include symmetric proximal muscle weakness, malaise, fatigue (worsening weakness as the day goes on or progressive weakness with exertion), dark-colored urine (suggests myoglobinuria) and/or fever,[1454] and possibly headaches.[1455] Symptoms can also include gluten encephalopathy (severe headaches, brain fog, slow thinking and cognitive difficulties such as memory loss). The damage to the brain can sometimes be seen in images generated by an MRI scanner).[1456]

This problem can affect bidirectional in the gut-brain axis pathway, in turn contributing to neuro-inflammation and cognitive dysfunction, making a person more vulnerable to dementia and Alzheimer's disease. Other neurological conditions include leg syndrome disorder, visceral hypersensitivity, hearing loss, and a variety of psychological disorders such as depression, anxiety, ADHD, autism, and schizophrenia.[1457]

Effect on General Health

A number of other health issues can arise due to gluten intolerance or sensitivity including inflammation, diarrhea, constipation, abdominal pain, bloating, weight loss, dysfunctional metabolic state, multiple-systems atrophy, migraine headaches, and joint pain.

Leaky Gut and Celiac Disease

Non-celiac gluten sensitivity can trigger neuroinflammation, gut-brain axis dysfunction, leaky gut, and vulnerability for dementia.[1458] Both CD and NCGS can cause leaky gut which allows pathogenic molecules to leave the intestinal system and pass through the defective mucosal gap into the blood stream.

These pathogens include overgrowths of intestinal bacteria or fungus (gut dysbiosis), such as the pathogenic gram-negative bacteria such as Bacteroides, Staphylococcus, Salmonella, Shigella [1459] and sulfate-reducing bacteria such as Desulfovibrio.[1460] [1461] In addition, reduced levels of friendly species such as Enterococcus, Bifidobacteria, and Lactobacillus are seen.[1462] [1463] [1464] [1465]

Nutritional deficiencies. The damaged villi associated with celiac disease are impaired in their ability to absorb a number of important nutrients, including vitamins B6, B12 (cobalamin) and folate, as well as iron, calcium and vitamins D and K.[1466]

Folate and/or cobalamin deficiency. Untreated celiac disease patients often have elevated levels of homocysteine, associated with folate (B9) and/or cobalamin deficiency (B12).[1467] [1468] In one study 41 percent of the patients studied were found to be deficient in B12, and 31 percent of these B12-deficient patients also had folate deficiency.[1469] Either B12 or folate deficiency leads directly to impaired methionine synthesis from homocysteine, because these two vitamins are both required for the reaction to take place. This induces abnormally high homocysteine (hyper-homocysteinemia).[1470] Supplementation with B9 caused homocysteine levels in CD patients to drop, but not supplementing with B12.[1471]

Anemia. Anemia is one of the most common manifestations of celiac disease outside of the intestinal malabsorption issues.[1472] [1473] Although both B9 and B12 can cause anemia, **iron deficiency** which does not response to iron therapy, appears to be the most important factors.[1474]

Molybdenum deficiency is rarely considered in diagnoses, as it is only needed in trace amounts. However, molybdenum is essential for at least two very important enzymes – sulfite oxidase and xanthine oxidase. Sulfite oxidase converts sulfite to the more stable sulfate. Sulfite is often present in foods such as wine and dried fruits as a preservative. Sulfate plays an essential role in the sulfated proteoglycans that populate the extracellular matrices of nearly all cell types.[1475][1476][1477]

Impaired sulfite oxidase activity leads to both oxidative damage and impaired sulfate supplies to the tissues, such as the enterocytes in the small intestine. The excess presence of sulfur-reducing bacteria such as Desulfovibrio in the gut is associated with celiac disease.[1478][1479]

Selenium deficiency is associated with celiac disease,[1480] and plays a significant role in thyroid hormone synthesis, secretion, and metabolism. Selenium deficiency is therefore a significant factor in thyroid diseases.[1481][1482]

Causes of Celiac Disease

Genetic. From a genetic perspective, only persons with the genotype HLA-DQ2 or HLA-DQ8 can develop celiac disease.[1483] Overall thirty to forty percent of the population carries either HLA-DQ2 or -DQ8. Many other genetic predispositions have been identified in recent years that play a smaller role (about three to four percent overall, versus about fifty percent for HLA-DQ2/8), other influences are now thought to be potential precipitating factors for celiac disease, including early and massive gluten exposure, bowel infections, and drugs.[1484]

Related Conditions

Other conditions are often found along with celiac disease. Some are potential markers for CD (e.g. Hashimoto's thyroiditis), others may be either a cause or a result of CD.

Autoimmune thyroid disease is associated with celiac disease.[1485][1486] Up to 43 percent of Hashimoto's thyroiditis patients showed signs of mucosal T-cell activation, typical of celiac disease.[1487]

Indole and kidney disease. Kidney disease is often associated with increased levels of celiac disease autoantibodies.[1488]

Dermatitis herpetiformis is a chronic itchy, blistering skin condition that affects about ten percent [1489] to seventeen percent [1490] of people with celiac disease.

Refractory celiac disease is diagnosed when symptoms and deterioration of intestinal villi persist despite treatment and a gluten-free diet.[1491] However, most cases of apparent celiac disease are due to consumption of hidden gluten in various processed foods.[1492] Psychological diseases have been linked to gluten intolerance. For example, some people with schizophrenia have been found to be gluten intolerant and improved on a gluten-free diet.[1493]

Symptoms

More than half of all diagnosed cases have no or few typical symptoms. Instead, the patient may suffer from conditions such as iron anemia, osteoporosis, osteomalacia (bone softening), dermatitis herpetiformis, mouth ulcers, headaches, joint pain, dysfunction spleen, musculoskeletal and neurological disorders, endocrinopathies, or skin diseases.[1494] [1495] [1496] and must be detected through screening tests.[1497]

Other atypical symptoms may include anorexia, delayed puberty (amenorrhea), difficulty concentrating, tooth-enamel defects, or short stature / growth retardation.[1498]

The most common symptoms of CD are:

- Diarrhea (experienced by about 79 percent of patients)[1499]
- Bloating (73 percent of patients)[1500] and gas, one of the most common symptoms
- Fatigue
- Weight loss, a sharp drop in weight, affecting 23 percent of patients[1501]
- Nausea and vomiting
- Constipation
- Depression, self-reported by 39 percent of patients[1502]

Diagnosis

Celiac Disease Diagnosis

Celiac disease is one of the better characterized diseases of the immune system. The affected patients all have the following:[1503]

- a genetic predisposition (either HLA-DQ2 or HLA-DQ8);
- a well-defined precipitating factor (gluten); and
- elevated levels of specific antibody proteins against tissue transglutaminase, which is a human enzyme.

Initially, diagnosis tries to determine whether symptoms could be due to another cause such as food intolerances, intestinal infections, or irritable bowel syndrome.

- **Serology blood test** looks for specific antibodies which exist as a result of an immune reaction to gluten.[1504]
- **Genetic blood test** to see if white blood cell antigens HLA-DQ2 or HLA-DQ8 are present.[1505] Genetic testing is the only test that is accurate if the patient has been avoiding gluten. The most sensitive and most accurate test is the IgA-tTG test (transglutaminase immunoglobulin A). Other recommended tests included total IgA and IgA-EMA. If IgA is deficient, then IgC/IgA-DGP is often added.

- Confirming the diagnosis once took years. Now the technology exists for doctors to look at the inside of the small intestine to confirm whether there is damage to the villi lining the intestine. **Endoscopy.** Via a long tube with a tiny camera an upper gastrointestinal endoscopy permits seeing the inside of the small intestine and take a tiny biopsy for analysis for damage to the villi.[1506] A **capsule endoscopy** uses a tiny wireless camera inside a small capsule that you swallow to take pictures of your entire small intestine. The camera takes thousands of pictures transmitted to a recorder.[1507]

Gluten Opioids

Gluten also contains some morphine-like compounds called gluten exorphins which can mask the effects of gluten on the intestinal wall.[1508] [1509] This can be tested by measuring antibodies to gluteomorphin and prodynorphin. Withdrawal is similar to opioid drugs including depression, mood swings and abnormal bowel movements.

Gluten Sensitivity

Some people may have a sensitivity rather than intolerance to gluten. They may experience many of the symptoms of celiac disease even though they do not have the genetic fingerprint.

Gluten sensitivity diagnosis

Although conventional medicine says there are no specific tests for gluten sensitivity (GS), there are some tests that can help determine GS:

- IgA anti-gliadin antibodies (these are found in about 80 percent of people with Celiac disease)
- IgG anti-gliadin antibodies
- IgA anti-endomysial antibodies
- Tissue Transglutaminase antibodies
- Total IgA antibodies

One potential problem with testing is that gluten is made up of several hundred peptides and gliadin is made up of twelve different sub-fractions. Most modern-day testing focuses on only the alpha-gliadin (one of the twelve sub-fractions) and therefore there is considerable room for error and false negative tests.

There is a laboratory (Cyrex Lab) that that is now testing for these sub-fractions and may help to minimize false negatives. Cyrex also offers array4 tests to check for gluten cross-reactivity with other grains.

Another test is ELISA, which places the blood of a person with gluten sensitivity into a dish of various neurological tissues and then inspecting the dish for an immune response. These tests though can often result in negative results, even though the person may still have a gluten sensitivity. A test should screen for an immune reaction to the alpha, omega, and gamma branches of gliadin as well as glutenin and deamidated gluten.

A more complete gluten antibody screening should include:

- Alpha gliadin
- Omega gliadin
- Gamma gliadin
- Wheat germ agglutinin (WGA)
- Gluteomorphin
- Prodynorphin
- Transglutaminase-2 (TG2)
- Transglutaminase-3 (TG3)
- Transglutaminase-6 (TG6)

Lectins

Some people may be gluten sensitive but do not react to the gluten portion of wheat, but instead react to the lectin portion. In wheat lectins are called wheat germ agglutin (WGA), which is found in whole wheat or sprouted wheat. WGA can pass through the blood-brain barrier and attach to the myelin sheath which is the protective coating of the nerves. It can also inhibit nerve growth factor which is critical for neuron growth and health.[1510]

Treatment Approach

Diet

Diet is the primary approach to bringing relief from both celiac disease and gluten sensitivity.

- **AVOID all varieties of wheat** (whole wheat, wheat berries, graham, bulgur, farro, farina, durum, kamut, bromated flour, spelt, etc.), as well as rye, barley and triticale, and all pasta except gluten-free pasta.
- **Grains free of gluten** include: amaranth, buckwheat, brown rice, millet, rice, sorghum and teff, as well as quinoa which is a seed, tapioca.
- **Gluten is hidden in some foods**. For example, tofu is gluten-free though most soy sauce is not. See the list of hidden sources of gluten toward the beginning of this chapter.

There are a number of therapeutic measures which may be helpful.

- **Probiotics**. Along with testing for the nutrients and conditions described above, probiotic treatment with Bifidobacteria has been shown to alleviate symptoms associated with celiac disease[1511] [1512] because it reduces inflammation.[1513] Live cultures of Bifidobacterium lactis may promote healing of the gut in conjunction with the gluten-free diet, or might even allow the celiac patient to consume modest amounts of gluten without damaging effects.[1514]
- **Vagus nerve** stimulation, may be available through a few non-invasive devices.[1515]
- **Alpha 7 nicotinic receptor agonists**[1516] which can ameliorate inflammation, are used to treat conditions such as Alzheimer's.[1517]

- **Corticotropin-releasing factor receptor 1** antagonist may ameliorate neuroinflammation and oxidative stress in NCGS.[1518]
- **Short chain fatty acids** may help regulatory T-cell induction as well as blood-brain barrier integrity.[1519] [1520] These include acetate, propionate, and butyrate which are found in fiber-rich foods.

- **DPP-IV** helps digest gliadin and casein and regulate the immune response for those with gluten sensitivity (does not work as well for those with celiac disease).[1521] [1522]
- **Antioxidants and flavonoids** can reduce inflammation due to gluten exposure.[1523] [1524] These include lycopene and quercetin which have been shown to prevent immune activation from gluten.[1525] Apigenin inhibits gut microflora from triggering inflammation.[1526] [1527] Luteolin inhibits LPS-induced inflammation in the gut lining.[1528] [1529] [1530]

Chapter 13. Diet and Brain Health

The typical American diet lacks enough raw or slightly steamed vegetables and fruits to supply digestive enzymes, and it is a diet without enough antioxidants to support proper digestion, enzyme production, or normal metabolic activity. As a result, we age more quickly than necessary and the risk of disease onset increases. The nutrient composition of processed foods in the Western diet can also negatively affect the brain and contribute to the development of degenerative diseases.[1531] [1532]

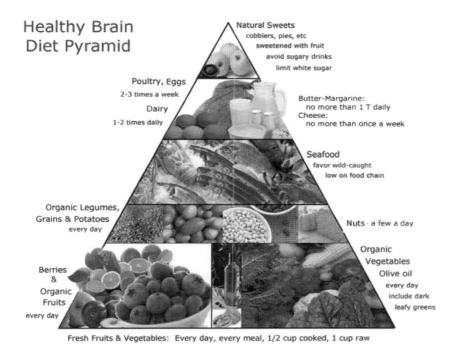

Healthy Brain Diet Pyramid

Natural Sweets
cobblers, pies, etc
sweetened with fruit
avoid sugary drinks
limit white sugar

Poultry, Eggs
2-3 times a week

Dairy
1-2 times daily

Butter-Margarine:
no more than 1 T daily
Cheese:
no more than once a week

Seafood
favor wild-caught
low on food chain

Organic Legumes,
Grains & Potatoes
every day

Nuts · a few a day

Organic
Vegetables
Olive oil
every day
include dark
leafy greens

Berries
&
Organic
Fruits
every day

Fresh Fruits & Vegetables: Every day, every meal, 1/2 cup cooked, 1 cup raw

One study that looked at 18,080 people found that a diet high in fried foods and processed meats is associated with lower scores in learning and memory.[1533] In a similar study with over five-thousand people it was found that a diet high in red meat, processed meat, baked beans and fried food was associated with inflammation and a faster decline in reasoning over ten years.[1534]

The Mediterranean style diet, that is rich in vegetables and seafood, has in studies, been shown to protect against cognitive decline. [1535] [1536]

A Plant-Based Diet

We believe a plant-based diet is a healthy diet. It consists mainly of plant-based foods, along with small portions of preferably organic, consciously produced animal products, such as free-range, grass-fed meats. Vegetarians on a strict plant-based diet need to routinely check their levels of certain nutrients that are difficult or not possible to obtain from plants and supplement where deficient. Be particularly careful of getting enough of vitamin B12, zinc, and iron.

Our recommended diet incorporates the following principles listed below. It is very similar to the MIND diet – a diet that combines the Mediterranean diet and a heart-healthy diet.

- **The Alkalizing diet** avoids the foods that cause inflammation, including high amounts of processed food, refined carbohydrates, poor-quality oils, and high levels of salt.
- **The Mediterranean diet** is alkaline in nature and avoids processed and refined foods; it is rich in vegetables and fruit.
- **Balance Essential Fatty Acids** of omega-3 and omega-6
- **Phytate reduction** to enhance better absorption of nutrients.

Note: See details of the MIND diet in the diet section of this book.

Go Organic

Evidence is increasing that the nutritional value of fruits and vegetables is closely linked to the quality of the soil they are grown in. Evidence is also increasing that non-organic foods are not the same as organically grown foods. Non-organically grown foods contain residues of herbicides and pesticides.[1537] Organic food contains significantly higher levels of polyphenols that are important for health.[1538] To quote an example. Organically grown tomatoes have seventy-nine percent more quercetin,[1539] twenty percent more lycopene, thirty percent more vitamin C, twenty-four percent more total phenolics, twenty-one percent more flavonoids, and five percent more in vitro antioxidant activity.[1540] Organic tomato juice contains much more beta-carotene, rutin, flavonoids, and quercetin compared to non-organic. The differences in nutritional constituents of tomatoes may vary according to growing season as the organic crop of a different season may have higher levels of vitamin C and quercetin.[1541]

A meta-analysis of research on organic compared to conventional dairy products found that the organic dairy products contained significantly higher amounts of protein, ALA, omega-3 and omega-6 oils, and other nutrients;[1542] there was also a higher ratio of omega-3 to omega-6.[1543] Other research suggests that organic foods may be higher in vitamin C, iron, phosphorus, and magnesium, and many organic foods may have higher levels of anthocyanins, flavonoids, and carotenoids.[1544] One more thing. Organic farming delivers greater ecosystem services and environmental benefits,[1545] making it the most sustainable farming method.[1546]

Favor These Foods

Pure Water

Drink plenty of pure water every day, preferably spring water or filtered water. As the filtering process removes many trace minerals exacerbating dehydration, it is essential that you add a supplement contain a full-spectrum of electrolyte-forming trace minerals to your water. Some nutritionists recommend half an ounce to an ounce of water per pound of body weight. But, you should drink what seems normal and natural. Water is essential for almost every cell activity. Being even slightly dehydrated reduces your metabolic efficiency. Chronic dehydration can lead to problems like kidney stones.[1547] If you often feel hungry, it might just be that you are dehydrated. As a bonus, if you are trying to lose weight, drinking a glass of water before meals will help you feel more "full". Drink 1/4 cup of water at a time (when not exercising). This is the amount of water the kidneys easily absorb and process at one time. Excess water intake will stress the kidneys.

Recommended. In general, try to keep water near you and sip it from time to time.

Caution:. Tap water may include the following toxins: arsenic, aluminum, fluoride, pesticides, over-the-counter drugs, and/or disinfectant byproducts. Recommended home filters include reverse osmosis filters, ion exchange filters, or granular carbon and carbon block filters. If you use a filter that removes all minerals, such as for distilled water and RO (reverse osmosis), you should consider adding the trace-minerals. Only a small amount is needed per glass of water.

Carotenoids from Vegetables and Fruits

The largest percentage of the diet in terms of quantity, should be vegetables and then fruits. Focus on lots of dark leafy-green vegetables, other colorful vegetables, and a few selection of fruit daily. These vegetables are rich in carotenoids, especially lutein and zeaxanthin, which are the colored pigments that your eyes need to function well. These macular carotenoids are associated with cognitive function in pre-adolescent children,[1548] young adults,[1549] and older adults.[1550] These xanthophylls (a carotenoid found in yellow fruit and vegetables and the Mediterranean diet) have the ability to limit oxidation and inflammation and therefore improve cognition and reduce the risk of dementias such as Alzheimer's.[1551] Dietary sources of xanthophylls include lutein and zeaxanthin in green leafy vegetables and corn, and β-cryptoxanthin in pumpkins, papayas, and peppers.

Carotenoids are the pigments found in plants, where they function as internal sunscreens, protecting the plants from solar radiation. Carotenoids are antioxidants that help protect the body from oxidative damage. Found throughout the body, some can cross the blood-brain barrier. Even if you don't like vegetables such as collards, kale, and spinach, you can add them to soups, puree them in green drinks, juice them with other fruits and vegetables, or add them to salads. Nightshade-family vegetables and fruit can cause inflammation for some; these include tomatoes, white potatoes, eggplant, okra, pepper, goji berries, sorrel, and tomatillos.

Recommended. Aim to eat 1/2 cup cooked or one cup uncooked vegetables at almost every meal, every day. Be sure to include dark leafy-green vegetables.

Whole Grains for Protein, Fiber, and Minerals

Whole grains supply protein, fiber, minerals, and some B vitamins (not B12). No single grain is healthier than any other. Each grain supplies a unique blend of nutrients. Therefore, enjoy a wide variety of whole grains. There is a good deal of debate as to whether organic and non-organic grains are equivalent, but there has been evidence that the quality of the soil in which grains are grown makes a difference. Whole grains are complex carbohydrates. They take a little longer to digest and help you maintain an even energy balance. They break down into glucose slowly. The slower the rate at which glucose is created, the more stable is your blood sugar. Food combining proponents recommend that grains be eaten with healthy fats and vegetables. Grains are best digested in an alkaline environment found in a diet high in such foods a green leafy and other vegetable, and very low in refined carbohydrates and sugar, meat and dairy.[1552]

Researchers report that whole grains, as opposed to processed (white or hulled) grains, are directly linked to better cognitive function[1553] and better able to ward off conditions such as accelerated cognitive decline,[1554] high blood pressure and heart disease.[1555]

Recommended. We recommend that you eat whole grains every day and vary your selection. Markets now offer a wide selection of different types of grains. Try them all.

Legumes

Legumes are a great source of protein, carbohydrates, fiber, minerals, and vitamins. They are higher in protein than other vegetables and generally low in fat. They're a good source of B-vitamins (but not B12) and contain antioxidant phytonutrients such as isoflavones and lignans. They partner well with whole grains because they are low in an essential amino acid, lysine. Cognitive performance in the elderly has been associated with a diet including legumes and other plant proteins.[1556] [1557]

Recommended. We recommend at least 1/2 cup of legumes, at least two times a week, preferably served in the same meal with whole grains, cereals and seeds. Soak them, if possible, or sprout them to reduce phytates. Phytates or Phytic acid impairs the absorption of iron, zinc and calcium and may promote mineral deficiencies.[1558]

Herbs and Spices

Use herbs and spices to completely or partially substitute for salt or sugar. They contain many phytonutrients such as carotenoids and polyphenols.

Recommended. Use herbs and spices daily for all meals. If you can, grow them fresh.

Nuts and Seeds for Healthy Fats, Protein, Vitamins, Minerals

Nuts and seeds provide healthy fats, protein, vitamins, and minerals, including vitamin E, zinc, and essential fatty acids.

- Walnuts provide high amounts of anti-inflammatory plant-based omega-3 fats, along with high amounts of copper, manganese, molybdenum, and biotin; they also contain powerful free-radical scavenging antioxidants. Walnuts appear to delay age-related cognitive impairment[1559] [1560] and protect memory[1561] as well as protect retinal health.
- Almonds contain plenty of vitamin E, magnesium, and protein, and help lower blood pressure and cholesterol levels while promoting weight loss and reducing hunger. In laboratory animal testing almonds were found to protect memory retention and increases acetylcholine levels in the brain.[1562] An interesting study looked at the "post-lunch dip" in cognition function and found that the addition of almonds reduced the "dip" in memory.[1563]

- Pecans contain more than nineteen vitamins and minerals, and research has shown they may help lower LDL cholesterol and promote healthy arteries.[1564]
- Pistachios are high in lutein, beta-carotene, and gamma-tocopherol (vitamin E) compared to other nuts (all excellent nutrients for eye health). An extract of the pistachio leaves is being explored for its ability to counteract oxidative stress diseases such as AD.[1565]
- Seeds such as sunflower seeds are rich in vitamins and minerals, including vitamin E, copper, B vitamins, manganese, selenium, phosphorus, and magnesium, which support heart health and the immune system.
- Pumpkin seeds offer a wide variety of nutrients, including zinc, magnesium, manganese, copper, and protein.

Recommended. We recommend a *few* nuts or seeds daily, especially walnuts and almonds. Vary the kind of nuts or seeds for good balance.

Other Protein

For vegetarians, good protein sources include fermented soy products such as tempeh, which per ounce provides more protein than beef. One study found that high tofu intake (but not tempeh, which is fermented) is associated with worse memory in elderly men and women in Indonesia,[1566] China,[1567] and Hawaii.[1568] The consumption of unfermented soy-based foods is negatively correlated with cognitive decline.[1569] And, soy isoflavones alone (in capsule form) do not improve cognition in the elderly with AD.[1570] For non-vegetarians, fatty fish like salmon (wild only) provide essential omega-3 fatty acids in addition to protein as well as smaller fish like herring and sardines that are lower on the food chain and tend to contain lower levels of toxic heavy metals than larger fish such as tuna.

Fats

A diet high in healthy fats includes cold pressed, extra virgin olive oil for your salads and using low heat for cooking, as well as eating wild caught salmon, sardines, mackerel for example is recommended. Avoid using vegetable oils in cooking in high heat, and using saturated fats (such as coconut oil or butter) increases neurogenesis.[1571]

Essential Fatty Acids

Omega-3s. The essential fatty acids, EPA and DHA are important for brain health as well as general well-being. DHA is critical for healthy brain function.[1572][1573][1574] Due to the easy availability of processed food in Western societies today, the consumption of saturated fatty acids and trans-fatty acids has greatly increased (as well as the significant increase in the amount of grains/carbohydrates eaten), while that of DHA has decreased.

Increasing evidences suggests that the omega-3 fatty acids are important for cognitive functioning and memory[1575] especially in those people who are deficient in omega-3s.[1576] Its benefits may arise from the fact that vasodilator function (relaxation of blood vessels) is enhanced.[1577] Studies show regular intake of EPA and DHA improves brain size compared to those with low intakes. One 2014 eight-year study of more than 1100 women showed brain size of two centimeters larger for those with large intake compared to the population with lower intake. The hippocampus, where we gain new memories, was 2.7 percent larger in women whose EPA/DHA levels were twice that of the comparative population.[1578] Another study suggested intake of omega-3 fatty acids from fish oil improves the brain's glymphatic system which is responsible for helping the brain remove waste debris, including amyloid protein that has been associated with Alzheimer's disease.[1579] [1580] [1581] Other studies conclude that essential fatty acids in the diet may have beneficial effects on learning, as demonstrated with studies of spatial recognition learning in rodent models of Alzheimer's disease.[1582] [1583] [1584]

Note. In general, it is preferable to obtain omega-3 derivatives from food sources (fish and sea-food) because of the prevalence of aldehydes in some commercially available supplements which have been shown to be mutagenic, cytotoxic, and inflammatory.[1585] In addition, commercially prepared supplements sometimes contain saturated and/or oxidized fats.[1586] If you must take omega-3 as a supplement, keep it refrigerated.

Omega-6. Although omega-6 fats are essential, the modern Western diet contains far more omega-6 fatty acids than necessary.[1587] The recommended ratio of omega-6 to omega-3 fatty acids in the diet is 4:1 or less. However, the Western diet has a ratio between 10:1 and 50:1 due primarily to the excess carbohydrates and sugars in the common diet, particularly white starches and sugars, vegetable oils and foods containing trans-fatty acids. In excess, those diet factors contribute to insulin resistance, oxidation of blood lipids, and silent, systemic inflammation. One study showed evidence that America's extreme omega-3/6 fat intake imbalance raises people's risks for dementia, including Alzheimer's.[1588]

Fasting

Research shows that caloric restriction or intermittent fasting slows aging, improves brain health and prolongs life.[1589] [1590] [1591] One study in fifty healthy adults showed that intermittent fasting for one month significantly decreased levels of inflammatory markers.[1592] One small study revealed that eight weeks of alternate-day fasting reduced levels of "bad" LDL cholesterol and blood triglycerides by twenty-five and thirty-two percent respectively.[1593] One study in mice showed that practicing intermittent fasting for eleven months improved both brain function and brain structure.[1594] Other animal studies have reported that fasting could protect brain health and increase the generation of nerve cells to help enhance cognitive function.[1595] [1596] Because fasting may also help relieve inflammation and it could also aid in preventing neurodegenerative disorders. In particular, studies with animals suggest that fasting may protect against and improve outcomes for conditions such as Alzheimer's disease and also Parkinson's.[1597] [1598]

Reduce These Foods

A characteristic feature of most of the foods we suggest you limit or avoid is their ability to create inflammation in the body. As discussed earlier, scientists are coming to understand that systemic inflammation is a contributing cause to eye disease and to most chronic health conditions such as heart disease, diabetes, lung issues, bone health, depression, cancer, and emotional disorders.[1599]

Similarly, these foods increase oxidative stress in the body. Overload of free radicals causes oxidative stress and plays a major role in the development of chronic and degenerative illness such as cancer, autoimmune disorders, aging, rheumatoid arthritis, cardiovascular and neurodegenerative diseases. Oxidative stress encourages excitotoxity, increased free radicals, inflammation, and changes to synapses in development of Alzheimer's[1600][1601] and Parkinson's.[1602]

Refined Carbohydrates

Avoid or minimize refined carbohydrates such as the white versions of bread, pasta, rice, and sugar. Most of their food value is removed when the nutrient-rich outer husks are removed in processing. Furthermore, they deplete the body of essential enzymes and minerals needed to break down these foods. For those prone to chronic inflammatory conditions, these foods are quite acidic (as opposed to alkaline) and exacerbate inflammation and oxidative stress.[1603]

In the past, carbohydrates were classified as either simple (such as sugar and fructose) or complex (such as those that contain fiber, vitamins, and minerals). More recently, the glycemic index has become more relevant because it rates foods by how quickly they break down into sugar in the body. It ranks carbohydrates on a scale from 0–100, based on how quickly and how much they raise blood sugar levels after eating.

Glycemic Index

A high glycemic index diet is linked to increased amyloid burden in adults who are still cognitively normal (amyloid positive), increasing Alzheimer's risk[1604][1605] and may reduce cognitive functioning in adults (findings are inconclusive).[1606] A high glycemic index also increases the risk of diabetes[1607] (type 1 diabetes is linked to cognitive impairments)[1608] heart disease,[1609][1610] and obesity.[1611][1612][1613] A glycemic index of 70 or above is considered high.[1614]

Low glycemic index foods have an index of 55 or less. A low glycemic index diet has anti-inflammatory benefits.[1615] These foods include lentils, cashews, kidney beans, black beans, garbanzo beans (used to make hummus), oranges, apples, almonds, walnuts, peanuts (though these can be inflammatory and should be avoided for anyone with an inflammatory condition), carrots, bran cereals, all leafy-green vegetables, quinoa, millet, wild caught fish, free-range beef, and eggs.

Medium glycemic index foods have an index of 56–69 and include whole grain breads, rice cakes, oatmeal, brown rice, and whole grain pasta.

High glycemic index foods have an index of 70–100 and include all refined carbohydrates (white flour, rice, pasta), sugars, refined breakfast cereals, baked potato, pretzels, French fries, couscous, millet, muesli, sugar sweetened soft drinks, fruit juices, melons, pineapple, corn tortilla, sweet corn, rice, udon noodles, and sugar added salad dressings.

Recommended. Favor whole grains over refined grains. Favor complex carbohydrates such as sprouted, multigrain breads and pastas.

Note. The glycemic index of food on your plate depends on several factors. For example, you can decrease the glycemic level by adding lemon juice or by increasing the proportion of low glycemic food in a meal. The longer starches are cooked, or the riper the fruit, the higher their index.[1616] Adding extra-virgin olive oil also reduces glycemic index, markedly more than low-fat butter in a meal.[1617]

Sweeteners

Sugar and the Brain

With consumption of soft drinks and candy, Americans consume an enormous amount of sugar, the equivalent of more than seven tablespoons daily. This amount of sugar is about 355 calories. We are in the midst of a crisis of obesity in the U.S. and the consumption of sweet foods is part of the problem.

The brain uses more energy than any other organ in the human body and glucose is its source of fuel. In the adult brain, neurons have the highest energy demand,[1618] requiring continuous delivery of glucose from blood. The main process by which this is accomplished is called glycolysis. Glucose provides precursors for neurotransmitter synthesis and ATP to fuel their actions. Glucose is also required for the brain's energy demands unrelated to signaling.[1619]

However, too much glucose is toxic to brain cells. This is a problem worsened by the fact that regular intake of sugar has drug-like effects in the reward center of the brain, creating a desire for more sugar. High blood glucose levels can negatively affect the brain in a number of ways:

1. It reduces functional connectivity of the default mode network, that system of the brain which links the individual with the outside world.[1620] Such altered functionality is associated with cognitive impairments.
2. It can cause the brain to atrophy or shrink[1621] as does deteriorating brain glucose metabolism[1622]
3. It can lead to cerebral small vessel disease which restricts blood flow in the brain which can result in cognitive difficulties and, if severe enough, can cause vascular dementia.[1623]

High Blood Sugar

The body needs insulin to carry glucose into the brain. Excess sugar (and refined carbohydrate intake) over time can result in insulin insensitivity (requiring the body to make more insulin) contributing the type-2 diabetes. The effects of glucose and other forms of sugar on the brain may be the most profound in diabetes.

Research strongly supports the fact that people without diabetes but with above normal blood sugar levels have an increased risk of developing dementia.[1624] There is a relationship between the breakdown of glycolysis and Alzheimer's disease,[1625] the severity of which is linked to the severity of Alzheimer's pathology. Lower rates of glycolysis and higher brain glucose levels correlate to more severe plaques and tangles in the brains of people with the disease. Enzymes, amino acids serine, glycine, and alanine are essential parts of glycolysis, and are lower in Alzheimer's cases compared to normal brain tissue samples.[1626] In addition, lower enzyme activity is associated with more severe Alzheimer's pathology in the brain and the development of symptoms.

Hypoglycemia is a common complication of diabetes caused by low glucose levels in the blood. This can lead to loss of energy for brain function and is linked to poor attention and cognitive function.

Inflammation

Sweeteners of all kinds contribute to inflammation. Sugar is one of the most acidic foods, and excess sugar in one's diet is considered a leading contributor to disease, such as type-2 diabetes, cardiovascular disease, high blood pressure (hypertension), cancer, and dementia.[1627]

Why Reduce Sugar

There are many reasons to reduce sugar intake.

- **Metabolic stability**. When you eat or drink something sweet, it gives a quick surge of energy. However, the consequence of glucose entering the bloodstream so quickly is that the body's ability to maintain stability is compromised.
- **Stable blood sugar levels**. With some attention to our diet, we can help balance blood sugar. This is especially true in type-2 diabetes (adult onset), which sometimes can be managed by diet alone. It is rarely true of type 1 diabetes (juvenile onset).
- **Stronger immune system**. Individuals with higher sugar consumption had shorter telomeres in their white blood cells as compared to those with lower sugar consumption (telomeres are the caps at the end of each strand of DNA that protect our chromosomes, like the plastic tips at the end of shoelaces).[1628]
- **Reduced glycation.** Glycation is the binding of sugar and protein molecules in one's body, and is part of the natural aging process. When the sugar molecule binds inappropriately to a protein, it forms a new compound called "advanced glycation end-products (AGE's)." AGE's cause ongoing inflammation and react with body tissues to produce free radicals and reactive oxygen species that damage healthy cells if not neutralized.

Recommended

Limit your sweets and avoid sugary drinks and sodas. In general, an alkaline diet will be a low sugar diet and will be anti-inflammatory. Avoid high glycemic index foods. Stevia is a great alternative to sugar and has been shown to be very safe.[1629] It is an herb that is not sugar (has zero calories) and works by stimulating the sugar receptors in the tongue. Stevia is two-hundred times sweeter than sugar taken in the same dosages, so a small amount (even 3-5 drops in plain yogurt for example) goes a long way. Too much stevia gives food a bitter taste.

Reduce AGE's. In addition to the above, avoid grilled and charred foods, fried foods, and slow cook your food or lightly steam your vegetables. Avoid vegetable oils for cooking in high heat. Olive oil is fine in low heat, saturated fats such as butter and coconuts oil have high heat tolerance which means that these oils when used in cooking maintain stability whereas oils such as vegetable oils have poor heat tolerance and can be quickly turned into an unhealthy oil high in free radicals when used in cooking. Complex carbohydrates and high fiber foods reduce the production of AGE's in the body. Foods that help clear one's body of AGE's include kale, collard greens, spinach, broccoli, cauliflower, citrus fruits, peaches, most berries, tomatoes, carrots, as well as green tea, grapeseed extract, carnosine, and vitamin B6.

Avoid artificial sweeteners. Sugar and artificially sweetened beverage intake have been linked to cardiometabolic risk factors, which increase the risk of cerebrovascular disease and dementia. Artificially-sweetened soft drinks are associated with an increased risk of ischemic stroke, all-cause dementia, and AD dementia.[1630][1631] Some of the adverse effects on the central nervous system caused by the intake of aspartame are headaches, mood changes, insomnia and seizures.[1632] Other effects include confusion, personality disorders, dizziness and visual difficulty.[1633] In mice studies, chronic aspartame consumption resulted in a longer time for the mice to locate the reward within the T-maze, which showed impaired long-term memory retention.[1634][1635][1636]

Ironically, although people consume artificial sweeteners in an attempt to reduce caloric intake and control or lose weight, studies actually show that consumption results in increased weight and has been attributed to obesity.[1637][1638] One reason may be that consumption of foods and fluids containing high-potency sweeteners interfered with the ability to detect sweet taste, thereby affecting energy regulation (and possibly increasing the desire for more sweets, or stimulating the desire for sugar).[1639]

Fats

For your oils, use extra virgin, first-cold pressed olive oil in a dark bottle on your salads and for low heat cooking. If necessary, for high heat only, use saturated fats such as coconut oil, butter, or ghee. But note that saturated fatty acids (in excess) and trans-fatty acids are may increase the risk of AD[1640][1641][1642][1643][1644] and affect cognition[1645] which could be due to decreased BDNF-related synaptic plasticity.[1646] Epidemiological studies have implicated diets rich in saturated fat with the development of Alzheimer's disease.[1647][1648] In mouse models, high-fat diets increase the deposition of amyloid beta peptides.[1649][1650][1651][1652]

Fried Foods

Fried foods provide almost no nutritional value and present digestive challenges. This is especially true of foods containing trans-fatty acids, which can cause diarrhea. Fried foods and foods containing trans-fatty acids substantially increase free radicals in the body that cause the breakdown of healthy cells. Excess intake of fried foods is tied to increased risk of diabetes and heart disease. One study found that people who ate fried food at least once per week had a greater risk of type 2 diabetes and heart disease, and the risk increased as the frequency of fried food consumption increased. On a per-calorie basis, trans fats appear to increase the risk of chronic heart disease more than any other micronutrient.[1653] In one study, the participants who ate fried foods 4–6 times per week had a 39 percent increased risk of type 2 diabetes, and those who ate fried foods seven or more times per week had a 55 percent increased risk.[1654]

Recommended.

- Limit fried foods, especially deep-fried foods.
- Avoid man-made fats (corn oil, safflower oil, trans fats, and hydrogenated vegetable oils, including canola oil).
- Avoid trans-fatty acids. These are oils that have added hydrogen incorporated to turn their liquid state into a solid, e.g. margarine. Avoid hydrogenated oils, trans-fatty acids, and saturated fats, which also disrupt the digestive process.

Processed Foods

Breads, frozen meals, canned foods, and other foods that have been created in "food factories" tend to be loaded with artificial sweeteners, flavor enhancers, and a host of preservatives. Many such chemicals have been gradually phased out as the food industry yields to scientific research, proving their detrimental-to-health qualities. A good example is the use of many different chemicals used to color food.[1655]

But there are a number of food additives that are banned in Europe that are still permitted in the U.S. These include, but are not limited to, Olestra, brominated vegetable oil, BHA/BHT, azodicarbonamide, rBGH or rBST hormones, and neonicotinoid pesticides.[1656] New chemicals are created frequently as substitutes for those that are no longer permitted. When you are in the grocery store about to buy pre-prepared foods, look at the label. If the food label includes any number of unidentifiable chemicals, you would be wise to avoid it or do some research. And if the first three ingredients are a refined grain, sweetener, or hydrogenated oil, it is best to pass it by.[1657]

Recommended. Cook from scratch whenever possible. Many healthy meals take no longer to prepare than frozen meals and are considerably better for you.

Additives

Processed foods all contain additives. These are ingredients that are designed to keep food from spoiling, to supply an inexpensive source of flavor, or to provide texture. Some of these additives include the following:[1658]

High fructose corn syrup. High fructose corn syrup is one of the worst culprits. This sweetener causes intracellular depletion of adenosine triphosphate (ATP). ATP is the primary biochemical that delivers energy throughout the body. ATP depletion due to damaged mitochondria or increased free radicals triggers neurodegenerative diseases.[1659] When a cell needs energy, the process of breaking down ATP releases energy. High fructose corn syrup causes nucleotide turnover (these are the structural components of compounds such as DNA). It increases generation of uric acid that may have a critical role in causing diabetes and obesity.[1660] There are a number of sweeteners that are chemically similar to high fructose corn syrup that may be labeled as fructose, invert sugar, honey, evaporated cane juice, sugar, and sucrose.[1661] Even when used in moderation, these are a primary or contributing cause of cardiovascular disease, cancer, liver failure, and tooth decay.[1662] They are implicated in metabolic syndrome,[1663] memory problems,[1664] and much more.

Phosphates. Many food additives contain phosphates, which increase danger for those with kidney disease and may contribute to heart disease, bone loss, and other chronic conditions.[1665] These are often added as flavor enhancers. Phosphates that occur naturally in food are fine as the body absorbs them incompletely. However, added inorganic phosphates can significantly increase the blood phosphate level. The main problem is damage to the blood system, causing malfunctioning of tissue that lines the blood vessels and the accumulation of plaque.[1666]

Sulfites. When added as a preservative, sulfites attack B1, especially under acid conditions.[1667] The relationship between B1 (thiamine) deficiency and dementia is well established; thiamine is required for proper glucose metabolism.[1668]

Emulsifiers. These help oil and water-based liquids stay mixed together in foods. When you add a bit of mustard to your vinaigrette, you are adding an emulsifier. Early research reports that lab animals given chemical emulsifiers added weight, added fat, had poor blood sugar control, and had more severe elimination problems. These artificial emulsifiers include gums, polysorbates 60 and 80, lecithin, and carboxymethylcellulose.[1669]

Hidden allergens. Potential allergens are hard to identify because they are undeclared, and they are the biggest cause of food recalls. Baked goods are the biggest source. The most common hidden allergens are milk, wheat, soy, and sometimes nuts.[1670]

Recommended. If you buy pre-prepared foods, read the label carefully, and avoid those with a long list of additives, preservatives, artificial flavorings, and colorings.

Caffeine

Caffeine appears to have a protective effect against cognitive impairment.[1671] However, quercetin, not caffeine in coffee and tea is the primary source of the neuroprotective benefit.[1672] Caffeine is a stimulant found in cocoa beans, coffee beans, black and green tea. Smaller amounts of caffeine intake have been found to have potential health benefits, e.g. coffee contains antioxidant phenols and reduces the risk of developing neurodegenerative disease and other health conditions, including type 2 diabetes mellitus and liver disease.

At the same time, on the negative side, coffee can increase serum homocysteine and cholesterol levels and therefore has adverse effects on the cardiovascular system[1673] and may have negative effects for some eye conditions (such as glaucoma, which is affected by high blood pressure) with excessive consumption.[1674] A 2019 meta-analysis of seven research studies suggests that caffeine can either increase or decrease symptoms in dementia patients depending on the other health issues of each individual.[1675]

Chinese medicine perspective on coffee

Coffee is yang in nature. It regulates Liver Qi (energy) and clears the Gallbladder, resulting in its ability to protect against formation of gallstones and alleviating constipation. Coffee moves Qi and Blood, invigorates, and disperses (meaning that it has a diuretic effect and helps move energy and fluids in the body).

The benefits and risks of drinking coffee depend on each person's constitution and the environment they live in. For people living in a cold environment, coffee can be very warming. For those living in a hot environment, it may create too much heat. In Chinese Medicine it is advised that excessive amounts of coffee will agitate the liver yang. Symptoms can include headaches (typically on one side of the head or in or above the eyes), breaking blood vessels on the outside of the eyes (sclera), elevated eye pressure (IOP), red eyes, visual disturbances, ocular migraines, possible changes in eyesight, ringing in the ears, dizziness, dry mouth, heavy feeling, insomnia, and increases in blood pressure. It can stimulate internal wind with symptoms that can include the following: pain that moves around, itchy skin conditions, dizziness/vertigo, tremor or spasms, sudden appearing rashes, sudden onset of headache or migraine with vertigo, or possibly sudden onset of disease.

For people that are yang deficient (low in energy and generally cold overall), moderate amounts of coffee can be therapeutic to warm the body and stimulate yang. Excessive amounts can eventually have the opposite effect by depleting the adrenals. Coffee is warm, sweet, and bitter. The slight sweetness of coffee also makes it mildly tonifying and nourishing. The primary bitter taste has the action of drying and dispersing. It can also clear heat, which helps balance out the very warm nature of coffee. It reduces the risk of colon cancer as it moves Qi and Blood in the large intestine.

In traditional Chinese medicine, food is divided into five natures: cold, cool, neutral, warm, and hot. Coffee brings warmth and heat to the body. So, a person who tends to have too much heat should avoid coffee or keep it at a minimum. Common symptoms of chronic heat include feeling hot, sweating all the time, being grumpy, having a swollen tongue, and often being constipated. Coffee can be helpful for those who tend to be cold and/or damp. Common symptoms of having a cold constitution include being pale, having cold hands and feet, sensitivity to cold temperatures, feeling weak, and having poor circulation. Dampness tendencies include being overweight, particularly around the stomach, distended stomach, sticky mouth, greasy tongue, swelling, water retention, loose stool, and/or nodule masses (lymph nodes).

Recommended. Limit yourself to one cup of coffee, tea, cocoa daily, and it is best unsweetened.

Alcohol

Alcohol reduces protective glutathione levels because it interferes with liver functioning. Although red wine has been touted for its antioxidant benefit and heart health, "moderate" consumption has been associated with an increased risk of breast cancer[1676] and heavy drinking increases the risk of many diseases, including circulatory, respiratory, digestive, and metabolic system conditions.[1677] A meta-analysis of twenty research studies determined that in adults younger than sixty, modest consumption (6 g/day to 12.5 g/day) of alcohol has a protective effect against dementia and excessive drinking (more than 38 g/day) elevates the risk.[1678] The lower rate (6 g/day) had the best protective effect.

Recommended. Limit alcohol consumption to one half glass of red wine daily.

The MIND Diet

The MIND diet is a hybrid of the Mediterranean diet (MeDi) and the DASH (heart-healthy) diets. It differs from the MeDi only in that it includes foods that promote cognitive health. It slows cognitive decline found with aging[1679 1680] and provides better verbal memory in later life.[1681] It may help prevent or slow the development of Alzheimer's,[1682 1683 1684] Parkinson's,[1685] the rate of cognitive decline,[1686] and other cognitive impairments.[1687]

Our healthy brain diet includes the suggested diet components of the MIND diet: green leafy vegetables, nuts, berries, beans, whole grains, fish, and poultry.
- Green leafy vegetables: at least six servings a week
- Other vegetables: at least one other vegetable every day
- Nuts: just a few nuts, at least five times a week
- Berries: especially blueberries, at least twice a week
- Beans: at least three times a week
- Whole grains: a variety of whole grains at every meal
- Fish: at least once a week
- Poultry (like chicken or turkey): at least twice a week

And to reduce:
- Red meat
- Butter and margarine – not more than one tablespoon daily
- Cheese – not more than once a week
- Pastries and sweets – not more than five times a week
- Fried and fast foods – not more than once a week

Comparison of Modern Diets

Other diets may be worth exploring. Every individual is different, and the dietary needs of one person can be vastly different from another. For ease, we have broken the diets into two primary categories: omnivorous and plant-based diets. Simply, the omnivorous diets include animal products while the plant-based diets include little.

Omnivorous Diets

The Atkins Diet

The Atkins diet is a popular low-carbohydrate, high-protein weight-loss diet created by the late cardiologist Robert Atkins, M.D. The diet, which advocates consuming only high amounts of proteins and fats, such as meat, poultry, seafood, eggs, butter, oils, and cheeses, along with high-fiber vegetables, at first promotes rapid weight-loss through the metabolic process called ketosis, which is the burning of fat, rather than carbohydrates for fuel. As the diet progresses, foods like beans/legumes, fruits, and whole grains can be added. The diet is extremely strict in staying away from starchy and sugary carbs, including bread, pasta, chips, cookies, and candy. It recommends a wide range of vegetables. One advantage of the Atkins diet is that it prohibits most, if not all foods with gluten, which tend to be high in carbs. People on Atkins, therefore, eat less gluten than people who eat the standard American diet.

Health Risks/Rewards

The advantage of the Atkins diet is that is particularly good for people sensitive to gluten. There is some evidence of a connection between celiac disease (and possibly non-celiac gluten sensitivity) and several types of cognitive impairment such as "Alzheimer's, vascular, and frontotemporal dementia.[1688] It is helpful in controlling body weight, and possibly helpful in reducing dementia, diabetes/metabolic syndrome/insulin resistance, acid reflux (GERD), acne, headaches, heart disease, and cancer.

The disadvantage of this diet is that a high protein diet is not ideal for many people, and the diet does not focus enough on eating the right, healthy oils and staying away from those that should be avoided. If the body is chronically depleted of carbohydrates, it exposes the liver to additional stress, as the liver produces glucose from fats and proteins instead of carbohydrates.[1689] Toxic amounts of ammonia can be produced, and the immune system can become compromised. Proteins are said to not metabolize "cleanly". A byproduct of protein metabolism is ammonia, which is not thoroughly eliminated through urine. Adequate intake of water is also essential since protein metabolism requires water to break down amino acids and to process and eliminate nitrogen. While the diet has proven effective for weight loss, opponents have gone as far as to condemn it as outright dangerous because of its high level of saturated fat intake, which has been linked to everything from high cholesterol and kidney problems to cancer.[1690] In addition, a goal of rapid weight loss is neither safe nor sustainable.

Note. Clinical trials of a modified Atkins diet to induce ketogenesis in patients with early AD or mild cognitive impairment found that where urinary ketones evidenced ketogenesis (the diet was difficult for most participants to follow consistently), there was a significant increase in memory-related testing scores and general vitality.[1691]

Blood Type Diet

Designed by Dr. Peter J. D'Adamo, this diet is based on the theory that the foods we eat react chemically with our blood type, and therefore, can either improve health or make a person more susceptible to certain disease. He states that blood type is a key genetic factor, and as such, is a factor in both health and disease.

He notes, for example, that people with blood type O can efficiently digest protein and fat, but their metabolism of carbohydrates tends to produce fats and triglycerides. Consequently, they have a lower risk for heart disease but a higher risk for developing stomach ulcers and thyroid disorders. In addition, type O is prone to the "fight or flight" response, resulting in emotional imbalances, including bouts of excessive anger. Type O's benefit from regular brisk exercise as a tonic for the entire system.[1692]

Health Risks/Rewards

The blood type diet could be effective because the foods recommended attempt to address underlying issues by blood type, thereby supporting overall health in a more individualized way. This diet might result in, for example, reducing emotional stress for type O people and improving digestion, which would make more nutrients available. It may be that eating incorrectly for one's blood type may increase inflammation, a key contributing cause of dementia. One example is that type O people can safely eat chicken without increasing inflammation, but with type B and AB people, chicken increases inflammation.[1693]

One risk is that strict adherence to the diet may ignore other factors such as genetics, environmental concerns, and so forth. A comprehensive review of the literature found no evidence to support the validity of the blood type diet.[1694][1695]

This doesn't mean that the diet doesn't work, but it may not work for everyone. For example, another study found that adherence to the type A diet was associated with lowered BMI, blood pressure, cholesterol, triglycerides, insulin, and other biomarkers. It found similar improvements for diet AB (except BMI), and the type O diet was linked to lower triglycerides. These researchers, however, concluded that while the diets were favorable for some people, **those results were not associated with blood type.**[1696]

Note. One three-year study associated AB blood type with a higher risk of dementia, but the research has not yet been replicated.[1697] AB is also linked to a higher risk of heart disease.[1698]

Ketone Diet

The ketogenic diet is a high-fat content diet in which carbohydrates are nearly eliminated so that the body has minimal dietary sources of glucose. People generally go on this diet to lose weight, though it may also help reduce triglycerides and increase good (HDL) cholesterol, as well as reduce blood sugar and insulin levels. Fatty acids are the primary source of cellular energy production by peripheral tissues and also the brain. In the absence of glucose, the preferred source of energy (particularly of the brain), are the ketone bodies that are used as fuel in extrahepatic tissues. The diet is composed of 80–90 percent fat, with carbohydrate and protein constituting the remainder of the intake.

The diet provides sufficient protein for growth, but insufficient amounts of carbohydrates for the body's metabolic needs. Energy is largely derived from the utilization of body fat and by fat delivered in the diet. These fats are converted to the ketone bodies beta-hydroxybutyrate, aceto-acetate, and acetone, which represent an alternative energy source to glucose. [1699] [1700]

There is evidence from uncontrolled clinical trials and studies in animal models that the keto-genic diet can provide symptomatic and disease-modifying activity in a broad range of neuro-degenerative disorders including Alzheimer's disease and Parkinson's disease, and may also be protective in traumatic brain injury and stroke. Although the mechanisms are not yet well de-fined, it is plausible that neuroprotection results from enhanced neuronal energy reserves, which improve the ability of neurons to resist metabolic challenges, and possibly through other actions including antioxidant and anti-inflammatory effects. It may as well have beneficial disease-mod-ifying activity applicable to a broad range of brain disorders characterized by neuron death.

There are reasons why the ketogenic diet might be helpful. The therapeutic implications of ke-tone bodies include the effects of ketone bodies in pathological conditions: ketosis, ketogenic diet, redox states, insulin resistance, and mitochondrial metabolism.[1701] [1702]

- The ketogenic diet might protect against amyloid beta toxicity. Direct application of beta-hydroxybutyrate in concentrations produced by the ketogenic diet has been found to protect hippocampal neurons from toxicity induced by amyloid beta(1–42).[1703] It increases gluta-thione peroxidase activity in rat hippocampus.[1704]
- It may enhance levels of γ-aminobutyric acid (GABA) levels, with a consequent increase in GABA-mediated inhibition. [1705]
- Enhancement of antioxidant mechanisms represents an additional potential mechanism of neuroprotection. For example, ketone bodies have been shown to reduce the amount of coenzyme Q semiquinone, thereby decreasing free radical production.[1706]
- A high carbohydrate intake worsens cognitive performance and behavior in patients with Alzheimer's disease.[1707]
- The ketogenic diet also increases production of specific mitochondrial uncoupling proteins (UCPs)[1708] and may also protect against various forms of cell death.[1709]
- A high-fat diet has been associated with effects on inflammatory mechanisms.[1710] [1711]

Note. The primary difference between the paleolithic diet and ketogenic diets (though very sim-ilar) is that ketogenic diet focuses on manipulating the three macronutrients (fat, carbs, and pro-tein) for those keeping score. The paleo diet is more about the food choices. You eliminate dairy, grains and processed foods, but balance the macronutrients any way you want.

Health Risks/Rewards

It is possible that the ketogenic diet could ameliorate Alzheimer's disease by providing greater amounts of essential fatty acids than normal or high carbohydrate diets. The diet is considered an anti-inflammatory diet due to the low carbohydrates and sugar and high fat content. It reduces insulin levels. Higher levels of circulating insulin have been linked to increased inflammation and has been implicated to be causative to neurological and brain disease. This diet also may promote weight loss.

However, consuming a high-fat diet to sustain ketosis can be detrimental to your long-term health. Many high-fat foods that are low in protein and carbohydrates, such as butter, lard, coconut, and egg yolks, are high in saturated fat, which can increase your risk of heart disease. Additionally, high-fat diets may cause injury to brain cells that help control your body weight. The diet also does not focus enough on only eating healthy fats, and avoiding most vegetable oils, fried food, bacon, etc. It is also a difficult diet to maintain. High level of ketones can result in ketosis, which overtime can become dangerous when ketones build up. High levels of ketones lead to dehydration and change the chemical balance of your blood. Negative symptoms of ketosis include short-term fatigue and performance, bad breath, suppressed appetite, digestive issues, and insomnia. A low-carb diet may also increase your risk of high cholesterol, kidney problems, and osteoporosis.

Additionally, a ketone diet may not provide enough glucose the brain needs to function optimally. The primary (almost sole) source of energy the brain needs comes from glucose, which is typically derived from carbohydrates (complex carbohydrates preferred) derived from one's diet. The backup system is ketones produced from the liver if not enough glucose is available, but this is done more on an emergency basis and is not optimal.

Metabolic Typing Diet

Designed by William L. Wolcott, this diet addresses biochemical individuality. The same foods and their nutrients can have different effects in different bodies. Metabolic means the chemical processes that occur within a living organism in order to maintain life. Metabolic typing regards an individual's genetics as the key factor in the digestion and "processing" of foods and utilization of nutrients.[1712] The assumption is that one type of diet can help prevent disease in one person, while the same diet may promote disease in another. The metabolic typing diet analyzes many different aspects of a person's physiological makeup, including blood type, in order to specify a diet appropriate for that person's biochemical and metabolic tendencies. While there are three "basic" metabolic type categories: the protein type, the carbo type, or the mixed type, adjustments need to be made in coming up with the best diet.[1713]

Health Risks/Rewards

Similar to the blood type diet, the metabolic type diet can be effective because the diet is more individualized by body type, which maximizes the nutritional benefits of the foods recommended according to metabolic type, thereby supporting overall brain and body health. One of the diets for the protein type is rich in organ meats and saturated fats and is thus more likely to increase the risk of heart disease and other conditions.[1714] Although the diet can be helpful for weight loss, research is lacking as to the long-term effectiveness and safety.[1715]

Mediterranean Diet

While the Mediterranean (MeDi) is markedly beneficial, with consistent results with respect to many health conditions, the MIND diet, described above, appears to be better for long term cognitive protection.[1716] The MeDi may be summarized this way.[1717]

- High in vegetables and some fruit (particularly those low in sugar)
- Emphasizes whole grains, legumes, and nuts.
- Uses herbs and spices, instead of salt, to flavor foods.
- Replaces butter with high quality, first-cold-pressed extra virgin olive oil. [1718]
- Fish and poultry are recommended not more than twice a week, and red meat twice per month.
- A glass of red wine (preferably organic) with dinner is even permitted. [1719]

Studies have shown that the Mediterranean diet may reduce the incidence of dementia (including a meta-analysis of 32 studies)[1720] [1721] and Alzheimer's disease.[1722] [1723] [1724] [1725] The MeDi is slightly associated with reduced Parkinson's progression,[1726] and early symptoms of Parkinson's. [1727] [1728] It significantly reduces the risk of heart disease,[1729] type 2 diabetes, cancer, some vision conditions, such as macular degeneration.[1730] [1731]

There is some controversy as to whether it reduces amyloid beta accumulation,[1732] [1733] [1734] but it does appear to improve neuroimaging biomarker profiles.[1735] [1736] Researchers also note that the anti-inflammatory and antioxidant polyphenols in the diet reduce the risk of microglia-mediated neuroinflammation.[1737]

Health Risks/Rewards

The Mediterranean diet is excellent for most people and many studies substantiate its benefits for brain and heart health. However, it may be more difficult for vegetarians or vegans due to added meat, chicken, or fish. Brain supporting foods should be added to this diet. See the description of the MIND diet above.

The Ornish Spectrum Program

More of a lifestyle program than a diet, this program emphasizes a low-fat, low-sugar, plant-based diet, along with regular exercise, stress reduction, and social support through relationship building. Although cardiologist Dean Ornish, designed the program specifically for heart health, he says the program works to improve health for anyone; and research has shown that it can reverse heart disease, type 2 diabetes, and even early-stage prostate cancer.[1738]

The nutrition part of the diet consists of fruits, vegetables, whole grains, and legumes (organic soy in particular) with an emphasis on whole unprocessed foods. In its strictest form, animal protein is limited to egg whites and nonfat dairy foods, and there are no added oils. Less than ten percent of calories come from fat. The diet starts with complex carbohydrates, fruits, and veggies. That makes it high in fiber and low in calories. Critics take issue with the low-fat component of the program and note that early (reversal) stages of the diet could be considered restrictive.

Health Risks/Rewards

The beneficial dietary aspect of this program is that it is rich in vitamins, minerals, antioxidants, and fiber, and it is low in sugar, saturated fats, and cholesterol, especially compared to high-protein/low-carb diets. Additionally, because the focus includes lifestyle actions toward improving heart health, the Ornish Spectrum program will not only boost circulation, but will also reduce stress.

However, the diet tends to be lower in other nutrients that are predominantly found in animal foods, such as vitamin B12, iron, and zinc, as well as omega-3 fatty acids. For this reason, Dr. Ornish recommends supplementing with a multivitamin[1739] and we recommend including omega-3 supplementation (such as a tablespoon of whole ground flax seed daily) or a fatty fish like salmon at least once a week.

Paleolithic Diet

This program is based on the hunter-gatherer diet of protein from lean meats, fruit (not too much and particularly those low in sugar, such as berries), and vegetables. There is essentially no dairy or grain in this diet. When you are following the paleo diet, you eat foods that were hunted or gathered far in the past, such as meats, fish, nuts, leafy-green vegetables, regional vegetables, and seeds.[1740] Here's how the modern version of the diet works.

- Consume organic and range-fed meats and wild caught fish.
- To obtain minerals, eat the animal bone marrow, and consume the organs.
- If you consume grains, they should be minimal and unrefined, including cereals, breads, and pastas (preferably soaked and sprouted).
- Add abundant organic vegetables and moderate amounts of organic fruit.
- Add additional carbohydrates for those who need them (athletes, physical laborers, etc.). These include complex carbohydrate-containing vegetables (winter squash, carrots, potatoes).
- Certain nuts, seeds, and legumes are recommended (roasted pumpkin seeds, soaked flax meal, almonds, peas, dried lentils, green beans, and edamame). Additional protein can also be obtained from soy products such as organic tofu, natto, tempeh (higher in protein by weight than meat), and miso.
- Eat algae, sea vegetables, and spirulina—rich sources of minerals and antioxidants.

Health Risks/Rewards

This diet has the potential to be very healthy. It can be high in antioxidants with a focus on fruits and vegetables, nuts and seeds, lean meats and fish, and oils from fruits and nuts, such as olive or walnut oil. It is important to understand that the paleolithic diet contains approximately three times more plants than our typical Western diet today. It is also a good anti-inflammatory diet and it may improve triglyceride and cholesterol levels as well as blood pressure, which are all risk factors for cognitive decline.

However, no research has established whether the paleo diet can prevent or slow dementia or cognitive impairment, although it may improve metabolic measures such as triglyceride and cholesterol levels and blood pressure.[1741] The primary risk of this diet is that it may not include enough vitamin D, calcium, and carotenoids like lutein and zeaxanthin. And the high levels of saturated fats increase the risk of heart disease.[1742] Risks also come from wild game that may contain disease. For example, a Canadian study found that chronic wasting disease, a problem for deer herds, could be transmitted to primates.[1743] A rare bacterial disease from eating rabbit meat is tularemia, rabbit fever.[1744]

South Beach Diet

The South Beach diet was created by cardiologist, Dr. Arthur Agatston and dietician, Marie Almon. It focuses on the control of insulin levels and the benefits of consuming unrefined or complex carbohydrates versus simple carbohydrates, which can cause rapid spikes in blood sugar levels that result in cravings and other deleterious health effects.

Dr. Agatston believed that low-fat regimens were not effective over the long term for preventing heart disease. It was initially designed to help patients lower their risk of developing heart disease, but it rapidly became popular as a diet for losing weight. The South Beach diet focuses on selecting the "right" carbohydrates, including whole grains, specific fruits and vegetables, and fats such as canola oil.[1745]

There are three phases in the diet with the goal of reaching one's ideal weight, and then keeping that ideal weight by maintaining healthy eating and lifestyle habits encouraged in the program. The diet differs from the Mediterranean diet, most substantially in the first two phases where it emphasizes lean proteins and non-starch vegetables. This means no fruit or fruit juices, sugar, or alcohol, but also no "starches" such as bread, rice, potatoes, pasta, baked goods, etc. In the third, or maintenance phase of this diet, these types of foods can be added back in, so long as guidelines are met surrounding them, and the person continues to drop 1–2 pounds per week, until their ideal weight is achieved.[1746]

Health Risks/Rewards

The South Beach diet is high in antioxidants with the focus on intake of fruits and vegetables, lean meats, healthy oils, and whole grains. It focuses on the "right" carbohydrates, based on their glycemic index. Its potential to reduce weight, lower high blood pressure, and reduce blood fat and cholesterol levels do support cognitive health. Heart disease and diabetes are two contributing causes of cognitive decline. This diet, however, does not include known cognition-supporting foods nuts and berries, nor does it limit oils to olive oil.

Plant-Based Diets

Vegan and Vegetarianism

All vegetarian diets promote the value of consuming plant-based foods as one's primary source of nutrition. Technically, a vegan diet would not include animal foods or products containing animal sources. However, because of the rise in interest in health and plant-based diets in the U.S., and to reflect our nation's shift in consciousness away from consuming certain types of animal products, many variations of the plant-based diet have been named. Below is a list of "vegetarian" diets in order of least plant-based to the most.

Caution: It is important for those on a strict plant-based diet to routinely check their levels of nutrients that are difficult to obtain from plants and to supplement, if and when required. These nutrients include, but are not limited to, vitamin B12, zinc, and iron. Vegetarians also need to make sure they are getting enough protein.

- **Pollo-vegetarians** eat poultry but omit red meat.
- **Pesco-vegetarians** add fish to their diet, but do not typically consume other meats. This diet is common in Asia, where hundreds of millions live on rice, fish, and vegetables.
- **Lacto-vegetarians** eat dairy products (but not eggs) along with other plant-based foods.
- **Lacto-ovo vegetarians** consume eggs and dairy products with other plant-based foods.
- **Vegans** abstain from eating animal products, including honey: plant-based foods only.
- **Ethical vegans or total vegetarians** not only live solely on plant-based foods, but also abstain from using products derived from animals, such as silk, leather, and wool.

The Vegan Diet

Veganism is more than just a diet. People who adopt the lifestyle may not do it for health reasons only, but for social, environmental, and ethical reasons. As noted above, a vegan does not eat anything that is animal based, including eggs, dairy, and honey. It is also common for vegans to avoid using any animal products (or those products tested on animals), out of concern for the welfare of all living creatures; these people may describe themselves as ethical vegans.

Health Risks/Rewards

The advantage of the vegan (and vegetarian) diet is an overall lower risk of disease. Numerous studies show that eating animal fats and proteins raises a person's risk of developing lifestyle diseases, such as cancer, diabetes, arthritis, hypertension, heart disease, obesity, and a number of other conditions.[1747] It is well documented that a whole-food, plant-based diet provides an abundance of nutrition and is crucial for reducing inflammation, a precursor to disease.

The McDougall Program

The McDougall Program is also more of a lifestyle plan than just a diet. Created by physician, and nutrition expert John A. McDougall, M.D., the program is a one-hundred percent plant-based (vegan) diet that includes whole grains and whole-grain products (such as pasta, tortillas, and whole-grain bread), a wide assortment of vegetables and fruit, plenty of spices, and usually only small amounts of sugar and salt to enhance the flavor; it also emphasizes regular exercise, as simple as a daily walk.

What sets this program apart from other plant-based programs is the exclusion of all oils, including olive oil, safflower oil, and corn oil. McDougall notes, "Oils are nothing more than liquid fats that increase obesity, which in turn, depress the immune function and contribute to the most common chronic diseases."

Health Risks/Rewards

The dietary aspect of the program is rich in vitamins, minerals, antioxidants, and fiber, with similar benefits to the Dean Ornish diet. The disadvantage for some is that this diet eliminates healthy oils, which have been shown in many research studies to help reduce heart disease, support brain and joint health, reduce inflammation, and support brain health. Furthermore, for some people, gluten is an inflammatory protein. Also, the protein contained in corn is a highly cross-reactive protein, which means that for some individuals, corn can be as proinflammatory as gluten. Very low consumption of beneficial omega-3 oils found in olive oil, fish, nuts, and seeds can contribute to health problems.

Chapter 14. Nutrient Groups for the Brain

Antioxidants, amino acids, essential fatty acids, minerals, and medicinal and culinary herbs provide essential nutrients to keep our brains healthy and protect against neurodegenerative conditions. This chapter discusses the general characteristics of these nutrient groups.

- Antioxidants
  - Enzymes
  - Phytonutrients
  - Vitamins
  - Vitamin-like nutrients
- Amino acids
- Essential fatty acids
- Herbs and whole foods
- Minerals

The next chapter provides details on specific nutrients from these groups which have a beneficial impact on brain health, neuroprotection, and reducing risk of neurodegeneration.

Antioxidants

Antioxidants are a basic tool to delay or manage dementia such as Alzheimer's because they aid in reducing the free radicals that damage the brain cells.[1749] Antioxidants include a number of phytochemicals that fight oxidation. They include phytonutrients (bioflavonoids, carotenoids, polyphenols, and indoles), enzymes (glutathione and super oxide dismutase), and vitamins and vitamin-like nutrients (vitamins A, B, C, E, CoQ10, alpha lipoic acid).

Since oxidative stress and inflammation appear to be involved in brain aging and in neurodegenerative diseases,[1750] it is theorized that increased consumption of antioxidants may be effective in preventing or ameliorating these changes. The neuroprotective effects of strawberry, bilberry, black currant, blackberry, blueberry, and mulberry, have been well documented.[1751][1752]

Neuroinflammatory processes in the brain are believed to play a crucial role in the development of neurodegenerative diseases, especially due to increased production of reactive oxygen species.[1753][1754] The free radical scavenging function of antioxidants is central to managing or preventing dementia because of the wide-spread damage caused by oxidation ranging from DNA mutation to neuroinflammation.

Polyphenols

Polyphenols[1755] are the largest group of phytonutrients and have been reported to have strong antioxidant activities in both in vitro and in vivo.[1756][1757] They are a group of over five-hundred phytochemicals which are naturally occurring micronutrients in plants. These act as powerful antioxidants to protect our health by neutralizing free radicals that occur with pollution, smoking, eating rancid foods, and as a byproduct of normal metabolism. It is also thought that polyphenols support the sympathetic nervous system,[1758] and reduce inflammation[1759] which is in turn linked to a lower risk of several chronic diseases.

The polyphenols are being closely investigated for their ability to prevent and treat neurodegenerative conditions. For example, the polyphenols curcumin, resveratrol, and tea catechins are of great interest to researchers because of their antioxidant capacity, cell signaling support, anti-inflammatory action, chelation ability, and neuroprotection – all of which are mechanisms associated with dementia.[1760][1761]

Top food sources in the polyphenol category include: apple, apple juice (pure), blackberry, blackcurrant, black chokeberry, black elderberry, black tea, celery seed, chestnut, cloves, cocoa powder, coffee (filtered), dark chocolate, flaxseed meal, green tea, hazelnut, highbush blueberry, globe artichoke heads, lowbush blueberry, Mexican oregano, plum, pomegranate juice (pure), red raspberry, red wine, soy yogurt, star anise, strawberry, sweet cherry, and whole grain rye bread.

Also high in polyphenols are black beans, black olives, broccoli, pecans, red onion, soy milk, and spinach.

Types of Polyphenols. Polyphenols include flavonoids, phenolic acids, stilbenes, coumarins, tannins, and lignans.

Flavonoids

Many epidemiological studies have shown that regular flavonoid rich fruit intake is associated with delayed Parkinson's disease, Alzheimer's disease, ischemic diseases, and aging effects.[1762][1763][1764][1765] There are more than six-thousand types of flavonoids, the largest group of phytonutrients. These plant-based biochemicals often contribute to the color of plant parts. They are divided into several groups: flavones, flavanols, flavanones, isoflavones, anthocyanidins, chalcones, and catechins, along with more subgroups. Each of these subgroups and each type of flavonoid carries its own distinct set of actions, benefits, and originating foods.

Flavonoids penetrate and accumulate in the brain regions involved in learning and memory, especially the hippocampus. They have neuroprotective benefits and neuromodulatory proteins that promote neurogenesis, neuronal function, and brain connectivity. They accomplish this through blood-flow improvement and angiogenesis (new blood vessel growth) in the brain and sensory systems. Studies indicate flavonoids offer the brain protective benefits with respect to normal aging, dementia, and stroke.[1766]

Most of the beneficial effects of flavonoids on cognition in animal models have been related to their antioxidant activity and their ability to control neuronal function, survival, synaptic plasticity, and long-term potentiation.[1767]

Flavonoids are being investigated as an aspect of nutritional interventions for dementia and mild cognitive impairment due to their antioxidant and anti-inflammatory capacity, as well as neuroprotective and metabolic function support.[1768] [1769] [1770] The knowledge of the biological actions of flavonoids assists in the development of new drugs for Alzheimer's and other neurological conditions.[1771] They play a role in controlling synaptic plasticity, reducing neuroinflammation, neurogenesis in the hippocampus, modulation of gut microbiota, and inhibition of pathological proteins.[1772]

Most vegetables are high in flavonoids, particularly those green and red in color. They are found in a wide variety of plant-based foods, particularly citrus fruits such as bananas, oranges, grapefruit, lemons, limes, vegetables, legumes, red wine, and green tea. Berries have a particularly high content of flavonoids, the best being red, blue, and purple berries. Darker and riper berries tend to have higher flavonoid value. Blackberries and black grapes are high in the flavonoids, epicatechin and catechin. Raspberries, cherries and red grapes may be high in anthocyanidins and cyanidin (best if consumed raw with the skin on), as well as beans including black and kidney beans, fava, and pinto beans, nuts (particularly walnuts, pecans, pistachios, cashews, and soybeans).

Vegetables in the nightshade family are also high in flavonoids including vegetables such as peppers, potatoes, tomatoes, and eggplants, but for many these should be avoided where chronic inflammation exists or skin conditions such as psoriasis and eczema. Other foods high in flavonoids are capers and chocolate, and spices like dill, thyme, and parsley.

Some studies showed improved cognitive function for those who regularly consumed chocolate (we recommend 85% or higher dark chocolate).[1773] [1774] Another example of the power of flavonoids is that cognitive function also increases with consumption of caper extract. Animals receiving caper bud extract exhibited decreased neurodegeneration in the hippocampus with a potential protective effect for learning and memory.[1775]

Phenolic acids

The beneficial effects of phenolic acids are well documented. They may be effective against Alzheimer's due to their anti-acetylcholinesterase and butyrylcholinesterase inhibiting action, and against amyloid beta peptide fibril formation.[1776] [1777] [1778] They play a role in reducing depression, neuroinflammation, heart disease, cell death, Parkinson's, Huntington's, ALS, and other neurological conditions.[1779]

Phenolic acids include compounds found in coffee, tea, apples, plums, pears, kiwi, grapes, mangos, cherries, as well as in vegetables including the yellow onion (highest content), cherry tomatoes, celery, broccoli, red cabbage, curly kale, artichokes, potato, rhubarb, seeds, whole wheat (including buckwheat, rye, oats, barley), rice and corn, legumes such as beans, soybeans (highest content), peas, spices (with highest content being in parsley and capsicum pepper).

Stilbenes

Stilbenes are a small group of plant chemicals. Resveratrol is probably the best-known and the most studied of them. Stilbenes such as resveratrol offer neuroprotective properties with antioxidant, anti-inflammatory, and anti-amyloid effects.[1780] Resveratrol is "a potent activator of SIRT1, and thus may mimic caloric restriction to prevent disease of aging."[1781] It plays a role in decreasing amyloid beta accumulation and toxicity, preventing damage to the hippocampus, depresses microglia activation.[1782]

There are only two stilbenes of note: resveratrol and pterostilbene. Resveratrol is a powerful antioxidant found in red wine, blueberries, cranberries, and peanuts. Consuming these foods has been linked to better heart health. Pterostilbene is found in high amounts in antioxidant-rich foods like blueberries, cranberries, and grapes, and has a higher bioavailability than many of its cousin antioxidants.

Lignans

Lignans are found in legumes, cereals, grains, fruits, algae, and some vegetables. The lignans found in Chinese magnolia (Schisandra chinesis, used in traditional Chinese medicine) have been linked with decreased cognitive impairment and improved learning and memory in AD animals.[1783] The mechanism may involve regulation of APP, neurotransmitter, and inflammatory metabolism, the antioxidant system, and formation of neurofibrillary tangles.[1784]

In other research, a lignan found in Norway spruce, 7-hydroxymatairesinol, was tested in a rodent model of Parkinson's, which slowed deterioration of the striatal dopaminergic neuron terminals (but not the cell bodies). Nonetheless motor activity improved.[1785]

The best sources of lignans include flax and sesame seeds. Whole flax seed, (rather than milled, which has much less lignan) is helpful in reducing LDL cholesterol[1786] which is the fatty type of cholesterol that goes on to form plaque. Poor circulation is a risk factor for neurodegenerative conditions, as are high levels of cholesterol in blood.[1787]

Coumarins

Coumarins are found in many plants, such as sweet woodruff, sweet grass, vanilla grass, and sweet clover. One of their bioactivities is their ability to become anti-Alzheimer's. They are also anti-inflammatory, antioxidant,[1788] antiviral, antimicrobial and antidepressant.[1789] Their value as a tool for AD is that they inhibit acetylcholinesterase.[1790] Their anti-coagulant capacity makes them a tool where blood thinners and clot-dissolvers are needed.

Tannins

One group of tannins, proanthocyanidins that are found in lentils, grape seed, apples, and cocoa seeds. This beneficial actions reduces oxidation of LDL cholesterol, protecting against chromosomal damage,[1791] and is a powerful antioxidant.[1792] These are functions that help reduce the risk of dementia and related conditions.

Amino Acids

Amino acids are biochemical compounds that combine to create proteins. The two are the building blocks of life. Furthermore, when proteins break down through digestion or other processes, they separate out into amino acids again.[1793] There are a number of ways of classifying amino acids. One way is to identify them by whether the body can produce them or whether they must come from food; these are the essential amino acids that cannot be made by the body. Two groups of essential amino acids, aromatic and acidic, are needed for proper brain function.

The aromatic amino acids include tryptophan, tyrosine, phenylalanine that are biosynthetic precursors for the neurotransmitters, serotonin, dopamine, and norepinephrine. Single meals, depending on their protein content, can rapidly influence uptake of aromatic amino acid into the brain, directly modifying their conversion to neurotransmitters. If these amino acids are not available in required amounts, this will directly affect the release of neurotransmitters from neurons, resulting in reduction in brain function.

Nonessential amino acids are produced by the body. Seven of them are used by the brain and enter the brain at varying rates: glycine, proline, serine, alanine, cysteine, aspartate, and glutamate. Serine and alanine are essential for the brain. Serine makes glycine, alanine makes glutamate and aspartate.[1794]

Of these the acidic amino acids, glutamate, and aspartate, are themselves brain neurotransmitters. Glutamate, for example is required, but excess glutamate (as from adding monosodium glutamate (MSG) to food) becomes toxic to nerve cells.[1795]

Essential Fatty Acids

Of the omega-3s, EPA and DHA are essential for both brain health and general well-being. DHA is especially important for brain health. It is needed for cognitive functioning and memory.[1796] Although omega-6 fats are essential (GLA provides the healthy, anti-inflammatory type of omega-6) the modern Western diet contains far more omega-6 fatty acids than necessary.[1797] The recommended ratio of omega-6 to omega-3 fatty acids in the diet is 4:1 or less. However, the Western diet has a ratio between 10:1 and 50:1 due primarily to the excess carbohydrates and sugars in the common diet, particularly white starches and sugars, vegetable oils and foods containing transfatty acids. Omega 7s are an overlooked, lesser known essential fatty acid which are helpful against the metabolic disorders that underlie diabetes, cardiovascular disease, obesity, and cancer. Omega-7 found in salmon, anchovies and olive oil is important as an anti-inflammatory agent.

Vitamins and Minerals

When we think of good nutrition, we most commonly think of vitamins and minerals, and with good reason. Acting together, they perform hundreds, perhaps thousands of roles in the body. In good supply, they build and protect bones, provide immune support, repair damage on both the macro and cellular level, and they convert food into energy. Thirteen vitamins are considered essential. These are vitamins A, C, D, E, K and eight B vitamins: thiamine (B1), riboflavin (B2), niacin (B3), pantothenic acid (B5), pyroxidine (B6), biotin (B7), folate (B9) and cobalamin (B12). Four of them (A, D, E, and K) are fat-soluble and are stored in fatty tissue. And the body produces some of them naturally: D from sunlight, and K produced by bacteria in the intestinal system.

Essential minerals for the body and the brain fall into two main groups, those that comprise much of the body's mineral supply, and those that are present only in trace amounts, but which are essential for healthy functioning. The balance of minerals, enzymes, and various neurobiological compounds form the basis of the health brain.

Herbs and whole foods

A wide variety of both medicinal and culinary herbs and whole foods are important sources of antioxidants, amino acids, essential fatty acids, minerals, vitamins and vitamin-like biochemicals found in plants. Some are traditionally used, with knowledge of their specific capacities going back thousands of years. Many of these traditional medicinal herbs as well as more common phytonutrients are being researched extensively for both their value in addressing neurodegenerative conditions, and for their value in the process of exploring why neurodegenerative conditions occur.

Chapter 15. The Nutrients

These are the nutrients which appear, based on peer-reviewed research, to be most important for protecting the brain from neuroinflammation and neurodegeneration, and reducing the risk of dementia and related conditions. What is important is that you enjoy a mostly plant-based diet with a wide variety of polyphenols and other biocompounds that provide these nutrients and that you get plenty of exercise and manage other conditions that may contribute to the onset of dementia.

If you would like to read abstracts of the studies that we've referenced, an easy place to do so is at PubMed (ncbi.nlm.nih.gov/pubmed), the research database of the National Institutes of Health. We've tried to include the newest research as of fall, 2019. You can search there for newer research on dementia and nutrients that catch your interest.

This section discusses a wide range of nutrients. Of those, pay special attention to the following:

- Ashwagandha
- Baicalein
- Bacopa monnieri

Acetyl-l-carnitine. (500mg per day best taken on an empty stomach). Acetyl-l-carnitine is the short-chain ester of carnitine, an amino acid that crosses the blood-brain barrier and guards against oxidative damage.[1798] It supports the mitochondria (energy producers in our cells), and lowers the increased oxidative stress associated with aging and has neuroprotective properties against oxidative stress) that can lead to amyloid-beta peptides, a principal component of plaques.

It protects against neurotoxic insults and may be an effective treatment for certain forms of depression.[1799] N-acetyl-carnitine may improve fatigue in the elderly,[1800][1801] and may raise the levels of nerve growth factor and increase the activity of acetylcholine, a neurotransmitter that is critical to healthy brain function and is substantially lost in Alzheimer's disease.[1802]

A small double-blind placebo-controlled twelve-week trial, using 2250 to 3000mg daily found that neuropsychological tests (MMSE, CGI, etc.) were markedly better than placebo, and did not depend on the baseline cognitive impairment. The researchers recommend it for early stages of Alzheimer's and vascular dementia.[1803]

Acetyl-l-carnitine supports neurogenesis in the brain resulting in improvements in memory and learning (due to increased synaptic neurotransmission)[1804] as well as mental status and cognitive function.[1805][1806][1807][1808][1809]

N-acetyl-L-cysteine is also the chemical precursor to glutathione and is a safe antidote for cysteine/glutathione deficiency.[1810]

Food sources: beef, milk, codfish, and chicken breast.

Acetyl-cysteine (NAC) (500mg – 1500mg per day) is one of the precursors for glutathione produced in the liver which is essential for brain and overall health. It is an excellent scavenger against reactive oxygen species (ROS),[1811] reducing cell death,[1812] which stimulate tau hyperphosphorylation.[1813] In addition to reducing inflammation and fighting free radicals, NAC stabilizes mitochondria in Alzheimer's patients.[1814] NAC at dosages of 50 or 100 mg/kg can significantly reduced tau positive cells in all the regions of the hippocampus, thereby minimizing neuronal loss and cognitive deficits.[1815] N-acetyl-L-cysteine is also the chemical precursor to glutathione and is a safe antidote for cysteine/glutathione deficiency.[1816]

Alpha lipoic acid. (150mg per day in "R" form (the most biologically available) or 300mg per day in combination of both "S" and "R" forms). ALA has been called the "universal" antioxidant because it boosts glutathione levels in cells already within a normal range, and has potent antioxidant actions, reducing oxidative stress.[1817 1818 1819 1820]

The alpha R form is the one most easily utilized by the body. Supplementation with alpha lipoic acid inhibits progress of tau protein toward fibrils of plaque, reduces cognitive decline, lipid peroxidation, inflammation, and tau-induced iron overload.[1821]

Its therapeutic potential for different neurogenerative diseases,[1822 1823 1824] including Alzheimer's[1825 1826] is due to noted improved mitochondrial function in Alzheimer's,[1827 1828] and Parkinson's patients.[1829 1830] It protects against age-related cognitive dysfunction for those with AD and other neurodegenerative conditions.[1831 1832 1833 1834 1835] Studies aiming to assess the neuroprotective effects of LA on behavioral outcomes show that LA can reduce memory deficits in different behavioral paradigms of AD.[1836 1837 1838]

A small 12-month placebo-controlled trial compared treatment with omega-3 and alpha lipoic acid with placebo and omega-3 alone finding little change in rate of decline, but because of the small sample the authors felt further investigation was warranted.[1839]

Food sources for ALA: leafy greens like spinach, broccoli tomatoes, and Brussels sprouts, beef liver, rice bran, yams, and potatoes. Intake of ALA, contained e.g., in nuts, might also directly contribute to the beneficial effects of Mediterranean diet on cognition and brain plasticity.[1840 1841]

Amla (Emblica officinalis) (500mg per day) belongs to the family Euphorbiaceae. It is an important ayurvedic medicinal herb and its fruits contain powerful antioxidant components: tannins and tannoids, vitamin C and bioflavonoids. Its anti-inflammatory, antioxidant, and other properties makes it ideal for synergistic value in enhancing other nutrients and medicinal herbs.[1842] Because it helps to enhance memory and reduce memory impairment, formulations containing it may have a role in managing conditions such as Alzheimer's and other impaired-memory conditions.[1843] Amla also possesses anti-cholinesterase[1844] activity which further suggests its potential for treatment of cognitive impairments induced by cholinergic dysfunction.[1845]

Apigenin (50mg once or twice daily) has been known to promote neurogenesis. It also has demonstrated anti-inflammatory, anticarcinogenic, and free radical-scavenging activities. In a mouse study, it protects brain neurovascular coupling against amyloid beta, reduces oxidative stress of cerebral cortex, protects cerebrovascular function, improves learning and memory capabilities, maintains neurovascular unit integrity, modulates microvascular function, increases regional cerebral blood flow, reduces neurovascular oxidative damage, and improves the cholinergic system. [1846] In another study, apigenin was shown to reduce inflammation and apoptosis (cell death) in the brain for those with AD.[1847]

Food sources: This little-known flavonoid is found in many fruits and vegetables including grapefruit, celery, and parsley.

Ashwagandha (Withania somnifera, 500mg twice per day with meals). Also known as Indian winter cherry or Indian ginseng, the root extract is another very important ayurvedic medicinal herb used as a nerve tonic[1848][1849][1850] and to handle stress.[1851][1852] It boosts the immune system,[1853] has strong antioxidant properties, may reduce inflammation (by inhibiting release of proinflammatory cytokines from microglial cells in vitro[1854]), and reduces neuronal cell death.[1855][1856][1857][1858] It may stimulate dendrite formation,[1859][1860] stimulate neurite outgrowth,[1861][1862][1863] and improve synaptic function.[1864][1865]

It is reported to increase immediate and general memory,[1866] and learning.[1867][1868] And in mouse models of AD, it reverses behavioral deficits, plaque load, and accumulation of beta-amyloid peptides[1869] that are linked to memory deficit.[1870] Aqueous extracts have been shown to increase acetylcholine content and choline acetyl transferase activity in rats. This might partly explain its cognition-enhancing and memory-improving effects.[1871][1872] It affects how the liver processes low-density lipoprotein, which increases beta amyloid in the blood, and decreases it in the brain.[1873] Studies of molecular modeling show its components (anamides A and C) bind to beta-amyloid and prevent fibril formation.[1874][1875] Neuronal cell death triggered by amyloid plaques was also blocked by with ashwagandha anamides.[1876][1877][1878]

As part of a complementary treatment strategy in neurodegenerative diseases such as Parkinson's, Huntington's, and Alzheimer's, ashwagandha supports daily living without adverse effects by reducing anxiety[1879] (in 88% of subjects)[1880] improving reaction time, task performance,[1881] and the ability to concentrate.[1882] The leaves also have nootropic (substances that may improve cognitive function) potential with multiple benefits including reversing Alzheimer and Parkinson pathologies, protecting against environmental neurotoxins, and enhancing memory.[1883]

Astaxanthin (AXT) (6–12 mg per day) crosses the blood-brain barrier.[1884] It is a potent antioxidant with a biological activity many times higher than that of alpha-tocopherol and beta-carotene.[1885] Benefits include: cardiovascular health, metabolic syndrome, treatment of gastric ulcers, and cancer, all of which have elements of inflammation and/or oxidative stress in their pathogenesis. Researchers find that it can specifically modulate microglial function,[1886][1887] by reducing oxidative stress and damage, which results in neuroprotective mechanisms.[1888][1889]

It reduces oxidative stress in vitro,[1890] oxidative biomarkers,[1891][1892][1893] oxidative damage in the aging hippocampus,[1894] and in the central nervous system.[1895] It may also influence synaptic plasticity through inducing an upregulation in BDNF.[1896][1897][1898] AXT supports cognition,[1899] learning, memory, and reaction time.[1900] It reduces neurotoxicity in cell culture models of Alzheimer's where PC12 cells were protected from cytotoxicity induced by amyloid beta fragments.[1901][1902] (PC12 cells are cells labs use that are able to reproduce for research and are useful as a model for studying neural differentiation and neurosecretion.) Not only can AXT treatment promote neurogenesis but it offers direct protection to insulted cells and limits the resulting sequence of cell death.[1903]

Sources: Natural AXT is produced from algae, yeast, and crustacean byproduct.

Avocado promotes healthy blood flow, helps lower blood pressure (a risk factor for cognitive decline), and reduces the risk of heart disease as it increases HDL-cholesterol concentrations.[1904] There is evidence for increased oxidative damage to macromolecules in a number of neurodegenerative diseases, and avocados have a large amounts of phytochemicals especially antioxidants.[1905] Avocados are cholesterol-free and loaded with the antioxidant lutein, monounsaturated fats, fiber, and other nutrients, and they are high in potassium and contain a wide range of other vitamins and minerals.[1906] Avocados and avocado oil are high in monounsaturated oleic acid, a heart-healthy fatty acid that is believed to be one of the main reasons for the health benefits of olive oil.

Bacopa monnieri (Brahmi, 250mg two times per day). Bacopa's active components, the saponins bacoside A and B, provide the beneficial effect on neurophysiological function.[1907][1908] Traditionally, brahmi has been used to improve memory[1909][1910] and cognitive function,[1911] and its   antioxidant capacity protects against oxidative stress.[1912][1913] Bacopa improves acetylcholinergic function, (protecting nerve cells from cell death)[1914] one of the brain's key neurotransmitters by decreasing muscarinic cholinergic receptor binding (one of two major receptors being targeted in Alzheimer's research) in the frontal cortex and hippocampus.[1915] It also protects membranes from damage in animal studies and in healthy humans.[1916][1917][1918]

In the hippocampus, bacopa supports the activity of enzymes (protein kinases) that regulate protein activity that may contribute to its ability to improve cognitive capacity, especially decision making, memory, creativity, and motivation.[1919] This neuroprotective effectiveness may be closely related to reducing inflammation[1920][1921][1922] which may account for its anti-arthritis activity.[1923]

In addition to the neuro-beneficial effects, bacopa reduces stress[1924] and anxiety.[1925] There are reports of improvement in healthy patients in ability to remember new information,[1926] in ignoring irrelevant information,[1927] and in verbal learning, memory acquisition, and delayed recall.[1928]

Baicalein is not available as a separate supplement though it is in certain herbal combinations. It is found in skullcap extract, (200-800 mg in multiple doses, once in the morning and once again at night) Baicalein is a flavonoid compound extracted from dried roots of traditional Chinese medicine scutellaria baicalensis (huang qin) and is widely used as an antioxidant and anti-inflammatory agent without side effects. It is found in relatively high amounts (compared to other plants) in the roots of scutellaria baicalensis georgi (skullcap).[1929]

Baicalein and the structurally similar **baicalin** act on the central nervous system[1930][1931] and can inhibit the activity of neurons that raise anxiety,[1932][1933] and can cross the blood brain barrier.[1934] Baicalein is a major component of flavonoids with anti-neuroinflammatory properties against damage caused by ischemia and reperfusion[1935][1936] (the process of restoring blood flow after a heart attack or stroke). It is a potent free-radical scavenger with antiallergic, anticarcinogenic, antiviral, and antibacterial properties.[1937] In mouse studies, baicalin improves cognitive function through this anti-neuroinflammatory activity and thus is a potential candidate for the treatment of Alzheimer's disease,[1938] improved amyloid beta-induced learning and memory deficit, damage to the hippocampus, and neuron cell death.[1939] It promotes neurogenesis in damaged sections of the brain, including in the hippocampus.[1940] It has been of great interest to investigators due to its versatility as a therapeutic agent for neurological diseases.[1941] In addition to its value in treating Alzheimer's it may be that indirect action on impaired insulin signaling and glucose metabolism accounts for the protective effect.[1942] Baicalein has a wide safety of margin and appears to be able to cross the blood-brain barrier (BBB),[1943] and may play a role in healing the BBB by reducing permeability.[1944]

Food sources: common fruits and vegetables such as onions, parsley, as well as oranges, tea, chamomile, and wheat sprouts.

Blueberries are flavonoid-rich fruit intake associated with delayed Parkinson's, Alzheimer's, ischemic diseases, and the effects of aging.[1945][1946][1947] The blue anthocyanin flavonoid pigment they contain can cross the blood-brain barrier so that it helps support neurogenesis and BDNF levels. Researchers note that these flavonoids increase spatial working memory, as well as modulating neural plasticity in the hippocampus, and improved cognitive behavior.[1948][1949] Supplementation with wild blueberry juice improves paired associate learning and word list recall.[1950] In another study supplementing with a formulation containing blueberry (including resveratrol), green tea, carnosine, vitamin D3, and biovin (grape extract), resulted in significantly increased processing speed.[1951]

Blueberries may help neurodegenerative diseases due to their ability to improve neurotransmission, protect against brain injury, stroke, and hinder certain neurotoxins and excitotoxicity.[1952][1953][1954][1955][1956][1957][1958] In other studies, scientists have discovered mechanisms to explain why blueberries can improve memory and restore healthy neuronal function to aged brains.[1959][1960][1961][1962] Black currants, blackberries, and bilberries exert similar effects.[1963][1964][1965]

Boswellia (Indian frankincense, 500mg per day) can inhibit the creation of a pro-inflammatory compound (leukotriene) biosynthesis in the most common type of white blood cells (neutrophilic granulocytes) by inhibiting the 5-LOX enzyme which transforms fatty acids into leukotrienes. In that way it inhibits various inflammatory diseases that are promoted by leukotrienes.[1966] The main bioactive compound of boswellia are boswellic acids which can cross the blood-brain barrier; their strong anti-inflammatory ability may be helpful in the early stages (and recovery from) stroke.[1967]

Broccoli is a member of the cruciferous family which also includes cabbage, kales, Brussel sprouts, and cauliflower. It contains significant amounts of powerful antioxidants. Its benefits include providing potent antioxidants, regulating enzymes, and controlling apoptosis (cell death), and vitamins E, C, K, and minerals such as iron, zinc, selenium, and the polyphenols kaempferol, quercetin glucosides, and isorhamnetin.[1968]

Cat's Claw (Uncaria tomentosa, 20mg-60mg daily) has been shown to prevent the activation of the transcription factor NF-kB and it directly inhibits TNF-alpha production by up to 65-85 percent,[1969][1970][1971] helping to reduce inflammation. Transcription factors are proteins that control the rate of genetic information transfer from DNA to RNA. The NF-kB transcription factor family of proteins are involved in immune and inflammatory responses, developmental processes, cell growth, and cell death.[1972]

Catechin is a flavonoid that can cross the blood brain barrier. It has powerful anti-inflammatory benefits. It is suggested that these bioactive tea components might be useful for neuronal degeneration treatment in the future.[1973] Green tea is a popular source for catechins.

Note. Decaffeinated green tea combined with ashwagandha, rhodiola, and panax ginseng and choline help to promote improved focus and increased energy while enhancing endurance and stamina.

Food sources: apricots, blackberries, black grapes, blueberries, black grapes, brewed black tea such as Darjeeling, peaches, raspberries, strawberries, chocolate, and red wine.

Celastrus paniculatus (Celastraceae family, 60mg per day) is of interest to researchers in neurodegenerative conditions such as Alzheimer's disease.[1974] Due to its antioxidant properties it prevents nerve cell damage against hydrogen peroxide toxicity[1975][1976] and glutamine induced toxicity.[1977] It helps improve memory performance.[1978][1979] Celastrus increases cholinergic activity that contributes to its ability to improve memory performance[1980] and cognitive function.[1981] Additionally, celastrus has antidepressant properties probably due to interaction with dopamine-D2, serotonergic, and GABA receptors. It is also an MAO-A (an enzyme) inhibitor, and can reduce blood corticosterone levels.[1982][1983]

Centella asiatica (gota kola, 700mg - 1400mg per day) is flavonoid-rich and belongs to the family Apiaceae. Gota kola is one of the important rejuvenating herbs for nerve and brain cells and is believed to be capable of increasing intelligence, longevity, and memory[1984][1985] It may also be helpful for AD, reverse amyloid beta toxicity in the brain,[1986][1987] and modulate mitochondrial oxidative stress[1988] and cell death.[1989][1990] Some of the compounds in gota kola are seen to reduce damage to nerve dendrites and nerve spine densities due to amyloid beta.[1991] It is also seen to reduce mitochondrial dysfunction[1992] in the hippocampus and improve memory and decision making in mouse models of AD.[1993] Studies on a few healthy human adults have shown promising cognitive-enhancing effects of gotu kola extracts.[1994][1995]

Chocolate (dark) and cocoa powder are packed with a few brain-boosting compounds, including flavonoids, caffeine, and antioxidants, and are high in flavonoids that may enhance memory and also help slow down age-related mental decline. It may support both visual acuity and cognitive function, explained by increased cerebral blood flow and induced retinal blood flow changes.[1996]

Choline (425mg for women–550 mg per day for men). Choline is an essential nutrient that is naturally present in some foods and available as a dietary supplement, is a water-soluble vitamin-like essential nutrient, and is a constituent of lecithin (present in many plants and animal organs).

Studies indicate that choline is recycled in the liver and redistributed from the kidney, lung, and intestine to the liver and brain when choline supply is low.[1997] Although some choline can be produced by the body, it is not enough to support healthy brain function so needs to be added through food (and supplements if needed).[1998]Choline is a source of methyl groups needed for many steps in metabolism and makes acetylcholine[1999][2000][2001] in our brains. Acetylcholine is an important neurotransmitter for memory, mood, muscle control, and other brain and nervous system function.

Choline also plays important roles in modulating gene expression, cell membrane signaling, lipid transport and metabolism, and early brain development.[2002][2003] Inside cells choline is converted to phosphatidylcholine and is used in the building and rejuvenation of cell membranes, especially in the brain.[2004] Choline, methionine, and folate metabolism interact at the point that homocysteine is converted to the essential amino acid methionine.[2005]

Higher choline intake is related to better cognitive performance.[2006] It is associated with various aspects of focus, stamina, and learning. Some Alzheimer's patients are reported to have acetylcholine as much as ninety percent lower than average, so memory loss may be closely linked to its deficiency.[2007]

Food sources: caviar, brewer's yeast, shiitake mushrooms, poultry, fish, shellfish, beef liver, dairy foods, eggs, wheat, rice, red potatoes, spinach, beets, legumes, Brussel sprouts and other cruciferous vegetables, and sunflower seeds.

Coffee. Coffee contains caffeine and antioxidants. Drinking coffee over the long term is linked to a reduced risk of neurological diseases, such as Parkinson's and Alzheimer's.[2008][2009][2010][2011] One meta-analysis found that subjects with the highest daily coffee consumption had a significant twenty-seven percent reduction in their risk for developing Alzheimer's disease (but only AD), compared with lower- or non-coffee drinkers.[2012] A newer meta-analysis[2013] however, included 34,282 participants, and found significant differences not only in Alzheimer's, but also in other cognitive threats.

Mice with Alzheimer's disease given caffeinated coffee showed improved immune responses in their brains that may help to clear beta-amyloid.[2014] One study showed that moderate drinkers during midlife (3-5 cups per day) has a sixty-five percent reduced risk of onset of dementia later in life.[2015] In addition, for those with mild cognitive impairment who had high caffeine plasma levels due to drinking three to five cups of coffee per day avoided having the dementia progress for the next two to four years.[2016]

A ten-year prospective cohort study in Europe showed that older men who consumed coffee had a ten-year loss of cognitive function of 1.2 points on a standard mental status examination, while non-coffee drinkers had an additional 1.4-point loss, a significant worsening of cognitive function.[2017] These benefits could be attributed to the high amounts of antioxidants[2018][2019] and other compounds in coffee rather than the caffeine content. A minor component of coffee unrelated to caffeine, eicosanoyl-5-hydroxytryptamide (EHT), provides protection in a rat model for AD. Dietary supplementation with EHT for six to twelve months resulted in substantial improvement in AD symptoms and pathology including reduced cognitive impairment, tau hyperphosphorylation, and elevated levels of cytoplasmic amyloid beta protein. EHT may also lower the risk on AD onset.[2020] Another animal study indicated that EHT improves the cognitive capacity of Parkinsonian mice linked to reduced fibril aggregation and phosphorylation, improved nerve health, and reduced neuroinflammation.[2021] A number of non-caffeine components of coffee have been tested as to their ability to inhibit amyloid-beta and tau aggregation. Researchers tested three instant coffee extracts (light roast, dark roast, and decaffeinated dark roast) and six compounds found in coffee: caffeine, chlorogenic acid (the major polyphenolic acid in coffee beans), quinic acid, caffeic acid, quercetin, and phenylindane. They discovered the following:[2022]

- All of the instant coffee extracts inhibited fibrillization and also promoted a-synuclein oligomerization. Oligomerization refers to the process of converting a compound into a structure that consists of oligomers, molecules with few repeating units.
- Dark coffee roast extracts were more effective oligomerization inhibitors than light roast.
- Pure caffeine had no effect.
- The coffee components chlorogenic acid, caffeic acid and quercetin inhibited amyloid beta fibrillization.
- Quercetin inhibited amyloid beta oligomerization.
- Caffeic acid and quercetin promote the aggregation of α-synuclein at higher concentrations. This could have a neuroprotective effect by promoting Lewy body formation and reducing concentrations of these toxic oligomers in the brain.
- Phenylindane was the only component that inhibited both amyloid beta and tau fibrillization as well as amyloid beta oligomerization.

In general, we do not recommend drinking more than two to three cups of coffee per day as it does have an effect on cortisol levels. There are many other natural herbal ways to increase energy including ginseng (American and Chinese), green tea and gingko biloba, ginger, and schisandra. Decaffeinated coffee is a good alternative since it still contains the valuable anti-inflammatory and antioxidant flavonoids and other compounds such as EHT,[2023] caffeic acid, quercetin, and phenylindane.[2024]

Note: From a Chinese medical perspective, those that tend toward having excess heat should avoid coffee. Although coffee's vasoconstrictor properties (due to caffeine) are minimal, it may be contraindicated for those with macular degeneration, Raynaud's, coronary artery disease, etc. as it does reduce blood flow to the brain, retina, and throughout the body.[2025][2026][2027][2028] Decaffeinated coffee may be a better option for these people.

Convolvulus pluricaulis (shankapushpi, no specific dosage)an Ayurvedic herb is available in powder form. It is used as a memory enhancing agent and may be useful for treatment of Alzheimer's[2029] in part, because it inhibits amyloid beta fibrillation.[2030] Several kinds of convolvulus extracts increase memory function and learning ability.[2031][2032] It contains a number of secondary metabolites such as steroids, anthocyanins, flavonol glycosides, and triterpenoids that support memory and other cognitive-related functions.[2033] Researchers have identified one of the extracts (from n-butanol), that inhibits symptoms of neurodegeneration (such as weight loss, grip strength, gait dysfunction, and locomotor problems), and in addition to improves the metabolic profile in the striatum and cortex — all of which accelerate the brain's antioxidant defense system.[2034] Convolvulus petal extract has been reported to reduce anxiety.[2035] This herb also has the potential to improve memory and decrease cholesterol.[2036]

Copper is used by the brain help control nerve signals. Too low or too high copper levels can seriously affect brain functions.[2037] It plays an essential role in nerve synopsis and regulates homeostasis of proteins. This is particularly relevant to neurological disorders such as Alzheimer's where copper and protein dyshomeostasis may contribute to neurodegeneration.[2038]

Plasma copper levels in and free serum copper levels are both elevated in aging and in brains with AD.[2039][2040] Elevated free copper negatively correlates with cognition, predicts the rate cognitive decline,[2041] and promotes amyloid beta aggregation.[2042]

Food sources of copper: avocado, chick peas, dried fruit (prunes), fermented soy foods (tempeh) goat cheese, liver, oysters (cooked), raw kale, spirulina, shiitake mushrooms, cashew nuts, sesame seeds, lobster, leafy greens, and dark chocolate.[2043]

CoQ10 (ubiquinol form, 100mg -200mg per day) is a potent antioxidant that promotes cellular energy production in heart, brain, and muscle tissue. Production of CoQ10 reduces in the body as one ages up to seventy percent in heart muscle,[2044] and also is affected by intake of statin drugs[2045][2046] by possibly up to forty percent.[2047][2048] It is concentrated in high energy organs such as the brain.[2049][2050][2051] CoQ10 is a neuroprotective antioxidant that reduces oxidative stress,[2052] amyloid pathology,[2053] and behavioral dysfunction. CoQ10 helps prevent cell death[2054] and is anti-inflammatory.[2055] It is essential for healthy mitochondrial function[2056] suggesting its benefit for Parkinson's patients.[2057]

Note. Anyone on statin drugs should be supplementing with CoQ10.

Food sources: organ (heart, liver, and kidney) and other meats (pork, beef, and chicken), fatty fish (trout, herring, mackerel, and sardines), spinach, cauliflower, broccoli, oranges, strawberries, soybeans, lentils, and peanuts.

Curcumin (Curcuma longa, 500mg–1200mg per day). Curcumin is the yellow herb turmeric often used in Indian and Middle Eastern cooking to make curry spice. It has powerful antioxidant and anti-inflammatory properties,[2058][2059][2060] and can cross the blood-brain barrier reducing oxidative stress around neurons and glial cells that is significantly associated with brain aging and injury.[2061] It decreases LDL oxidation and fights free radicals that trigger nerve deterioration[2062] in conditions such as Alzheimer's,[2063][2064][2065][2066] Parkinson's,[2067][2068] and neurodegenerative disease.[2069][2070] Curcumin has been shown to improve cognitive function in the aging population.[2071][2072] Other studies show that curcumin boosts brain-derived neurotrophic factor (BDNF) and may help delay age-related mental decline and dementia.[2073][2074]

Curcumin consumption supports the immune system in clearing amyloid protein[2075][2076][2077] by binding to it and preventing it from misfolding into fibrils to form tau tangles.[2078][2079] In AD mice given low doses of curcumin, levels of beta-amyloid decreased by around forty percent compared to control. In addition, low doses of curcumin also caused a forty-three percent decrease in the plaque burden that beta-amyloid has on the brains of AD mice. Surprisingly, low doses of curcumin given over longer periods were more effective than high doses in combating the neurodegenerative process of AD.[2080]

Food sources are primarily the spice curry, often used in Indian and Indonesian food. For best absorption, a curcumin supplement should have either piperine (a pepper extract) added and/or phospholipids such as lecithin to improve bioavailability. An older study showed that adding 20mg of piperine to 2g of curcumin improved its bioavailability markedly.[2081] About five percent of turmeric is curcumin and about five percent of black pepper (by weight) is piperine. Even 1/20th of piperine improves bioavailability. Curcumin is also fat soluble, so cook your turmeric and black pepper (freshly ground) briefly in oil before adding.

Note. Although a six-month pilot showed that curcumin doses up to 4g daily were safe,[2082] curcumin taken in high dosages may be toxic, so higher doses than what is recommended above should only be done under a health care professionals care. For some people, higher dosage in the amount suggested above may result in some numbness, so start with a lower amount first then work you way up to the higher dosage depending on how you feel. It may also have slight blood thinning properties so should not be taken without your doctors' supervision if on blood thinners. Curcumin is not recommended for persons with biliary tract obstruction because it stimulates bile secretion. It is also not recommended for people with gallstones, obstructive jaundice, and acute biliary colic. Curcumin supplementation of 20-40 mg have been reported to increase gallbladder contractions in healthy people.[2083] [2084]

Dehydroepiandrosterone (DHEA, 25mg per day). Dehydroepiandrosterone (DHEA) and its sulfate (DHEA-S) are two active hormones (androgens) mainly produced by the adrenal glands. DHEA is the most abundant steroid hormone in humans, has biological effects throughout the body, and is produced by the gonads, adrenal glands, and by the brain. It is a neurosteroid (brain steroid).[2085] The body uses DHEA to produce other hormones such as estrogen and testosterone, but production declines with aging. It has strong antioxidant activity and supports nerve health; DHEA-S is supports executive function and memory. It has its own receptors in cells in the brain.[2086]

In cases of depression, low DHEA levels are seen along with brain volume shrinkage. High cortisol/low DHEA ratios are linked to smaller hippocampal volume in people with major depression.[2087] Low levels seen in older women with mild-to-moderate cognitive impairment (a likely precursor to Alzheimer's), were improved by taking 25mg/day resulting in increased cognitive scores and daily living skills, along with improved verbal test scores.[2088] Researchers attribute its ability to reduce depression to increasing neurogenesis when it stimulates a specific receptor (sigma-1).[2089]

Studies show that people with higher DHEA levels have less mental confusion, lower anxiety, and a less negative mood.[2090] The only way to get more DHEA than your adrenal glands produce is to take a DHEA supplement.

Note. As DHEA is a hormone, discuss dosages with your doctor before adding as a supplement. Cholesterol-lowering medications (statins) reduce DHEA content and therefore accelerate the aging process.[2091]

2-dimethylaminoethanol (DMAE, 150 mg per day as dimethylaminoethanol bitartrate). DMAE is a free-radical scavenger and a precursor of choline, which in turn supports increased production of the neurotransmitter acetylcholine.[2092] DMAE is sometimes taken as centrophenoxine resulting in better absorption because the active molecule is bound to an absorption enhancer.[2093] Another form, dimethylaminoethanol pyroglutamate (DMAE p-Glu) reduces memory impairments in animals.[2094]

It may possibly reduce accumulation of amyloid beta in the brain by stabilizing cell membranes[2095] which has been considered one of the main mechanisms of aging.[2096] However, only anecdotal evidence exists of a direct amyloid beta link.

Food sources: salmon, anchovies, and sardines.

Dopamine is an essential neurotransmitter that is associated with the sense of reward, motivation, memory, attention, and it also regulates body movements.[2097][2098] Low dopamine levels are linked to reduced motivation, and enthusiasm along with fatigue and apathy,[2099] inability to concentrate, forgetfulness, moodiness, insomnia, and sugar cravings.

Studies show that increasing the amount of tyrosine and phenylalanine in the diet can increase dopamine levels in the brain, which may promote thinking and improve memory. Natural ways to promote dopamine include eating protein (tyrosine and phenylalanine)[2100][2101][2102] which are found in protein-rich foods like almonds, turkey, beef, eggs, dairy, bananas, beans, soy and legumes. You can also increase dopamine by reducing the amount of saturated fat, supplementing with probiotics, consuming velvet beans (also known as Mucuna pruriens), exercise regularly, and get enough sleep.

Dopamine is depleted in Parkinson's patients, and therapy has included replacing it with levodopa[2103] or dopamine agonists. Imbalances in dopamine (due to addiction, over-medication, extended medication) can result in dopamine dysregulation syndrome with symptoms of hallucinations, panic attacks, etc.[2104][2105]

Folate (folic acid/vitamin B9, 1,000mcg–5,000mcg per day). Folate is needed to support choline in the body, so a deficiency in folate may affect brain support.[2106] Adequate levels of folate are essential for brain function, and folate deficiency can lead to neurological disorders, such as depression[2107] and cognitive impairment.[2108]

Folate supplementation either by itself or in combination with other drugs has proved helpful in cases of AD or dementia.[2109][2110][2111][2112] In a six-month double-blind placebo-controlled study of AD patients who were given 1mg of folic acid to supplement their prescription cholinesterase inhibitors, improved outcomes were noted with respect to changes in homocysteine levels.[2113]

Folate helps with DNA repair, inhibits DNA breakage, and bolsters DNA methylation. Folic acid and vitamin B12 are required for the synthesis of methionine and s-adenosylmethionine (SAM), the common methyl donor required for the maintenance of methylation patterns in DNA.[2114] From an epigenetics point of view, folic acid deficiency inhibits re-methylation of SAM and s-adenosyl homocysteine (factors in chromosome instability).[2115]

Foods that supply folate: citrus fruits, cruciferous vegetables, eggs, fortified grains, legumes, green beans, green, leafy vegetables, nuts and seeds, radishes, turnips, and wheat germ.

Garlic (optimized, 1200mg per day) has over 1,000 research publications regarding its health benefits over the last decade. Its use for healing goes back to the Egyptian times in 1550 BC. The health benefits of garlic and its preparations have been widely recognized for prevention and treatment of cardiovascular disease and other metabolic diseases, cancer, and diabetes.[2116] Many of the research results from early years are mixed.[2117] [2118] This may be because a variety of extracts were tested and some, such as aged garlic extracts, are more efficient.

One common cause of a wide variety of neurodegenerative conditions is cerebrovascular dysfunction.[2119] Garlic's support for the cardiovascular system is well documented has much potential as a prevention of and therapy for dementia. It has been observed to reduce thrombosis, high blood pressure, atherosclerosis, high cholesterol, suppresses LDL oxidation,[2120] [2121] [2122] [2123] and it supports healthy platelet function.[2124] [2125] Fibrinolysis (the process of preventing blood clots that occur naturally) is also enhanced by garlic, resulting in dissociation of clots and thrombi[2126] [2127] by 36–130 percent over a three-week to three-month period in healthy patients as well as patients who had a heart attack.[2128] [2129]

Garlic is a potent antioxidant and is reported to be effective against diseases of which oxidative stress is a cause.[2130] It boosts the levels of natural glutathione,[2131] [2132] [2133] is an important cellular detoxifier, and as much as 5-10 grams of garlic extract boosts the immune system.[2134] [2135] [2136]

Aged garlic stands out as having superior beneficial effects, (600mg per day) including hepatoprotective, neuroprotective, and antioxidant,[2137] while other preparations may actually stimulate oxidation.[2138] With respect to Parkinson's it is neuroprotective,[2139] reduces neuroinflammation,[2140] [2141] and reduces motor dysfunction.[2142]

With respect to Alzheimer's, aged garlic ameliorates amyloid beta caused neurotoxicity and cognitive impairment.[2143] Aged garlic extract restricts several of the cascades related to synapse deterioration and neuroinflammation,[2144] improves cognitive impairment and neurodegeneration caused by amyloid beta accumulation,[2145] [2146] regulates cholinergic function,[2147] improves short-term recognition memory in lab animals, and slows the inflammatory response.[2148]

Aged garlic extract also increased intracellular glutathione levels.[2149] It offers support for the cardiovascular system,[2150] reduces blood pressure,[2151] inhibits platelet aggregation effectively,[2152] and reduces elevated homocysteine levels.[2153] It boosts the immune system[2154] thereby supporting cancer patients,[2155] and has a place in immunotherapy.[2156] [2157]

Note: Garlic does have blood thinning properties so if you are on any blood thinning medications, check with your doctor first before taking garlic.

Ginger root (500mg – 800mg per day). Ginger has been used for thousands of years for the treatment of ailments, such as colds, nausea, arthritis, migraines, and hypertension. It is reported to decrease age-related oxidative stress biomarkers.[2158] It contains a very high level of total antioxidants surpassed only by pomegranate and some types of berries.[2159] Orally given, ginger extract (100 mg/kg body weight) normalizes nitrous oxide levels and glutathione levels, and also decreases the level of lipid oxidation.[2160] [2161] One of the many health claims attributed to ginger is its purported ability to decrease inflammation, swelling, and pain. [6]-gingerol,[2162] a dried ginger extract, and a dried gingerol-enriched extract[2163] were each reported to exhibit analgesic and potent anti-inflammatory effects. In another study, ginger has been suggested to be effective against inflammation, osteoarthritis, and rheumatism.[2164] These anti-inflammatory benefits may be useful in preventing and treating dementia.

Otherwise healthy menopausal women often begin to show signs of cognitive impairment such as poor working memory.[2165] Cognitive function improved in healthy middle-aged women given 800mg daily. While reduced dosages (400mg or less) had little benefit, working memory significant improvement with the 800mg dosage.[2166] In this study improvements were noted in power and continuity of attention as well as quality and speed of memory.[2167]

Ginger extract inhibits beta-amyloid peptide-induced cytokine and chemokine expression in cultured THP-1 monocytes.[2168] It is found to reverse behavioral dysfunction and AD-like symptoms in AD rats.[2169] Combined with peony root it inhibits amyloid beta accumulation and pathology in AD mice.[2170]

Gingko Biloba (120mg – 240 mg per day). Gingko is an age-old herb for supporting circulation[2171][2172] kidney function, [2173] and overall health. Combined with other nutrients (Polygala tenuifolia and Lycii fructus) researchers have noted neuroprotective results with beneficial effects on memory, cognitive function and reduced cell death.[2174] Combined with quercetin it supports neurogenesis although it does not prevent dementia.[2175]

Although research is mixed as to its benefits for memory[2176] and Alzheimer's prevention, there is some evidence that gingko increases neurogenesis,[2177] raises BDNF (brain derived neurotrophic factor) levels,[2178] enhances cognitive function,[2179] (temporarily in healthy subjects),[2180] and appears to consistently improves attention, some executive processes and long-term memory.[2181] It ameliorates mild to moderate dementia in AD patients. This is perhaps due to hormone sensitivity regulation, endocrine improved homeostasis, and proteolysis of tau protein before plaque formation.[2182]

Its usefulness as an anti-AD agent may be that it provides a synthesis of antioxidant, anti-inflammatory,[2183] and other relevant factors.[2184] Gingko is more effective than placebo for Alzheimer's, vascular dementia, and mixed dementia,[2185] and compared to the drug donepezil, ginkgo yielded similar results for helping patients with mild AD.[2186] Although gingko does not appear to prevent AD, one European large-scale study[2187] revealed delays in conversion to AD in patients treated for at least four years with gingko extract.[2188] It found that working memory improved and concluded that as many as 20.7 percent of working memory (WM) tests in chronic Gingko Biloba Extract trials had yielded significant results in working memory improvement.

Ginkgo or ginkgo extract (especially Egb761® a standardized extract) supports healthy brain function[2189][2190][2191][2192] in a number of ways including enhancing peripheral and cerebral circulation,[2193] providing neuroprotection through antioxidant capacity,[2194][2195][2196] influencing neurotransmitter systems critical for cognition, and improving working memory.[2197][2198][2199] It promotes nerve transmission rate, improves the neurotransmitter synthesis, and normalizes acetylcholine receptors in the hippocampus, the area of the brain most affected by Alzheimer's disease.[2200] A 2017 review of the literature suggests modest expectations, but indicates that it is effective for people with mild dementia when given in doses greater than 200mg/day for at least five months.[2201]

Note that gingko does have slight blood thinning properties so consult your doctor first if on any blood thinning medications before adding as a supplement.

Ginseng, Panax (500mg – 1,000mg per day of ginseng root extract). Ginseng has been shown to improve learning and memory, reduce apoptosis, inhibit neuroinflammation,[2202]improve neuro-plasticity, support neuronal growth, offer neuroprotection,[2203][2204] and repair damaged neuronal networks.[2205][2206] Ginseng extract supports neurogenesis in the hippocampus,[2207][2208] brain recovery due to stroke,[2209][2210][2211] has cholinergic properties,[2212][2213] inhibits amyloid beta neurotoxicity, inhibits cell death,[2214] reduces reactive oxidation stress, and has anti-inflammatory effects.[2215] It has been demonstrated to induce significant regeneration of nerve axons and dendrites damaged by amyloid beta(25-35) as well as recovery from memory loss.[2216] A study of molecular modeling demonstrates that its active components, withanamides A and C, bind to amyloid beta and inhibit fibril development.[2217]

Other studies confirm ginseng as being effective for reducing depression, an increasing major clinical challenge for those with dementia and AD.[2218][2219][2220] Depression can result, in time, in progressive damage to nerve cells.[2221] This neuronal cell damage, coupled with a neuroinflammation-induced reduction in neurogenesis, can result in hippocampal cell death.[2222][2223] Ginseng demonstrated similar levels of efficacy as the commercially available antidepressant, fluoxetine.[2224]

Ginseng is effective in reducing the negative effects of stress[2225] and may have the potential to improve anxiety.[2226] Ginseng and ginsenosides improve learning and memory by enhancing brain plasticity and increasing neurogenesis, thereby affecting neuronal density in hippocampus.[2227] Ginsenosides have been identified as an effective treatment for organ damage and cell death, as well as for immunological and metabolic conditions.[2228][2229][2230] One twelve-week study showed significant improvement in cognitive function in an AD control group from supplementation with Korean red ginseng.[2231][2232] The benefits gradually declined after supplementation ceased.[2233]

Ginseng is an effective antioxidant, improves vasomotor function and prevents blood clots. These effects positively improve cardiovascular health.[2234][2235] It reduces the effects of oxidative stress in the brain (in mitochondria[2236]) and may remove free radicals generated by amyloid beta.[2237][2238][2239][2240][2241]

Note: For some people ginseng can cause overstimulation. Start with a small dose, gradually increase, and check with your health provider.

Glucose. When we think of glucose, we usually think of the results of too much sugar. However, in right amounts, glucose is essential. Carbohydrates (and sugars) are converted to glucose in the body. Glucose crosses the blood-brain barrier and is critical for health brain function (thirty percent of the brain energy comes from glucose). The brain only uses what it needs at any time so excess glucose is converted to glycogen and stored for future use. In the adult brain, neurons have the highest energy demand,[2242] requiring continuous delivery of glucose from blood. In humans, the brain accounts for two percent of the body weight, but it consumes twenty percent of glucose-derived energy.[2243] Glucose provides energy precursors for neurotransmitter synthesis[2244] and the ATP (energy storage molecule) to fuel their actions as well as other brain non-signaling activities. Signaling, neuronal computation, information processing,[2245] learning,[2246] and long-term memory formation all depend on glucose.[2247]

Not all sugar is equal. For example, three tablespoons per day of honey provides all the glucose the brain needs for optimal brain energy (the equivalent would be eating sixteen pounds of chocolate chip cookies per day). Excess sugar has resulted in a crisis of obesity in this country, diabetes, and heart disease. Corn syrup is the most common sugar used in cheap desserts and one of the worst for the body.

Food sources of preferred sugars: Red beets, fruit (both regular and dried), turnips, spring onion, rutabaga, honey, maple syrup.

Glutathione (GSH) (900 mg per day in capsule form or 200mg per day in sublingual or intraoral form which is preferred). Glutathione is referred to as the "anti-aging antioxidant" because it is one of the few nutrients that can neutralize the full spectrum of different types of free radicals in one's body, and is one of the body's most potent antioxidants.[2248] It is comprised of three amino acids: glycine, glutamine, and cysteine. Glutathione is the most prevalent antioxidant in the brain. It is the richest non-protein thiol molecule in tissues and possesses the ability to prevent cerebral reactive oxygen species (ROS) accumulation.[2249]
Reduced GSH levels are seen in aging and in diseases with where oxidative stress is a factor, including AD.[2250][2251] Lower glutathione levels are associated with greater brain amyloid plaque buildup[2252] in the temporal and parietal regions.[2253][2254][2255]

In the brain glutathione plays an essential role in protecting astrocytes and neurons. Each type of cell prefers unique extracellular precursors for glutathione which plays a role in these cells ability to dispose of outside harmful peroxides.[2256] Glutathione therapy has good potential to help reduce cognitive impairment due to its antioxidant capacity acting in the brain.[2257]

Glutathione levels may be a good noninvasive biomarker of early Alzheimer's.[2258] Glutathione exists in both reduced (GSH) and oxidized (GSSG) states. GSH levels are decreased and GSSG levels are increased, consistent with increased oxidative stress.[2259] The ratio of GSSG to GSH is used as a marker of redox thiol status and oxidative stress. There is a linear correlation between increased GSSG levels and decreased cognitive status of AD patients using the Mini Mental Status examination (MMSE).[2260] Research has also linked glutathione to a number of non-ROS detoxification processes as well as immune cell function and the regulation of induced cell death.[2261]

Goji berry (wolfberry or Lycium barbarum) (500mg once or twice per day). Goji berry has been used in Chinese medicine for over 2,000 years. It contains powerful antioxidants to reduce oxidative stress and has strong neuroprotective and neurogenesis supporting properties.[2262][2263]

Oxidative damage of biomolecules increases with age and is postulated to be a major causal factor of various degenerative disorders.[2264][2265] Goji berry has great potential in the treatment of Parkinson's disease[2266] and may help stimulate nerve growth in the brain to support learning and memory,[2267] as well as preventing the formation of amyloid-beta.[2268] Goji berry extract protects against nerve injury and loss caused by beta amyloid peptides, glutamate excitotoxicity, ischemic attack, and other neurotoxic effects. It is used to reduce symptoms in AD mice and enhance neurogenesis in the hippocampus, which in turn enhances memory and learning ability.[2269] Drinking goji berry juice may improve energy, mood, and digestive health.[2270] Similar to other berries, goji berries contain high amounts of zeaxanthin and lutein,[2271] [2272] as well as vitamins A and C, and contains a spectrum of proanthocyanidins, anthocyanins, flavonoids, and carotenoids.

Grapeseed extract (GSE, 300mg per day). Grapeseed extract is very high in flavonoids called proanthocyanidins which some believe could prevent cognitive decline. Its antioxidant ability[2273] may help to reverse damage to the hippocampus caused by seizures that threaten mitochondrial function.[2274] It has been shown to have neuroprotective effects by inhibiting DNA damage in the brain in the case of stroke.[2275]

Flavonoids tend to be neuroprotective toward conditions like Alzheimer's through a combination of antioxidant and anti-inflammatory properties.[2276] GSE's antioxidant and anti-inflammatory flavonoids, (especially gallic acid)[2277] inhibit aggregation[2278] [2279] [2280] of amyloid beta peptides into neurotoxic soluble amyloid beta.[2281] [2282] [2283]

Green, leafy vegetables such as such as kale, spinach, collards, lettuce, and broccoli are rich in brain-healthy nutrients like vitamin K, lutein, folate, and beta carotene. Studies show regular consumption of green, leafy vegetables slows cognitive decline. Specifically, phylloquinone, lutein, and folate are likely the source of the effect on cognitive decline.[2284] [2285] [2286] A meta-analysis examining research involving 21,175 people found that the consumption of fruit and vegetables was significantly and inversely related to cognitive decline and disorders.[2287]

Guggul (Commiphora wighitti, C. mukul and related species) is a traditional Ayurvedic medicinal herb that contains ferulic acids, phenols and non-phenolic aromatic acids that powerfully neutralize free radicals. Guggul may be useful for the treatment of AD[2288] and other oxidative stress-related diseases.[2289] It activates the BDNF signaling pathway and enhances neurogenesis in the hippocampus.[2290] [2291] Its memory enhancing[2292] and anti-dementia activity is due to reduction in acetylcholinesterase contents in the hippocampus[2293] as well as cholesterol-lowering, and antioxidant properties which protect against models of dementia induced by toxins.[2294]

Hesperidin (100mg – 500mg per day) promotes nerve cell differentiation and survival,[2295] and also enhances the neuroprotective capacity of astrocytes, by inducing them to secrete soluble factors involved in neuronal survival in vitro, and increasing the number of neural progenitors.[2296] It reduces cognitive impairment, oxidative stress, and cell death in animal models of Alzheimer's[2297] and inhibits amyloid fibril formation.[2298]

Food sources of hesperidin: Citrus fruits including grapefruit, as well as apricots, plums, and bilberry. Vegetables containing hesperidin include green and yellow peppers, peas, green leafy vegetables, and broccoli. Whole grains, such as buckwheat, also contain hesperidin.

Huperzine A is a naturally occurring compound found in a moss species that acts as a cholinesterase inhibitor improving neurotransmitter levels. A growing body of evidence has demonstrated that HupA could effectively reverse or attenuate cognitive deficits in rodents, primates, and humans.[2299] It has been shown to increase neurogenesis by 25-41percent through the increase in the survival rate of neural progenitor cells and it helps keep early neurons from dying off prematurely.[2300] However, research results are mixed. Some studies are poorly designed and there is a lack of long-term safety information. [2301] [2302] But, it may be useful as part of an AD treatment strategy because some studies show that it improves cognitive performance, behavioral dysfunction, memory, and offers neuroprotection.

Note. While some small studies indicate that HupA may be valuable in an AD treatment strategy, the Alzheimer's Association recommends not taking huperzine A, especially if you're taking a prescribed cholinesterase inhibitor, such as donepezil (Aricept), rivastigmine (Exelon) or galantamine (Razadyne). Taking both could increase your risk of serious side effects.[2303]

Iron deficiency is often characterized by brain fog and impaired brain function, and has been linked to oxidative stress and neurodegenerative diseases. It plays an important role in neuronal processes such as myelination, synaptogenesis, behavior, and synaptic plasticity.[2304]

Lecithin (1200mg – 3600mg per day) is composed of mostly omega-3 and omega-6 fatty acids, and makes up to thirty percent of the dry weight of the brain. The fat layer covering the myelin sheath that protects nerve cells is mostly lecithin. Lecithin increases the absorption of fat-soluble vitamins such as vitamin A and supports overall brain activity. Lecithin improves most types of memory, including visual and verbal memory. A derivative, phosphatidylserine, combined with phosphatidic acid supports memory, cognition, daily activity skills, and mood in elderly patients with dementia and AD.[2305] It exhibits anti-cholinesterase and free radical scavenging ability.[2306]

Lithium has been used to promote healthy mood for some time.[2307] But now research indicates that lithium helps inhibit the GSK3 enzyme in a model of Alzheimer's, which affects tau protein phosphorylation.[2308] Phosphorylation is a biochemical process where phosphate combines with an organic compound. Phosphorylated tau proteins can contribute to age-related cognitive decline and memory health. Inhibiting GSK3 may also help maintain healthy glucose levels already within normal range in the brain.[2309] Lithium also promotes autophagy the healthy breakdown of tau and amyloid beta proteins. And, in animal studies lithium helped maintain memory health and cognitive performance.[2310]

Lotus root extract (no specific dosage, usually part of a multi-herbal formula) is the edible rhizome of a plant, Nelumbo nucifera and promotes neurogenesis.[2311] Lotus root is high in vitamins B6 and C. Researchers have observed a protective effect against amyloid beta protein-caused cell death in a vitro model of AD[2312] and other neurodegenerative conditions.[2313]

Lutein (12mg – 20mg per day) benefits vision as well as the brain. Its neuroprotective ability comes from its role as an antioxidant. Lutein protects the brain against oxidation, and along with zeaxanthin help maintain the health of the brain, enhance blood flow to the part of the brain that supports cognitive function, and improves the integrity of the brain's white matter tracts. In the brain it is found in highest concentrations in the areas where DHA and high oxidative stress occurs, and where it is well positioned to protect against lipid oxidation.[2314] [2315] [2316] [2317]

Lutein levels in the brain can be indicated by lutein levels in the retina (correlated with retinal macular pigment density).[2318] Lutein accumulates in the brain and its content in neural tissue has been positively correlated with cognitive function.[2319] [2320] [2321] Therefore, lutein may be a useful biomarker of lutein concentrations in brain tissue. This relationship may explain the significant correlation found between macular pigment density and cognitive function in healthy adults.[2322] [2323] [2324] Macular pigment density also has been found to be significantly related to multiple measures of temporal processing speed, [2325] [2326] an important aspect of sensory and cognitive function. Some studies assert that among the carotenoids, only lutein (or lutein plus zeaxanthin) are consistently associated with a wide range of cognitive measures including executive function, language, learning and memory.[2327] [2328] A four-month double-blind, placebo-controlled trial in older women revealed that those who were supplementing with 12mg per day of lutein and 800mg per day of DHA had markedly improved verbal fluency scores, as well as improvements memory and learning.[2329] [2330]

Lutein plus zeaxanthin and lycopene correlate inversely with Alzheimer's mortality.[2331] Higher levels of the macular pigments (lutein, zeaxanthin, and mesozeaxanthin) are linked to improvements in cognition (vision only) in Alzheimer's patient.[2332] But, data from the large six-year AREDS study reported that there was no statistically significant correlation between lutein/zeaxanthin and cognitive function.[2333]

Xanthophylls are carotenoids found in foods such as fruits and vegetable this give them their color and are powerful antioxidants and show up as color yellow in foods. Xanthophylls, like lutein, stabilize membranes and are known to accumulate in cell membranes and nerve axons[2334] because they have both water-repelling and water-attracting qualities.[2335] Lutein has high solubility in membranes and strongly influences membrane properties including fluidity, ion exchange, oxygen diffusion and membrane stability,[2336] and may influence interneuronal communication through effects on gap junctions.[2337]

Note: See also the discussion of zeaxanthin; the combination of lutein and zeaxanthin offers great protective potential.

Food sources: Yellow and orange foods, corn, eggs, and dark green vegetables including kale, spinach, collards, mustard greens, dark green lettuce, Brussels sprouts, and broccoli.

Luteolin (not the same as lutein) is an antioxidant flavonoid with strong anti-inflammatory[2338] [2339] and antidepressant effects as well as capacity to increase neurogenesis[2340] and BDNF.[2341] [2342] [2343] In addition, it inhibits microglial IL-6 release, microglial activation, and microglia-induced nerve cell death.[2344] [2345] [2346] [2347] [2348] It offers neuroprotection, and improves memory. When made more bioavailable through methylated luteolin forms, it could possibly be developed into effective treatments for neuropsychiatric disorders and brain fog.[2349]

Food sources: Celery, thyme, peppermint, sage, oregano, green peppers, bell peppers, radicchio, celery seeds, and chamomile tea.

Lycopene (3mg per day). Lycopene has demonstrated greater antioxidant abilities compared with the other carotenoids, such as beta-carotene, lutein, and zeaxanthin.[2350] Lycopene has been shown to exhibit neuroprotective effects by reducing oxidative stress,[2351] suppressing production of inflammatory cytokines, and reducing accumulation of amyloid plaques.[2352] [2353] This process inhibits the neuroinflammatory cascade that leads to neuroinflammation.[2354] Lycopene has been shown to attenuate cognitive deficits by improving inflammation in the gut–liver–brain axis as well improving glycolipid metabolism.[2355] These are mechanisms by which lycopene provides neurocognitive protection as well as inhibition of neuronal apoptosis and restoration of mitochondrial function.[2356]

Food Sources: Several types of fruit including tomatoes and watermelon

Magnesium (l-threonate, 3,000–6,000mg per day). Magnesium is one of the most essential minerals in the human body, connected with brain biochemistry and the fluidity of neuronal membrane. A deficiency can lead to depression[2357] and both too high and too low magnesium serum levels are linked to increased risk of dementia from all causes.[2358] It is the second most abundant intracellular mineral after potassium, and is involved in over six hundred enzymatic reactions including energy metabolism and protein synthesis, and plays an important physiological role particularly in the brain, heart, and skeletal muscles.[2359]

Magnesium status is of interest to researchers because it has antioxidant and neuroprotective properties. Magnesium is essential for learning and memory,[2360] and has been shown to support brain plasticity for optimal learning, memory, and cognitive function. It enhances both short-term synaptic facilitation and long-term potentiation and plays a role in preventing Alzheimer's.[2361] A unique compound called magnesium-L-threonate boosts brain magnesium levels by an approximate fifteen percent.[2362] It suppresses action of the enzyme responsible for beta amyloid deposits by an impressive eighty percent.[2363]

High levels of magnesium in both blood serum and cerebral spinal fluid in Parkinson's patients were noted in a 2018 meta-analysis, and the researchers noted that it is considered a risk factor for Parkinson's.[2364] Although measuring magnesium is a fast way of checking magnesium status, blood levels have little correlation with total magnesium. Most magnesium is inside cells or bone; only 1% of body magnesium is present in extracellular fluids, and only .3% in blood.[2365] Normal levels of magnesium are good for the brain and overall health, help reduce inflammation and builds healthy bones.

Food sources: Avocados, dark chocolate, nuts (including almonds, cashews, and Brazil nuts), legumes, tofu, seeds (including flax, pumpkin, and chia seeds), spinach, soy milk, whole wheat bread, yogurt, oatmeal, banana, and salmon.

Melatonin (1mg – 3mg before bedtime). Melatonin is a potent antioxidant[2366] that boosts the immune system by improving efficiency of other naturally produced and supplemental antioxidants.[2367] It increases glutathione levels,[2368] and its antioxidant[2369] and immune system boosting effect is intensified by vitamin C,[2370] or vitamins C and E.[2371] Melatonin is produced at night by the pineal gland and helps regulate sleep. It is a hormone derived from the amino acid tryptophan and its production declines with age.[2372] It may be therapeutic for elderly people with age-related dementia with disrupted sleep issues[2373] include AD patients.[2374] Age-related cognitive impairment may be directly correlated to reduced melatonin levels.[2375] [2376] [2377] Melatonin increases and helps regulate neurogenesis,[2378] [2379] [2380] [2381] supports the brain's normal antioxidant protection and helps inhibit factors that can lead to cognitive decline.[2382] [2383] [2384]

Note. Exposure to blue light (computers and mobile devices) inhibits the production of melatonin.[2385]

Moringa oleifera, (no specific dosage, usually in a multi-herbal formula) **is** an important medicinal herb in India. It is one of the nootropic (may improve cognitive ability) herbs that has been identified for possible value in treating Alzheimer's.[2386] It contains antioxidant vitamins C and E, and the flavonols quercetin and kaempferol.[2387] The seed extract has neuroprotective properties against brain damage in stroke, restored cognitive impairment, promoted neurogenesis in the hippocampus, and improved cholinergic function.[2388][2389] In several animal studies it positively altered transmitters used in the memory process and supported memory.[2390][2391] In animal models of Alzheimer's it alleviates homocysteine-caused AD-like pathologies and cognitive impairments.[2392] Similarly, in an animal model of Parkinson's it modulates inflammation, oxidative stress, and cell death.[2393]

Mulberry (Mori fructus, 500mg per day). Mulberry is a common plant used in Chinese medicine, where it is classified as a blood tonic, and helps stimulate neurogenesis.[2394] It is anti-inflammatory[2395] antioxidant, and reduces oxidative stress.[2396] Anthocyanin, the flavonoid pigment in mulberry fruit, may protect against cerebral stroke.[2397] Samjunghwan, a traditional medicine comprised of Mori fructus, Samjunghwan, a traditional medicine comprised of Mori fructus, Lycii radices cortex, and Atractylodis rhizome alba, provides significant protection of rat cortical neurons from amyloid-beta neurotoxicity against mitochondria cell death pathways.[2398] This suggests helpfulness in AD. Researchers find that components in root bark of white mulberry may be the most promising preventative and therapeutic agents for Alzheimer's.[2399] Some components are identified as having neuroprotective quality by supporting glutathione and reducing free radicals.[2400]

Mushrooms have been used since ancient times in Chinese, Korean, Japanese, Egyptian, and European cultures for their nutritional, healthful, and healing properties.[2401] They are high in nutrients including copper, phosphorus, vitamins D, B2 and B3 and selenium, an antioxidant that helps protect cells against damage. Potent antioxidants in mushrooms include: polysaccharides, polyphenols, phenolic acids, flavonoids, vitamins, tocopherol, ascorbic acid, niacin, ergosterol, and carotenoids.[2402][2403] Mushrooms have long been used not only as food but also for the treatment of various ailments. Numerous studies have shown both within in vitro and mammal studies to have potential roles in the prevention of many age-associated neurological diseases including Alzheimer's and Parkinson's. These include the following mushrooms: Lions mane (Hericium erinaceus), Reiki (Ganoderma lucidum), Sarcodon scabrosus, Antrodia, Rhodopsin, Pleurotus giganteus, Maitake (Grifola frondosa), and many more.

A number of mushrooms have been reported to stimulate neurite growth.[2404] Aqueous extract of L. rhinocerotis sclerotium,[2405] L. rhinocerotis mycelium,[2406] Ganoderma neo-japonicum,[2407] and Pleurotus giganteus[2408] induce neuronal differentiation and stimulate neurite outgrowth of PC12 and N2a cells. (PC12 cells are cells labs use that are able to reproduce for research and are useful as a model for studying neural differentiation and neurosecretion. N2a are fast growing mouse cells again used for research to study the neural differentiation mechanism and neurite growth.) A methanol extract of Cordyceps militaris (5–20 mg/mL) is able to increase new nerve projections (neurite sprouting), an expression of an enzyme that is responsible for synthesis of the neurotransmitter acetylcholine (ChAT expression in differentiated N2a cells).[2409]Administration of another mushroom species, C. militaris, also restores toxin-induced memory deficit in vivo. In addition, various mushrooms may reduce beta amyloid-induced neurotoxicity and have anti-acetylcholinesterase, nerve growth factor (NGF) synthesis, neuroprotective, antioxidant, and anti-(neuro)inflammatory effects.[2410]

Precautions: Not all mushrooms are edible and many can be toxic, so do not pick wild mushrooms, unless know what you know exactly what you are doing. From a Chinese medical perspective, mushrooms may cause bloating and be difficult to digest for those prone to "dampness." Symptoms include poor digestion and absorption, water retention, phlegm, edema (fluid retention), and discharges, feelings of heaviness and dizziness, and/or feelings of heaviness and dizziness.

Mushroom, Antrodia camphorate is found in Taiwan, is used to protect against a wide range of health conditions. It normalizes high blood pressure, supports liver and kidney health, is neuroprotective, and inhibits cell death in neurons (by suppression of JNK and p38 activities).[2411] Fermented (with deep ocean water) may inhibit the toxicity of amyloid beta peptide.[2412] A derivative, antroquinonol, improved learning and memory, reduce amyloid beta in the hippocampus, and reduced abnormal increase in astrocytes (caused by cell death of nearby neurons) in a mouse model of AD.[2413] These effects were most pronounced in the fruiting body rather than the mycelium.[2414] In a mouse model of Parkinson's, Antrodia polysaccharides and triterpenoids significantly improved the striatum's dopamine levels, and could reduce neuroinflammation levels.[2415]

Mushroom, Maitake (Grifola frondosa, hen of the woods) is an edible and tasty mushroom that grows in large clusters like the fluffed tail feathers of a hen[2416] with potential for managing neuroprotective diseases.[2417][2418] A combination of maitake and shiitaki mushrooms was the most effective for immune system support, followed by maitake and then shiitaki alone.[2419]

Mushroom, lion's mane (Hericium erinaceus, yamabushitake) is a culinary and medicinal mushroom well established as a food source for brain and nerve health and is often used in vegetarian diets to replace meat in cooking. It triggers neurite outgrowth and regeneration of damaged nerves. It has been shown to help protect against the onset of dementia and may reduce the risk of neurodegenerative disease-induced cell death. [2420]

Fifty to eighty-year-old Japanese men and women diagnosed with mild cognitive impairment were given oral dosages of four 250 mg tablets containing ninety six percent of yamabushitake dry powder three times a day for sixteen weeks. They experienced improvements in cognitive function during the duration of the trial with no adverse effects.[2421] In other research extracts promoted nerve growth factor gene expression in the hippocampus,[2422][2423] and nerve cell support.[2424] Of several medicinal mushrooms tested, only lion's mane extract promoted nerve growth factor mRNA expression (depending on concentration) and enhanced nerve growth factor protein.[2425] The confirmed pharmacological actions in the central nervous system demonstrate that improvements are possible in ischemic stroke, Parkinson's disease, Alzheimer's and depression.[2426]

In mice, a diet enhanced with lion's mane mushroom supported locomotor activity, (did not change spatial memory), but did yield improvements in recognition memory, a function of the hippocampus.[2427] Enriched with erinacine A (major bioactive diterpenoid compounds extracted from cultured mycelia of lion's mane) this combination safely shows promise in treating neurodegenerative diseases including Alzheimer's and Parkinson's disease.[2428] Lion's mane has been found to help repair nerve damage, reduce anxiety and depression, protect against ulcers, manage diabetes, and exhibit antimicrobial action.[2429]

Mushroom, Pleurotus giganteus is an edible mushroom popular in Malaysia.[2430] It may offer hepato-protective effects (ability of a chemical substance to prevent damage to the liver)[2431] and is said to promote nerve and brain health.[2432] Its component, uridine, stimulated neurite outgrowth in vitro.[2433]

Mushroom, reishi (Ganoderma lucidum, Ling Zhi) is a white-rot fungus viewed as a traditional Chinese tonic for promoting health and longevity. Although the use of Ganoderma lucidum as an elixir has been around for thousands of years, studies offer validation. The main active constituents, including polysaccharides, triterpenes, and peptidoglycans, are found in the fruit body, mycelium, and spores.[2434] Reishi mushrooms are strong antioxidants[2435] that inhibit reactive oxygen species and their lipid oxidation. An ethanol extract augments cellular antioxidant defense through activation of the transcription factor, Nrf2/HO-1.[2436] Transcription factors are proteins that convert DNA into RNA. Reishi also inhibits neurodegeneration,[2437][2438] promotes nerve cell differentiation,[2439][2440] and performs other neuro-supportive effects that could slow down the progress of Alzheimer's or Parkinson's.

Mushroom, Sarcodon scabrosus is a bitter mushroom that (in animal models) can reduce or even prevent age-related neurodegenerative disease by inducing neurite growth, differentiation, and prevent. Studies suggest that it induces neurite growth, neuronal differentiation and prevents cell death.[2441][2442]

Mushroom, shiitake (Lentinula edodes) is an edible mushroom with powerful immune-system stimulation capacity, which is even more potent when combined with maitake mushroom glucan extract.[2443] Shiitaki mushroom reduces high cholesterol, and acts as an antioxidant, antitumor and antibacterial agent.[2444]

Mushroom, tiger milk (Lignosus rhinocerotis) is an edible mushroom from Malaysia and Southeast Asia, is valued for producing vitality, alertness, and in several animal studies overall wellness.[2445] It is used to reduce fever, inflammation, and treat respiratory disorders.[2446] In mice, it caused a 38.1 percent increased neurite-bearing cells,[2447][2448] and in a similar study it produced an induced maximum neurite outgrowth of 20.8 and 24.7 percent in brain and spinal cord.[2449] It is even more effective when combined with gingko biloba.[2450] Combined with curcumin resulted in 27.2 percent enhanced neurite outgrowth compared to curcumin alone.[2451] Researchers note that tiger milk mushrooms can be considered as an alternative in non-communicable diseases but that validation studies with human trials are needed.[2452]

Nattokinase (NK, 100mg – 200mg per day, best taken between meals) is a fermented soybean product that has been consumed as a traditional food in Japan for thousands of years, and is suggested to contribute significantly to the longevity of Japanese people.[2453][2454] It is a safe, effective enzyme for those who need a potent blood-clot dissolving protein for the treatment for cardiovascular diseases[2455][2456][2457] and hypertension.[2458] The effects of NK are similar to the well-known blood thinner, aspirin. Nattokinase improves blood flow by inhibiting platelet aggregation and thrombus formation,[2459] was reported to have an effect on several types of thrombosis.[2460][2461][2462] NK shows a clear neuroprotective effect in stroke patients.[2463]

NK exhibits little to no side effects, with studies indicating that an oral administration of NK can be absorbed by the intestinal tract.[2464] It may also reduce Alzheimer's disease risk[2465] because it is capable of degrading amyloid fibrils.[2466] Researchers are exploring its anti amyloid, antifribrinolytic and antithrombotic activity (all important in inhibiting AD) through nanoparticle delivery.[2467] In an animal model of AD, this NK nanonutraceutical reversed toxin-induced behavioral and neurochemical changes through antioxidant effect, which suggests a benefit in reducing cognitive impairment linked to Alzheimer's.[2468]

Nuts and berries. The synergy and interaction of the nutrients in nuts and berries is noted for reduction of oxidative stress, inflammation, vascular reactivity, platelet aggregation, and enhanced immune function – all of which support brain health.[2469] These are easily applied therapeutic foods in the treatment and prevention of age-related brain dysfunction.[2470][2471]

Berries, of course, are much valued for their high antioxidant levels and the combination of the two foods makes a perfect brain tonic. Especially favor blueberries, bilberries, blackberries, mulberries, and goji berries.

Good nuts include walnuts, hazelnuts, Brazil nuts, peanuts, almonds, cashews, flax seed, sunflower seeds, sesame seeds, and un-hydrogenated nut butters such as peanut butter, almond butter, and tahini. In general, intake of nuts showed good results in better overall cognition at older ages.[2472]

Oleuropein (in olive leaf extract, 500mg per day with or without food, olives, and virgin olive oil). Oleuropein, a polyphenolic compound has therapeutic potential against Alzheimer's disease. Oleuropein[2473][2474][2475] and especially oleuropein aglycone[2476][2477] binds to amyloid beta peptide interfering with its aggregation process (by inhibiting tau protein),[2478] and instead favors the formation of nontoxic disordered aggregates. Olive leaf extract contains polyphenols which exert antioxidant, anti-inflammatory, anti-cancer, antimicrobial, antiviral, anti-atherogenic, hypoglycemic, hepatic-, cardiac- and neuro-protective effects.[2479][2480][2481][2482][2483][2484][2485] It also helps protect the brain and central nervous system from the neuroinflammation and oxidative stress-caused damage leading to strokes and age-related degenerative conditions such as AD and PD.[2486]

Olive oil (extra virgin olive oil, first cold press). Virgin olive oil, also containing oleuropein are inversely correlated with the incidence of some forms of cancers (colon, breast, and skin cancer).[2487][2488][2489] It has anti-angiogenesis properties (meaning helps prevent the growth of unwanted blood vessels).[2490] Another phenolic compound, oleocanthal, is a minor olive oil constituent. It is a strong antioxidant with anti-inflammatory action that helps boost the production of key proteins and enzymes that may help prevent Alzheimer's disease. Oleocanthal improves removal of amyloid beta protein from neurons[2491] through the process of autophagy[2492] and may be useful as an adjunct to other therapies.[2493]

Omega-3 fatty acid (2,000mg – 3,000mg per day) may be helpful in AD onset, but supplementation is not enough for AD treatment.[2494] Omega-3s can influence brain elasticity thereby effecting central nervous system functioning.[2495] About sixty percent of your brain is made of fat, and half of that fat are omega-3 fatty acids.[2496] Your brain uses omega-3s to build brain and nerve cells, and these fats are essential for learning and memory.[2497] [2498] In healthy older people they have been found to improve executive functions, learning, memory, gray matter volume, and white matter microstructure.

Essential benefits include being anti-inflammatory, which supports its role in delaying or preventing cognitive decline in early stages of AD.[2499][2500][2501] In lab animals it is seen to improve cerebral blood flow and lower triacylglycerol levels.

Omega-3 fatty acids have been found to improve general clinical function in patients with mild or moderate AD, mild cognitive impairment.[2502][2503][2504][2505][2506][2507] They dramatically increase BDNF (brain-derived neurotrophic factor) levels, stimulating neurogenesis, increased brain size, neural growth, and general neuroprotective benefits.[2508][2509][2510] More specifically, omega-3s increase neurite growth, enhance neuronal cell transmission, and neurotransmitter release.[2511][2512][2513][2514][2515] One study reported that by taking fish oil as a source of EFAs, it could reduce the risk of onset of AD. For those without the *ApoE4* gene,[2516] other studies found that eating fish two-three times per week reduced the risk of AD onset by fifty percent over four years.[2517][2518] And, another study showed that those who ate fish one or more times per week showed lower levels of amyloid plaque and neurofibrillary tangles compared to those who did not include fish in their weekly diet. Dietary deficiency of omega-3 fatty acids in humans has been associated with increased risk of other mental disorders, including attention-deficit disorder, dyslexia, dementia, depression, bipolar disorder, and schizophrenia.[2519][2520]

Food sources: A diet that includes regular consumption of wild-crafted fish is the best way to get the omega-3 fatty acids (compared to taking fish oil, which may have become rancid or oxidized),[2521] though high-quality fish oil supplements are a good substitute for daily consumption of access to a regular fish diet is not available. For vegetarians, the best source is fresh flax seed meal, which also contains the antioxidant and heart-healthy alpha linolenic acid.[2522]

A is the most important omega-3. (300mg – 600mg per day for prevention, 900mg – 1800mg per day, therapeutic dosage). For brain health, DHA is the most important omega-3 fatty acid but the average American consumption of DHA is only about 100-200mg per day.[2523] DHA (docosahexaenoic acid) comprises one third of the essential fatty acids that make up sixty percent of our brain. Brain synapses have a higher concentration of DHA than almost any other tissue in the body. Is an essential nutrient and a nutraceutical for brain health and diseases[2524] and is essential for neurotransmission and supports critical neuroprotectins for nerve signaling.[2525][2526] Neuroprotectins are proteins that form the structure within brain cells and the connective tissue between brain cells.[2527] DHA is also essential for energy regulation in the body and brain, regulating key enzymes needed for feeding energy to cells. [2528]

DHA and the blood brain barrier. High DHA intake (with high plasma DHA), however, is not necessarily linked to high brain DHA levels, suggesting that DHA stability changes in the elderly.[2529] Some scientists report that lysophospholipid (LPA) form of DHA is more effective in getting DHA to the brain and that the blood-brain barrier does not transmit DHA in the more common form of supplements.[2530][2531] More research is needed to confirm whether this is correct.

DHA and mild cognitive impairment. In one study older adults with minimal cognitive impairment took DHA, melatonin, and tryptophan as an emulsion for twelve weeks, and underwent a battery of cognitive, behavioral, and nutritional tests. Their memories, mental status, and verbal fluency all improved significantly.[2532]

DHA and memory. Within the brain itself, the hippocampal region, most closely related to memory, show the greatest DHA concentrations[2533][2534][2535] and both blood flow to this region and neurogenesis there increase following supplementation.[2536][2537] DHA concentrates in the structures involved in forming new memories, such as synaptic membranes and tiny outgrowths called neurites.[2538][2539] DHA supplementation provides a synergistic boost to regular exercise. Studies show that exercise along with DHA supplementation in animals performed better on memory tasks than do those receiving either treatment alone.[2540][2541]

DHA and AD. DHA might have a beneficial impact in neurodegenerative diseases like Alzheimer's.[2542][2543][2544][2545] Those at risk for AD, and those with cognitive impairments often have a DHA deficiency.[2546][2547] Researchers suggest that the mechanism for the benefit may be in reduced oxidative damage in microglia cells, and upregulation of antioxidant stress pathways.[2548] AD patients have significantly lower levels of DHA in the neurons of their hippocampus[2549] suggesting that a lack of DHA makes people more vulnerable to the disease, and/or that the brain's attempts to heal itself deplete its cellular stores of DHA.[2550] Changes in DHA levels in CSF fluid were inversely correlated with CSF levels of total and phosphorylated tau.[2551] The multiple beneficial effects of DHA supplementation may depend on severity, gene type, and other dietary habits.[2552]

In an AD mouse model, animals on a DHA-enriched diet had seventy percent less amyloid-beta than controls.[2553] DHA is found to protect against synaptic loss[2554] and protect cell-signaling survival pathways from cell death.[2555] One nine-year study showed that those with high levels of DHA have a forty-seven percent reduced risk of AD onset.[2556] In both the Chicago[2557] dietary fat intake study and the Rotterdam Study,[2558] risk of incident dementia found by the researchers showed a sixty percent reduction in the incidence of Alzheimer's disease in those eating at least one fish-containing meal a week.

DHA Supplements.

New evidence suggests that high/low DHA concentrations in blood are not correlated to high/low concentrations in the brain, and that taking DHA supplements doesn't necessarily increase it in the brain due to constraints of the blood-brain barrier. It appears to be more related to the degree of homeostasis of DHA in the brains of elderly people.

A lysophospholipid (LPA) form of DHA may be more effective. LPA is extracted from egg yolks, bovine brain, and soybeans.

DHA and neurogenesis. Low DHA levels are also linked to low levels of brain and cellular growth factors such as brain-derived growth factor (BDNF).

DHA roles and metabolism.

- DHA is a major regulator of intracellular calcium oscillations,[2559][2560] which regulate a vast array of cellular functions including: mitochondrial function, gene activation, oxidative stress response, neurotransmitter release, neuron migration, and maturation.[2561]
- DHA enhances outgrowth of connections between neurons, improved transmission of electrical pulses across synapses, and protects against the physical and biochemical changes associated with Alzheimer's disease.[2562][2563][2564][2565] It metabolically advances to DEA (N-docosahexaenoyl ethanolamide) in accomplishing that.[2566] Brain synapses have a higher concentration of DHA than almost any other tissue in the body.[2567]
- DHA has potent anti-inflammatory properties that protect and support the critical production of neuroprotectins.[2568][2569][2570] Neuroprotectins are powerful anti-inflammatory and molecules that protect cells from apoptosis (cell death).[2571]
- Animal studies show learning and memory deficits with DHA deficiency; studies of the animals' brains demonstrate inflammatory and oxidative damage to neurons. All of these issues resolve when adequate DHA intake resumes.[2572][2573]
- DHA is essential in the energy regulation in the body and brain, that is regulating key enzymes essential for feeding energy to cells. Research suggests a strong link between DHA levels and neurodegeneration because up to sixty percent of the energy consumed by the brain is linked to enzymes such as the Na(+)K(+)ATPase enzyme.[2574]

Vegetarians tend to be woefully deficient in DHA and this puts them at a higher risk of cardiovascular disease and possibly AD, so we recommend supplementing daily with a high-grade algae formula. vegetarians supplemented with algae-based DHA enjoy the same drop in cardiovascular risk factors as do non-vegetarians consuming fish oil. Oil such as flaxseed can help but is not used as efficiently in the body.

For vegetarians, seaweed and algae, nuts, chia, flax and hemp seeds, brussels sprouts, walnuts, edamame, algal oil (from algae), perilla oil (from perilla seeds) are all excellent sources of DHA.

Consuming about three grams daily of fatty fish offers a 19-23 percent reduction in the risk of mild cognitive impairment, a condition associated with later progression to Alzheimer's disease. People who eat still larger amounts of fatty fish may experience protection of up to 75 percent.[2575]

Food sources: fatty fish such as anchovies, salmon, herring, mackerel, tuna, sardines, and halibut, and algae. Vegetarians can supplement DHA in the form of algae or flaxseed meal.

Other fatty acids, such as alpha-linolenic acid and stearidonic acid are precursors of EPA and DHA in the body and can be converted to EPA and DHA by the body, although the process is not as efficient as getting EPA and DHA directly from food and supplements. Those fats can be derived from land-based foods such as nuts, seeds, and oils.

EPA. According to some researchers the benefits of EPA (eicosapentaenoic acid) tend to be more for depression[2576] and for the heart and circulatory system. However, others feel that EPA has a neuroprotective role and the interaction between EPA and DHA may be important. Like DHA, in order to increase EPA levels in the brain, a lysophosphatidylcholine (LPC) form is most effective, and enriches both EPA (100-fold) and DHA (two-fold) in the brain. [2577] The reason is that the blood-brain barrier requires the LPC form rather than free EPA in the triacylglycerol form.[2578]

Omega-6 fatty acid (GLA, 360 mg to 2,000 mg daily). The most common omega-6 fat is gamma linoleic acid (GLA), produced in the body by linoleic acid, which can be converted into arachidonic acid (ARA) and may be, in turn, converted into inflammation-promoting compounds. However even a high intake of linoleic acid does not increase inflammatory responses.[2579]

GLA provides the healthy, anti-inflammatory type of omega-6. It is found in very small amounts in some leafy greens and nuts, while the pro-inflammatory fats linoleic acid and arachidonic acid are present in ample amounts in vegetable oils and chicken, and eggs and meat, respectively. GLA is found in certain oils, such as evening primrose oil and borage oil. When consumed, much of it is converted to another fatty acid called dihomo-gamma-linolenic acid (DGLA).

Sources: Natural sources of GLA include borage oil (17-25%), black currant oil (15-20%), and evening primrose oil (7-10%).[2580]

Omega-7 fatty acid (sea buckthorn, 250mg per day) is an overlooked, lesser known essential fatty acid with some significant benefits. It is helpful against the metabolic disorders that underlie diabetes, cardiovascular disease, obesity, and cancer. Omega-7 supplements the benefits of omega-3s with respect to the cardiovascular system and blood lipid levels. It can help break the cycle of high blood sugar, elevated lipid levels, inflammation, and excess fat gain[2581] as well as enhance insulin sensitivity.[2582][2583][2584] Omega-7 has been shown to cause an increase in fat breakdown and an increase in the enzymes involved in fat burning for energy.[2585]

Researchers found that patients taking an omega-7 supplement for thirty days experienced a forty-four percent reduction in inflammation biomarkers such as C-reactive protein. This demonstrated that such supplementation decreased inflammation and blood lipids, restoring their risk status to those of normal individuals.[2586] Sea buckthorn significantly increases the level of beneficial high-density lipoprotein (HDL) cholesterol fraction[2587] that may help to prevent cardiovascular diseases in healthy people.[2588]

Phosphatidylserine (PS, 100mg – 400mg per day) is a fatty substance that is made up of both amino acids and fatty acids. It covers and protects the neural cells in the brain and is essential for brain function. The majority of the fats in brain cell membranes are composed of phosphatidylserine. The omega-3 fatty acids EPA and DHA work synergistically with PS to provide the building blocks for healthy cell membranes. PS is critical to healthy cell membranes and brain tissue in the hippocampus.[2589]

PS may improve cognitive and memory functions.[2590] Phosphatidylserine is also essential for the brain to properly metabolize glucose (sugar) providing brain energy resources.[2591] PS is critical to healthy cell membranes and brain tissue in the hippocampus. It can cross the blood-brain barrier with beneficial effects to biochemical alterations and structural deterioration in nerve cells. It supports both short-term and long-term memory, improves the ability to retrieve memories, reason and resolve problems, and supports focus and attention.[2592] It supports good neurotransmission more than merely transmitting nerve signals; it increases the number of receptor sites on cell membranes.[2593]

Supplementing with 100mg of phosphatidylserine and 80mg phosphatidic acid produced from soy lecithin was found to absorb well, and resulted in having positive effect on memory, mood, and cognition among elderly test subjects.[2594] In one study, elderly women with depressive disorders were treated with a placebo for fifteen days and then with a PS supplement for thirty days. They experienced a consistent improvement of depressive symptoms, memory and behavior.[2595] Another study showed similar results with elderly subjects suffering from depression given 300 milligrams of PS every day for thirty days who experienced an average of seventy percent reduction in the severity of their depression.

Note: Omega-3 deficiency also causes a thirty-five percent reduction in brain PS levels. This may strongly correlate to depression levels, so supplementing with omega-3 fatty acids along PS may be effective for depression.

Food sources for PS: Soy lecithin (best food source), Atlantic herring and mackerel, tuna, chicken leg without the bone, mullet, veal, beef, bovine brain, chicken liver, anchovy, sardines, whole grain barley, organ muscles and meats, and soybeans.

Pinocembrin (PCB, no specific dosage, may be part of a multi-antioxidant formula) is the most abundant flavonoid in propolis (from bee pollen) and has been shown to have neuroprotective effects in vivo and in vitro. PCB reduces neurotoxicity in the brain as well as cell death rate related to mitochondrial function.[2596]

Note. We do not recommend taking bee pollen since it often contains pesticides, especially agricultural insecticides such as chlorpyrifos and acetamiprid.[2597]

Piperine is an active ingredient of black pepper and is included in many supplements, especially with curcumin, where it strongly improves curcumin absorption[2598] and improves gastrointestinal functional. Piperine supports neurogenesis, BDNF levels, and cognitive functioning.[2599]

Polygalae radix (35–45mg per day) is the root of Polygala tenuifolia willd, and has commonly been used for the treatment of amnesia and anxiety in traditional Korean medicine. It is typically found typically as part of herbal formulas such as Kai-xin-san[2600] and Bushen Tiansui,[2601] both of which are found to be effective tools against Alzheimer's.

Pomegranate juice is a source of the polyphenol, punicalagin, which is a strong anti-inflammatory agent that may reduce amyloid beta plaque levels.[2602 2603] It also contains potent antioxidants and anti-atherogenic agents (tannins, anthocyanins) reducing the risk of heart disease.[2604] One study found that mice fed pomegranate juice learned faster and had significantly less build-up of beta amyloid in their brains.[2605] Other mice studies showed reduced activity of NFAT (nuclear factor of activate T-cell), decreased the beta amyloid secretion of TNF (tumor necrosis factor),[2606] and inhibited cholinesterase.[2607] Researchers are investigating the pomegranate components, uro-lithins, which give rise to these effects.[2608]

Pumpkin Seeds contain powerful antioxidants that protect the body and brain from free radical damage.[2609]

Pycnogenol (maritime pine bark) is an extract from the bark of the French maritime pine with known antioxidative and neuroprotective effects. It has been suggested for potential use in the prevention or in early stages of mild cognitive impairment and AD.[2610]

Pycnogenol is one of the most potent antioxidant compounds currently known.[2611] It is fifty to one hundred times more potent than vitamin E in neutralizing free radicals and it helps to recycle and prolong the activity of vitamins C and E. It supports vascular health,[2612] healthy circulation,[2613][2614][2615] helps inhibit inflammatory factors[2616][2617][2618] and has potent antioxidant properties.[2619][2620][2621]

It has been found to reduce oxidative stress and improve cognitive function in healthy adults (age 35-55),[2622] and to improve memory in the elderly.[2623] It decelerates development of am-yloid plaque and improves spatial memory in a mouse model of Alzheimer's.[2624] Other lab animals, pretreated with pycnogenol and vitamin E were better protected from toxic insult to cognitive per-formance and oxidative damage in the hippocampus, and also experienced boosted levels of glu-tathione—all of which suggest a promising approach for treatment of oxidative stress-related neu-rodegeneration.[2625] These results have been replicated in human cell lines.[2626][2627] Similarly, pycno-genol protected Parkinsonian mice from neuroinflammation and neurodegeneration.[2628]

Food sources: wine, grapes, apples, cocoa, tea, nuts, and some berries.

Pyrroloquinoline Quinone (PQQ, 10mg – 20mg per day) is a small quinone compound family which influences multiple cellular pathways, including the production of nerve growth factor and providing neuroprotection. It is reported to improve learning ability and may also enhance working memory. It can increase cerebral blood flow in the prefrontal cortex. Increasing blood flow to the brain could help protect against cognitive decline and dementia in the elderly, espe-cially in attention and working memory.[2629]

PQQ may have neuroprotective properties[2630] against Alzheimer's, Parkinson's, and cognitive injuries. It protects the brain against neurotoxicity induced by other powerful toxins, including mercury and oxidopamine, toxins that are suspected to cause Alzheimer's and Parkinson's.[2631][2632] It prevents ag-gregation of alpha-synuclein and amyloid-beta, proteins associated with Parkinson's and Alzheimer's diseases,[2633][2634] offers neuroprotection for memory and cognition in aging animals and humans,[2635] stim-ulates mitochondrial biogenesis,[2636] decreases oxidative damage,[2637] and was shown to reduce inflamma-tion in one of the first studies to replicate results from animal studies to results in human studies. This study also replicated results in PQQ's ability to affect mitochondrial-related metabolism.[2638] PQQ also improves brain electrophysiological function after traumatic brain injury, decreasing lactate dehydrogen-ase content in astrocytes exposed to glutamate.[2639]

Food sources of PQQ: banana, cabbage, carrot, celery, egg yolk, fava beans, field mustard, green tea, green pepper, kiwi, miso, fermented soybeans orange, papaya, parsley, potato, spinach, sweet potato, and tomato.

Quercetin (250-500mg 1-2 times per day) is an antioxidant and anti-inflammatory flavonoid. Like other antioxidants it has wide ranging benefits including reducing the risk of neurodegenerative disorders, cancer, cardiovascular diseases, allergic disorders, thrombosis, atherosclerosis, hypertension, and arrhythmia.[2640] It reduces DNA damage, and increases glutathione in cell lines used for research (SH-SY5Y cells).[2641]

Quercetin limits brain cell death due to chronic inflammation[2642] that often leads to both Alzheimer's and Parkinson's diseases.[2643][2644][2645] Furthermore, it protects brain cells against excitotoxicity, the damage done by repeated excitatory electrical impulses observed in Alzheimer's and other neurodegenerative diseases.[2646][2647][2648][2649]

Due to its potent antioxidant effects, quercetin may reduce toxicity of the dangerous and abnormal accumulated amyloid-beta proteins[2650] preventing brain cell death in animal models of Parkinson's disease[2651] by activating the brain's natural Nrf2 antioxidant defense system.[2652][2653][2654][2655][2656] Quercetin neutralizes free radical that attack mitochondrial membrane.[2657][2658][2659] Quercetin protects brain cells against excitotoxicity, the damage done by repeated excitatory electrical impulses observed in Alzheimer's, Parkinson's[2660] and other neurodegenerative diseases.[2661][2662][2663][2664]

Food sources: citrus fruits, apple, onion, parsley, berries, green tea, and red wine.

Radix puerariae (Pueraria lobata, no specific dosage, usually part of a multi-herbal formula) has multiple health benefits. The active component, puerarin, has been shown to dilate arteries and help lower blood pressure. It can protect learning and memory from impairment induced by toxins,[2665] ischemic brain injury,[2666] amyloid beta peptide,[2667] and chronic alcoholism.[2668]

Resveratrol (150mg per day) is an anti-inflammatory and antioxidant compound found in red grapes and red wine. Resveratrol helps promote and maintain optimal health and longevity,[2669] is linked to insulin balance,[2670] reduces inflammation,[2671] and supports cardiovascular health.[2672] Resveratrol appears to be helpful against AD mechanisms.[2673][2674][2675] It encourages enhanced mitochondrial function, modulates metabolic regulators linked to neurological disorder onset[2676] and improves a number of biomarkers associated with Alzheimer's. It is shown in comparative research, to reduce membrane permeability in the blood-brain barrier (although it crosses the blood-brain barrier)[2677][2678] and the accumulation of amyloid beta clumpings in the brain.[2679] It supports brain plasticity,[2680] enhances mitochondrial function[2681] and neurite outgrowth and the stimulation of mitochondrial biogenesis.[2682]

Food sources: apples, red grapes and wine, blueberries, mulberries, strawberries, cranberries, grape juice, dark chocolate, peanuts, pistachios.

Resveratrol with **Quercetin** (150mg-250mg transresveratrol with 150mg-300mg quercetin daily). Resveratrol is more effective combined with quercetin. In one study, the combination significantly improved memory performance of healthy overweight adults compared to placebo.[2683] The combination is especially effective for reducing obesity (by influencing to gut microbiota),[2684] a risk factor for neurodegenerative conditions.

Rhizoma anemarrhenae (zhimu, no specific dosage, usually part of a multi-herbal formula) contains active constituents include the saponins sarsasapogenin, smilagenin, neogitogenin, and markosapogenin. Zhimu protects learning and memory against toxic insult,[2685][2686] cholesteremia and ischemic brain injury,[2687] improves the speed of acetylcholine synthesis and density of M-type Ach receptors,[2688][2689] and scavenges free radicals.[2690] Saraspongenin is an especially promising compound for AD treatment, and a hybrid of it and trizolyl has been created in the search for AD drugs.[2691]

Rhodiola rosea extract (200–600mg per day) roots contain high levels of phytochemicals such as flavonoids, monoterpenes, triterpenes, and phenols with anti-inflammatory, neuroprotective,[2692] anticancer, cardioprotective, and anti-depression properties.[2693] It helps to reduce fatigue and promotes alertness in healthy subjects.[2694]

Researchers have found that in animal studies rhodopsin or its crude extract protects learning and memory[2695][2696][2697] from toxic insults,[2698] increases acetacholine content, reduces cholinesterase activity in the brain, increases antioxidation activity,[2699] reduces cognitive impairment (probably due to enhancement of neural-signaling chemicals in the brain such as dopamine and acetylcholine),[2700][2701] and protects against cell death.[2702]

Rosemary (R. officinalis. 150–700mg per day) improves cognitive deficits,[2703] is antidiabetic,[2704][2705] anti-inflammatory, antioxidant,[2706] antithrombotic,[2707] antidiuretic,[2708] and antiulcerogenic.[2709][2710] It is also antibacterial,[2711] anti-cancer,[2712] antinociceptive (pain-killing),[2713][2714] and its constituent, carnosol, protects the liver from oxidative stress.[2715]

Rutin (450mg per day) is a glycoside of the flavonoid quercetin, and is also known as vitamin P. It can cross the blood brain barrier, and has powerful anti-inflammatory benefits. Rutin has been shown to have an extensive array of pharmacological applications due to its numerous properties including antioxidant, anti-inflammatory, cardiovascular, neuroprotective, antidiabetic, and anticancer activities.[2716][2717]

Rutin has a potential protective role in neurogenerative disorders, such as AD,[2718][2719][2720] due to its beneficial effects as a potent antioxidant.[2721][2722][2723] Also notable is its effect on processing and clumping of amyloid beta, and ability to change to the oxidant-antioxidant balance linked to nerve cell death.[2724]

Food sources: Apricots, buckwheat, cherries, figs, grapes, grapefruit, green tea, plums, and most citrus fruits including oranges.

Salvia miltiorrhiza bunge (danshen, red sage, 600mg per day) contains over 160 distinct antioxidant polyphenols.[2725] It promotes blood flow and removal of toxins. In China it is frequently used for cardiovascular and hematological disorders.[2726] It may enhance cognition and protect against neurodegenerative disease.[2727] It has a strong effect in increasing neurogenesis.[2728] Danshen can improve cholinergic functions in the central nervous system[2729] by inhibiting inflammatory reaction (by halting the breakdown of the chemical messenger acetylcholine or ACH).[2730] One of its compounds, salvianolic acid B, has a strong effect in increasing neurogenesis, and may be useful in fighting cognitive impairment after stroke and other neurodegenerative problems.[2731]

A literature review summarizes the research with two active components of S. miltiorrhiza, salvianolic acid A, and salvianolic acid B. A blocks aggregation of, and disaggregates AB42 fibers in SH-SY5Y cells, reduces learning and memory impairments in lab animals, and might inhibit the activity of B-secretase.[2732] B is the most active antioxidant from danshen, which protects cells from amyloid beta toxicity, reduces mitochondrial stress and preserves synapse density.[2733] Other danshen active compounds, danshensu, tanshinone I, tanshinone IIA, and cyptotanshinone, exhibit similar qualities against AD in the lab setting.[2734]

Note. May be contraindicated when on blood thinning medication such as coumadin (warfarin).

Salvia officinalis (culinary sage) enhances memory retention by interacting with muscarinic and cholinergic pathways that are involved in learning and memory.[2735] Small pilot studies find it effective in treating memory loss in elderly patients.[2736] Like danshen, culinary sage contains large amounts of antioxidant and anti-inflammatory polyphenols.[2737]

Selenium (200mcg per day) is one of the precursors for glutathione production in the liver, and is essential for neutralizing free radicals. Selenium deficiency is associated with cognitive decline[2738] [2739] and DNA hypomethylation.[2740] [2741] It can modulate DNA and histones to activate methylation-silenced genes,[2742] may have anticarcinogenic properties through modifications of epigenetic processes in the cell.[2743] However, an eight-year study involving 3786 subjects which observed the effects of vitamin E and/or selenium found no evidence of reduced risk of dementia[2744] even though selenite is an inhibitor of tau hyperphosphorylation.[2745] Very high or very low levels of selenium may play a role in the pathogenesis of Parkinson's.[2746] The brain does have the highest priority to receive and retain selenium even in the face of its deficiency, and dysfunction of selenoprotein is linked to Parkinson's.[2747]

Food sources: Brazil nuts, yellow fin tuna, chicken, beef, ham, beans, sunflower seeds, brown rice, and oats.

S-adenosyl-l-methionine (SAM-e, 1200–2200mg per day). SAM-e is a natural biochemical that boosts the production of phosphatidylserine (PS), discussed above. It supports protein methylation which, if impaired, leads to brain deterioration. Some conditions such as metabolic syndrome reduce SAM-e levels,[2748] and its availability to cells determines its ability for protein methylation.[2749] Metabolic syndrome is identified as a group of symptoms linked to cardiovascular disease and type two diabetes. SAM-e may be more effective than placebo and equal in efficacy to tricyclic antidepressants (amitriptyline, amoxapine, desipramine, doxepin, imipramine, nortriptyline, protriptyline, and trimipramine) for treating major depressive disorder when administered either intravenously or intramuscularly.[2750] However SAM-e is relatively expensive and unstable; taken orally, l-methionine can increase SAM-e levels in the brain.[2751]

Food sources: Spirulina, asparagus, mustard greens, green peas, cauliflower, okra, spinach, broccoli, sesame seeds, oats, soy (tofu), brazil nuts, sunflower butter, sweet corn, garlic. Avoid diets with large amounts of lamb, beef, or pork, which are high in methionine and which also can elevate homocysteine, contributing not only to cardiovascular disease, but neurodegeneration.

Seratonin is a biochemical produced in the brain by nerve cells, and is essential for signaling. It is found mostly in the digestive system, in blood platelets, and throughout the central nervous system. Low levels of serotonin in the brain may cause depression, anxiety, and sleep trouble.[2752]

Mood may influence social behavior, and social support is one of the most studied psychosocial factors in relation to health and disease,[2753] possibly resulting in mimicking symptoms of dementia. Ways to increase serotonin is through regular exercise, having a healthy diet, getting plenty of sunshine and meditating regularly, as well as increasing tryptophan (5HTP) and Vitamin B6.

Foods highest in tryptophan: Meat, cheese, fish/crab, salmon, turkey, spirulina/seaweed, spinach, pineapples, bananas, dates, eggs, oats, nuts, and seeds.

Serrapeptase (120,000IU or 36mg per day split up between meals). The enzyme serrapeptase is proteolytic (breaks down food into energy) derived from the silkworm and commonly used in Japan and Europe for its anti-inflammatory, anti-edemic and analgesic effects. It may have anti-atherosclerotic effects (similar to nattokinase), also due to its properties to break down blood clots (fibrinolytic) and break down dairy foods (caseinolytic).[2754] It basically works by helping the body break down protein debris in the vessels and tissues.

Note: Serrapeptase might interfere with blood clotting, so some researchers worry that it might make bleeding disorders worse. If you have a bleeding disorder, check with your healthcare provider before using serrapeptase.

Taurine (750–1,000mg per day) is an antioxidant amino acid with neuroprotective effect. It used in every cell of the body, and levels in the body decrease with age. Taurine may be helpful for Parkinson's and depression.[2755][2756][2757] Patients with PD have low taurine plasma levels, which is aggravated by the drug levodopa, which may further deplete taurine.[2758] In Alzheimer mice, taurine improved cognitive impairment by binding to oligomeric amyloid beta.[2759] It offers support through a variety of mechanisms.[2760]

This nutrient plays an important part in overall brain health by helping the body create new brain cells by activating "sleeping" stem cells. In animals, taurine also increases the survival of new neurons, resulting in an increase in adult brain cell creation.[2761][2762][2763] Its antioxidant and anti-inflammatory capacity, along with modulating signaling pathways, timing[2764][2765][2766][2767][2768] and ability,[2769] are useful in neurodegenerative conditions. It can even favorably mimic the actions of certain neurotransmitters, such as GABA, used by the body for learning.[2770][2771] Taurine helps keep the arteries supple and flexible,[2772] supports the endothelium (delicate lining of blood vessels), [2773][2774][2775] and supports heart muscle strength.[2776]

Food sources: Highest levels are in shellfish, especially scallops, mussels, and clams. High amounts of taurine can also be found in the dark meat of turkey and chicken, and turkey bologna, sea algae, brewer's yeast, and breast milk.

Tea, green and black (704mg per day, equal to three cups of green tea, or 338mg EGCG/day)[2777]. Both green and black tea contain flavonoid catechins that help protect the aging brain, reduce the incidence of dementia, AD, and PD,[2778] reduce amyloid beta accumulation in mice,[2779][2780] and reduce cognitive decline.[2781][2782][2783] Both forms of tea contain other active components which may contribute to reduced risk of cardiovascular disease, [2784] (cholesterol levels[2785] and hypertension)[2786] [2787], stroke (21% reduced risk with three cups daily),[2788] cancer,[2789][2790][2791] and dementia.[2792][2793]

Tea offers potent antioxidant protection[2794][2795][2796][2797]that reduces oxidative stress caused by inflammation.[2798][2799] It has neuroprotective properties,[2800][2801][2802][2803][2804][2805] and positively influences mitochondrial health, intracellular signaling pathways, intracellular messengers, transcription factors and healthy gene expression.[2806] These factors account for tea's support of thinking, problem solving, and reasoning.[2807]

Epigallocatechin gallate (EGCG) is the most important of the tea catechins. It enhances healthy cell reproduction, metabolic function, liver function, normal body weight, and cardiovascular health. It helps cognitive health, supports the immune system.[2808]

Theanine (l-theanine is its chemical mirror image, and is most often tested). Theanine increases serotonin, and dopamine in the brain, as well as BDNF. It is able to cross the blood-brain barrier. L-theanine reportedly modulates alpha brain-wave activity and play a role in tasks requiring attention, as well as to provide benefit to mental states in healthy adults.[2809] L-theanine administered orally increases BDNF in the hippocampus over three to four weeks, [2810][2811][2812][2813] and there is mounting evidence of a neuroprotective effect.[2814][2815][2816] In a recent study l-theanine treated AD patients experienced reduced stress-related symptoms, such as sleep disturbances as well as cognitive improvements in verbal fluency and executive function.[2817]

Trytophan and 5-HTP (5-HTP, 50–300mg, 1-3 times daily) are chemical precursors to serotonin and help increase serotonin levels which may, in turn, have neurogenesis benefits in mice.[2818] 5-HTP is often used to help with depression and as a sleep aid.

Vitamin A (Palmitate, 1,000–5,000mcg per day). Retinoid acid, the biochemical formed by vitamin A, is a neurotransmitter in the brain. It regulates a number of gene products and modulates neurogenesis, neuronal survival, and synaptic plasticity.[2819] Levels of vitamin A and its precursor, beta-carotene, are lower in AD patients. They have been clinically shown to slow the progression of dementia, and in vitro studies, to inhibit the development, and negative effects of amyloid beta fibrils. In animal models of AD, injections of vitamin A into the peritoneum decreased brain amyloid plaque deposition and tau phosphorylation, reduced nerve degeneration, and improved spatial learning and memory.[2820] Vitamin A is needed to convert light into an electrical signal that can be sent to the brain. One of the first symptoms of vitamin A deficiency can be night blindness, known as nyctalopia.[2821]

Vitamins B1, B2, B3, B6, B9, and B12 deficiencies are found in Alzheimer's patients but the mechanisms and direct causal relationship are still under investigation. They are essential for supporting nerve function, neurotransmission, lowering homocysteine levels, supporting essential enzyme transactions, and supporting overall brain and heart health. Deficiencies in these vitamins mimic dementia symptoms, increase homocysteine levels, and result in mood disorders including depression.[2822] High levels of homocysteine levels may cause or contribute to AD onset, and can be reduced by supplementing with high levels of these B vitamins. Of all the B-vitamins, vitamins B1 (thiamine), B3 (niacin), and B12 (cobalamin), are most clearly associated with deterioration in mental state.

In one study 133 participants were given a daily combination of three B vitamins (0.8 mg folic acid, 20mg vitamin B6, 0.5mg vitamin B12). The researchers determined that the combination appeared to slow cognitive and clinical decline in people with mild cognitive impairment, in particular in those with elevated homocysteine.[2823] Another study suggested that the accelerated rate of brain atrophy in elderly with mild cognitive impairment can be slowed by treatment with homocysteine-lowering B vitamins.[2824]

Vitamin B1 (thiamine) is critical for memory formation.[2825] Low levels of B1 are found in AD patients and excess B1 reduces AD-like symptoms.[2826] Wernicke-Korsakoff syndrome, which includes symptoms of dysfunctional coordination, confusion, hallucinations, and memory loss, is caused by B1 deficiency.[2827] A B1 deficiency can also result in loss of appetite,[2828] [2829] and heart failure due to poor pumping capacity. This is often the result of alcoholism, [2830] even in the cases where there is enough overall nutritional food intake, as the alcohol affects proper thiamine metabolism.

Food sources of B1: Sunflower seeds, navy and black beans, barley, dried and green peas, lentils, pinto and lima beans, oats. *Foods that deplete thiamine include*: tea, coffee, alcohol, and raw fish.

Vitamin B3 (niacin) Two rare neurologic syndromes are caused by niacin and thiamine deficiencies. Niacin deficiency is a known cause of pellagra, a disease characterized by symptoms of dementia, diarrhea, and dermatitis that can be resolved through niacin supplementation.[2831] [2832]

Disease effects on the central nervous system begin with neurasthenia (an ill-defined medical condition characterized by lassitude, fatigue, headache, and irritability, associated chiefly with emotional disturbance), followed by symptoms of psychosis, including disorientation, memory loss, and confusion. Pellagra can result from alcoholism and gastrointestinal disease and is endemic to populations that consume maize or sorghum as the primary food.

Food sources: Avocado, brown rice, lamb, liver, chicken breast, green peas, potatoes, tuna, turkey, salmon, anchovies, sardines, shrimp, pork ground beef, peanuts, and whole wheat.

Vitamin B6 (pyridoxine) is used in Alzheimer's therapy. Vitamin B6 participates in more than 140 essential enzymatic reactions, including protein metabolism, conversion of tryptophan to niacin, and neurotransmitter function.[2833]

Food sources: Cereals, pistachios, sunflower seeds, banana, garlic, beans, vegetables including cabbage and spinach, liver, brewer's yeast, brown rice, beef, chicken, sweet potato, potato, tuna, turkey, eggs, royal jelly.

Vitamin B12 (cobalamin, 1,000mcg per day). Deficiency of B12 has been linked to mental decline often mistaken for dementia. Vitamin B12 deficiency is common with older age, occurring in more than twenty percent of persons sixty-five years and older,[2834] and as the result of increased prevalence of gastritis and other digestive conditions that interfere with absorption.[2835] Causes of B12 deficiency can result from impaired absorption, pernicious anemia, and diets deficient in B12.[2836]

Vitamin B12 is essential for the production of neurotransmitters,[2837] support of brain cell health, and healthy levels of homocysteine (which have been implicated with onset of AD).[2838] [2839] [2840] Vitamin B12 works synergistically with vitamin B6 and folate to regenerate (methylate) the amino acid methionine, which helps to maintain already healthy homocysteine levels within the normal range.[2841] [2842] [2843] [2844] [2845]

Cobalamin deficiency may cause cognitive deficits and even dementia. In Alzheimer's disease, the most frequent cause of dementia in elderly persons, low serum levels of vitamin B12,[2846] may be misleading. Study findings suggest that cobalamin deficiency may cause a reversible dementia in elderly patients.[2847] In one study of 107 senior adults (not in nursing homes), those found with B12 deficiencies had the greatest brain loss volume.[2848] The research is mixed as to whether B12 deficiency, along with high homocysteine and low folic acid) is a risk factor for AD.[2849 2850 2851 2852]

Studies have connected deficiencies in Vitamin B12 to cognition, mood, depression,[2853] and a neurologic syndrome characterized by cognitive and psychiatric disturbances, degeneration of the spinal cord, and peripheral nerves.[2854 2855] These can be resolved by high-dose vitamin B12 therapy.[2856 2857] Deficiencies in Vitamin B12 also contribute to risk of atherosclerosis, heart attack, stroke,[2858] pernicious anemia,[2859] and psychiatric and neurological disorders.[2860] Studies also show that people with anemia are at a higher risk of developing dementia.[2861 2862]

A diet rich in taurine, cysteine, folate, B12 and betaine may reduce AD risk,[2863] and daily supplementation of oral 400μg folic acid plus 100μg vitamin B12 improves cognitive functioning in memory performance after 24 months.[2864] B12 may lessen the risk of AD.[2865]

Common foods high in vitamin B12: Sardines, beef, clams, tuna, fortified cereals and nutritional yeast, trout, salmon, fortified soy, almond and rice milks, milk and dairy products, and animal liver and kidneys.

Vitamin D (5,000IU per day. D2 or D3 are best absorbed,[2866]). An estimated forty-seventy-five percent of all adults are vitamin D deficient. This may be because vitamin D is only naturally present in a few foods. Normal plasma levels of Vitamin D (between 75-100nmol/L) has been shown to help maintain healthy cognitive levels and prevent premature death. Healthy blood levels of D correspond to better scores on cognitive health tests and better maintenance of cognitive ability in aging individuals.[2867 2868 2869 2870] Low levels of Vitamin D have been implicated in a range of health problems and premature death.[2871] Researchers have suggested low vitamin D levels as increasing risk of AD: from deficiency (lower than 25nmol/L)[2872] to insufficiency (levels of 25-50 nmol/L)[2873] being high risk factors for cognitive decline. However, a 2019 meta-analysis found that when other risk factors (such as cardiovascular disease, cancer, physical activity, cholesterol levels, and alcohol intake) are taken into account, those levels were not statistically significant or associated with AD.[2874] Additionally, clinical interventional studies do not link increased D levels with improved cognition.[2875] Nonetheless, vitamin D does benefit and protect the brain by activating macrophages which break down and remove debris in the brain, including excess beta-amyloid deposits.[2876 2877 2878]

Food sources: About 20-30 minutes (depending where you live) of daily exposure to sunlight, consume oily fish like salmon, tuna, swordfish or mackerel, cod liver oil, as well as milk, eggs, and cheese.

Vitamin E (200–800mg per day) is a potent antioxidant that has been shown to cross the blood-brain barrier.[2879 2880] The most bioavailable form is the alpha-tocopherol form,[2881] but a <u>combination</u> of the different forms may be even more effective (four tocotrienols: alpha, beta, gamma, and delta). For example, in one study concentrations of alpha-tocopherol were correlated with higher amyloid-beta plaque burdens when gamma-tocopherol levels were low and plaque was less when gamma-tocopherol was high (in combination with alpha-tocopherol).[2882]

Vitamin E has many benefits for brain health[2883 2884 2885] including slowing down cognitive decline in patients with AD (with memantine)[2886] or B vitamins (folic acid. .8mg, B6 20mg, B12 .5mg over two years),[2887] and related disabilities,[2888] having neurogenesis properties, reducing effects of free radical and oxidative stress, reducing the risk of developing AD[2889 2890 2891] (in patients over age eighty[2892]), improving cognitive functioning (along with vitamin C, in a six-year study,[2893] and in a ten-year study[2894]), improving performance in perceptual speed, as well as in lowering neuritic plaque density.[2895] And in a two-year study of patients with moderately severe AD reducing level of care needs.[2896] People who consume higher vitamin E-containing foods and who also do not experience inflammation or oxidative stress exhibit reduced cognitive decline[2897 2898] (as much as a thirty-five percent reduced rate of decline)[2899] when tested with standard mental state tests.[2900 2901 2902]

E combined with B vitamins, vitamins E and C also work well together to prevent oxidative damage in the brain. Vitamin E neutralizes and removes free radicals, while vitamin C deactivates free radicals that manage to pass through the lipid membrane, and also reactivates the antioxidant properties of vitamin E.[2903] Those eating diets high in vitamin E and C may have a lower risk of developing AD (vitamin E >15 mg/day). Another study identified better cognitive performance after combined use of vitamins E, C, and NSAIDs.[2904]

Ninety percent of the population does not consume the RDA of 15mg/day but average closer to half that value—around 7mg/day.[2905] Patients with less than half the recommended daily vitamin E have poorer cognitive ability than those with higher intake levels.[2906] Women with lower levels of Vitamin E showed brains being two years older compared to women with normal vitamin E.[2907] There are markedly lower levels of vitamin E in the cerebrospinal fluid and blood of AD patients.[2908 2909 2910 2911 2912] In other long-term studies supplementing with 2,000IU of vitamin E helped slow the progression of Alzheimer's disease (AD) by about nineteen percent annually over 2.3 years.[2913]

Note on sources. There are mixed results on vitamin E. However, an eight-year study involving 3786 subjects who observed the effects of vitamin E and/or selenium, found no evidence of reduced risk of dementia.[2914] There are also possible safety issues in taking high dosages of vitamin E, but there have been no reports of adverse effects of high levels of vitamin E from food sources.[2915] The dietary form of vitamin E significantly reduces the negative effects of reactive oxygen and nitrogen species in the body and brain cells.[2916] But, high doses from supplements can cause blood coagulation problems.[2917]

Note. Supplementation with vitamin E should not exceed 400IU –800IU per day unless under a doctor's supervision as it can thin the blood, particularly in patients on blood thinning medications.

Food sources: Wheat germ, raw swiss chard and collard greens, cooked mustard greens, red pepper, raw spinach, cooked asparagus, avocado, sunflower seeds, almonds, hazelnuts, peanuts and peanut butter, salmon, rainbow trout, mango, kiwi fruit, and pumpkin.

Vinpocetine (lesser periwinkle plant, Vinca minor, 30mg(3x10mg)–60mg(3x20mg) per day) enhances cerebral blood flow by dilating blood vessels and reducing blood viscosity. It readily enters the bloodstream after oral supplementation.[2918] The higher dose is effective but not statistically significant.[2919] It is widely used in Japan and many European countries to treat a number of cerebrovascular diseases. Promising evidence from the laboratory suggests that vinpocetine protects brain tissue from the oxidative stress caused by amyloid beta[2920] Also, because vinpocetine blocks receptors involved in AD development,[2921] vinpocetine supplements have a potential role in preventing Alzheimer's. It may play a role in Parkinson's therapy because in animal studies it increased the activity of noradrenergic pathways in the locus coeruleus.[2922]

Studies show it improves blood supply to the brain,[2923 2924 2925 2926] by inhibiting an enzyme (phosphodiesterase type 1) and reducing intracellular calcium levels, which dilates vessels and reduces blood viscosity enabling brain blood vessels to relax.[2927 2928 2929] Vinpocetine has cognitive enhancing effects resulting in improved abilities to retain and recall information[2930 2931] and improved ability in daily activity.[2932] It increases oxygen and glucose use by the brain,[2933 2934] maintains optimal energy of healthy brains,[2935 2936] maintains healthy levels of some neurotransmitters[2937 2938] promotes healthy attention, short-term memory (in animals)[2939] and concentration[2940] [2941 2942 2943] (in healthy human volunteers)[2944] and has an inhibitory effect on inflammation.[2945 2946]

Other benefits include being helpful in patients with urgency, urge incontinence, and possibly other kinds of incontinence,[2947 2948] improvements in hearing as well as in "ringing" of the ears, or tinnitus, following trauma to the ear.[2949]

Walnuts (Raw or Roasted) are a great brain food with a high concentration of DHA with more antioxidants (diarylheptanoids, quinones, polyphenols, flavones and terpenes) compared to other nuts.[2950 2951 2952] They are high in vitamin E, melatonin and polyphenols, especially in their papery skin.[2953] These components not only protect brain cells from oxidative stress and neuroinflammation[2954] but also improve messaging, neurogenesis, and enhance isolation of insoluble toxic protein clumps.[2955 2956] Walnuts are a good nut in heart-healthy diets because they reduce oxidative stress,[2957] particularly after eating a meal high in LDL "lousy" cholesterol.[2958]

Zeaxanthin (2-12mg per day) combined with **lutein**. Like lutein, zeaxanthin is an antioxidant carotenoid found in yellow to orange colored vegetables. Both are part of the xanthophyll family which are able to immerse themselves in fatty brain cell membranes, crossing between the cell's exterior and interior environments.[2959] This stabilizes cell structures and protects against oxidative stress from inside and outside the cell. Research studies show that the combination helps maintain cognitive function memory, and executive (prioritizing and decision-making) function. Higher blood levels of zeaxanthin and lutein are associated with better processing speed[2960] and enhancing brain blood flow in the parts of the brain involving cognitive functions[2961] resulting in improved integrity of the brain's white matter tracts. White matter, found in the subcortical part of the brain, contains dense nerve fibers, Increased activation in this part of the brain, responsible for cognition and memory, was the result in a one-year study of older patients taking the combination (2mg zeaxanthin plus 10mg lutein) compared to controls.[2962]

Food sources: Saffron, goji berries, egg yolks, maize, orange peppers, dark, leafy green vegetables, kiwi fruit, grapes, peas, spinach, oranges, tangerines, and zucchini.

Zinc (40-60mg per day, when supplementing, copper should be taken as well in a 15:1 zinc to copper ratio). Zinc is essential for nerve signaling[2963] and synaptic function.[2964][2965] It inhibits oxidative stress and neurotoxicity,[2966] enhances cognition,[2967] supports cardiovascular and neurological health, and helps maintain vision in the elderly.[2968] Zinc is needed for hippocampus-dependent learning and memory.[2969][2970] In the brain zinc is located mostly in the retina of the eye, and in hippocampal vesicles (sacs) near synapses. Zinc is required at the synapse for the signaling function of axons (mossy fibers) of small neurons (granule cells)[2971][2972] and is released when the synapses are stimulated.[2973]

Zinc deficiency is widespread, especially in the elderly,[2974] and is linked to the stress response,[2975] immune dysfunction,[2976][2977] cognitive[2978] and learning impairment, and memory loss.[2979][2980][2981] Low levels in the brain are linked to many neurological problems including, neurodegenerative conditions such as Alzheimer's, Parkinson's, Huntington's disease, amyotrophic lateral sclerosis, and prion disease.[2982] Deficiency is also linked to mood disorders such as depression.

Serum zinc declines with age in people for unknown reasons. AD patients are relatively zinc deficient compared to age matched controls.[2983] Although zinc levels are lower in AD and Parkinson's patients so far there is no direct causal link.[2984] Amyloid plaque binds to zinc, most likely resulting in additional neuron death.[2985] But zinc supplementation can be helpful. In a six-month double-blind study in patients age seventy and over, zinc supplementation was shown to protect against cognition loss.[2986]

Note. Because a deficiency in zinc can mimic AD symptoms, blood levels should be checked by your doctor. <u>High dosages of zinc can be toxic</u> and paradoxical can play a role in initiating and inhibiting oxidative stress and neurotoxicity.[2987]

Food sources: Oysters, crab and lobster, eggs, dairy like cheese and milk, dark chocolate, meat and poultry, vegetables such as mushrooms, spinach, broccoli, kale, and garlic, legumes such as hummus, chickpeas, lentils, edamame, and black beans, nuts and seeds, whole grains.

Chapter 16. Nutrients: Absorption, Taking Nutrients

Different delivery systems—tablet, softgel, liquid, subligual, etc.—have different rates of absorption. The rates of absorbance vary greatly according to different researchers, but what seems to be more important is how fast they reach the body. Most nutrients, like vitamins, are not taken with time-specific requirements, and so the delivery method may not be critical.

In short, liquids and soft gels are the easiest to take, and reach the blood stream most quickly compared to pills, tablets, and hard-shell capsules. They do a better job of protecting the nutrients from degradation due to oxidation, light, or UV radiation, but have a shorter shelf life.[2988]

- Pills or tablets: 10-39% absorption, slowest to be absorbed[2989]
- Capsules: 20- 3% absorption, slow to be absorbed. Hard shell capsules make it easier to delivery time-released drugs, or dual-action drugs.[2990]
- Transdermal Patch: 45%, absorbed slow and continually
- Soft gels: More quickly absorbed. Liquid gel capsules are coated with a gelatin that is easily digested, allows smaller particles which further speeds absorbance. They protect active ingredients effectively and protect nutrients from oxidation and degradation, light, and UV radiation. They tend to have shorter shelf life than tablets.[2991]
- Sublingual (droppers): 85-90% absorption, quickly absorbed[2992]
- Intramuscular injection: 90% absorption, very quickly absorbed[2993]
- Intraoral Spray (under the tongue): 95% absorption, very quickly absorbed[2994]
- Liquid extracts: 98%absorption, very quickly absorbed[2995] [2996]
- Intravenous: 100% absorption, immediately absorbed[2997]

Note: If you are taking time-released medications or supplements, do not crush tablets or open capsules.

Take the most important nutrients under the tongue if available. It's not how much you take but how much your body tissues absorb that is important. Intraoral and sublingual absorption has become a viable solution with the introduction of liposomes.[2998] Liposomes are little fat containers that can hold nutrients and provide an efficient transport system that allows for maximum absorption by the body. These fat containers bypass the stomach and take a quicker route by slipping through the sub-mucosal membrane under the tongue and directly into the bloodstream. With a greater concentration of nutrients in the blood, more nutrients reach their intended destination, thereby requiring a lower dosage intake.

These are issues that can negatively impact absorption:

- **Antibiotics.** People who have been on long term antibiotics have reduced absorption as good bacteria in the gut needed to help breakdown food is killed. If taking antibiotics, take acidophilus supplements between dosages. This will help build up the good bacteria in the digestive tract destroyed by the antibiotics. It is especially important for elderly patients to take acidophilus on a regular basis.

- **Aging**. The aging population has fewer enzymes and HCL needed to break down food.
- **Inflammation**. Inflammatory conditions[2999] and diabetes (which can impact the vagus nerve causing food to stay in the stomach longer (gastroparesis [3000]) often affects good digestion as well and therefore lessens nutrients taken into the body.
- **Taking medications** that reduce stomach acid with reduce one's ability to absorb nutrients through the digestive tract (and also increase the risk of anemia). A wide range of medications can affect how well one digests and absorbs nutrients from food. Check with your doctor or online for further information. Drugs that may injure the lining of the intestine, such as tetracycline, colchicine, or cholestyramine.

The intraoral spray or sublingual method of delivery is very helpful for individuals who have difficulty swallowing pills or capsules and is also cost effective since a lower dosage of nutrients is needed.

Remember, more nutrients in a pill or capsule is not necessarily better. Ask what is important:

- How well can we insure the intake of recommended "therapeutic dosages?"
- What is the quality of the nutrients?
- Are nutrients buffered and time-released?
- Are they combined with other nutrients?

As practitioners, we know how much nutrients we want patients to take therapeutically, but what we do not know is how much of the nutrients prescribed are absorbed into the patients' bloodstream through their digestive tracts. We do know that as one gets older, one's absorption rate through the intestinal tract reduces, sometimes significantly, particularly when combined with serious health conditions, or particular digestive disorders such as ulcers, diverticulitis, gastric problems, acid reflux, etc.

Other factors that affect absorption include the following:

- **Stress** restricts the flow of blood in the body by tightening muscles and restricting the free flow of fluids. Meditation, yoga, tai chi, or even daily walks in nature can all help reduce stress significantly.
- **Eating slowly.** We should be eating our food slowly and thoughtfully. Try never to eat on the run, and don't eat while working. Make eating a special time.
- **Exercise** helps the body rid itself of harmful toxins that build-up daily. Even a brisk walk of only twenty minutes per day can have a major impact in protecting the brain.
- **Positive thinking**. In Chinese medicine, excessive thoughts of anger, worry, resentment, grief, and fear all have significant effects on the free flow of "energy" in our body. Excess anger and/or stress often imbalances the Liver, which then causes the Stomach and Spleen meridians to be affected, impacting both the ability to absorb nutrients as well as distribute the nutrients throughout the body.
- **Eating healthy food**. Our bodies crave fresh food, particularly fruits, vegetables, and grains. These foods provide energy to our bodies in the form of vitamins, minerals, and

natural enzymes. Excessive intake of "dead" food such as fast foods, or highly processed foods, requires our bodies to use its own enzymes and energy to digest food in an attempt to separate whatever limited nutrients may be available. Eat fruits and vegetable raw or slightly steamed for best absorption. Carrots and tomatoes that are cooked offer a higher availability of antioxidant than eaten raw.

- **Other causes** of poor absorption include: chronic inflammatory conditions such as celiac disease, Crohn's disease, chronic pancreatitis, or cystic fibrosis. Diseases of the gallbladder, liver, or pancreas, parasites, Lyme disease, radiation therapy.

Here are some of the signs of malabsorption:

- Certain sugars: You may have bloating, gas, or explosive diarrhea.
- Protein: You may have dry hair, hair loss or fluid retention, or possible edema due to fluid retention.
- Fats: Stools that are soft and bulky or may be light-colored and foul-smelling. Stools are difficult to flush and may float or stick to the sides of the toilet bowl.

Tips for Taking Vitamins and Maintaining Good Digestion

- If possible, take vitamins with food. Digestive enzymes are stimulated when eating and aid in nutrient absorption.
- Limit fluids during meals to improve digestion. Especially avoid cold or iced drinks when eating.
- If possible, use liquid and/or sublingual vitamins. They are the most easily assimilated by the body. Soft gels are the next best choice.
- A small amount of apple cider vinegar, taken just prior to a meal, will stimulate production of digestive juices.
- Vitamin A and Lutein compete for absorption, so take separately.
- Vitamin C enhances the absorption of iron found in plant foods (eating iron-rich foods with tea or milk has the opposite effect). Vitamin C is best absorbed when in ascorbate form (attached to a mineral, typically usually calcium, magnesium, and/or sodium) and with some combination of bioflavonoids and/or additional minerals.
- Vitamin D is important for calcium absorption (particularly vitamin D3 as the better absorbed form),.
- Vitamins A, D, E, K are all fat soluble so best taken with a little fat such as with fish oil.

Chapter 17. Alternative Modalities

Aromatherapy

Aromatherapy, employing essential oils, is another popular method in the Ayurvedic system. Through this therapy different scents enter the sensory system and affect physiological and psychophysiological functioning.

Essential oils are natural aromatic plant compounds that offer a variety of healthy benefits. Aroma components from natural products have been used for mental, spiritual, and physical healing since the beginning of recorded history. Many ancient civilizations, including Egypt, China, and India, have used aromatherapy as a popular complementary and alternative therapy for more than thousands of years.[3001] Essential oils and fragrance compounds have been used for the treatments of various psychological and physical disorders such as headaches, pain, insomnia, eczema, stress-induced anxiety, depression, and digestive problems.[3002 3003]

In humans, about three-hundred active olfactory receptor genes are devoted to detecting thousands of different fragrance molecules through a large family of olfactory receptors of a diverse protein sequence. The sense of smell plays an important role in the physiological effects of mood, stress, and working capacity. Electrophysiological studies reveal that fragrances affect spontaneous brain activity and cognitive functions, which are measured by an electroencephalograph (EEG). Studies suggest a significant role for olfactory stimulation in the alteration of cognition, mood, and social behavior.[3004 3005]

Essential oils work differently than prescribed medications. Essential oil therapy uses plant extracts, often applied to the skin, to help in many ways, including relief of tension and anxiety, improvement of sleep, reduction of pain, enhancement of circulation, improvement of digestion, and more.

They help us connect more deeply to our healing capabilities. They work with the body to stimulate our immune systems, helping us to heal not just the symptoms, but the causes behind our diseases and disorders. Because plant essences contain such a rich and complex blend of naturally occurring minerals, vitamins and more, they can adapt to the ever-changing organisms that affect our health, keeping them in balance and improving our ability to connect to our own biology.

Essential Oils and Dementia

Although one 2016 review suggests that aromatherapy is no better than placebo in helping to manage dementia,[3006] there is some evidence that aromatherapy using various essential oils may have some potential for improving cognitive function, especially in patients with AD.[3007 3008 3009 3010] Used with massage, they may help to calm agitated people with dementia.[3011] One study looked at the effects of massage with a cream containing lavender, sweet marjoram, vetiver, and patchouli on dementia patients in a residential care facility. They saw a decrease in "dementia-related behaviors."[3012] The intervention, massage with the cream, was performed five times per day, so this intervention required quite a bit of caregiver time.[3013] Another study used fewer applications of a cream containing Melissa, which also demonstrated a decrease in agitation behaviors in their clients with severe dementia.

In a typical study of patients with AD aromatherapy showed significant improvement in total touch dementia assessment scale (TDAS) scores. Result of routine laboratory tests showed no significant changes, suggesting that there were no side-effects associated with the use of aromatherapy. The conclusion of the study was that aromatherapy an efficacious non-pharmacological therapy for dementia. Aromatherapy may have some potential for improving cognitive function, especially in AD patients.[3014]

Another study reviewed seven studies on aromatherapy with 428 participants. The conclusion of the study was that aromatherapy was effective for reducing agitation for those with dementia.[3015] Another eight-week study used aromatic massage, and concluded that this method can be an effective and safe intervention to alleviate specific agitated behaviors and depressive mood in individuals with dementia.[3016] A 2001 random control study tested the relaxing effects of an aromatherapy massage on disordered behavior in dementia. The results showed preliminary evidence of a measurable sedative effect of aromatherapy. Aroma therapy has also been found effective for use on the elderly for pruritus, skin pH, skin hydration and sleep (in long-term care hospitals).[3017]

Aromatherapy (through inhalation) has also shown great potential as a safe, therapeutic treatment option for depression.[3018] It also has shown to help in promoting sleep in the elderly with dementia suffering from sleep disturbances.[3019] [3020] [3021]

Essential Oil Protocol

Medicinal essences are both harmonizing and healing, and the more deeply we connect to nature and our bodies, the more effectively the essences will do their job. They are a versatile powerhouse and offer us many gifts, without side effects. Use them with care.

Application

Topical. We recommend that essential oil dilutions should be applied topically[3022] as dementia is often accompanied by a decrease in olfactory function. While it is true that anosmia, the inability to smell, does not prevent essential oils from having effects through inhalation,[3023] aromatherapeutic massage can help people additionally through the touch aspect of the massage.[3024] While some practitioners state that essences must always be blended in a carrier oil and should never be put directly on the skin, we have found that the greatest medicinal power is achieved by using the essences undiluted. The most powerful and medically effective way to apply medicinal essences is topically: directly on the skin, undiluted, or neat.

When using essences on the skin, sometimes it can be important to apply or layer them in a certain order. Oils which have a yang or hot quality like oreganos or clove bud tend to be skin irritants and should be used with great care on the skin. Using a "cold-hot-cold" format allows you to safely apply such essences almost anywhere on the body. We recommend beginning and ending with an essence that has a yin, or cool quality. Apply the sensitive or hot essence(s) in between, using slightly fewer drops to assure that the area they cover is within the "boundaries" of the area covered by the initial yin essence.

- Heating essences: oregano, clove bud, ginger, turmeric
- Cooling essences: ylang ylang, peppermint, spearmint

Skin Reactions

While for the most part essences do not have side effects, they may cause skin irritation, either because of a reaction to the essence itself or because the essence triggers a detoxification reaction (which is a good thing!). Always do a test patch when using a new essence and consider skin type (fair skinned more sensitive than most) when selecting and applying essences. Tip for those with sensitive skin: the soles of the feet are full of receptors and can usually take any essence.

However careful we are, almost everyone will have a skin reaction one time or another when using essential oils. This is because the skin is a major dumping ground for hidden toxicities that are stored in the tissues, and the essences are great detoxifiers. If the skin reaction is extreme, either use some essences to help neutralize the skin reaction or reduce the dosage until the skin reaction clears.

Please try to keep the essences away from the mouth, eyes, and mucous membranes. But do not be alarmed if a few drops do get in one of these sensitive areas; while it might be quite uncomfortable for fifteen to thirty minutes, it will not do any damage. To alleviate the discomfort, you can apply a pure oil like olive oil or coconut oil to the area to neutralize the irritating effect of the essence.

Steam inhalation. Several drops may be added to bath water, or to a steamer (designed for that use).

Air disbursement. Diffuse through a room using an aromatherapy device that gently warms a pad with a few drops of essential oil on it. A few drops can be placed on a cotton ball and put next to a bed, or sprayed lightly on bed linens, or a few drops applied directly to clothing.

Important Essential Oils for Brain Health

For brain health, the most important essential oils include lavender, frankincense, and vetiver. Other medicinal and aromatic plants that address symptoms of dementia such as agitation, insomnia, and depression in both patients and fatigue and burnout in caregivers include bergamot, caraway, eucalyptus, geranium, juniper, lavender, lemon, lemongrass, mint, orange, peppermint, pine, rosemary, sage, tea tree, thyme, and ylang-ylang.

In particular, the essential oils of **lemon balm and lavender** are the most used aromatherapeutic treatments for behavioral and psychological symptoms in dementia.[3025] [3026] [3027]

Note: For some herbs, the qualities imparted by consuming them are also available from the aroma alone. You can review the qualities of herbal supplements taken by mouth in the previous Nutrients chapter.

Some top aromatherapy herbs are:

Bergamot can be used to relieve anxiety,[3028] agitation, mild depression, stress, and relieve insomnia (in a study, combined with lavender and ylang ylang).[3029] To use bergamot oil, place a few drops in a bath, use as a massage oil, diffuse through a room, or use a spray on clothing or linens. [3030] [3031] Researchers feel it is also helpful for chronic pain because of its active components.[3032]

Ginger oil promotes good digestion, improves loss of appetite, reduces postoperative nausea[3033] and reduces constipation. As a massage (with rosemary oil) it produces longer sustained relief from osteoarthritis pain than plain massage.[3034] Ginger oil can be applied directly to the skin as an abdominal massage, inhaled, diffused, sprayed, or placed on a compress.

Non-aroma benefits: Numerous studies in animals show that ginger can protect against age-related decline in brain function,[3035] [3036] [3037] improve reaction time and working memory.[3038] It also helps improve digestion,[3039] and may drastically lower blood sugar levels and improve heart disease risk factors.[3040]

Frankincense is from the genus Boswellia. It has many benefits including reducing inflammation[3041] and can play a role in regulating signaling pathways related to inflammation, immune response, and tissue regeneration.[3042] It helps balance mood and can help minimize irritability, impatience, hyperactivity, and restlessness.

Non-aroma benefits: Reduction of inflammation,[3043] helps reduce symptoms of osteoarthritis and rheumatoid arthritis,[3044] helps reduce pain and improves mobility,[3045] has anti-anxiety and depression-reducing properties, helps increase learning (short-term memory, and long-term memory in rats whose dams received aqueous extract of B. serrata orally during the gestation period).[3046]

Lavender helps calm and balance strong emotions[3047] and may be useful in Alzheimer's-type dementia care.[3048] [3049] [3050] [3051] It has been used to help with depression, and anxiety (because it inhibits receptor binding).[3052] It also helps with anger, and irritability because it reduces cortisol.[3053] It improves a sense of relaxation and coronary blood flow (also due to reduced plasma cortisol),[3054] and can help with some cases of insomnia when used with ylang ylang and bergamot.[3055] A Chinese study of patients with AD concluded lavender could be used as an excellent adjunctive therapy for the management of agitation, with positive effects shown from seventeen AD patients exposed to lemon and rosemary essential oil in the morning and lavender and orange essential oils in the evening. The hypothesis concluded that the mixed lemon and rosemary aromas activate the sympathetic nervous system in order to improve concentration and memory in the morning, and the mixed lavender and orange aromas activate the parasympathetic nervous system, thus making the patients quiet in the evening.[3056] It is believed that inhaled lavender acts via the limbic system, particularly the amygdala and hippocampus.[3057]

Non-aroma benefits: An orally administered lavender oil preparation, Silexan, improved associated symptoms such as restlessness, disturbed sleep, and somatic complaints and had a beneficial influence on general well-being and quality of life.[3058] [3059] A major component of lavender, linalool, is reported to inhibit glutamate.[3060] Exposure to lavender effectively improved spatial memory deficits induced by dysfunction of the cholinergic system.[3061] In an animal model of Alzheimer's disease, a water-diffused extract injection effectively reversed spatial learning deficits.[3062]

Lemon Balm (Melissa officinalis) has been shown to help calm and relax people who are dealing with anxiety and insomnia, improve memory and ease indigestion. Lemon balm oil can be dropped into a bath, inhaled directly, diffused, sprayed, or applied directly to the skin as a massage oil. Lemon balm applied as massage twice a day for four weeks, reduced agitation in AD patients without significant side effects.[3063]

Non-aroma benefits: In a study of lemon balm extract and patients with Alzheimer's as measured through the eleven-item cognitive subscale of the Alzheimer's Disease Assessment Scale (ADAS-cog) and the CDR-SB, cognition improved and agitation was reduced in a four-month period.[3064] The effectiveness of M. officinalis in AD could be explained by some cholinergic activities that have been detected in its extracts, which is also shared by sage and Ginkgo biloba.[3065]

Peppermint can be used to stimulate the mind and calm nerves at the same time. It is best used in the morning. Peppermint oil can be inhaled directly, diffused in a room, used as a massage oil, sprayed in the air, or even placed in a bath. One study including 144 young adults demonstrated that smelling the aroma of peppermint oil for five minutes prior to testing produced significant improvements in memory,[3066] and brain function. Another study found that smelling these oils while driving increased alertness and decreased levels of frustration, anxiety, and fatigue.[3067]

Rosemary helps improve the mind and spirit, by stimulating the mind and calming nerves at the same time. It also eased constipation and symptoms of depression. Best used in the morning, peppermint oil can be inhaled directly, diffused in a room, used as a massage oil, sprayed in the air, or added to bath water. One dosage recommendation is to mix three drops of rosemary oil with ½ teaspoon of coconut oil and rub on upper neck or use in a diffuser for one hour per day.

In healthy adults, lavender is calming, and for example, reduces reaction time, while rosemary enhances memory performance, but slows speed of memory.[3068] In another study, rosemary and lemon oils in the morning and lavender and orange in the afternoon helped to improve personal orientation related to cognitive function.[3069] In a Japanese study of healthy volunteers, both concentrated and less concentrated aromas of lavender and rosemary reduced cortisol levels (the stress hormone).[3070]

Sage (Salvia officinalis) plants are traditionally noted for their antioxidant effects and ability to enhance 'head and brain' function, improve memory, quicken the senses, and delay age-associated cognitive decline.[3071]

Ylang Ylang produces relaxation effects and helps[3072] ease depression while also promoting good sleep, both for patients with AD and the caregivers.[3073] Ylang Ylang is often combined with lemon oil and can be placed in a bath, inhaled, diffused, or sprayed. It has been also reported to have blood pressure lowering effect suggesting its potential use in managing hypertension.[3074]

Note: Other uses of essential oils are found in the appendix.

Ayurvedic Medicine

In recent years, there is renewed interest in the use of phytochemicals for the treatment of dementia, since pharmacological treatment of dementia through the use of drugs (haloperidol, risperidone, aripiprazole, olanzapine, cholinesterase inhibitors, memantine, and benzodiazepines) is often inadequate and has many side effects.[3075] [3076]

Ayurvedic medicine has been used for over 1400 years for a broad range of health conditions including neurodegenerative diseases (and dementias). New research in the West combined with Ayurvedic medicine may help increase nerve growth factors and neurotrophic factors and reduce inflammation and oxidative damage, providing strong support for the use of herbal therapy for AD.[3077]

Several ayurvedic herbs have been studied and shown to support the nervous system and help restore memory.[3078] They show promise in reversing the AD pathology and may enhance memory and rejuvenate cognitive functions.[3079] [3080] These herbs contain compounds such as lignans, flavonoids, tannins, polyphenols, triterpenes, sterols, and alkaloids, that show a wide spectrum of pharmacological activities, including anti-inflammatory, anti-amyloidogenic, anti-cholinesterase, hypolipidemic, and antioxidant effects.[3081] [3082] [3083] Some of the ayurvedic medicinal herbs modulate the neuro-endocrine-immune systems and are also rich sources of antioxidants and anti-inflammatory compounds. [3084] [3085]

See the Nutrients chapter for more information on the following ayurvedic medicinal herbs:

- **Ashwagandha** (Withania somnifera, fam. Solanaceae), or Indian ginseng, is a common herb used in Ayurvedic medicine as an adaptogen or anti-stress agent. Components within this herb components produce anti-stress, antioxidant, and immunomodulatory effects in acute models of experimental stress. [3086] [3087] [3088] [3089] [3090]
- **Brahmi (Bacopa monnieri)** is memory enhancing, anti-inflammatory, analgesic, antipyretic, sedative, and an antiepileptic agent, which acts as a nootropic (repairing damaged neurons and improving brain function). It protects neural cells of the prefrontal cortex, hippocampus, and striatum against cytotoxicity and DNA damage implicated in AD. Bacosides increase glutathione peroxidase and chelate iron.[3091]
- **Gotu kola** (Centella asiatica). Asiaticoside derivatives from gotu kola (asiatic acid and asiaticoside) are capable of cell death due to oxidative damage and/or amyloid beta toxicity. There are broad potential implications for its use in treating neurodegenerative conditions due to its ability to repress mitochondrial dysfunction.[3092]

- **Guggulu** (commiphora wightii) contains potent scavengers of superoxide radicals and can be important for the treatment of neurodegenerative diseases that are associated with oxidative stress,[3093] as well as addressing the link between cholesterol,[3094] amyloid precursor protein processing and membrane interactions[3095] and AD.[3096][3097]
- **Shankhpushpi** (Convolvulus pluricaulis) is a common plant in India that helps improve memory and cognitive function.[3098][3099][3100] Its metabolites contribute to its nootropic and memory enhancing properties, along with its other pharmacological activities.[3101][3102]
- **Curcumin** is a compound in turmeric (in curry powder) with antioxidant, anti-inflammatory, anti-cancer, and neuroprotective abilities. It crosses the blood brain barrier and binds with amyloid beta and inhibits its aggregation,[3103][3104] as well as fibril and oligomer formation.[3105][3106] The absorption rate and bioavailability of curcumin can be increased by consuming it with black pepper (Piper nigrum).[3107]

Craniosacral Therapy

Craniosacral therapy may be another way to help treat Alzheimer's disease. The craniosacral system, which comprises bone and the meningeal system in the brain and spinal cord, helps to transmit the flow of cerebral spinal fluid throughout the central nervous system, and tends to get compromised in middle age as much as fifty percent. Craniosacral therapy is a gentle touch method to manipulate the joints in the cranium or skull, parts of the pelvis, and the spine to treat disease, developed in the 1970s by John Upledger, a doctor of osteopathy, as a form of cranial osteopathy.

Craniosacral therapy helps restore and maintain the healthy flow of cerebrospinal fluid (CSF) which functions as a sink for brain extracellular solutes (waste). This may include solutes that build-up in the brain resulting in amyloid beta. Clearance through paravenous flow (transport of solutes has been observed in the spaces surrounding cerebral arteries and veins) may also regulate levels of the proteins in the brain that are involved with neurodegenerative conditions.[3108][3109]

The glymphatic system is a waste clearance pathway for the central nervous system, and may play a significant role in clearing waste build-up in the brain. It is most active during sleep and may have implications in headache and in neurodegenerative diseases associated with pathologic protein aggregation including Parkinson's disease and Alzheimer's disease.[3110]

The glymphatic system functions much like the lymphatic system but is managed by the glial cells within the brain. Glial cells are non-neuronal brain cells with several regulatory and protective roles including destruction of pathogens and removal of dead nerve cells.[3111]

One twelve-week 2008 pilot study showed regular craniosacral treatments statistically significantly reduced agitation, including aggressive behavior, both physically and verbally in patients with AD. The working theory by some is that this technique helps heavy metals move across the blood brain barrier, and this resourcing of the body is part of what helps decrease dementia symptoms in the above study.[3112]

Traditional Chinese Medicine

Traditional Chinese medicine (TCM) has been in practice for over 3,000 years, and is time proven as an effective approach to helping manage disease and reduce pain. In effect, Chinese medicine helps to maximize the body's natural healing process by approaching each person as a unique individual and developing treatment strategies as relates to imbalances in one's unique body. In other words, three patients may enter an acupuncturist's practice with the same symptoms and even Western diagnosis but end up getting three different acupuncture (and herbal) treatments.

There are reports of dementia and forgetfulness in the oldest medical book in China,[3113] written more than 2000 years ago. The TCM sages and practitioners mapped seventy-one lines along which energy flow in the body, called meridians that are the same for everyone. TCM identifies certain organs (which we here capitalize for clarity) as major systems. Of the seventy-one meridians, twenty are most commonly used; a dozen refer to organs along with another eight "extraordinary" meridians. Each meridian has its own function for how it maintains health within the body. When any of the meridians stay out of balance, ultimately pain and/or disease occurs.

We recommend working with a Chinese medical practitioner to determine the best treatment options regarding herbs and acupuncture. In Chinese medicine, each person is viewed as a unique individual. Some treatment strategies will vary for those with the same diagnosis and symptoms. Strategies based on the meridian patterns shown as being out of balance related to each person's health conditions. We DO NOT recommend purchasing Chinese herbal formulas on your own without consulting a qualified practitioner.

The Spleen, Kidney, and Heart organ systems influence intellect. Certain meridians, and acupuncture points further influence the brain directly. The two main approaches for helping with Alzheimer's Disease is through herbs and acupuncture. A primary herb used is Huperzine A (see the Nutrients chapter for a full description), although it is not recommended for patients taking other Alzheimer's medication.

- **Kidney meridian**. In TCM theory, the Kidney rules over the endocrine system and is responsible for overseeing growth, reproduction, and storage of Qi (energy) to support all the other meridians in the body. It-is the main meridian for brain function and support. Primary prevention of age-related cognitive issues involves safeguarding the Kidney yin, yang, and jing (adrenals, hormone balance, and genetic endowments) throughout the life span with a healthy diet, lifestyle, and avoidance of toxins. The cognitive functions of the brain are said to be regulated by the heart (the kidney provides the substance, the heart the regulation of activity), which influences long-term memory and recall and is damaged by emotional and chemical over-stimulation.
- **Heart meridian** rules circulation, Shen (spirit), and cognitive functions of the brain. If the heart is "agitated" or thrown into imbalance by patterns such as "Excess Phlegm," it can affect memory, cognition, and wisdom.

- **Spleen meridian** influences short-term memory, analytical thinking and concentration and is damaged by worry and poor nutrition.
- **Du meridian** (which runs up the front middle of one's body), benefits attention problems associated with ADD/ADHD, and autism. The Du meridian enters the brain to influence all neurological activity by nourishing, stimulating, or calming the brain and spirit.

Your Chinese medical practitioner may consider the following herbs to determine the optimal treatment strategy as follows:

- **Kidney and brain support**. Kidney essence astringents such as rose fruit and schizandra; and qi and blood tonics that ultimately help nourish the essence such as astragalus, polygonatum, and tang-kuei are frequently recommended to benefit the brain.
- **Heart**. zizyphus, biota, polygala, and acorus are considered important for treating heart disorders affecting memory and cognition.
- **Patent formulas** that nourish energy or qi of the heart: Bu Nao Wan (Brain Tonic Pills) or Jian Nao Wan (Healthy Brain Pills)

Meridian Patterns

There are twenty primary meridians most often looked at by TCM practitioners/acupuncturists in determining the best treatment strategies for senile dementia, here are the most common patterns that may come up in intake and evaluation:

Spleen qi deficiency, with phlegm and stagnating blood obstructing orifices to brain.

The Spleen (meridian) in Chinese medicine is the Yin organ paired with the Yang Stomach meridian, and among other things is responsible for digestion, transformation, and transportation, meaning the breakdown of nutrients in the body and the transport of those nutrients throughout the body.

Signs and symptoms of Spleen qi deficiency can include difficulty in waking up and/or brain fog when waking up in the morning, acid reflux, loss of appetite, bloating and gas particularly after eating, hemorrhoids, diabetes, or eating disorders.

Emotional signs of Spleen imbalance: Excess worry and overthinking which can harm the spleen and cause a lack of appetite, fatigue/exhaustion and/or inhibited qi flow causing insomnia or lack of mental clarity. Note that excessive work, studying or reading can damage the spleen.

Foods to eat. Pumpkin and other squash, root vegetables including sweet potato, yam and taro, miso soup, mustard leaf, quinoa, lentils, oats, tofu (tempeh is the best for protein), chicken, cherries, dates, figs, grapes in moderation, Longan lamb, licorice (DGL), and black strap molasses in moderation.

Foods to avoid. Refined carbohydrates (white foods) such as white bread, pasta, rice, bread, and sugar (multigrain forms of these food are much better), fried foods, iced drinks, citrus fruits, pork, bananas, dairy, yeast-based foods such as beer, bread (organic sprouted breads are better).

When to eat. Restrict eating late at night, overeating, or over combining too many different foods in one meal.

Liver qi stagnation, with qi entanglement, phlegm accumulation, and stagnating blood.

One of the primary functions of the Liver (meridian) is to maintain the free flow of energy and blood circulation throughout the body.

Signs and symptoms of Liver Qi Stagnation include: difficulty in swallowing, sensation of a lump in the throat, stuffiness in the chest, sighing a lot, hiccups, stomach ache worsens with anger, digestion issues, bitter taste in the mouth, constipation, oversleeping, and irregular or painful periods.

Emotional signs of Liver Qi stagnation: Gets angry easily (often inappropriately), easily frustrated, mood swings, irritability, or depression.

Foods to eat. Celery, cucumber, lightly steamed vegetables, for protein chicken, mussels or beef (or tofu or tempeh for vegetarians), green microalgae such as chlorella or blue green algae help detoxify the liver, wheat grasses, sprouts, pungent foods, coconut milk, watercress, all the members of onion family (including scallions), mustard greens, turmeric, garlic, basil, bay leaf, cardamom, rosemary, marjoram, cumin, fennel, bay leaves, dill, ginger, black pepper, saffron, horseradish, rosemary, mint, and lemon balm. Anti-Qi stagnation foods include: cherries, peaches, strawberries, pine nuts, turnip, cauliflower, broccoli, Brussels sprouts, cabbage, bitter and sour foods that detoxify the liver include mung beans and their sprouts, seaweed and kelp. Foods good for liver stagnation include lettuce, cucumber, watercress, millet, plums, beets. Chlorophyll rich foods are mushrooms, radish, and daikon.

Foods to avoid. Rich foods, large meals, fried foods, excessive dairy, processed foods, large amounts of meat, spicy food. Also, keep sugar and coffee down to a minimum, excess eggs, nuts, seeds, and vegetable oils. Eat fruit separately from meals to ease digestion.

When to eat. Eat the last meal of the day by 6 to7pm to allow maximum energy to go to regeneration of the liver and gallbladder during their peak time of 11pm-3am.

Hot phlegm clogging the orifices

Signs and symptoms. Swelling of the lymph glands, ovarian cysts, thyroid nodules, breast lumps that are not hardened, thickened fluid obstructing the bursa of the joints, digestive disorders including nausea, vomiting, and greasy stools. Lung phlegm can result in coughing, asthmatic breathing, and expectoration of sputum. Stomach phlegm causes nausea, vomiting, and fullness.

Emotional signs. Easily angered, irritable, dementia, mania.

Foods to eat. Seaweed, radish, apple peel, grape fruit, lemon peel, pear, persimmon, tangerine peel, licorice, elderflower tea, grapefruit juice, peppermint or ginger tea, blueberries, hawthorn berries, goji berries and yellow fruits in moderate quantities, pear juice.

Foods to avoid. Dairy, spicy food, grains, nuts, sugar, excess salt, fatty meats, fried food, orange juice, excessive carbohydrates, raw salads, and uncooked foods (best to lightly steam your vegetables).

Spleen and kidney yang deficiency, with phlegm and stagnating blood obstructing the orifices to the brain.

Signs and symptoms. Cold limbs and easily feeling cold, desire for warm drinks and food, sluggish digestion, intermittent constipation, and diarrhea with undigested food, easily tired or fatigued, edema, clear and abundant urination, lower back soreness, slow metabolism, weight gain, weakened immune system, ease of catching colds.

Emotional signs. Excess worry or fear, lack of initiative.

Foods to eat. Generally eat warming food, quinoa, oats, spelt, sweet, mustard greens, parsnip, onion, leeks, scallion, parsley, radish, squash, sweet potato, kale, turnip, watercress, winter squash, mushrooms, chestnuts, sunflower seeds, sesame seeds, pistachio, walnut, sweet, brown rice, cherries, litchi, dates, peaches, apricots, raspberry, strawberry, cranberries, chicken, anchovy, lobster, mussel, shrimp, trout, lamb, venison, kidneys (both beef and lamb), black and aduki beans, basil, caper, thyme, cayenne, cinnamon bark, clove, fennel seed, dill, garlic, basil, anise, caraway, ginger, nutmeg, cumin, clove, horseradish, rosemary, jasmine tea, and ginseng tea.

Foods to avoid. Limit eating raw food, cooling grains (rice, corn, buckwheat, and rye are acceptable as they are neutral), cayenne, all hot peppers, black pepper (alright in small doses), dairy, sweeteners (barley malt, rice syrup and molasses are exceptions). Try not to skip meals and get plenty of rest, iced cold drinks with food.

Deficiency of liver yin and kidney yin, with phlegm and stagnating blood obstructing the orifices

Signs and symptoms. High blood pressure, diabetes, cold, lower back pain, dry mouth particularly at night, dry throat, night sweats, thirst, constipation, dizziness, forgetfulness, malar flush (plum-red discoloration of the high cheeks), nocturnal emissions, desire to lie down and sleep, ringing in the ears, constipation, dark, scanty urination, premature ejaculation.

Foods to eat. Potato, squash, zucchini, sweet potato, asparagus, string beans, beets, yam, alfalfa sprouts, oats, barley, millet, asparagus, kelp, potato, seaweed, sweet potato, yam, spinach, celery, carrots, parsley, tomato, kelp, spirulina, wheatgrass, seaweed, mushrooms (including wood ears & tremella), black sesame seed, black, mung and aduki beans, clams, oysters, chicken, duck, apples, mango, peaches, melons, mulberry, grapes, cherries, peaches, plums, coconut, raisins, molasses, oils including olive oil, flaxseed, tofu, tempeh, miso, almond, nuts and seeds, organic cow or goat yogurt, sea salt, one broth soups, licorice, cucumber, sauerkraut, pear For non-vegetarian, meats help build Yin.

Foods to avoid. Citrus fruits, coffee and black tea, vinegar, pickles, chilies, cinnamon, ginger, garlic, dairy, cloves, onions, shallots, leeks, basil, wasabi, curry, alcohol, pepper.[3114]

Qi and blood stagnation, obstructing the orifices to the brain

Signs and symptoms. Vomiting of blood, nosebleeds, painful periods, irregular menstruation, clotting and dark menses, abdominal pain, abdominal masses, body tension, cramping, or pain. For blood stagnation, you may feel tension, cramping, or pain. Blood stagnation is often involved in dysmenorrhea, ovarian cysts, endometriosis, fibroids, cardiac events, and some cancers.

Emotional signs. Feeling of "stuckness," depression, anger, or frustration.

Foods to eat. Cooked or roasted vegetables, root vegetables, eggplant, onion, garlic, scallion, ginger, vinegar, eggplant, shiitake, hawthorn berry, foods and herbs that move Qi & Blood (onions, garlic, saffron, horseradish, shallots, leeks, chives, pepper, ginger, cayenne pepper, and chili pepper, turmeric, nutmeg, oregano, basil, rosemary, and cinnamon). Use only healthy fats such as first cold pressed, extra virgin olive oil, coconut oil, avocado oil (avocados), nuts. For protein, eat lean meat, fish, or chicken. For vegetarians, include tempeh, legumes, almonds, walnuts, unsalted pumpkin, or sunflower seeds. Pay attention to breathing and posture while eating. Eat only until you feel 70-80% full.

Foods to avoid. Cold and damp foods. Limit dairy and avoid fried foods, cold foods (such as iced water, smoothies, or ice cream), as well as refined foods, raw fruits, vegetables, and salads (lightly steam your vegetables), refined sugar, fatty food (pizza, fast food, chips, and red meat).

Insufficiency of kidney-yin and yin-blood: vascular dementia, tinnitus, diabetes,

One study reported that the prevalence of vascular dementia in the elderly is approximately 1.2 to 4.2 percent and it accounts for 10–50 percent of dementia cases.[3115] The brain areas involved were in cognition, memory, and behavior leading to a progressive cognition decline, functional ability impairment, and behavioral problems.

Signs and symptoms:

- Yin deficiency: Dry mouth, night sweats, frequent urination, low back pain, high blood pressure, fatigue, paleness, shortness of breath, and scanty menstrual flow.
- Blood deficiency: Palpitations, shortness of breath, headaches and dizziness, swelling and soreness of the tongue and mouth, restless legs, pale skin, fatigue, increased anxiety, eye floaters, loss of hair, dry eyes, nails and hair, body aches, numbness and weak tendons that are easily injured, insomnia, heart palpitations and irregular heart-beat, excessive dreaming, arthritis, difficulty falling and/or staying asleep, a feeling of floating and disembodiment.

Emotional signs:

- Yin (Kidney) deficiency: Being fearful, weak willpower, insecure, aloof, isolated.
- Blood deficiency: Anxiety, difficulty relaxing, easily stressed, possibly excess anger and psychological disorders.

Foods to eat. Blood building foods include: whole grains, lightly sautéed vegetables and soups, good sources of protein (such as tempeh, eggs, beans, chicken, fish, grass fed meat), seeds and nuts, pumpkin, quinoa, leafy greens, oatmeal, beets, sea vegetables, spirulina /blue green algae, nutritional yeast. Helpful supplements are iron (taken with vitamin C for better absorption), and vitamin B12.

Foods to avoid. Excess drinking (and drugs), overconsumption of meat, damp, cold and raw foods.

Research

Several Chinese herbs activate multiple signaling pathways involved in neurogenesis, including notch, wnt, sonic hedgehog, and receptor tyrosine kinase pathway.[3116] These herbs contain active components such as polysaccharides that impact cognition and other brain functions.[3117]

Acupuncture can inhibit toxic protein accumulation, normalize glucose metabolism, and provide neuroprotective effects.[3118] It has a positive influence on synaptic adaptability, increases neurotropic factors, protects the blood-brain barrier, protects against cell death, inflammation, and oxidative stress.[3119]

Alzheimer's. Herbs such as Herba Epimedii, Coptis chinensis franch, Rhizoma curcumae longae, green tea, Ganoderma, and Panax ginseng act as potential AchE inhibitors.[3120] They have multi-target characteristics, as opposed to single-target drugs, permitting impact on the multiple factors of (oxidation, inflammation, cell death, etc.) linked to Alzheimer's.[3121][3122]

Several studies have looked at the use of acupuncture in treating Alzheimer's symptoms. The more recent studies are investigating why acupuncture may be quite helpful.[3123][3124] In a randomized, controlled, parallel-group study of over twelve weeks with a twelve week follow-up. It was found that acupuncture treatment improved cognitive function more effectively than donepezil.[3125] A meta-analysis of acupuncture plus herbal medicine reported that although some studies were weak, acupuncture plus herbal medicine may have advantages over western drugs.[3126]

Parkinson's. Some Chinese herbal medicines are useful as an adjunct to help improve both motor and non-motor symptoms, permit lower doses of dopaminergic drugs, and reduce dyskinesia.[3127][3128] A meta analysis of twelve randomized controlled trials with 869 participants who had idiopathic (unknown cause) Parkinson's found greater improvement (compared to conventional medicine only) when Chinese medicinal herbs were included in treatment.[3129] Researchers are exploring modifications of TCM herbal medicines specifically for Parkinson's (and other neurological disorders), such as modifying the Chunggan decoction to the Gami-Chunggan formula.[3130]

The use of acupuncture to treat Parkinson's symptoms such as movement function[3131] and pain[3132] is also promising. Points commonly chosen are GB34, ST36, GV16, LR3, GV20, GV14. Researchers have been testing which acupuncture points are most effective.[3133] A meta-analysis of thirty-five studies[3134] and another of forty-two studies[3135] reports that there are practical and positive implications. A pilot found improvement but no difference between acupuncture and sham acupuncture in fatigue measurements.[3136] (Note, these two 2017 meta-analysis may be analyzing the same research.) Another meta-analysis reviewed nearly one-thousand articles, finding twenty-five of them to be acceptable and nineteen of them to be high quality. This study also concluded that acupuncture for Parkinson's has significant beneficial effects.[3137]

Post traumatic stress disorder. Researchers identified TCM patterns most likely to be beneficial in treating PTSD with its symptoms including depression, anxiety, insomnia, and chronic pain. The most likely patterns were "Heart Shen disturbance caused by Heat, Fire, or a constitutional deficiency; Liver Qi stagnation; and Kidney deficiency. Secondary patterns identified were outcomes of long-term Liver Qi Stagnation-Liver overacting on Spleen/Stomach, Liver Fire, Phlegm Fire, Phlegm-Damp, and Heart Fire and constitutional deficiencies in the Heart, Kidney, and Spleen organ systems."[3138]

Acupuncture is at least as effective as drug therapy for chronic post-traumatic headaches.[3139] In animal studies of PTSD it modulates stress response caused by signaling pathways[3140] and over-expression of certain biochemicals contributing to the stress response.[3141] Researchers are analyzing selection of acupoints for treatment and the main acupuncture points used include GV20, EX-HN-1, GV 24, GB 20, HT7, PC6, LR3, and SP6. These points refer to "smoothing liver and governor vessel to regulate the spirit as priority and assisted by nourishing kidney and supporting yang to peace the spirit, as well as strengthening spleen and helping qi to smooth meridians."[3142]

In addition, using acupressure of acupuncture points, the Emotional Freedom Technique (EFT) is especially suitable for PTSD treatment of a number of neurologic markers.[3143] An eight-week study of Transcendental Meditation in treating veterans with PTSD reported "reductions in PTSD symptoms, experiential avoidance, and depressive and somatic symptoms, as well as increases on measures of mindfulness and quality of life." Gains were either maintained or continued to improve through the twenty-month follow-up.[3144] [3145] Another study found that after three months use of psychotropic medications decreased among vets with anxiety and PTSD who practiced Transcendental Meditation.[3146]

Chronic traumatic encephalopathy. While we found no research on CTE and TCM, the guidelines above may be applicable on a case by case basis. However, acupuncture is useful in treating traumatic brain injury according to the first meta-analysis ever completed of forty-nine studies involving 3511 patients, and so may be effective in limiting CTE development. The researchers reported that these studies were generally of poor quality because they had too small sample sizes, and other limitations. But, these studies nonetheless suggested that acupuncture produced superior effects in restoring consciousness in cases of traumatic brain injury.[3147]

Dementia. In a meta study investigating TCM in vascular dementia, the researchers reported that although the evidence was of poor quality, the results were generally good. They identified

NaoMaiTai, NaoXinTong, and TongXinLuo as especially promising.[3148] TCM was found to decrease the pneumonia risk in patients with dementia.[3149]

Acupuncture therapy, in animal studies of vascular dementia, appears to provide benefits through multiple factors including improving synaptic plasticity, cognitive function, and protection from oxidative stress, cell death, and neuroinflammation.[3150] A 2019 review of acupuncture and acupressure techniques for dementia behavioral and psychological symptoms of dementia found that there were statistically significant improvements in activities of daily living (75% improvement), agitation (100%), anxiety (67%), depression (100%), mood (100%), neuropsychological disturbances (67%), and sleep disturbances (100%).[3151]

Yoga and Brain Health

Yoga, originally from India, has become a popular form of exercise and entertainment in the West. Yoga is now practiced in bars with steins of beer replacing water bottles. There is goat yoga, yoga on paddleboards, hip hop yoga, yoga with kittens and puppies and the list goes on. Advertisements and magazines feature young fit women in spandex performing pretzel-like feats of flexibility and strength. This is what has come to represent yoga in the popular imagination.

However, Yoga has been around for thousands of years and is not described thus in classic literature. The Yoga Sutras, by Sage Patanjali, was compiled prior to 400CE, but the philosophy and practices it describes are said to be thousands of years older. The Sutras, a synthesis and organization of knowledge about yoga from older traditions, are organized into four chapters. The first chapter is all about the mind, how to experience transcendence of thought, the benefits of doing so, and the states of consciousness that can be attained. The second chapter describes the practices of yoga, or the eight limbs that lead to the transcendent states of consciousness described in the first chapter. The third chapter describes the powers that come from attaining yogic states, and the fourth chapter is about liberation, attaining enlightenment. In fact, the Yoga Sutras are ALL about the mind, and how yoga can optimize the human experience and reduce suffering. The only yoga posture described in the Sutras is a steady, comfortable seat. In second sutra of the first chapter, Patanjali defines yoga as control over the mind:

Yoga citta vrtti nirodha

Yoga is the cessation of the modifications, or fluctuations, of the mind. *Sutra 1.2*

Chapter one describes the activities of the mind, structural changes in the mind, the mind's potential for distraction and focus, as well as cognition, mood, residue of experience and conditioned patterns of thinking and behavior. It describes how distracted conditions of the mind lead to suffering. The purpose of yoga is to prevent the misery that is not yet come. It is an ancient method of preventative medicine.

Heyan duhkham anagatam

The misery which is not yet come is to be avoided. *Sutra 2.16*

Both media articles and complementary medicine researchers often make a distinction between yoga and meditation. However, meditation is defined as the seventh limb of yoga in the Sutras. It is not something outside of yoga or different from yoga. The eight limbs of yoga are the Yamas (self restraints) and Niyamas (observances), Āsana (physical postures), Prāṇāyāma (breath control), Pratyāhāra (control of the senses), Dhāraṇā (concentration), Dhyāna (meditation) and Samādhi (a transcendent state of consciousness).

The first five limbs purify action, and the last three are the mastery of the mind. The last three limbs can be viewed as a continuum of consciousness. When concentration becomes one pointed it is meditation. When meditation goes beyond the one-pointed focus, the mind becomes expansive, limitless, where there is no awareness of the body or individual self, a feeling of oneness with ALL. In Samadhi there is no pain or suffering.

The eight limbs of yoga provide a comprehensive set of practices to address the whole human being. While western medicine looks at the person as a sum of parts and different specialists focus on different parts, yoga provides a holistic model of human health, which is a balance across all levels of being, defined as the five Kośas, or sheaths. The Kośas are divided into three bodies – the physical body, the subtle body, and the causal body.

- The physical body has one sheath, Anandamaya Kośa. Ana means food, and this is the food sheath. We are what we eat. A yogic diet is one that causes the least amount of harm to the body, animals, and the planet. Ahimsa, or non-harming is the very first Yama. A whole-foods plant-based diet causes the least amount inflammation in the body. Diet and physical yoga practices, the third limb, Āsanas, optimize the health of the physical body.

- The subtle body has three sheaths – Pranamaya Kośa – the energy sheath, Manomaya Kośa – the mental sheath, and Vijnanamaya Kośa – the wisdom sheath, the inner witness. The practices for the subtle body include the fourth through seventh limbs of yoga. These practices bring balance and harmony to the whole being.

- The causal body has one sheath – Ananandmaya Kośa, the body of bliss. What yoga tells us is that this bliss body is part of who we are, our birthright. While pain may be an inevitable part of life, suffering is optional. We just need to remove the obstacles to realizing our true self and experience the body of bliss within.

Yoga says these sheaths are extremely permeable. An imbalance or disturbance in one will affect the others. For example, chronic pain and illness can lead to depression or disturbances in Manomaya Kośa, the mental and emotional sheath. Conversely, disturbances in the mind can lead to physical pain. Yoga recognizes the importance of maintaining a positive mindset and describes the problems that arise from failing to do so. The practice of Pratipaksha Bhavana is a practical and effective way to eliminate negative thoughts in the mind.

Pratipaksha bhavana

When negative thoughts disturb, cultivate the opposite thoughts. *Sutra 2.33*

Negative thoughts, such as himsa (hurtfulness) whether done, caused to be done, or approved – arising from greed, anger, delusion (whether) mild, medium, intense – have unending fruition in suffering and pain; Thus the yogi should cultivate the opposite thoughts.

Western science is in the relatively early stages of gaining empirical evidence of the mind-body connection and its role in disease and healing, something yoga has known for millennium. A 2018 review of over 3,500 research studies by a team of scientists led by Amy Gimson, a researcher at the University of Southampton's Faculty of Medicine in the United Kingdom, found that moderate to severe anxiety may lead to dementia in later years.[3152]

Herb Benson, who pioneered research on the relaxation response, has found that meditation can actually change gene expression.[3153] The body of scientific research is growing, and pointing to the effectiveness of yoga for preventing or improving disease, and in particular, brain health.

What Scientific Research Says about Yoga and Brain Health

Yoga practices were developed for the purpose of maximizing health and wellbeing. Dr. Timothy McCall has kept a list of research[3154] that has shown yoga to be effective in over one-hundred diseases, and the list keeps on growing. What other drug or medical intervention has been shown to be effective in over one hundred diseases? While the ancient (and modern) yogis just felt the positive effects of yoga and knew from their experience that it works, modern medical practitioners and researches want to know why.

An interesting meta-analysis looked at twenty-one neuroimaging studies of about 300 people while they were meditating. The analysis found eight brain regions consistently altered in meditators: the hippocampus (memory) and seven other regions of the brain associated with cognition (frontopolar cortex/BA 10), body awareness (sensory cortices and insula), emotional regulation (anterior/mid cingulate and orbito-frontal cortex), and communication within and between brain regions (superior longitudinal fasciculus and corpus callosum).[3155]

Yoga and Stress

Yoga is emerging as an evidence-based, complementary, and integrative therapy for stress and in particular, for chronic long-term stress which has been shown to have a significant negative effect on the nervous system and endocrine system. Long-term stress may contribute to or worsen a myriad of health problems including cardiovascular disease, diabetes, digestive disorders, sleep disorders, depression, and anxiety. Although scientific understanding of the mechanisms of how yoga benefits stress is still evolving, recent research has shown that yoga decreases stress as a result of modulation of the central nervous system (CNS). This includes the brain and spinal cord and the peripheral nervous system that is comprised of the somatic nervous system and the autonomic nervous system (ANS).

The ANS unconsciously regulates physiologic functions and is further divided into the sympathetic nervous system and parasympathetic nervous system that work together to maintain homeostasis. The sympathetic nervous system (SNS) mobilizes the body for action and is often referred to as "flight, fight, freeze" response whereas the parasympathetic system (PNS) returns the body to a resting state and is referred to as "rest and digest." The hypothesis is that stress causes the SNS to become overactive and downregulates the PNS which can result in an increase in heart rate and blood pressure, sleep disturbances, digestive issues, and mental health problems. When stuck in the SNS the stress hormones keep pumping, causing inflammation and disease. Yoga is thought to benefit stress primarily by decreasing the overactivity of the SNS and by stimulating the PNS. This decreases the stress response and promotes a calm and relaxed state. We need balance for a healthy productive life.

It is well-known that the SNS is activated during vigorous exercise and that with regular cardiovascular activity, one can improve his/her baseline resting state. Yoga includes both vigorous and restorative physical practices, along with breathing and meditation practices. Following the more energizing practices with relaxation not only brings balance to the ANS but the relaxation that follows is often felt more deeply. Leading to a return to a restful state with a lower heart rate, blood pressure and circulation returning to digestive and reproductive organs.

Yoga, GABA, and Brain Health

Gamma-amino butyric acid (GABA) is an amino acid that acts as a neurotransmitter in the central nervous system, inhibits excess neuron activity and has a calming effect. Low levels of GABA are associated with anxiety, insomnia, PTSD and Alzheimer's disease. Yoga has an indirect effect on the parasympathetic nervous system, gamma-amino butyric acid (GABA) and allostatic load, or the cumulative effect of stress on the body over time.[3156]

The main peripheral pathways of the parasympathetic nervous system are within the vagus nerve, the tenth cranial nerve, which transmits signals between the body (heart, lungs, and digestive organs) and the central nervous system. Yogic breathing practices such as Ujjayi slow the breath down, increasing the length of the exhale and increase airway resistance and restore autonomic nervous system balance (possibly as a direct result of vagus nerve stimulation in the diaphragm), and also by increasing GABA in the brain. This would explain the positive emotional states, cognitive benefits and the decrease in the stress response felt after a yoga practice.

A previous landmark randomized control trial study by Chris C. Streeter's research group showed that there were no substantial increases in GABA levels over the twelve-week study for either the yoga or the walking group. However, there was an acute increase in GABA in the thalamus immediately after the one hour yoga session that was not evident in the walking group. The increase in GABA following the yoga sessions was positively correlated to improved mood and decreased anxiety. This supports the hypothesis that the difference is that yoga stimulates the vagus nerve through slower breath rates while walking does not have the same effect.[3157]

Research has shown that dysfunction in the GABAergic system may contribute to mild cognitive impairment and Alzheimer's disease. GABA and Glutamate are the main inhibitory and excitatory neurotransmitters in the human brain and may influence Amyloid beta, the main component of the amyloid plaques found in Alzheimer brains. One explanation is that low GABA levels prevent inhibition of glutamate and over time, glutamate over activity promotes cell death, including healthy brain cells.[3158]

Under stress the brain initiates a cascade of events that involves the hypothalamic-pituitary-adrenal (HPA) axis. The hypothalamus releases corticotropin-releasing factor (CRF) that binds to CRF receptors on the anterior pituitary gland where adrenocorticotropic hormone (ACTH) is released. Then, ACTH binds to the receptors in the adrenal cortex that ultimately results in an increase in the production of steroid hormones called glucocorticoids, which include cortisol, (often referred to as the "stress hormone") and glucose, which increases blood sugar. Stress hormones signal to the hypothalamus that there is a physiological or psychological threat and the cycle continues. Regulation of HPA axis response is important for maintaining both mental and physical health. Diseases like depression, cognitive deficits, and Alzheimer's disease are associated with dysfunction of the HPA axis. Prolonged activation of the HPA axis and high cortisol levels are thought to contribute to inflammation by impairing the glucocorticoid receptors which reduces the immune system's ability to respond to cortisol and lower inflammation.

Yoga, Inflammation and Disease

The primary neurotransmitter released by the parasympathetic nervous system via the vagus nerve is acetylcholine. This affects the cardiovascular system by dilating blood vessels, decreasing heart rate, increasing gastrointestinal peristalsis, toning the urinary tract, and regulating breathing. Acetylcholine not only plays an important role in learning and memory but it fights inflammation, autoimmunity, and degeneration by lowering inflammatory markers and increasing T cells which are important for the immune response. It also modulates the function of hypothalamus, thus influencing the control of body temperature (thermoregulation), sleep, food intake, the function of endocrine glands, and ability to adapt to stress.

Those with Alzheimer's disease have a decrease in acetylcholine. Medically, AD is treated with an acetylcholinesterase inhibitor, an enzyme that prevents the breakdown of acetylcholine. Increasing acetylcholine availability is thought to modulate the expression and production of the pro-inflammatory and anti-inflammatory cytokines, which include immunoregulatory proteins such as interleukin and interferon.

Yoga practices that include physical poses (asanas), breathing techniques (pranayama), and meditation have substantial health benefits due to their ability to minimize sympathetic nervous system responses and reduce inflammation associated with stress. A study by Janice K. Kiecolt-Glaser, a psychoneuroimmunologist, and her research team compared inflammatory and endocrine responses of novice and expert yoga practitioners with two controls to address the underlying mechanisms associated with yoga's potential ability to reduce stress.[3159]

The hypothesis for this study was that experienced yoga practitioners (those who practiced yoga regularly for two years) would have lower levels of inflammation, and smaller autonomic, endocrine, and inflammatory responses to the stressors than novices (those who participated in yoga classes or home practice with yoga videos for six to twelve sessions). Novices and experts did show a group difference in interleukin-6, an indicator of inflammation and increase in positive affect. The research found no differences in the stress biomarkers but this may be due to primarily to the limitations in the study design, especially the limitations on introducing more advanced yoga practices in order to accommodate the novices.

A more recent study investigated physiological and immunological markers of stress and inflammation before and after a three-month yoga retreat that included daily physical postures, controlled breathing practices, and seated meditations during which the participants focused on mantra repetition, breath, emptying the mind, focusing on bodily sensation, and eating a vegetarian diet. The researchers found that yoga had a positive effect on immunologic markers of stress and inflammation, primarily with increases in the plasma levels of BDNF, a neuromodulator that plays an important role in learning, memory and the regulation of complex processes such as inflammation, immunity, mood regulation, stress response and metabolism as well as changes in cortisol (which is part of the HPA axis), which suggests improved stress resilience. The participants also reported improvements in overall wellbeing that may also be explained by lifestyle change, including diet.[3160]

These studies show that yoga practices can have positive effects on the body's chemistry and overall health, including brain health.

Yoga and Neuroplasticity

Neuroplasticity refers to the ability of neurons (nerve cells) and neural pathways to change and adapt the brain by forming new neural connections throughout life. Neuroplasticity allows the neurons in the brain to adjust in response to new situations or to changes in their environment and to compensate for injury and disease. Repeated thoughts and behaviors get stronger, including unhealthy ones. New and healthy thoughts and behaviors can rewire the brain and become predominant with practice while older, less healthy habits begin to fade. A regular yoga practice has the potential to promote positive changes in the brain and consequently, in the mind.

A landmark study in 2005 by Sara Lazar and her research team showed for the first time that meditation promotes neuroplasticity. This research was the first to show that those who practiced meditation long-term had cortical thickening in the areas of the brain associated with attention, sensory processing and interoception (awareness of internal physiological processes). Furthermore, the study suggests that meditation might reduce age-related cortical thinning.[3161]

Yoga and Dementia Conditions

Kriya Yoga (KY) has been reported to have benefits important for cognition rendering it helpful as part of an AD therapy program.[3162] [3163] In one study it was compared to Memory Enhanced

Training (MET) and in another study as to their effectiveness in improving mild cognitive impairment.[3164] Participants were tested for cognitive functioning and mood at baseline, the conclusion of the study at twelve weeks and again at twenty-four weeks. Interventions for both groups were highly structured and comprehensive. The KY group included tuning in, warm up, breathing techniques, yoga, meditation, relaxation, and chanting at home. The MET group included memory education, strategies, home practice, and non-cognitive factors such as self-confidence, anxiety, and negative expectations. Both the KY group and the MET group showed improvement in verbal and visual memory but the KY group had a greater effect on executive functioning, mood, and resilience.

Mindfulness-Based Stress Reduction (MBSR). In an eight-week controlled study, meditation naïve participants received audio recordings for a guided daily mindfulness practice that consisted of a body scan, yoga and sitting meditation. Researchers found increased activity in the posterior cingulate cortex, the temporo-parietal junction, the cerebellum, and the hippocampus. These areas are associated with emotion regulation, self-referential processing, perspective taking and memory.

There were no significant changes on the Alzheimer's Disease Assessment Scale-Cognitive Subscale (ADAS-cog) from baseline, but there were qualitative interviews that revealed that participants enjoyed the program and described improvements in mindfulness, wellbeing, interpersonal skills, acceptance/awareness of Mild cognitive impairment (MCI) and decreased stress. The results from the functional MRI showed that the MBSR group had significantly improved functional connectivity in the default mode network (DMN) and experienced less atrophy in the hippocampus, both areas affected by AD.[3165 3166]

The DMN is a set of brain regions that show highly correlated brain activity when the brain is at rest as opposed to connectivity during tasks that require focused attention. The significance of the DMN is not well-understood. It may serve many functions. However, it is thought that it is a part of the process of how autobiographical memories are retrieved. Hippocampus atrophy has been correlated to impairment in memory, especially the formation of new memory, as well as with the presence of tau protein that builds up in AD.

Mindfulness. The concept of mindfulness includes some yoga practices including awareness of the body and breath, and meditation practices, but it strips out yoga philosophy and all spirituality to make it more acceptable to western health providers and practitioners. While mindfulness is not a complete lifestyle practice, studies have shown that focusing and controlling thoughts can help improve cognition.

One study assessed the effects of mindfulness interventions for patients and caregivers in an 8-week program with pre and post-test analyses including quality-of-life, mood and sleep and as well as having participants rate their experience.[3167] The sessions were ninety minutes long with a progression of mindfulness practices starting with attention to breathing and progressing to attending to bodily sensations, followed by movement, loving kindness and meditation. The researchers added features from Dialectical Behavioral Therapy and from Acceptance and

Commitment Therapy. Participants had homework (including audio exercises) and kept a log. The results from the post-test for both patients and caregivers showed an increase in quality of life, reduced anxiety, depression, and improved sleep. Patients with MCI/AD reported improved coping, increased energy, greater focus, acceptance of the illness and found that the overall experience of the program was helpful. Caregivers said that they felt more compassionate toward their family member, more aware of aspects of their own life that helped with stress, anger and fear related to MCI/AD.

A mixed-method longitudinal study from Australia with persons with MCI and family support persons (FSP) investigated whether mindfulness practices can improve cognitive function, psychological health, mindfulness, and activities of daily living.[3168] MCI participants and their FSPs participated in an eight-week group-based mindfulness training program which included a one-year follow-up using a pre- and post- intervention design. In the ninety-minute weekly group sessions participants engaged in a formal practice with body scans, breathing techniques and in sustained attention and loving kindness meditation practices. They were also encouraged to practice informally by extending attentiveness to everyday activities such as mindful eating and walking, reading, and solving puzzles.

Preliminary results reported that those who meditated more showed greater improvements in cognitive and everyday activity functioning and may have potentially ameliorated the cognitive and functional decline of neurodegenerative MCI[3169] In addition, those who rated their informal mindfulness practice higher than average showed greater improvement in trait mindfulness. The benefits of improved functioning and prevention in neurogenerative MCI participants extended to the FPSs as well. Caregivers are high risk for MCI themselves so decreasing the caregiver burden and providing additional supports may serve to decrease the incidence of MCI in FPSs as well.

Transcendental Meditation (TM, Program)[3170] includes instruction in a mental practice, classes for intellectual understanding, and lifetime follow-up. Optional additions are breathing technique (pranayama), yoga postures (asanas), and in-residence long meditation practice. It has been found to be effective in treating symptoms such as anxiety[3171][3172] found in Alzheimer's patients. It is effective in reducing stress, depression and burnout.[3173] fMRI studies find that blood flow is increased in the brain, especially in the anterior cingulate and dorsolateral prefrontal cortices (attention centers) with decreased blood flow in pons and cerebral (arousal centers).[3174] It safely lowers blood pressure.[3175][3176] It appears to have a significant beneficial effect on immune cells due to its effect on the neuroendocrine axis and the immune system.[3177] It is effective as well in reducing the neurological and behavioral symptoms of post-traumatic stress disorder in veterans.[3178]

In addition, it is significantly effective in reducing compassion fatigue and burnout in caregivers.[3179] Community-dwelling caregivers of patients with dementia also benefited from improved cognitive function, mood, quality of life, and stress response although the sample was small.[3180]

Ancient Wisdom for Modern Times

Contrary to the popular perception of yoga as trendy exercise, yoga includes a comprehensive set of practices that address the physical, energetic, emotional, intuitive, and spiritual aspects of our being. The ancient yogis developed yoga practices to control the fluctuations of the mind to improve health and wellbeing at all levels of being, reduce suffering, and achieve one's highest potential through expanded awareness. The growing body of research evidence is demonstrating the efficacy of these practices.

The research studies cited above show that reducing stress benefits overall health and reduces disease and conditions linked to dementia. Yoga has been shown to be an effective practice for reducing stress.

The mindfulness studies highlight the benefits of increasing focus and awareness for improving cognition. Yoga practices require moment-to-moment presence, awareness, and focus.

The research studies consistently reported an improvement in quality of life scores (QOL), as well as improved cognition. Yoga is a complete lifestyle with practices to harmonize and balanced all layers of our being.

"Study the mind and engage in positive action. You choose your life based on your thoughts.

You change your life based on your thoughts."

Yogini Kaliji, Founder of TriYoga.

Chapter 18. Self-Help

Recommendations for Good Brain Health

1. **Eat without distractions.** Eat slowly without watching TV or being distracted by other activities.
2. **Eat a healthy diet** (alkaline diet with plenty of fruits and vegetables). Eating poor quality foods leads to poor brain function (see the Diet and Brain Health chapter.)
3. **Juicing for the brain:** Try to juice at least a few times a week. Here's a juicing recipe for the brain: (some combination of the following plus your favorite fruits and vegetables, not too many sweet fruits): green, leafy vegetables such as kale, broccoli, red beets, parsley, avocado, apples, blueberries (especially these), strawberry, bilberry, black currant, blackberry, mulberry, goji berries, citrus fruits such as lemon, apple, kiwi, grapes, pomegranate juice, prunes, walnuts, chia seeds, yogurt, ginger and honey.
4. **Eat hours before bedtime.** The gallbladder and liver (meridians in Chinese medicine) are most active between 11:00pm-3:00am and if the body's energies are being used for digestion, their repair function will not be at an optimal level.
5. **Maintain consistent furniture locations** and daily patterns if you have memory problems.
6. **Work closely with health care and social workers** for support.
7. **Reduce anxiety with meditation.** Some form of meditation daily will reduce anxiety and cortisol levels (flight and fight mode). Three studies reviewed all reported significant findings or trends towards significance in a broad range of measures. They included a reduction of cognitive decline, reduction in perceived stress, increase in quality of life, as well as increases in functional connectivity, percent volume brain change and cerebral blood flow in areas of the cortex.[3181]

    Daily practice of meditation helps improve attention, reduce depression, improve sleeping, cognitive function, and neural circuitry, and even increase grey matter in parts of the brain responsible for muscle control, and sensory perception such as seeing and hearing, memory, emotions, speech, decision making, and self-control.
8. **Reduce anxiety with other relaxation.** Set aside at least twenty minutes per day for some mindful relaxation (could be meditation, prayer, yoga, even a walk in the woods). Simply taking a few deep breaths engages the vagus nerve which triggers a signal within your nervous system to slow heart rate, lower blood pressure, and decrease cortisol.

    The next time you feel yourself in a stressful situation that activates your "fight-or-flight" response, close your eyes and take ten slow, deep breaths, and feel your entire body relax and decompress. Relax by listening to music. Watch a funny movie.
9. **Socialize with a friend** one or two times a week (can be for a drink, cup of coffee, dinner, movie etc.) In a 2016 study, researchers found that there was a 7.5 times greater risk and association between loneliness and the amount of amyloid deposited in the brain in cognitively normal adults.[3182]
10. **Keep learning**. A 2007 study with twenty-seven Dartmouth college students demonstrated that significant changes are occurring in adults who are learning. The structure of their brains

undergoes change in white matter. White matter is composed of bundles, which connect various gray matter areas (the locations of nerve cell bodies) of the brain to each other, and carry nerve impulses between neurons.[3183] This includes learning or playing an instrument, learning new subjects, doing daily memory exercises, crosswords, playing chess, etc. Mentally stimulating activities and certain brain-training programs are associated with lower brain amyloid levels and a decreased risk of AD.[3184] [3185]

11. **Exercise daily** which can include fast walking, swimming, tennis, or other sports, work-outs at the gym, yoga, etc. Not only does exercise strengthen the physical body, but it improves neurogenesis[3186] (the growth of new nerve cells). Regular exercise might even delay a rare form of early onset Alzheimer's disease. Two and a half hours of walking or other physical activity a week thwarted mental decline tied to autosomal dominant Alzheimer's disease (ADAD), a genetic form of Alzheimer's. Participants of the study did at least 150 minutes per week of walking, running, swimming or other exercise. They experienced lowered levels of key biological markers of Alzheimer's disease in their cerebrospinal fluid, including tau (a protein that builds up in the brains of people with Alzheimer's).[3187] Another study showed that people with a history of exercise that have the ApoE4 gene (increases the risk of AD onset 10-30 percent) did not develop dementia and has less *b*-amyloid in their brains.[3188]

Also consider the **type** of exercise. Interval walking is especially valuable. In this mode of exercise walkers perform three minutes of easy walking and three minutes of walking in which heart rates rise to about ninety percent of maximum for your condition. Researchers note that after twelve weeks, compared to continuous moderate walking, interval walkers showed significant improvements in both physical endurance and memory performance. The more fit, the more their memory improves.[3189] [3190]

12. **Practice good oral hygiene.** One study reviewed 549 articles on oral hygiene and concluded that older people with dementia had high scores for gingival bleeding, periodontitis, plaque, and assistance for oral care. In addition, candidiasis, stomatitis, and reduced salivary flow were frequently present in older people with dementia.[3191]

13. **Cultivate and encourage a positive attitude.** Having a positive attitude has been shown to increase one's average lifespan 7.5 years compared to a negative mental attitude.[3192]

Chapter 19. Harmful Drugs

Drugs that can cause or mimic the symptoms of dementia should be reviewed with your doctor if you are showing any signs of brain fog, memory and/or balance issues.

Anticholinergic Drugs

Anticholinergic drugs are those that block the neurotransmitter acetylcholine in the central and the peripheral nervous system).[3193] They are typically used to treat a variety of conditions such as urinary incontinence, overactive bladder, chronic obstructive pulmonary disorder (COPD), and certain types of poisoning. Although brain dysfunction systems can often disappear after discontinued use of these drugs, sometimes the damage is more permanent and can look like Alzheimer's disease[3194] and/or they may be associated with increased dementia risk.

A well-known risk with anticholinergic medications is acute impairment in specific aspects of cognition (e.g., working memory, attention, psychomotor speed) which has been demonstrated in single dose experimental studies[3195] and cohort studies.[3196] In addition, anticholinergics may be associated with global cognitive impairment.[3197] Volunteers using anticholinergic drugs had less brain volume and larger ventricles (the cavities inside the brain). Researchers also found that anticholinergic medications led to users' brains processing blood sugar (glucose) differently. This was a sign of brain activity in both the overall brain and in the hippocampus, a region that's tied to memory and which shows early effects of Alzheimer's disease.

Animal studies suggest that anticholinergic drugs may contribute to brain inflammation, a potential contributor to dementia.[3198]A 2018 study of 3434 participants 65 years or older with a diagnosis of dementia reviewed the most common anticholinergic drug classes used in order to determine the association between the duration and level of exposure to different classes of anticholinergic drugs and subsequent incident dementia. During a mean follow-up of 7.3 years, 797 participants (23.2%) developed dementia (637 of these [79.9%] developed Alzheimer disease). They investigated tricyclic antidepressants, first generation antihistamines and bladder antimuscarinics. The conclusion was that higher cumulative use of some anticholinergic medications is strongly associated with an increased risk for dementia.[3199] [3200]

The risk of dementia increased with greater exposure for antidepressant, urological, and anti-Parkinson drugs with scores of 3. This result was also observed for exposure fifteen to twenty years before a diagnosis.[3201] Another long-term study has similar conclusions. Dementia risk increased along with the cumulative dose. Taking an anticholinergic for the equivalent of three years or more was associated with a fifty-four percent higher dementia risk than taking the same dose for three months or less. The body's production of acetylcholine diminishes with age, so blocking its effects can deliver a double whammy to older people (acetylcholine is one of the most essential neurotransmitters for communication within the brain and rest of the body).[3202]

In 2008, Indiana University School of Medicine geriatrician Malaz Boustani developed the anticholinergic cognitive burden scale, which ranks these drugs according to the severity of their effects on the mind. They recommend avoiding drugs with ACB scores of 3 or above. Examples of these medications include: atropine (Atropen), belladonna alkaloids, benztropine mesylate (Cogentin), clidinium, cyclopentolate (Cyclogyl), darifenacin (Enablex), dicylomine, diphenhydramine (Benedryl),[3203] fesoterodine (Toviaz), flavoxate (Urispas), glycopyrrolate, homatropine hydrobromide, hyoscyamine (Levsinex), ipratropium (Atrovent), orphenadrine, oxybutynin (Ditropan XL), propantheline (Pro-banthine), scopolamine, methscopolamine, solifenacin (VES-Icare), tiotropium (Spiriva), tolterodine (Detrol), trihexyphenidyl, and trospium.

There are alternatives to these drugs. For example, "selective serotonin re-uptake inhibitors (SSRIs) like citalopram (Celexa) or fluoxetine (Prozac) are good alternatives to tricyclic antidepressants. Newer antihistamines such as loratadine (Claritin) can replace diphenhydramine or chlorpheniramine (Chlor-Trimeton). Botox injections and cognitive behavioral training can alleviate urge incontinence."[3204]

Note This study found that use of certain medications was more common in people later diagnosed with dementia. That doesn't mean these drugs caused dementia, so further research needs to be done.

Additional Commonly Used Types of Medications That Dampen Brain Function

Benzodiazepines. This class of medication is often prescribed to help people sleep, or to help with anxiety. They do work well for this purpose, but they are habit-forming and have been associated with developing dementia. A 2018 meta-analysis of twelve studies, reviewing more than 981 thousand individuals found an association between them and development of dementia, but was unable to distinguish between Alzheimer's, vascular dementia, long- versus short-acting benzodiazepines, and duration and dose exposures.[3205] Examples of these drugs include: lorazepam, diazepam, temazepam, alprazolam, and zolpidem (brand names Ativan, Valium, Restoril, and Xanax, and Ambien, respectively).[3206]

Antipsychotics and mood-stabilizers. In older adults, these are usually prescribed to manage difficult behaviors related to Alzheimer's and other dementias. These are also prescribed for serious mental illness such as schizophrenia. A 2015 study of nursing home residents with dementia concluded that antipsychotic discontinuation is most likely to succeed if it's combined with adding more social interventions and also exercise.[3207]

Opiate pain medications. These drugs overtime can impair memory over time. Commonly prescribed opiates include hydrocodone, oxycodone, morphine, codeine, methadone, hydromorphone, and fentanyl. (Brand names depend on the formulation and on whether the drug is mixed with acetaminophen.) Tramadol (brand name Ultram) is a weaker opiate with weaker prescribing controls.

For a further list of drugs that can impair memory, go to www.healthinaging.org/ medications-older-adults. Another excellent site for more information is https://betterhealthwhileaging.net/medications-to-avoid-if-worried-about-memory.

Summary. In summary, drugs have side effects. So, it is important to evaluate each drug with your doctor to best determine if the benefits are greater than the associated risks.

Appendix 1

	Alpha lipoic acid	Amla	Antho-cyanins	Apigenin	Beta-alaine & L-carnosine	Bacopa monnieri	Catechin	Celastrus panicu-latus	Cinnamon	Choline	Cocoflavo-noids & chocolate	Coffee
Crosses blood-brain barrier			X	X			X					
Brain plasticity &/or healthy brain support												
Supports brain cell neurogenesis &/or protects against dopaminergic nerve loss				X								
Increases brain dopamine concentration &/or reduces dopaminergic loss							X					
Supports BDNF and/or neurogenesis &/or plasticity					X	X			X		X	
Decreases neurogenesis												
Reduces cognitive decline &/or improves memory/ cognitive function	X	X		X		X	X	X		X		X
Helps reduce depression, improve mood							X	X				
Reduces or inhibits inflammation				X								X
Supports blood flow to the brain												X
Reduces oxidative stress &/or protects against neurotoxicity	X			X								
Helps prevent brain cell death				X								
Supports mitochondrial function / energy production	X											
Reduces anxiety, stress &/or improves sleep						X						
Protects myelin sheath &/or supports methylation												
Neuroprotective benefits							X	X				
Cleans up brain debris												
Reduces homocysteine levels												
Dementia-mimicking deficiencies												

Natural Brain Support

	Copper	Curcumin*	DHA	DHEA	DMAE	Dopamine	Folic acid	Glucose	Gotu kola	Grapeseed extract	Green tea	Gut microbia***	Hesperidin
Crosses blood-brain barrier		X	X					X					
Brain plasticity &/or healthy brain support	X		X					X		X			
Supports brain cell neurogenesis &/or protects against dopaminergic nerve loss		X								X	X	X	X
Increases brain dopamine concentration &/or reduces dopaminergic loss													
Supports BDNF and/or neurogenesis &/or plasticity		X	X						X	X		X	
Decreases neurogenesis													
Reduces cognitive decline &/or improves memory/ cognitive function		X	X	X	X	X	X	X		X	X	X	X
Helps reduce depression, improve mood						X	X					X	
Reduces or inhibits inflammation		X	X						X	X	X	X	
Supports blood flow to the brain													
Reduces oxidative stress &/or protects against neurotoxicity		X	X							X	X		
Helps prevent brain cell death			X					X	X				
Supports mitochondrial function / energy production	X	X	X					X		X	X		
Reduces anxiety, stress &/or improves sleep				X		X	X						
Protects myelin sheath &/or supports methylation							X					X	
Neuroprotective benefits		X	X	X			X						X
Cleans up brain debris													
Reduces homocysteine levels													
Dementia-mimicking deficiencies						X		X					

*Peperine enhances the benefits of curcumin   **Probiotics

236

Natural Brain Support

	Iron	Jyotish-mati	Lavender (oil)	Lecithin	Lotus root extract	Lutein	Magne-sium	Milk thistle extract	Moringa oleifera	Nattoki-nase	N-acetyl-cysteine	Olive oil	Omega 3*	Omega 6
Crosses blood-brain barrier						X					X		X	
Brain plasticity &/or healthy brain support	X			X			X							
Supports brain cell neurogenesis &/or protects against dopaminergic nerve loss					X	X	X	X						
Increases brain dopamine concentration &/or reduces dopaminergic loss														
Supports BDNF and/or neurogenesis &/or plasticity										X			X	
Decreases neurogenesis						X								
Reduces cognitive decline &/or improves memory/ cognitive function	X	X	X	X		X			X		X	X	X	
Helps reduce depression, improve mood			X										X	
Reduces or inhibits inflammation			X			X				X		X	X	X
Supports blood flow to the brain			X			X				X			X	
Reduces oxidative stress &/or protects against neurotoxicity	X					X			X		X		X	
Helps prevent brain cell death						X					X		X	
Supports mitochondrial function / energy production											X			
Reduces anxiety, stress &/or improves sleep			X										X	
Protects myelin sheath &/or supports methylation				X		X								
Neuroprotective benefits		X				X			X				X	
Cleans up brain debris														
Reduces homocysteine levels														
Dementia-mimicking deficiencies	X						X							
*Alpha Linoleic Acid, EPA & DHA														

Natural Brain Support

	Omega 7	Pante-thine	Black pepper	Phosphati-dylserine	Pinocem-brin	Radix puerariae	Rutin	Red sage*	Selenium	Seratonin	Serrapept-ase	Shankh-pushpi**
Crosses blood-brain barrier				X			X					
Brain plasticity &/or healthy brain support				X								
Supports brain cell neurogenesis &/or protects against dopaminergic nerve loss		X	X	X	X				X			X
Increases brain dopamine concentration &/or reduces dopaminergic loss												
Supports BDNF and/or neurogenesis &/or plasticity			X									X
Decreases neurogenesis												
Reduces cognitive decline &/or improves memory/ cognitive function			X	X					X	X		X
Helps reduce depression, improve mood				X						X		
Reduces or inhibits inflammation	X							X			X	X
Supports blood flow to the brain						X		X			X	
Reduces oxidative stress &/or protects against neurotoxicity				X							X	
Helps prevent brain cell death					X							
Supports mitochondrial function / energy production					X							
Reduces anxiety, stress &/or improves sleep				X				X				X
Protects myelin sheath &/or supports methylation								X	X			
Neuroprotective benefits				X								
Cleans up brain debris												X
Reduces homocysteine levels												
Dementia-mimicking deficiencies									X			

*Chinese sage or danshen   **Convolvulus pluricaulis

Natural Brain Support

	Trytophan & 5-HTP	Vitamin A	Vitamin B1	Vitamin B12	Zeaxanthin	Zhimu*	Zinc
Crosses blood-brain barrier					X		X
Brain plasticity &/or healthy brain support		X		X			
Supports brain cell neurogenesis &/or protects against dopaminergic nerve loss	X	X					
Increases brain dopamine concentration &/or reduces dopaminergic loss							
Supports BDNF and/or neurogenesis &/or plasticity							
Decreases neurogenesis					X		
Reduces cognitive decline &/or improves memory/ cognitive function			X	X	X	X	X
Helps reduce depression, improve mood				X	X		
Reduces or inhibits inflammation							
Supports blood flow to the brain					X		
Reduces oxidative stress &/or protects against neurotoxicity							
Helps prevent brain cell death							
Supports mitochondrial function / energy production							
Reduces anxiety, stress &/or improves sleep	X			X			
Protects myelin sheath &/or supports methylation							
Neuroprotective benefits		X					X
Cleans up brain debris							
Reduces homocysteine levels				X			
Dementia-mimicking deficiencies			X	X			X
* Rhizoma anemarrhenae							

Appendix 2. Soaking and Spouting Guide

For the average healthy person with a nutrient rich diet, here is a simple way to reduce phytates from your diet.

- Soak all nuts, seeds, legumes, and grains in warm un-chlorinated water. You can add about a tablespoon of something acidic to each cup to be soaked.[3208]
  - For grains, soak 7–8 hours or overnight.
  - Soft nuts, such as walnuts, pecans and cashews only need about four hours of soaking.
  - Grains, such as oats and corn, require longer soaking. Adding freshly ground rye flour or sourdough rye culture and some lemon juice or yogurt can help; keep in a warm place overnight. For each cup of grain, add a tablespoon of something acid, such as yogurt, raw apple cider vinegar, lemon juice, whey, or kefir.
  - Rinse in the morning before cooking.
- You can add unrefined salt into the water when you soak nuts to activate enzymes that neutralize enzyme inhibitors.
- Nuts that will be eaten later can be dehydrated on the lowest heat possible in the oven until completely dried. It is best to stir them occasionally and make sure they do not get burnt.

Nuts

- Almond: 8–12 hours soaking, 12 hours sprouting.
- Cashew: 2–6 hours soaking, does not sprout.
- Pecan: 4–7 hours soaking, does not sprout.
- Walnut: 4-7 hours soaking, does not sprout.
- Brazil, pistachio, pine nut: Do not soak, do not sprout.

Seeds

- Alfalfa: 8 hours soaking, 2–5 days sprouting.
- Flax: 8 hours soaking, does not sprout.
- Pumpkin: 8 hours soaking, 1–2 days sprouting.
- Sesame: 8 hours soaking, 1–2 days sprouting.
- Sunflower: 2 hours soaking, 12-18 hours sprouting.

Grains

- Buckwheat: 15 minutes soaking, 1–2 days sprouting.
- Barley: 6 hours soaking, 2 days sprouting.
- Corn: 12 hours soaking, add lemon, etc., 2–3 days sprouting.
- Millet: 8 hours soaking, 2–3 days sprouting.
- Oats: 6 hours soaking, 2–3 days sprouting.

- Quinoa: 2 hours soaking, 1–2 days sprouting.
- Rice: 9 hours soaking, 3–5 days sprouting.
- Spelt/Rye: 8 hours soaking, 2–3 days sprouting.
- Wheat/Kamut: 7 hours soaking, 2–3 days sprouting.

Legumes

- Adzuki: 8 hours soaking, 3–5 days sprouting.
- Chickpea: 12 hours soaking, 12 hours sprouting.
- Lentil: 8 hours soaking, 12 hours sprouting.
- Mung: 1-day soaking, 2–5 days sprouting.
- Other beans and dried peas: soak overnight, sprout 2–3 days.

Note. Times can vary, depending on water, room temperature, and freshness. Try not to use too much water, and don't soak too long as they can spoil (especially if kept warm). If they spoil, you can usually tell by the rancid odor.

Appendix 3. Benefits of Juicing

Food for Your Brain

Juicing provides a concentrated source of nutrients and antioxidants and is particularly important for those people with health conditions or even healthy people on the go that do not have the time to consistently eat a healthy diet. We recommend using only organic foods for juicing when possible.

Juicing Versus Smoothies & Green Drinks

Some of us don't juice because we don't have time, we don't have a juicer, we don't like the clean-up, or we just are not wild about juice. Although juicing allows us to have maximum usable nutrients, we can, instead, make smoothies using these same recipes. If you have a blender which turns raw fruits and vegetables to a smooth puree or near liquid consistency then you can make great smoothies and green drinks.

Making freshly juiced drinks of mostly organic fruit and vegetables is a critical part of the process of healing your eyes and body. The health of your eyes is tied to the health of your body. Juicing is a great way to get the freshest, purest nutrients into your body in the most easily digested manner, and in turn having those nutrients readily available in the quickest time. It can take only several minutes for nutrients from fresh juice to be utilized by your body. And once they are in your body, they are carried through the blood stream to all parts of your body including your eyes.

Benefits of Juicing

Enzyme Protection

Enzymes are the catalysts for your body's essential and effective functioning. They increase the rate of nearly all of the chemical reactions in every cell. A variety of glands and organs produce these enzymes in the process of regulating metabolism, circulation, respiration, reproduction, and the functioning of the brain. Within your digestive system specific enzymes help digest food. They break down food into smaller building blocks so that the body can absorb them rapidly. They are found in your saliva, your stomach, your intestinal tract, and the pancreas.

Enzymes convert proteins into peptides and amino acids which are the building blocks for muscles and hormone production. They convert fat into fatty acids and glycerol. They convert starches and sugars into glucose.

Enzymes are in fruits and vegetables and help in the breakdown of those foods by your body. But they become sluggish above 118 degrees F and deteriorate completely above 130 degrees F. [3209] Although opinions are mixed on this, we believe cooking in microwaves denatures protein and enzymes in the food. We prefer people heat their food on the stove or in the oven, but if one wants to use a microwave, it should be just for short periods of time to warm the food up so as not to denature the enzymes and proteins.

Juicing is a way to consume the maximum possible enzymes. It should be noted that some very highspeed juicers or blenders operate at such high speed that the temperature can rise about 188 degrees or even 130 degrees, and this high heat does destroy some of vitamins and enzymes in the juice.

Faster Digestion

When you consume solid foods, it takes up to two or three hours (more for meat, fish, and poultry) for your body to break it down into usable components. Although fiber is important for good health, the juicing process removes fiber making digestion faster, in approximately twenty to thirty minutes.[3210]

Concentrated Nutrients

Juicing concentrates the nutrients. By juicing the various recipes that we recommend you quickly introduce ample amounts of nutrients into your system, more than you could take in comfortably if you ate all of those fruits and vegetables whole.

Living Juice

Many people feel that to nourish your own life it is important to consume foods that are "alive". Juicing preserves this quality of life that is destroyed through cooking.

Juice for Health

There is ample research for almost every eye and health condition that demonstrates that diets high in fruits and vegetables are critical to good health and reduce the risk of disease.

Vegetable Protein

Fruit and vegetables contain more protein than you might think. Vegetables such as green beans, corn, artichoke, watercress, and the cabbage family (broccoli, cauliflower, brussels sprouts, etc.). have the most protein of the vegetables. And juices are an easy way to add additional protein such as brewer's yeast, wheat germ, or add whole grains to your juicing recipe.

Phytochemicals

Carotenoids and bioflavonoids, for example, are phytonutrients known as phytochemicals. These are chemical compounds that exist only in fruits and vegetables for the purpose of controlling their color and smell. The colors and smells attract pollinators, and, more importantly, the colors protect the plants from damaging UV radiation from the sun. Likewise, when you consume them, they help protect your health and vision. For example, lutein is found in yellow fruits and vegetables and is also in the macula of the eye, where it acts as potent antioxidant and internal sunscreen, protecting the most sensitive part of the eye from blue, violet, and ultra-violet light. Juicing is a wonderful way to get large quantities of phytochemicals that are readily absorbed into the body.

Other Nutrients

Incorporating dark green leafy vegetables in your juices or smoothies also provides nutrients such as B vitamins like folate which are methyl donors. The addition of methyl groups (CH3) to molecules (called methylation), helps many processes in our body such as producing neurotransmitters for brain function, repairing DNA, turning genes on and off, improving immunity and detoxification.

Juicing Tips

Follow your comfort. You may consume as much fresh juice as you wish, as long as you don't force it. Follow your comfort level. At least one-half to one pint daily is great. For therapeutic purposes, your healthcare professional might recommend larger amounts daily.

Note, if weak digestion: However, if you have weak digestion then juicing or smoothies may not beneficial for you. If you experience pain, gas, bloating or diarrhea, then reduce the amount and number of juices you drink. Do not add ice or frozen vegetables or fruit. Allow fresh fruits and vegetables to warm to room temperature before juicing. If symptoms persist you can substitute warm cooked vegetable soups or purees.

Freshness. You should drink your fresh juice as soon as you make it and not store it for later. Many enzymes and vitamins break down quickly once exposed to the air or sunlight.

Organic. Non-organic products contain pesticides, and not only on the surface of the skin. If you juice non-organic foods you are likely consuming concentrated amounts of those pesticides. Some feel that pesticides reside mostly in fiber, which is removed, but it is better to be safe.

Brain Juicing Recipe: Try some combination of the following plus your favorite fruits and vegetables, not too many sweet fruits: green, leafy vegetables such as kale, broccoli, red beets, parsley, avocado, apples, blueberries (especially these), strawberry, bilberry, black currant, blackberry, mulberry, goji berries, citrus fruits such as lemon, apple, kiwi, grapes, pomegranate juice, prunes, walnuts, chia seeds, yogurt, ginger and honey.

Equipment.

There are many excellent juicers. We recommend those that operate at a slow 80rpm, slowly enough to not create heat. Most juicing equipment works at 3600rpm or higher. The Omegas units are known as "masticating juicers". They chew up fruits and vegetables slowly, preserving nutrients and enzymes. The downside is slightly slower operating time and slightly longer cleanup.

Vitamix has a reputation for being an excellent machine; Nutribullet and Ninja are also good at much lower cost.

Note: These machines are not low speed and so they do generate heat and some nutrients and enzymes are lost. However, they are better than not making a refreshing nourishing drink at all. The Vidia vacuum blender removes air to prevent oxidation. It has a maximum speed of 20,000 rpm, not low speed. Other juicers are available on the market, so read reviews to determine the best one for you.

Appendix 4. About Essential Oils

Bergamot can be used to relive anxiety, agitation, mild depression, and stress. This mood elevating and calming oil can also be used to relieve insomnia.[3211]

Clary sage (Salvia sclarea) calms the mind and reduce feelings of anxiety. Clary sage oil can help alleviate stress by inducing a sense of well-being.[3212] It also has antibacterial properties,[3213] and acts as a natural antidepressant.[3214]

Frankincense has been used to promote healthy cellular functions. It helps balance mood by improving concentration and focus, and can help minimize irritability, impatience, hyperactivity, and restlessness. Frankincense helps relieve chronic stress and anxiety, reducing pain and inflammation, boosting immunity.[3215]

Ginger root is known to be helpful for anyone struggling with digestion issues.[3216] As aromatherapy, its effects are similar and it helps to reduce nausea,[3217] sea sickness, and heartburn, increases bowel movements, and cleans out the intestinal tract. It is very supportive for the kidneys and brings an overall yang (warming) energy to the digestive system. It is anti-bacterial[3218] and can also help with chronic fatigue, provide a storehouse of extra energy, and increase mental clarity.

Lavender is well known as a sleep aid.[3219] It is thought to be calming and able to balance strong emotions. It reduces nervous tension, relieves pain, disinfects the scalp and skin, enhances blood circulation, and treats respiratory problems. It has also been used to help with depression, anger, and irritability,[3220] and can help in some cases of insomnia.[3221] Lavender reported to be useful in the treatment of acute as well as chronic or intractable pain.[3222]

Lemon (and other citrus oils) provides uplifting effects on the body and mind, and promotes physical energy and reduces stress. It is shown to be antimicrobial against food pathogens and spoilage bacteria.[3223]

Lemon balm (Melissa officinalis) is also one of the most studied and more effective oils. Lemon balm reduces agitation[3224] and is shown to help calm and relax people who are dealing with anxiety and insomnia. It also improves memory and eases indigestion.

Marigold (Tagetes) helps relax the stomach's digestive process, reduces parasites, and worms in the stomach. It also offers mental clarity and works as a decongestant, anti-inflammatory, and anti-fungal agent (helps with candida).[3225]

Peppermint is one of the most popular essential oils used to stimulate the mind as well as support concentration, focus, memory, and overall mental performance.[3226] It calms the nerves at the same time and is best used in the morning. It is very supportive for the digestive system, relieving dyspepsia, nausea, distension, and flatulence, and is also effective at reducing inflammation, especially in the digestive tract and colon. It offers us the ultimate cooling and refreshment.

Energetically dry and cool, Peppermint can stimulate the nerves and brain and reduce fevers and flu symptoms.

Rosemary is highly anti-bacterial and an antioxidant.[3227] It helps improve sluggish digestion, and can reduce candida, chronic fatigue, and cardiac fatigue. It helps improve poor concentration and depression symptoms and can ease constipation and reinvigorate the appetite. Rosemary oil can be directly inhaled, diffused through a room, or used as a spray expectorant for coughs and bronchitis.[3228]

Saffron is antibacterial, blood purifying, antioxidant, decongestant, and memory enhancer.[3229] In Ayurvedic medicine it is an herb that pacifies all three doshas.

Spearmint is a liver cleaner, calms the nerves, freshens the mouth, and helps in overall detoxification. Spearmint is very yin, or cooling.[3230]

Spike lavender helps reduce stress relieves pain, helps with headaches, and has anti-inflammatory properties. It is similar to lavender but contains more camphor.[3231]

Tangerine helps support bile production and aids in draining the gallbladder. It is very relaxing and uplifting and is helpful for reducing insomnia.[3232]

Tea tree lemon is calming and uplifting, with strong anti-bacterial and anti-viral properties. It supports healthy skin, reduces candida and toe fungus.[3233]

Turmeric is a yang (warming) medicinal essence, is a great liver detoxifier and aids in clearing gallstones and colitis. It is very uplifting and contains high levels of antioxidants, has anti-inflammatory and antiseptic qualities, and is good for insomnia. Turmeric offers anti-cancer support, reducing tumors and cancers both internally and externally.[3234]

Verbena lemon aids digestion while reducing diarrhea and rectal inflammation. It supports deficiencies in the pancreas, liver, and gallbladder. It improves depression and reproductive health in both men and women.[3235]

Ylang Ylang oil can help ease depression while also promoting good sleep and relaxation.[3236]

Zanthoxylum is a highly sedative essence, supports digestion and helps decrease anxiety, toothaches, and gum disease.[3237]

How to Apply Medical Essential Oils

For digestive issues, apply four drops twice a day on the area of concern around the stomach and digestive tract. You can usually use two essences at a time, and utilizing one pair for about two weeks before moving to the next pair.

Auricular Use

Application behind the ears is great for head congestion, headaches, sinus problems, general malaise, and cold and flu symptoms. Use about five drops each of five to seven essences. Apply them on the area about midway behind the ear down to the bottom of the neck, layering over the eustachian tubes. Put the first essence behind one ear, then the other ear, and continue going back and forth until you have used all your selected essences. Use respiratory essences, antihistamine essences, antibacterial essences.

Oral Use

Oral use of essences should be approached with care and only done under the supervision of an experienced aromatherapist. The digestive process breaks down the essences, so oral usage is generally not as powerful as topical, but this method can be used in conjunction with topical application for an additive effect. The average absorption rate with oral usage is twenty to twenty-five percent.

Sublingual Use

Sublingual use (under the tongue) is more effective than swallowing the essence due to the higher level of receptors in this area. The average absorption rate there is thirty to thirty-five percent.. Do this only under the supervision of an experienced aromatherapist.

Inhalation

Using this protocol is a great application for sinus problems, respiratory congestion, lung infections, etc. Boil a cup or mug of water (preferably on the stove, not in a microwave), then add your essences. Some essences that are commonly used in this approach are eucalyptuses, pines, spruces, peppermints, laurel leaf, Himalayan soti, and tea tree. If you are using three or four essences, put about five to seven drops of each in the hot water and hold a towel over your head, making a tent over the cup, capturing the steam. Breathe deeply, inhaling the essences carried by the steam. When the water cools, drink it.

How Much to Use

Determining how many drops of essence to use is an art, not a science. "One size does not fit all." Every situation is different and must be considered individually. Also, the application method influences how much of the essence will be absorbed by the body. Here are some factors to consider.

How serious is the condition? For someone in a crisis situation you might use more than for "routine maintenance". A person's height and weight are important. The larger the person, the more drops one uses. A good place to start is eight to ten drops each of up to four or five essences if the person is of average height and weight. For a large or overweight person, the amount should be increased accordingly. For a small or underweight person, the amount should be decreased.

Other factors make a difference too. Consider the person's eating habits, exercise level, and emotional state. People with unhealthy lifestyles need larger amounts of the essences than people with healthy lifestyles. Age makes a difference. For elders, children, and infants, the amount used should be reduced. Since working with babies and children requires much judgment and discretion, it is best to consult an experienced medicinal aromatherapist until you have developed depth of knowledge in this area. Medicinal essences bring the body's systems into balance. Essences that work with blood pressure, bring it into balance. Essences that work with thyroid functioning bring it into balance; essences that are anti-bacterial only kill the harmful bacteria, bringing the body back into balance, all while supporting the immune system.

Appendix 5. The Blood-Brain Barrier

The blood-brain barrier prevents toxins and microorganisms from crossing from the blood stream into the tissue of the brain. At the same time, certain beneficial nutrients are capable of crossing this barrier. But generally, integrity of the blood-brain barrier is important and its compromise contributes to a number of neurodegenerative conditions.

Causes of a compromise in the blood-brain barrier include: chronic stress, excess alcohol usage, environmental toxic exposure, amyotrophic lateral sclerosis, uncontrolled diabetes, epilepsy, stroke, brain trauma and edema, candida overgrowth, systemic diseases such as liver and chronic inflammatory conditions (that can result in Vitamin B deficiency, elevated homocysteine levels), as well as having a poor diet and low level of antioxidants.

The blood-brain barrier does have mechanisms to repair itself. Ways to help this repair process include:

- **Glucocorticosteroid** (GC) treatment. GCs were shown to restore BBB integrity in patients with MS.[3238]
- **GABA** is a chemical messenger that is widely distributed in the brain. GABA's natural function is to reduce the activity of the neurons to which it binds. GABA serves to control the fear or anxiety experienced when neurons are overexcited. GABA crosses the blood-brain barrier. A simple test is to take 800-1,000mg of GABA and give yourself a two-to-three-hour window see whether it affects you. It is best to take GABA between 6 p.m. and 9 p.m., so you can sleep it off if it sedates you. If GABA causes relaxation, calming, and sedation don't keep taking it regularly, or you risk shutting your GABA receptor site and a retest won't be accurate.

    If GABA causes anxiety, irritability, or panic this also indicates a permeable blood-brain barrier. Eating some protein may help alleviate these symptoms. This GABA test is further explained in Datis Kharrazian's book, *Why Isn't My Brain Working?*

- **Yoga** in the form of meditation sessions can increase in GABA, positively correlated to improved mood and decreased anxiety, support the hypothesis that meditation stimulates the vagus nerve through slower breath rates.[3239]
- **Brain-healthy lifestyle.** All of the tips in the self-help chapter are important to protect the blood brain barrier: eat good, nutritious, non-inflammatory, antioxidant-rich food only when you are hungry, don't smoke, get enough sleep, reduce electromagnetic fields from cell phones, WiFi, cell towers, etc, get plenty of exercise, and reduce your stress load.

Note. In the event of having a known blood-brain barrier compromise, do not do chelation therapy as chelation can pull out toxins from the liver resulting in additional inflammation.

Appendix 6. Brain Supporting Formulas

From Naturaleyecare.com:

Brain Formulas

Advanced Eye and Vision Support Formula - whole food, organic, GMO free

Cognirev Extra Strength Intraoral Spray

Dr. Grossman's RX-Anti-Aging Formula

Dr. Grossman's Meso Plus Formula with Mirtogenol

MycoBotanicals Brain 60 vegcaps

Oceans 3™ - Better Brain 90 gels

Discounted Packages

Brain and Memory Support Packages 1

Brain and Memory Support Packages 2

Parkinson's Support Package 1

Parkinson's Support Package 2 with Stem Cell Support

Books

Natural Eye Care: Your Guide to Healthy Vision

Natural Parkinson's Care: Your Guide to Preventing and Managing Parkinson's

Please email us with any questions at info@naturaleyecare.com or call 845-475-4158

Appendix 7. Eyes and Dementia

The Optic Nerve and the Brain

The optic nerve actually is brain tissue. There is a remarkable correlation between nutrients that support the health of the retina and optic nerve and those that support healthy brain function. Some of these important nutrients for both eye and brain include: anthocyanins, apigenin, astaxanthin, curcumin, gingko biloba, ginseng, glutathione, lutein, omega-3 fatty acids, resveratrol, taurine, vitamin A, vitamin E, vinpocetine, zeaxanthin, zinc and more.

Common essential common food sources: avocado, blueberries (and other dark berries), cruciferous vegetables, eggs, dark chocolate, goji berries, green leafy vegetables, mushrooms (reiki, shiitake, lion's mane), olive oil, and red wine.

See the Nutrients chapter for more details.

Macular Pigment versus Alzheimer's

One way of measuring retinal health is to look at the thickness of the macular pigment, whose role is to protect the retina from damaging blue, and UV radiation from sunlight (and some electronic devices). Alzheimer's patients have significantly lower macular pigment (MP), and correspondingly, poorer visual function, when compared to control subjects of similar age.

It is known that patients with dementia and Alzheimer's have poor diets lacking in colored fruit and vegetables[3240][3241][3242] and it is these strongly antioxidant-rich foods that supply the carotenoids that make up the macular pigment. On average, AD patients consume fewer carotenoids than patients free of AD and they also have a thinner layer of macular pigment compared to controls. Enrichment of enrichment of macular pigment has been shown to improve visual function, in both diseased and non-diseased retina.

In one study, the supplementing AD patients with the carotenoids lutein (10mg), zeaxanthin (2mg) and mesozeaxanthin (10mg) showed a significant improvement in retinal health and visual acuity compared to non-AD patients. Patients exhibited significant increases in serum concentrations of lutein, zeaxanthin and mesozeaxanthin and in macular pigment (MP) with consequential improvements in visual function. The placebo groups exhibited no significant change in any of these outcome measures.[3243] Earlier studies showed benefits on macular pigment were not as successful with the addition of just mesozeaxanthin.[3244][3245] High serum concentrations of lutein and zeaxanthin are also associated with a lower risk of AD mortality in adults[3246] and that plasma antioxidants are depleted in those with MP or AD when compared to subjects with normal cognitive function.[3247]

Eye Disease and Brain Neurodegeneration Risk

There are several eye diseases which are considered risk factors for later-in-life neurodegenerative conditions, such as Alzheimer's. It's probably not that the eye disease causes the dementia, but that the conditions which cause the eye disease are also risk factors for brain neurodegeneration.

Open angle glaucoma, a leading cause of blindness, causes an increasing loss of peripheral vision. Risk factors include genetics, heavy use of computers (especially in nearsighted people), diabetes, high blood pressure, severe nearsightedness, and use of corticosteroids.

Patients who have been diagnosed with glaucoma are at higher risk (46% higher)[3248] of developing Alzheimer's, but not Parkinson's. Women with glaucoma have a greater risk than men, and people over sixty-five-years old have a greater risk than those younger than sixty-five.[3249]

Although some studies with few subjects do not show a connection, a new study with 15,317 subjects in a Taiwan cohort have found that normal- or low-tension glaucoma patients were four times as likely to develop Alzheimer's.[3250] [3251]

Optical coherence tomography of the eye can detect changes in the average thickness of the retinal nerve fiber layer, and ganglion cell complex which are associated with loss of brain volume that also provides clues about the connection with AD.[3252]

Macular degeneration (AMD), an eye disease which may be managed (in early stages) though careful attention to nutrition and lifestyle factors, causes an increasing loss of central vision as the macula portion of the retina deteriorates.

Patients with macular degeneration have a fifty percent higher risk of developing Alzheimer's.[3253] Researchers found no correlation between recently developed AMD, but those who have established AMD are at greater risk than people without AMD.

Diabetic retinopathy is the deterioration of the retina brought on by untreated diabetes. Patients with diabetic retinopathy are fifty percent more likely to develop Alzheimer's than controls whether the condition has developed recently or has been established for some time. [3254]

Cataracts. Researchers found no correlation between presence of cataracts and Alzheimer's incidence.[3255]

Vision Testing for Alzheimer's

It may be possible to detect very early stages of Alzheimer's disease by looking at the eyes fifteen to twenty years before clinical diagnosis. Cedars-Sinai has developed an optical imaging technique[3256] that may enable doctors to detect very early amyloid plaque buildup. A large clinical study of volunteers from Australia and the U.S. is investigating the possibilities for early detection.

Two other universities, the University of San Diego and Emory in Atlanta are testing whether the equipment recognizes plaque buildup in existing Alzheimer's patients. The problem is to figure out whether plaque observed in a retinal scan is correlated to plaque detected in a positron emission tomography (PET) scan. PET scans are invasive, use radioactive tracers, and are very expensive, so that this new technique is very promising.

Early results indicate that the non-invasive test can detect Alzheimer's with 100 percent sensitivity and 80.6 percent specificity. With one-hundred percent sensitivity the test doesn't overlook any actual positives by misidentifying them; 80.6 percent specificity means that the test rarely identifies something else as amyloid plaque. Sensitivity avoids false-negatives; specificity avoids false-positives.[3257] In other words, it errs on the side of caution.

Even more exciting is that current tests can't identify Alzheimer's until the disease is well progressed, but this new technique will allow diagnosis fifteen to twenty years before symptoms appear. This makes it possible to address the problem by other means early on.

Appendix 8. On the Horizon

Avenues of Investigation

5HT6 receptors on brain cells can 'lock' some neurotransmitters rendering them unavailable for communication between neurons. People with Alzheimer's have low levels of one of these receptors, acetylcholine. Limiting the activity of the 5HT6 receptor may increase acetylcholine levels and improve neuron-to-neuron communication.[3258]

Inflammation reduction. Neuroinflammation is the inflammation of neural tissue which is the body's attempt to heal an acute injury, but when excessive or chronic can result in the death of neuron cells both in the brain and central nervous system. It has long been known to play a role in AD. Beta-amyloid plaques and tau tangles both stimulate the immune response in the brain and, in response, over-active microglia produce compounds that can damage nearby cells.[3259]

Beta-secretase (BACE1). One of the enzymes that clips the APP gene (Protein Coding), BACE1, makes it possible for beta-amyloid to form. Therapies that interrupt this process may reduce the amount of beta-amyloid in the brain and ultimately intervene in the development of Alzheimer's disease.[3260]

Mechanisms of tau protein. Tau protein, a prime component of tau tangles, helps maintain neuron structure through tiny tube-like structures called microtubules that deliver nutrients throughout the neuron. Scientists are researching whether there are means to keep tau protein from collapsing and tangling, resulting in destruction of the microtubules and the neuron.[3261]

TPP1 gene. Amyloid beta aggregates can be enclosed by microglia and passed to lysosomes which break down excess materials in the body, but the process is slow. A new innovative target for treating AD appears to be the use of the lysosomal enzyme tripeptidyl peptidase 1 (TPPI) which destabilizes fibrillar amyloid beta by splitting it into parts.[3262]

Ongoing Research

Research is, of course, continually being updated. You can go to clinicaltrials.gov to see specifics on upcoming, ongoing, and completed research. Abstracts reporting research results are also available at pubmed.ncbi.nlm.nih.gov.

The following drugs are still in research and are not available to the public.

AADvac1 vaccine is being tested in a Phase 2 clinical trial with 185 patients with mild Alzheimer's disease. It stimulates the body's immune system to attack an abnormal form of tau protein that destabilizes the structure of neurons.[3263] A study published in 2020 reports that humanized tau antibodies promote tau update by microglia without increased inflammation.[3264] [3265]

Aducanumab is an antibody being studied as a potential drug that eases symptoms of Alzheimer's disease. Early studies showed decreased levels of beta-amyloid in the brains of study volunteers. Two Phase 3 studies have been completed and the FDA has authorized a study with patients. 2,400 patients who were enrolled in the previous studies are eligible and will receive 10 mg/kg of aducanumab monthly for 100 weeks.[3266]

The A4 Study (Anti-AB Treatment in Asymptomatic Alzheimer's Disease) is an ongoing prevention trial that will enroll 1,000 patients around the country who are currently asymptomatic but have a high chance of developing Alzheimer's in the upcoming years either because they have either a genetic predisposition, or a PET (positron emission imaging) scan revealed abnormal levels of beta amyloid plagues in the brain. The study was expected to complete in 2022[3267] but issues related to COVID-19 have delayed research.

The working hypothesis behind A4 is that by giving an anti-amyloid drug, solanezumab, to the volunteers during the preclinical stages of Alzheimer's, doctors will be able to delay any cognitive decline. Solanezumab which binds to amyloid, removes it from the brain, and eliminates it via the circulatory system.

Side effects from solanezumab may include mild chills, which are related to a reaction to the infusion. This is the first time that solanezumab will be tested on asymptomatic people, but not the first time it's been tested in humans

JNJ-54861911 is a BACE inhibitor that had been well tolerated by patients with preclinical or mild cognitive impairment. It is currently in a Phase 3 study to determine if it slows cognitive decline in people who do not have Alzheimer's symptoms but have elevated levels of beta-amyloid in the brain. The study is expected to be completed in 2024.[3268][3269] However, it has been linked to increases in liver enzymes.[3270]

Leukine (Sargramostim) is used to treat conditions in which white blood cell counts are low, such as in certain types of leukemia (a blood cancer) or in patients who received a bone marrow transplant. It is currently being investigated as a potential treatment for cognitive problems related to Alzheimer's disease, trial end date in May of 2020. It is also being tested as a treatment for COVID-19.[3271]

Phototherapy and stem cells. With senior populations growing, much research is focused on stem cells. A stem cell niche is the microenvironment in the extra cellular matrix in which a stem cell resides. This extracellular matrix stimulates regeneration on the cellular level. Stem cell production diminishes with age and after age seventy stem cell activity is scant. One of the most promising candidates for stem cell regeneration is the human copper-binding peptide GHK-Cu (glycyl-L-histidyl-L-lysine) a small, naturally occurring tri-peptide present in human plasma that also can be released from tissues in case of an injury.[3272] Complex influences in stem cells' microenvironment determine whether the stem cell will function normally, improving tissue repair and regeneration, or transform into a malignant cell. Stem cell senescence also depends on gene expression and microenvironmental cues. Both laboratory and gene studies suggest that GHK, a very safe molecule and low-cost molecule, could improve stem cell therapies.[3273]

This peptide discovered in 1973 by Pickart, has the highest concentration in young adults (age twenty-five and younger), when tissues have the most regenerative potential; however, it declines with age.[3274] The first indication that GHK affects stem cells came from mouse studies where GHK-Cu produced a very strong amplification of hair follicle size. A similar peptide, Ala-His-Lys-copper 2 , produced even stronger actions .[3275] Based on laboratory data and gene profiling data, GHK-Cu may be used to improve stem cell therapy and to help shift regeneration processes to healthy levels.

Tests are currently being conducted by the NFL on players that have had head injuries. These tests are using phototherapy to stimulate stem cell regeneration with GHK-Cu molecules incorporated into a photo biomodulation system. The body uses light (phototherapy) to initiate chemical reactions in the body. For example, red light has been used in infrared therapy. Lasers are a source of high energy light used in surgical procedures and phototherapy is now being used for non-surgical face lifts. There is a proprietary and patented form of phototherapy (brand name X39), that uses the body's own heat to activate the chemical reaction that triggers a specific response. This can be accomplished through a transdermal delivery system that is placed on the skin. Made from organic crystals, and when activated, it stimulates the nerves and acupuncture points on the skin. The frequency emitted has been tested with an FTIR machine for efficacy by the company who makes the patch. This is safer and more bioavailable than microneedle or oral methods of providing GHK-Cu.

The NFL Alumni Medical Research Foundation (dba of the NFL Alumni Foundation) has agreed to participate in its first study investigating the effects of a Non-invasive photo biomodulation therapy (Lifewave X39) on the brain function of players who had experienced a TBI during their career. A previous study by Psy Tec Labs with the same X39 used brain mapping to assess differences in brain function. All participants in this study showed dramatic changes in their scalp topographic maps reporting the amplitude of the P300 recording for each channel, and also in their coherence maps. According to their coherence maps, the majority of participants started with an overactive brain and their brain calmed down significantly after three weeks of wearing the X39 patch. Several participants reported various notable improvements and most participants reported feeling slightly better or a lot better at the end of their participation.[3276]

As the results of the NFL study are published we should have confirmation that this is a valid treatment for brain injury, stem cell regeneration and potentially help for memory loss. More information on this technology can be found at Lifewave.com/EOLDist.

Pimavanserin can "unlock: the 5HT2A receptor because it mimics a serotonin 'key'." However, pimavanserin has the opposite effect of serotonin: it reduces communication between neurons. This may have the effect of reducing the symptoms of dementia-related psychosis. A Phase 3 clinical trial significantly reduced risk of psychosis by 2.8 times compared to placebo. [3277] Developers will seek FDA application in 2020.[3278]

Testing Methods

Researchers are looking at using different scanning techniques of the brain to help determine dementia and AD diagnosis. These tests include:

A CT scan uses an x-ray method that makes hundreds of images while rotating 360 degrees around the area that is being studied. A computer processes these images to produce two dimensional cross-sectional images of the area, like slices from a loaf of bread.

MRI forms two-dimensional, cross-sectional images of the brain. But MRI relies on a powerful magnet rather than x-rays to capture the images. Because the technique is based on the amount of water in a given tissue, MRI provides a more refined and clearer view of the brain.

Functional MRI (fMRI) looks not only at the structure of the brain, but also at the metabolic processes taking place at the time of the scan.

Positron emission tomography (PET), are increasingly being used in the diagnosis of dementia. Until PET scan use, many people without amyloid beta accumulation were being treated for Alzheimer's incorrectly.[3279]

- FDG-PET measures how much glucose is being taken up by brain cells and gives information about the level of activity (function) in various areas of the brain that might be affected by various dementias. FDG-PET imaging examines how the brain is working metabolically because functionally brain cells depend on glucose for their energy supply by determining how much of a radioactive tracer attached to a glucose molecule is taken up by brain cells a radiologist can determine whether cells in specific brain areas are functioning normally

Clinical Trials

To locate related research near you, go to https://www.verywellhealth.com/leading-alzheimers-and-dementia-charities-and-organizations-4145316 or call at 212-204-4000.

Appendix 9. Brain Supporting Characteristics

Nutrients that Cross the Blood Brain Barrier

- Acetyl-L- Carnitine
- Apigenin
- Astaxanthin
- Baicalein
- Blueberries (anthocyanin colorant)
- Catechin
- Curcumin
- DHA
- Lutein
- N-Acetyl-cysteine
- Omega-3 fatty acids
- Phosphatidylserine
- Resveratrol
- Rutin
- Vinpocetine
- Vitamin A
- Vitamin E
- Zeaxanthin
- Zinc

Nutrients That Have the Potential of Breaking Down Amyloid Fibrils

- Apigenin
- Ashwagandha
- Centella asiatica
- Curcumin
- Coffee
- CoQ10
- DHA
- Extra virgin olive oil
- Gingko biloba
- Ginseng
- Grapeseed extract
- Magnesium
- Nattokinase
- Olive leaf extract
- Omega-3 fatty acids
- Pomegranate juice
- PQQ
- Vitamin A
- Vitamin E
- Walnuts (raw)

Nutrients That Help Prevent the Formation of Amyloid Fibrils (NF-κB, blocking amyloid beta (Aβ) production)

- Apigenin
- Ashwagandha
- Curcumin
- Ginger
- Ginseng
- Gotu kola (Centella asiatica)
- Green tea
- Olive leaf extract
- Omega-3 fatty acids
- Quercetin
- Radix puerariae
- Vinpocetine
- Vitamin A

Nutrients That Support Brain Cell Neurogenesis and/or Brain Plasticity

- Acetyl-l-Carnitine
- Ashwagandha
- Astaxanthin
- Baicalein
- Blueberries
- Curcumin
- DHA
- Gingko Biloba
- Ginseng
- Goji berry (aka wolfberry)
- Grapeseed extract
- Green tea
- Gut Microbia
- Hesperidin
- Iron
- Luteolin
- Lotus Root Extract
- Magnesium
- Melatonin
- Mulberry
- N-Acetyl-cysteine
- Omega-3 fatty acids
- Piperine (pepper)
- Phosphatidylserine
- Sage (aka danshen and salvia)
- Reiki mushrooms
- Resveratrol
- Rhodiola
- Shankhpushpi (Convolvulus pluricaulis)
- Taurine
- Theanine
- Trytophan and 5-HTP
- Vinpocetine
- Vitamin
- Vitamin E

Nutrients That Increase BDNF and May Increase Neurogenesis

- Alpha lipoic acid
- Ashwagandha
- Astaxanthin
- Beta-alanin and l-carnosine
- Blueberries
- Cinnamon
- Cocoflavonoids and chocolate
- DHA
- Gingko biloba
- Ginseng
- Goji berry (aka wolfberry)
- Gotu kola (Centella asiatica)
- Green tea
- Gut microbia
- Huperzine A
- Magnesium
- Magnolol
- Milk thistle extract
- Nattokinase
- Omega-3 fatty acids
- Pantethine
- Piperine (pepper)
- Phosphatidylserine
- PQQ
- Resveratrol
- Selenium
- Shankhpushpi (Convolvulus pluricaulis)
- Theanine
- Vinpocetine
- Vitamin D3

Nutrients/Foods That *Decrease* Neurogenesis

- High amounts of sugar, carbohydrates, and unhealthy fats (trans-fatty acids (as in most margarines and many chips, fried food)
- Excessive amounts of food (overeating) and especially late light eating.
- Foods that contribute to inflammation include: refined carbohydrate, fried foods, vegetable oil (when not organic, refined and in a dark bottle such as corn, safflower, soy, and cottonseed oils), refined (white) foods, dairy (for more many people)
- An acidic diet (which included the foods mentioned above).
- Alcohol consumption (of more than a beer or glass of red wine per night)
- Excessive caffeine
- Deficiencies in Vitamins A, B1, B9 (thiamine) and folic acid.

Nutrients Shown to Reduce Cognitive Decline for Those with AD

- Alpha lipoic acid
- Amla
- Apigenin
- Ashwagandha
- Astaxanthin
- Baicalein
- Brahmi (Bacopa monnieri)
- Celastrus paniculatus
- Choline
- Curcumin
- Coffee
- Convolvulus pluricaulis
- DHEA
- Folate (vitamin B9)
- Ginger
- Gingko biloba
- Ginseng
- Grapeseed extract
- Green tea
- Gut microbia
- Lecithin
- Lutein
- Luteolin
- Moringa oleifera
- N-acetyl-cysteine
- Omega-3 fatty acids
- Phosphatidylserine
- PQQ
- Pycnogenol
- Rhizoma anemarrhenae
- Rhodiola
- Selenium
- Vinpocetine
- Vitamin B1
- Vitamin B12
- Vitamin E
- Zeaxanthin
- Zinc

Nutrients That Reduce Brain Inflammation

- Apigenin
- Ashwagandha root
- Astaxanthin
- Baicalein
- Cat's claw
- Coffee
- CoQ10
- Curcumin

- Garlic
- Ginseng
- Green tea
- Gut Microbia
- Lutein
- Olive leaf extract
- Omega-3 fatty acids
- Omega-6 fatty acids (black currant seed and borage oils)
- Omega-7 fatty acids
- Pycnogenol
- Reiki mushrooms
- Resveratrol
- Rutin
- Sage (aka danshen and salvia)
- SAM-e
- Vinpocetine
- Zeaxanthin

Nutrients That Support Blood Flow to the Brain

- Apigenin
- Baicalein
- Coffee
- Garlic
- Gingko biloba
- Ginseng
- Gut microbia
- Lutein
- Mulberry
- PQQ
- Resveratrol
- Sage (aka danshen and salvia)
- Vinpocetine
- Zeaxanthin

Nutrients That Reduce Oxidative Stress to the Brain

- Alpha lipoic acid
- Apigenin
- Ashwagandha
- Astaxanthin
- Blueberries
- DHA
- Garlic
- Ginger
- Ginseng
- Goji berry (aka wolfberry)
- Grapeseed extract
- Guggulu
- Iron
- N-Acetyl-cysteine
- Melatonin
- Moringa oleifera
- Mulberry
- Phosphatidylserine
- PQQ
- Pycnogenol
- Quercetin
- Rutin
- Vinpocetine
- Vitamin E
- Zeaxanthin

Nutrients That Help Prevent Cell Death

- Apigenin
- Ashwagandha
- Baicalein
- CoQ10
- DHA
- Ginseng
- Gotu kola
- Luteolin
- Pinocembrin
- PQQ
- Quercetin

Nutrients That Help Prevent or Reduce Tao Build-up and Fibril Formulation

- Grapeseed extract
- Olive leaf extract
- Omega-3 fatty acids
- Vitamin A
- Vitamin E

Nutrients with Neuroprotective Benefits

- Acetyl-l-carnitine
- Alpha lipoic acid
- Astaxanthin
- Baicalein
- Brahmi (Bacopa monnieri)
- Blueberries
- Catechin
- Celastrus paniculatus
- Choline
- CoQ10
- Copper
- Curcumin
- DHA
- DHEA
- Folate (vitamin B9)
- Garlic
- Hesperidin
- Moringa oleifera
- Omega-3 fatty acids
- Phosphatidylserine
- Pomegranate juice
- PQQ
- Pycnogenol
- Quercetin
- Reiki mushrooms
- Rutin
- Taurine
- Theanine
- Vinpocetine
- Vitamin E

Nutrients that Promote Mitochondrial Support

- Astaxanthin
- Copper
- Curcumin
- DHA
- Ginseng
- Green tea
- Pinocembrin
- PQQ
- Quercetin
- Reiko mushrooms
- Resveratrol
- Rhodiola

Nutrients that Support Brain Synapse/Acetycholine System

- Glucose – The brain requires glucose, but too much is a neurotoxin
- Zinc

Nutrients that Reduce Stress and/or Anxiety, Fatigue

- Acetyl-l-carnitine
- Convolvulus pluricaulis
- Goji berries
- Rhodiola rosea
- Clary sage essential oil
- Lavender essential oil
- Lemon Balm essential oil
- Frankincense essential oil
- Patchouli essential oil
- Peppermint essential oil
- Rosemary essential oil
- Spearmint essential oil
- Tea tree lemon essential oil

Nutrients That Help Reduce Depression

- 5-HTP
- Baicalein
- Celastrus paniculatus
- Folate (vitamin B9)
- Ginger
- Ginseng
- Goji berry (aka wolfberry)
- Luteolin
- N-acetyl-cysteine
- Olive leaf extract
- Omega-3 fatty acids
- Phosphatidylserine
- Rhodiola
- Sage (aka danshen and salvia)
- SAM-e
- Trytophan and 5-HTP
- Vitamin B12
- Ylang Ylang (and poor sleeping)

Appendix 10. COVID-19 and the Brain

It is important to do all we can to avoid contracting COVID-19 (or, perhaps, similar viruses that may appear in the future). COVID-19 can cause a myriad of health issues, both during initial illness, and after supposed recovery. In addition to common respiratory symptoms, COVID-19 patients experience a wide variety of neurological, cognitive, psychological, and psychiatric symptoms, as well as a loss of sense of taste and smell for an unspecified period of time.

The brain contains several "types" of matter: white matter and grey matter. Grey matter contains many cell bodies and not many nerve cells. White matter includes many nerve cells. The long threadlike part of nerve cells are called axons. Their role is to convey nerve impulses throughout the regions of the brain, and through the grey matter. Axons are protected with a thin layer of myelin which insulates and protects them. They are whitish in color and because of their prevalence the parts of the brain containing many of them are known as white matter.

Damage to white matter affects learning and brain functions, and the ability to act as a relay and coordinating communication between different brain regions.

This is important because it appears that COVID-19 causes changes in white brain matter and development of white matter lesions, resulting in neuron hypoxia, a deficiency in the amount of oxygen reaching the tissues and dysfunction.[3280]

A number of both temporary and long-lasting symptoms have been noted:

- Symptoms include fatigue, shortness of breath, cough, joint pain, and chest pain.[3281]

- Symptoms also include for about 15% of patients, loss of taste ageusia) and/or smell (anosmia).[3282] These symptoms are often the first to appear in COVID-19 patients.[3283]

- Long term symptoms, of COVID-19 "long haulers" include: muscle pain or headache, fast or pounding heartbeat, loss of smell or taste, memory, concentration or sleep problems, rash or hair loss.[3284]

- COVID-19 can cause long term brain damage, even in young people. This includes strokes, seizures and Guillain-Barre syndrome, a condition that causes temporary paralysis[3285] when the immune system attacks the nervous system.

- SARS-CoV-2 has been detected in the cerebral-spinal fluid (CSF) of some patients. Patients have experienced post-COVID confusion, and inflammation in the brain (encephalitis).[3286]

- COVID-19 may also increase the risk of developing Parkinson's disease and Alzheimer's disease, even in young people,

Appendix 11. Resources

Recommended Books

Bredesen, Dale E. (2017). The End of Alzheimer's: The First Program to Prevent and Reverse Cognitive Decline.

Cortright, Brant , Ph.D. (2015). The Neurogenesis Diet & Lifestyle: Upgrade Your Brain, Upgrade Your Life.

Kharrazian, Datis. (2013). Why Isn't My Brain Working: A revolutionary understanding of brain decline and effective strategies to recover your brain's health.

Mosconi, Lisa. (2018). Brain Food: How to Eat Smart and Sharpen Your Mind.

Jennings, Timothy R. (2018). The Aging Brain: Proven Steps to Prevent Dementia and Sharpen Your Mind.

Related Organizations

Brain Disease Organizations

Alzheimer's Association Phone: 800-272-3900 https://www.alz.org/

Alzheimer's Research and Prevention Foundation (ARPF) Phone: 212-204-4000 https://www.verywellhealth.com/leading-alzheimers-and-dementia-charities-and-organizations-4145316

The American Brain Foundation (ABF) https://www.americanbrainfoundation.org/

Cure Alzheimer's Fund Phone: 781-237-3800 https://curealz.org/

The Fisher Center for Alzheimer's Research Foundation (FCARF) Phone: 800-259-4636 https://www.alzinfo.org/ Email: info@alzinfo.org

Lewy Body Dementia Association (LBDA) https://www.lbda.org/

Caregiver Organizations

Alzheimer's Foundation of America
Phone: 866-232-8484 https://alzfdn.org/ E-mail: info@alzfdn.org

The Alzheimer's Family Services Center
Phone: (714) 593-9630 https://afscenter.org/

National Alliance for Caregiving
Phone: (301) 718-8444 https://www.caregiving.org/resources

AARP
https://www.aarp.org/caregiving/local/info-2017/important-resources-for-caregivers.html

Other Books by Safe Goods Publishing

Natural Eye Care Series: Macular Degeneration	*$ 14.95*
Natural Eye Care Series: Glaucoma	*$ 14.95*
Natural Eye Care Series: Cataracts	*$ 14.95*
Natural Eye Care Series: Dry Eye	*$ 14.95*
Natural Eye Care Series: Floaters	*$ 14.95*
The Shattered Oak	*$ 14.95*
A Barnstormer Aviator	*$ 12.95*
Flying Above the Glass Ceiling	*$ 14.95*
Spirit & Creator (Spirit of St. Louis)	*$ 29.95*
Letters from My Son	*$ 22.95*
Nutritional Leverage for Great Golf	*$ 9.95*
Overcoming Senior Moments Expanded	*$ 9.95*
Prevent Cancer, Strokes, Heart Attacks	*$ 11.95*
Cancer Disarmed Expanded	*$ 7.95*
Eye Care Naturally	*$ 8.95*
Velvet Antler	*$ 9.95*

www.SafeGoodsPublishing.com

Endnotes

---

[1] Gray JD, Rubin TG, Hunter RG, McEwen BS. (2014). Hippocampal gene expression changes underlying stress sensitization and recovery. *Mol Psychiatry.* Nov; 19(11):1171-8.

[2] Wood ER, Dudchenko PA, Robitsek RJ, Eichenbaum H. (2000). Hippocampal neurons encode information about different types of memory episodes occurring in the same location. *Neuron.* Sep; 27(3):623-33.

[3] McEwen BS, Morrison JH. (2013). The brain on stress: vulnerability and plasticity of the prefrontal cortex over the life course. *Neuron.* Jul 10; 79(1):16-29.

[4] Radley JJ, Sisti HM, Hao J, Rocher AB, McCall T, Hof PR, et al. (2004). Chronic behavioral stress induces apical dendritic reorganization in pyramidal neurons of the medial prefrontal cortex. *Neuroscience.* 2004; 125(1):1-6.

[5] Liston C, Miller MM, Goldwater DS, Radley JJ, Rocher AB, et al. (2006). Stress-Induced Alterations in Prefrontal Cortical Dendritic Morphology Predict Selective Impairments in Perceptual Attentional Set-Shifting. *J Neurosci.* 2006 Jul 26; 26(30):7870-4.

[6] Ibid. Liston. (2006).

[7] Sandi C. (2013). Stress and cognition. *Wiley Interdiscip Rev Cogn Sci.* May; 4(3):245-261

[8] McEwen BS, Sapolsky RM. (1995). Stress and cognitive function. *Curr Opin Neurobiol.* Apr; 5(2):205-16.

[9] Squire, LR; Schacter DL. *The Neuropsychology of Memory.* Guilford Press. 2002.

[10] Lupien SJ, Wilkinson CW, Brière S, Ménard C, Ng Ying, Kin NM, et al. (2002). The modulatory effects of corticosteroids on cognition: studies in young human populations. *Psychoneuroendocrinology.* Apr; 27(3):401-16

[11] McEwen BS. (1999). Stress and hippocampal plasticity. *Annu Rev Neurosci.* 22():105-22.

[12] Lupien SJ, Lepage M. (2001). Stress, memory, and the hippocampus: can't live with it, can't live without it. *Behav Brain Res.* Dec 14; 127(1-2):137-58.

[13] Woolley CS, Gould E, McEwen BS. (1990). Exposure to excess glucocorticoids alters dendritic morphology of adult hippocampal pyramidal neurons. *Brain Res.* Oct 29; 531(1-2):225-31

[14] Sapolsky RM, Uno H, Rebert CS, Finch CE. (1990). Hippocampal damage associated with prolonged glucocorticoid exposure in primates. *J Neurosci.* Sep; 10(9):2897-902.

[15] Ibid. Sapolsky. (1990).

[16] Gould E, Tanapat P, McEwen BS, Flügge G, Fuchs E. (1998). Proliferation of granule cell precursors in the dentate gyrus of adult monkeys is diminished by stress. *Proc Natl Acad Sci U S A.* Mar 17; 95(6):3168-71.

[17] Lawrence MS, Sapolsky RM. (1994). Glucocorticoids accelerate ATP loss following metabolic insults in cultured hippocampal neurons. *Brain Res.* May 23; 646(2):303.

[18] Sapolsky RM, Pulsinelli WA. (1985). Glucocorticoids potentiate ischemic injury to neurons: therapeutic implications. *Science.* Sep 27; 229(4720):1397-400.

[19] Popoli M, Yan Z, McEwen BS, Sanacora G. (2011). The stressed synapse: the impact of stress and glucocorticoids on glutamate transmission. *Nat Rev Neurosci.* Nov 30; 13(1): 22–37.

[20] McEwen BS. (1999). Stress and hippocampal plasticity. *Annu Rev Neurosci.* 22():105-22.

[21] Roozendaal B, McEwen BS, Chattarji S. (2009). Stress, memory and the amygdala. *Nat Rev Neurosci.* Jun; 10(6):423-33.

[22] Joëls M, Fernandez G, Roozendaal B. (2011). Stress and emotional memory: a matter of timing. *Trends Cogn Sci.* Jun; 15(6):280-8.

[23] Ibid. Joëls. (2011).

[24] McEwen BS, Nasca C, Gray JD. (2016). Stress Effects on Neuronal Structure: Hippocampus, Amygdala, and Prefrontal Cortex. *Neuropsychopharmacology.* Jan; 41(1): 3–23.

[25] Blackburn D, Sargsyan S, Monk PN, Shaw PJ. (2009). Astrocyte function and role in motor neuron disease: a future therapeutic target? *Glia.* Sep;57(12):1251-64.

[26] Blackburn D, Sargsyan S, Monk PN, Shaw PJ. (2009). Astrocyte function and role in motor neuron disease: a future therapeutic target? *Glia.* 2009 Sep;57(12):1251-64.

[27] Wang D, Jacobs SA, Tsien JZ. (2014). Targeting the NMDA receptor subunit NR2B for treating or preventing age-related memory decline. *Expert Opin Ther Targets.* 2014;18(10):1121-30.

[28] Erickson KI, Voss MW, Prakash RS, Basak C, Szabo A, Chaddock L, et al. (2011). Exercise training increases size of hippocampus and improves memory. *AF Proc Natl Acad Sci U S A.* Feb 15; 108(7):3017-22.

[29] Queensland Brain Institute. What is synaptic plasticity? Retrieved Jul 17 2019 from https://qbi.uq.edu.au/brain-basics/brain/brain-physiology/what-synaptic-plasticity.

[30] Fietta P, Fietta P. (2007). Glucocorticoids and brain functions. *Riv Biol.* Sep-Dec;100(3):403-18.

[31] Ibid. Sandi. (2013). Wiley Interdiscip Rev Cogn Sci.

[32] De Felice FG, Lourenco MV, Ferreira ST. (2014). How does brain insulin resistance develop in Alzheimer's disease? *Alzheimers Dement.* Feb; 10(1 Suppl):S26-32.

[33] Montaron MF, Drapeau E, Dupret D, Kitchener P, Aurousseau C, Le Moal M, et al. (2006 White Matter versus Gray Matter. *Neurobiol Aging.* Apr; 27(4):645-54.

[34] McEwen B, Lupien S. Stress: hormonal and neural aspects. In: Ramachandran VS, editor. Encyclopedia of the human brain. Amsterdam: Elsevier; 2002. pp. 463–474. Memory formation under stress: quantity and quality. Schwabe L, Wolf OT, Oitzl MS *Neurosci Biobehav Rev.* 2010 Mar; 34(4):584-91.

[35] McEwen BS. (2015). "Chapter 34 – Stress". In Neurobiology of Brain Disorders. Pp 558-569.

[36] Dhabhar FS. (2009). Enhancing versus suppressive effects of stress on immune function: implications for immunoprotection and immunopathology. *Neuroimmunomodulation.* 16(5):300-17.

[37] Dhabhar FS, Malarkey WB, Neri E, McEwen BS. (2012). Stress-induced redistribution of immune cells--from barracks to boulevards to battlefields: a tale of three hormones--Curt Richter Award winner. *Psychoneuroendocrinology.* Sep; 37(9):1345-68.

[38] Ibid. De Felice. (2014). *Alzheimers Dement.*

[39] Bennur S, Shankaranarayana Rao BS, Pawlak R, Strickland S, McEwen BS, Chattarji S. (2007). Stress-induced spine loss in the medial amygdala is mediated by tissue-plasminogen activator. *Neuroscience.* Jan 5; 144(1):8-16.

[40] Lau T, Bigio B, Zelli D, McEwen BS, Nasca C. (2017). Stress-induced structural plasticity of medial amygdala stellate neurons and rapid prevention by a candidate antidepressant. *Mol Psychiatry.* Feb; 22(2):227-234.

[41] Vyas A, Mitra R, Shankaranarayana Rao BS, Chattarji S. (2002). Chronic stress induces contrasting patterns of dendritic remodeling in hippocampal and amygdaloid neurons. *J Neurosci.* Aug 1; 22(15):6810-8.

[42] Ibid. Vyas. (2002).

[43] Ibid. Lau. (2017).

[44] Krishnan V, Han MH, Graham DL, Berton O, Renthal W, Russo SJ, Laplant Q, et al. (2007). Molecular adaptations underlying susceptibility and resistance to social defeat in brain reward regions., *Nestler EJ Cell.* 2007 Oct 19; 131(2):391-404.

[45] Ibid. Erickson. (2011). *AF Proc Natl Acad Sci U S A.*

[46] Burggren AC, Shirazi A, Ginder N, London ED. (2019). Cannabis effects on brain structure, function, and cognition: considerations for medical uses of cannabis and its derivatives. *Am J Drug Alcohol Abuse.* Jul 31:1-17.

[47] Castilla-Ortega E, Ladron de Guevara-Miranda D, Serrano A, Pavon FJ, Suarez J, et al. (2017). The impact of cocain on adult hippocampal neurogenesis: Potential neurobiological mechanisms and contributions to maladaptive cognition in cocaine addiction disorder. *Biochem Pharmacol.* Oct 1;141:100-117.

[48] Abrous DN, Adriani W, Montaron MF, Aurousseau A, Rougon G, Le Moal M, et al. (2002). Nicotine Self-Administration Impairs Hippocampal Plasticity. *J Neurosci.* May 22 (9) 3656-3662.

[49] DeBry SC, Tiffany ST. (2008). Tobacco-induced neurotoxicity of adolescent cognitive development (TINACD): a proposed model for the development of impulsivity in nicotine dependence. *Nicotine Tob Res.* Jan; 10(1):11-25.

[50] Le Houezec J. (2003). Role of nicotine pharmacokinetics in nicotine addiction and nicotine replacement therapy: a review. *Int J Tuberc Lung Dis.* Sep; 7(9):811-9.

[51] Couey JJ, Meredith RM, Spijker S, Poorthuis RB, Smit AB, Brussaard AB, et al. (2007). Distributed network actions by nicotine increase the threshold for spike-timing-dependent plasticity in prefrontal cortex. *Neuron.* Apr 5; 54(1):73-87.

[52] Guillem K, Bloem B, Poorthuis RB, Loos M, Smit AB, Maskos U, et al. (2011). Nicotinic acetylcholine receptor β2 subunits in the medial prefrontal cortex control attention. *Science.* Aug 12; 333(6044):888-91.

[53] Virtual Genetics Education Centre, University of Leicester. DNA, genes and chromosomes. Retrieved May 5 2019 from https://www2.le.ac.uk/projects/vgec/schoolsandcolleges/topics/dnageneschromosomes.

[54] Ibid. Virtual Genetics Education Centre.

[55] Wikipedia. RNA. Retrieved May 5 2019 from https://en.m.wikipedia.org/wiki/RNA.

[56] Bhandari T. (2016). If genes don't turn off, brain's wiring gets screwy. Retrieved May 5 2019 from https://www.futurity.org/turn-off-genes-learning-1210412-2/.

[57] Bird A. (2007). Perceptions of epigenetics. *Nature.* May 24; 447(7143):396-8

[58] Rönn T, Volkov P, Davegårdh C, Dayeh T, Hall E, Olsson AH, (2013). A six months exercise intervention influences the genome-wide DNA methylation pattern in human ad ipose tissue. *PLoS Genet.* Jun;9(6):e1003572.

[59] Rivera CM, Ren B. (2013). Mapping human epigenomes. *Cell.* Sep 26; 155(1):39-55.

[60] Kanherkar RR, Bhatia-Dey N, Csoka AB. (2014). Epigenetics Across the Human Lifespan. *Front Cell Dev Biol.* 2 49

[61] Jones PA, Baylin SB *Nat Rev Genet*. 2002 Jun; 3(6):415-28

[62] Santos-Rebouças CB, Pimentel MM *Eur J Hum Genet*. 2007 Jan; 15(1):10-7.

[63] Feng J, Fan G *Int Rev Neurobiol*. 2009; 89():67-84.

[64] Lattal KM, Wood MA. (2013). Epigenetics and persistent memory: implications for reconsolidation and silent extinction beyond the zero. *Nat Neurosci*. Feb; 16(2):124-9.

[65] Phillips T. (2008). The role of methylation in gene expression. *Nature Education*. 1(1):116.

[66] Rose NR, Klose RJ. (2014). Understanding the relationship between DNA methylation and histone lysine methylation. Biochimica et Biophysica Acta. Dec;1839(12):1362-72.

[67] Wikipedia. Histone methylation. Retrieved May 5 2019 from https://en.wikipedia.org/wiki/Histone_methylation.

[68] Ibid. Phillips. (2008).

[69] Ibid. Rose. (2014).

[70] Wikipedia. Transcription factor. Retrieved May 3 2018 from https://en.wikipedia.org/wiki/Transcription_factor.

[71] Pembrey M, Saffery R, Bygren LO; Network in Epigenetic Epidemiology. (2014). Human transgenerational responses to early-life experience: potential impact on development, health and biomedical research. J Med Genet. Sep; 51(9): 563–572.

[72] Waterland RA, Jirtle RL. (2004). Early nutrition, epigenetic changes at transposons and imprinted genes, and enhanced susceptibility to adult chronic diseases. *Nutrition*. Jan; 20(1):63-8.

[73] Nestler EJ. (2014). Epigenetic Mechanisms of Drug Addiction. *Neuropharmacology*. Jan:76(0-0).

[74] Kirkpatrick B. (2016). Epigenetic Mark Might Make Some People More Prone to Drug Addiction. Retrieved May 5 2019 from https://www.whatisepigenetics.com/epigenetic-mark-might-make-some-people-more-prone-to-drug-addiction/.

[75] Robison AJ, Nestler EJ. (2011). Transcriptional and Epigenetic Mechanisms of Addiction. *Nat Rev Neurosci*. Oct 12;12(11):623-7.

[76] Ibid. Kanherkar. (2014). *Front Cell Dev Biol*.

[77] Csoka AB, Szyf M. (2009). Epigenetic side-effects of common pharmaceuticals: a potential new field in medicine and pharmacology. *Med Hypotheses*. Nov; 73(5):770-80.

[78] Renthal W, Nestler EJ. (2008). Epigenetic mechanisms in drug addiction. *Trends Mol Med*. Aug; 14(8):341-50.

[79] Liu H, Zhou Y, Boggs SE, Belinsky SA, Liu J. (2007). Cigarette smoke induces demethylation of prometastatic oncogene synuclein-gamma in lung cancer cells by downregulation of DNMT3B. *Oncogene*. Aug 30; 26(40):5900-10.

[80] Rehan VK, Liu J, Naeem E, Tian J, Sakurai R, Kwong K, et al. (2012). Perinatal nicotine exposure induces asthma in second generation offspring. *BMC Med*. 2012 Oct 30; 10():129.

[81] Shukla SD, Velazquez J, French SW, Lu SC, Ticku MK, Zakhari S. (2013). Multigenerational epigenetic effects of nicotine on lung function. Leslie FM *BMC Med*. Feb 4; 11():27.

[82] Shukla SD, Velazquez J, French SW, Lu SC, Ticku MK, Zakhari S. (2008). Emerging role of epigenetics in the actions of alcohol. *Alcohol Clin Exp Res*. 2008 Sep; 32(9):1525-34.

[83] Zakhari S. (2013). Alcohol metabolism and epigenetics changes. *Alcohol Res*. 35(1):6-16.

[84] Dabelea D, Mayer-Davis EJ, Lamichhane AP, D'Agostino RB Jr, Liese AD, Vehik KS, et al. (2008). Association of intrauterine exposure to maternal diabetes and obesity with type 2 diabetes in youth: the SEARCH Case-Control Study. *Diabetes Care*. Jul; 31(7):1422-6.

[85] Smith J, Cianflone K, Biron S, Hould FS, Lebel S, Marceau S, et al. (2009). Effects of maternal surgical weight loss in mothers on intergenerational transmission of obesity. *J Clin Endocrinol Metab*. 2009 Nov; 94(11):4275-83.

[86] Waterland RA, Michels KB. (2007). Epigenetic epidemiology of the developmental origins hypothesis. *Annu Rev Nutr*. 2007;27:363–388.

[87] Biniszkiewicz D, Gribnau J, Ramsahoye B. (2002). Dnmt1 overexpression causes genomic hypermethylation, loss of imprinting, and embryonic lethality. *Mol Cell Biol*. 2002;22(April (7)):2124–2135.

[88] Radtke KM, Ruf M, Gunter HM, Dohrmann K, Schauer M, Meyer A, et al. (2011). Transgenerational impact of intimate partner violence on methylation in the promoter of the glucocorticoid receptor. *Transl Psychiatry*. Jul 19; 1():e2

[89] Zucchi FC, Yao Y, Ward ID, Ilnytskyy Y, Olson DM, Benzies K. (2013). Maternal stress induces epigenetic signatures of psychiatric and neurological diseases in the offspring. *PLoS One*. 2013; 8(2):e56967

[90] Azad MB, Konya T, Maughan H, Guttman DS, Field CJ, et al. (2013). Gut microbiota of healthy Canadian infants: profiles by mode of delivery and infant diet at 4 months. *CMAJ*. Mar 19; 185(5):385-94.

[91] Koplin J, Allen K, Gurrin L, Osborne N, Tang ML, et al. (2008). Is caesarean delivery associated with sensitization to food allergens and IgE-mediated food allergy: a systematic review. *Pediatr Allergy Immunol*. Dec; 19(8):682-7.

[92] Hyde MJ, Mostyn A, Modi N, Kemp *PR*. (2012). The health implications of birth by Caesarean section. *Biol Rev Camb Philos Soc*. Feb; 87(1):229-43.

[93] McGowan PO, Sasaki A, D'Alessio AC, Dymov S, Labonté B, Szyf M, et al. (2009). Epigenetic regulation of the glucocorticoid receptor in human brain associates with childhood abuse. *Nat Neurosci*. Mar; 12(3):342-8.

[94] Meaney MJ. (2001). Maternal care, gene expression, and the transmission of individual differences in stress reactivity across generations. *Annu Rev Neurosci*. 2001;24:1161-92.

[95] Ibid. Meaney. (2001).

[96] Plotsky PM, Meaney M. (1993). Early, postnatal experience alters hypothalamic corticotropin-releasing factor (CRF) mRNA, median eminence CRF content and stress-induced release in adult rats. *J Brain Res Mol Brain Res*. May; 18(3):195-200.

[97] Ibid. Meaney. (2001).

[98] Weaver IC, Cervoni N, Champagne FA, D'Alessio AC, Sharma S, Seckl JR, et al. (2004). Epigenetic programming by maternal behavior. *J Nat Neurosci*. 2004 Aug; 7(8):847-54.

[99] Ibid. Weaver (2004).

[100] Hoffmann A, Spengler D. (2014). DNA memories of early social life. *Neuroscience*. 2014 Apr 4; 264():64-75.

[101] Rönn T, Volkov P, Davegårdh C, Dayeh T, Hall E, Olsson AH, et al. (2013). A six months exercise intervention influences the genome-wide DNA methylation pattern in human adipose tissue. *PLoS Genet*. 2013 Jun; 9(6).

[102] Sanchis-Gomar F, Garcia-Gimenez JL, Perez-Quilis C, Gomez-Cabrera MC, Pallardo FV, Lippi G. (2012). Physical exercise . an epigenetic modulator: Eustress, the "positive stress" as an effector of gene expression. *J Strength Cond Res*. Dec; 26(12):3469-72.

[103] Tari AR, Nauman J, Zisko N, Skjellegrind HK, Bosnes I, et al. (2019). Temporal changes in cardiorespiratory fitness and risk of dementia incidence and mortality: a population-based prospective cohort study. *Lancet Public Health*. Nov;4(11):e565-e574.

[104] Reynolds G. (2019). The Right Kind of Exercise May Boost Memory and Lower Dementia Risk. *New York Times*. Nov. 6, 2019.

[105] Kovacevic A, Fenesi B, Paolucci E, Heisz JJ. (2019). The effects of aerobic exercise intensity on memory in older adults. *Appl Physiol Nutr Metab*. Oct 30.

[106] Horowitz AM, Fan X, Bieri G, Smith LK, Sanchez-Diaz CI, et al. (2020). Blood factors transfer beneficial effects of exercise on neurogenesis and cognition to the aged brain. *Science*. Jul 10;369(6500);167-173.

[107] Tsankova N, Renthal W, Kumar A, Nestler EJ. (2007). Epigenetic regulation in psychiatric disorders. *Nat Rev Neurosci*. May; 8(5):355-67.

[108] Hardy TM, Tollefsbol TO. (2011). Epigenetic diet: impact on the epigenome and cancer. *Epigenomics*. Aug; 3(4):503-18.

[109] Waterland RA, Jirtle RL. (2003). Transposable elements: targets for early nutritional effects on epigenetic gene regulation. *Mol Cell Biol*. Aug; 23(15):5293-300.

[110] Carone BR, Fauquier L, Habib N, Shea JM, Hart CE, Li R. (2010). Paternally induced transgenerational environmental reprogramming of metabolic gene expression in mammals. *Cell*. 2010 Dec 23; 143(7):1084-96.

[111] Jennings BA, Willis G. (2015). How folate metabolism affects colorectal cancer development and treatment; a story of heterogeneity and pleiotropy. *Cancer Lett*. Jan 28; 356(2 Pt A):224-30.

[112] Gage, F. (1998). Neurogenesis of hippocampus. *Nat Med*. 4, 1313-1317

[113] Thangthaeng N, Poulose SM, Gomes SM, Miller MG, Bielinski DF. (2016). Tart cherry supplementation improves working memory, hippocampal inflammation, and autophagy in aged rats. *Age* (Dordr). Dec; 38(5-6):393-404.

[114] Holtzman DM, Mobley WC. (1994). Neurotrophic Factors and neurologic disease. *West J Med*. Sep; 161(3): 246–254.

[115] Blais M, Levesque P, Bellenfant S, Berthod F. (2013). Nerve growth factor, brain-derived neurotrophic factor, neurotrophin-3 and glial-derived neurotropic factor enhance angiogenesis in a tissue-engineered in vitro model. *Tissue Eng Part A*. Aug;19(15-16):1655-64.

[116] Kuhn HG, Dickinson-Anson H, Gage FH. (1996). Neurogenesis in the detate gyrus of the adult rat: age-related decrease of neuronal progenitor proliferation. *J Neurosci*. Mar 15; 16(6):2027-33.

[117] Hattiangady B, Shetty AK. (2008). Aging does not alter the number or phenotype of putative stem/progenitor cells in the neurogenic region of the hippocampus. *Neurobiol Aging*. Jan; 29(1):129-47.

[118] Li G, Fang L, Fernandez G, Pleasure SJ. (2013). The ventral hippocampus is the embryonic origin for adult stem cells in the dentate gyrus. *Neuron*. May 22;78(4):658-72.

[119] Yuan TF, Paes F, Arias-Carrion O, Ferreira Rocha NB, de Sa Filho AS, et al. (2015). Neural Mechanisms of Exercise: Anti-Depression, Neurogenesis, and Serotonin Signaling. *CNS Neurol Disord Drug Targets*. 2015;14(10):1307-11.

[120] Yao B, Christian KM, He C, Jin P, Ming GL, et al. (2016). Epigenetic mechanisms in neurogenesis. *Nat Rev Neurosci*. Sep;17(9):537-49.

[121] Jain KK. (2018). Neurotrophic factors. Retrieved Aug 2 2019 from http://www.medlink.com/article/neurotrophic_factors.

[122] Razavi S, Nazem G, Mardani M, Esfandiari E, Salehi, et al. (2015). Neurotrophic factors and their effects in the treatment of multiple sclerosis. *Adv Biomed Res*. 2015; 4:53.

[123] Vega JA, García-Suárez O, Hannestad J, Pérez-Pérez M, Germanà A. (2003). Neurotrophins and the immune system. *J Anat*. Jul; 203(1):1-19.

[124] Götz R, Köster R, Winkler C, Raulf F, Lottspeich F, et al. (1994). Neurotrophin-6 is a new member of the nerve growth factor family. *Nature*. Nov 17; 372(6503):266-9.

[125] Kerschensteiner M, Stadelmann C, Dechant G, Wekerle H, Hohlfeld R. (2003). Neurotrophic cross-talk between the nervous and immune systems: implications for neurological diseases. *Ann Neurol*. Mar; 53(3):292-304.

[126] Saarma M. (2000). GDNF - a stranger in the TGF-beta superfamily? *Eur J Biochem*. Dec; 267(24):6968-71.

[127] Stolp HB. (2013). Neuropoietic cytokines in normal brain development and neurodevelopmental disorders. *Mol Cell Neurosci*. Mar; 53():63-8.

[128] Li Y, Luikart BW, Birnbaum S, Chen J, Kwon CH, et al. (2008). TrkB regulates hippocampal neurogenesis and governs sensitivity to antidepressive treatment. *Neuron*. Aug 14; 59(3):399-412.

[129] Palmer TD, Takahashi J, Gage FH. (1997). The adult rat hippocampus contains primordial neural stem cells. *Mol Cell Neurosci*. 1997; 8(6):389-404.

[130] Huang EJ, Reichardt LF. (2001). Neurotrophins: roles in neuronal development and function *Annu Rev Neurosci*. 2001; 24():677-736.

[131] Jones KR, Fariñas I, Backus C, Reichardt LF. (1994). Targeted disruption of the BDNF gene perturbs brain and sensory neuron development but not motor neuron development. *Cell*. Mar 25; 76(6):989-99.

[132] Schwartz PM, Borghesani PR, Levy RL, Pomeroy SL, Segal RA. (1997). Abnormal cerebellar development and foliation in BDNF-/- mice reveals a role for neurotrophins in CNS patterning. *Neuron*. Aug; 19(2):269-81.

[133] Lindsay RM. (1988). Nerve growth factors (NGF, BDNF) enhance axonal regeneration but are not required for survival of adult sensory neurons. *J Neurosci*. Jul; 8(7):2394-405.

[134] Muramatsu R, Yamashita T. (2014). Concept and molecular basis of axonal regeneration after central nervous system injury. *Neurosci Res*. 2014 Jan; 78():45-9.

[135] Ichim G, Tauszig-Delamasure S, Mehlen P. (2012). Neurotrophins and cell death. *Exp Cell Res*. Jul 1; 318(11):1221-8.

[136] Gould E, Beylin A, Tanapat P, Reeves A, Shors T. (1999). Learning enhances adult neurogenesis in the hippocampal formation. *J Nat Neurosci*. Mar; 2(3):260-5.

[137] Young D, Lawlor PA, Leone P, Dragunow M, During MJ. (1999). Environmental enrichment inhibits spontaneous apoptosis, prevents seizures and is neuroprotective. *Nat Med*. Apr; 5(4):448-53.

[138] Wibrand K, Berge K, Messaoudi M, Duffaud A, Panja D, et al. (2013). Enhanced cognitive function and antidepressant-like effects after krill oil supplementation in rats. *Lipids Health Dis*. Jan 25; 12:6.

[139] Wu W, Wang X, Xiang Q, Meng X, Peng Y, et al. (2014). Astaxanthin alleviates brain aging in rats by attenuating oxidative stress and increasing BDNF levels. *Food Funct*. 2014;5:158–166.

[140] Nagahara AH, Tuszynski MH. (2011). Potential therapeutic uses of BDNF in neurological and psychiatric disorders. *Nat Rev Drug Discov*. Mar; 10(3):209-19.

[141] Moltenia R, Barnarda RJ, Yinga Z, Roberts CK, Gomez-Pinilla F. (2002). A high-fat, refined sugar diet reduces hippocampal brain-derived neurotrophic factor, neuronal plasticity, and learning. *Neuroscience*. 2002;112(4):803-14.

[142] Jovanovic JN, Czernik AJ, Fienberg AA, Greengard P, Sihra TS. (2000). Synapsins as mediators of BDNF-enhanced neurotransmitter release. *Nat. Neurosci*. 3:323–329.

[143] Mei F, Nagappan G, Ke Y, Sacktor TC, Lu B. (2001). BDNF facilitates L-LTP maintenance in the absence of protein synthesis through PKMζ. *PLoS One*. 2011; 6(6):e21568.

[144] Abidin I, Köhler T, Weiler E, Zoidl G, Eysel UT, et al. (2006). Reduced presynaptic efficiency of excitatory synaptic transmission impairs LTP in the visual cortex of BDNF-heterozygous mice. *Eur J Neurosci*. Dec; 24(12):3519-31.

[145] Soliman F, Glatt CE, Bath KG, Levita L, Jones RM, et al. (2010). A genetic variant BDNF polymorphism alters extinction learning in both mouse and human. *Science*. 12; 327(5967):863-6.

[146] Park H Poo, MM. (2013). Neurotrophin regulation of neural circuit development and function. *Nat. Rev. Neurosci*. 14, 7-23.

[147] Stranahan AM, Mattson MP. (2012). Recruiting adaptive cellular stress responses for successful brain ageing. *Nat Rev Neurosci*. Jan 18; 13(3):209-16.

[148] Ibid. Wu. (2014). *Food Funct*.

[149] Binder DK, Scharfman HE. (2004). Brain-derived neurotrophic factor. *Growth Factors*. 2004 Sep; 22(3):123-31.

[150] Acheson A, Conover JC, Fandl JP, DeChiara TM, Russell M, et al. (1995). A BDNF autocrine loop in adult sensory neurons prevents cell death. *Nature*. Mar 30; 374(6521):450-3.

[151] Maisonpierre PC, Le Beau MM, Espinosa R 3rd, Ip NY, Belluscio L, et al. (1991). Human and rat brain-derived neurotrophic factor and neurotrophin-3: gene structures, distributions, and chromosomal localizations. *Genomics*. Jul; 10(3):558-68.

[152] Shen Q, Goderie SK, Jin L, Karanth N, Sun Y, et al. (2004). Endothelial cells stimulate self-renewal and expand neurogenesis of neural stem cells. *Science*. May 28; 304(5675):1338-40.

[153] Heese K, Low JW, Inoue N. (2007). Nerve growth factor, neural stem cells and Alzheimer's disease. *Neurosignals*. 2006-2007; 15(1):1-12.

[154] De Munter JP, Melamed E, Wolters E. (2014). Stem cell grafting in parkinsonism--why, how, and when. *Parkinsonism Relat Disord*. Jan; 20 Suppl 1():S150-3.

[155] Rosser A, Svendsen CN. (2014). Stem cells for cell replacement therapy: a therapeutic strategy for HD? *Mov Disord*. Sep 15; 29(11):1446-54.

[156] De Miranda AS, Zhang CJ, Katsumoto A, Teixeira A. (2017). Hippocampal adult neurogenesis: Does the immune system matter? *J Neurol Sci*. Jan 15;372:482-495.

[157] Sierra A, Encinas JM, Deudero JJ, Chancey JH, Enikolopov G, et al. (2010). Microglia shape adult hippocampal neurogenesis through apoptosis-coupled phagocytosis. *Cell Stem Cell*. Oct 8; 7(4):483-95.

[158] Nimmerjahn A, Kirchhoff F, Helmchen F. (2005). Resting microglial cells are highly dynamic survelliants of brain parenchyma in vivo. *Science*. May 27; 308(5726):1314-8.

[159] Morrens J, Van Den Broeck W, Kempermann G. (2012). Glial cells in adult neurogenesis. *Glia*. Feb;60(2):159-74.

[160] Barkho BZ, Song H, Aimone JB, Smrt RD, Kuwabara T, et al. (2006). Identification of astrocyte-expressed factors that modulate neural stem/progenitor cell differentiation. *Stem Cells Dev*. Jun; 15(3):407-21.

[161] Song H, Stevens CF, Gage FH. (2002). Astroglia induce neurogenesis from adult neural stem cells. *Nature*. May 2; 417(6884):39-44.

[162] Barkho BZ, Song H, Aimone JB, Smrt RD, Kuwabara T, et al. (2006). Identification of astrocyte-expressed factors that modulate neural stem/progenitor cell differentiation. *Stem Cells Dev*. Jun; 15(3):407-21.

[163] Ventura R, Harris KM. (1999). Three-dimensional relationships between hippocampal synapses and astrocytes *J Neurosci*. Aug 15; 19(16):6897-906.

[164] Ashton RS, Conway A, Pangarkar C, Bergen J, Lim KI, et al. (2012). Astrocytes regulate adult hippocampal neurogenesis through ephrin-B signaling. *Nat Neurosci*. Oct; 15(10):1399-406.

[165] Oh J, McCloskey MA, Blong CC, Bendickson L, Nilsen-Hamilton M, et al. (2010). Astrocyte-derived interleukin-6 promotes specific neuronal differentiation of neural progenitor cells from adult hippocampus. *J Neurosci Res*. Oct; 88(13):2798-809.

[166] Palmer TD, Willhoite AR, Gage FH. (2000). Vascular niche for adult hippocampal neurogenesis. *J Comp Neurol*. Oct 2; 425(4):479-94.

[167] Shen Q, Wang Y, Kokovay E, Lin G, Chuang SM, et al. (2008). Adult SVZ stem cells lie in a vascular niche: a quantitative analysis of niche cell-cell interactions. *Cell Stem Cell*. Sep 11; 3(3):289-300.

[168] Gu Y, Janoschka S, Ge S. (2013). Neurogenesis and hippocampal plasticity in adult brain. *Curr Top Behav Neurosci*. 2013;15:31-48.

[169] Bernstein R. (2016). The Mind and Mental Health: How Stress Affects the Brain. Retrieved Jul 10 2019 from https://www.tuw.edu/content/health/how-stress-affects-the-brain/.

[170] Akiyama H, Barger S, Barnum S, Bradt B, Bauer J, et al. (2000). Inflammation and Alzheimer's disease. *Neurobiol Aging*. May-Jun; 21(3):383-421.

[171] Rogers J, Mastroeni D, Leonard B, Joyce J, Grover A. (2007). Neuroinflammation in Alzheimer's disease and Parkinson's disease: are microglia pathogenic in either disorder? *Int Rev Neurobiol*. 2007; 82():235-46.

[172] Landreth GE, Reed-Geaghan EG. (2009). Toll-like receptors in Alzheimer's disease. *Curr Top Microbiol Immunol*. 2009;336():137-53.

[173] Zonis S, Pechnick RN, Ljubimov VA, Mahgereftreh M, Wawrowsky K, et al. (2015). Chronic intestinal inflammation alters hippocampal neurogenesis. *J Neuroinflammation*. Apr 3;12:65.

[174] López-Otín C, Blasco MA, Partridge L, Serrano M, Kroemer G. (2013). The hallmarks of aging. *Cell*. Jun 6; 153(6):1194-217.

[175] Widomska J, Subczynski WK. (2014). Why has Nature Chosen Lutein and Zeaxanthin to Protect the Retina? *J Clin Exp Ophthalmol*. 2014 Feb 21; 5(1):326.

[176] Sarahian N, Sahraei H, Zardooz H, Alibeik H, Sadeghi B. (2014). Effect of memantine administration within the nucleus accumbens on changes in weight and volume of the brain and adrenal gland during chronic stress in female mice. *J Med Sci: Pathobiology*. 2014;17:71–82.

[177] Sapolsky, R.m., Uno, H., Rebert, C.S., and Finch, C.E. (1990). Hippocampal damage associated with prolonged glucocorticoid exposure in primates. *J Neuroci*. 10(9):2897-290.

[178] Bremmer JD. (1999). Does stress damage the brain? *Biol Psychiatry*. Apr 1;45(7):797-805.

[179] Gurvits TV, Shenton ME, Hokama H, Ohta H, Lasko NB, et al. (1996). Magnetic resonance imaging study of hippocampal volume in chronic combat-related posttraumatic stress disorder. *Biol Psychiatry*. Dec 1;40(11):1091-9.

[180] Gurvits TV, Lasko NB, Schachter SC, Kuhne AA, Orr SP, et al. (1993). Neurological status of Vietnam veterans with chronic posttraumatic stress disorder. *J Neuropsychiatry Clin Neurosci*. Spring;5(2):183-188.

[181] Sapolsky R. (1999). Stress and your shrinking brain. *Discover*. 20(3):113-122.

[182] Sun D. (2014). The potential of endogenous neurogenesis for brain repair and regeneration following traumatic brain injury. *Neural Regen Res*. Apr 1; 9(7): 688–692.

[183] Zheng W, ZhuGe Q, Zhong M, Chen G, Shao B, et al. (2013). Neurogenesis in adult human brain after traumatic brain injury. *J Neurotrauma.* Nov 15;30(22):1872-80.

[184] Hotting K, Roder B. (2013). Beneficial effects of physical exercise on neuroplasticity and cognition. *Neurosci Biobehav Rev.* Apr;37(9).

[185] Ma CL, Ma XT, Wang JJ, Liu H, Chen YF, et al. (2017). Physical exercise induces hippocampal neurogenesis and prevents cognitive decline. *Behav Brain Res.* Jan 15;317:332-339.

[186] Kempermann G, Gage FH. (1999). Running increases cell proliferation and neurogenesis in the adult mouse dentate gyrus. van Praag H, *Nat Neurosci.* Mar; 2(3):266-70.

[187] Mustroph ML, Chen S, Desai SC, Cay EB, DeYoung EK, Rhodes JS *Neuroscience.* 2012 Sep 6; 219():62-71.

[188] Pereira AC, Huddleston DE, Brickman AM, Sosunov AA, Hen R, et al. (2007). An in vivo correlate of exercise-induced neurogenesis in the adult dentate gyrus. *Proc Natl Acad Sci U S A.* Mar 27; 104(13):5638-43.

[189] Yoon MC, Shin MS, Kim TS, Kim BK, Ko IG, et al. (2007). Treadmill exercise suppresses nigrostriatal dopaminergic neuronal loss in 6-hydroxydopamine-induced Parkinson's rats. *Neurosci Lett.* Aug 9;423(1):12-7.

[190] Gold SM, Schultz KH, Hartmann S, Mladek M, Lang UE, et al. (2003). Basal serum levels and reactivity of nerve growth factor and brain-derived neurotrophic factor to standardized acute exercise in multiple sclerosis and controls. *J Neuroimmunol.* May;138:99–105.

[191] Kobilo T, Liu QR, Gandhi K, Mughal M, Shaham Y, et al. (2011). Running is the neurogenic and neurotrophic stimulus in environmental enrichment. *Learn Mem.* Aug 30;18(9):605-9.

[192] Schmolesky MT, Webb DL, Hansen RA. (2013). The Effects of Aerobic Exercise Intensity and Duration of Levels of Brain-Derived Neurotrophic Factor in Healthy Men. *J Sports Sci Med.* Sep;12(3):502-511.

[193] Griffin EW, Mullally S, Foley C, Warmington SA, O'Mara SM, et al. (2011). Aerobic exercise improves hippocampal function and BDNF in the serum of young adult males. *Physiol Behav.* Oct 24;104(5):934-41.

[194] Whiteman AS, Young DE, He X, Chen TC, Wagenaar RC, et al. (2014). Interaction between serum BDNF and aerobic fitness predicts recognition memory in healthy young adults. *Behav Brain Res.* Feb 1;259:302-12.

[195] Winter B, Breitenstein C, Mooren FC, Voelker K, Fobker M, et al. (2007). High impact running improves learning. *Neurobiol Learn Mem.* May;87(4):597-609.

[196] Tsai CL, Chen FC, Pan CY, Wang CH, Huang TH, et al. (2014). Impact of acute aerobic exercise and cardiorespiratory fitness on visuospatial performance and serum BDNF levels. *Psychoneoruendocrinology.* 41:121-131.

[197] Van Praag H, Christie BR, Sejnowski TJ, Gage FH. (1999). Running enhances neurogenesis, learning, and long-term potentiation in mice. *Proc. Natl. Acad. Sci. U. S. A.* 96:13427–13431.

[198] Khatri P, Blumenthal JA, Babyak MA, Craighead WE, Herman S, et al. (2001). Effects of exercise training on cognitive functioning among depressed older men and women. *J Aging Phys Act.* 9:43–57.

[199] Saraulli D, Costanzi M, Mastrorilli V, Farioli-Vecchioli S. (2017). The Long Run: Neuroprotective Effects of Physical Exercise on Adult Neurogenesis from Youth to Old Age. *Curr Neuropharmacol.* 15(4):519-533.

[200] Van Praag H, Lucero MJ, Yeo GW, Stecker K, Heivand N, et al. (2007). Plant-derived flavanol (–) epicatechin enhances angiogenesis and retention of spatial memory in mice. *J Neurosci.* May 30;27:5869–5878.

[201] Loprinzi PD, Ponce P, Zou L, Li H. (2019). The Counteracting Effects of Exercise on High-Fat Diet-Induced Memory Impairment: A Systematic Review. *Brain Sci.* Jun 20;9(6):E145.

[202] Han TK, Leem YH, Kim HS. (2019). Treadmill exercise restores high fat diet-induced disturbance of hippocampal neurogenesis through B2-adrenergic receptor-dependent induction of thioredoxin-1 and brain-derived neurotrophic factor. *Brain Res.* Mar 15;1707:154-163.

[203] Wu A, Ying Z, Gomez-Pinilla F. (2008). Docosahexaenoic acid dietary supplementation enhances the effects of exercise on synaptic plasticity and cognition. *Neuroscience.* Aug 26; 155(3):751-9.

[204] Vaynman S, Ying Z, Gomez-Pinilla F. (2004). Hippocampal BDNF mediates the efficacy of exercise on synaptic plasticity and cognition. *Eur J Neurosci.* Nov; 20(10):2580-90.

[205] Ibid. Gould. (1999). *J Nat Neurosci.*

[206] Ibid. Gould. (1999).

[207] Sisti HM, Glass AL, Shors TJ. (2007). Neurogenesis and the spacing effect: Learning over time enhances memory and the survival of new neurons. *Learn Mem.* 14:368-375.

[208] Poulose SM, Miller MG, Scott T, Shukitt-Hale B. (2017). Nutritional Factors Affecting Adult Neurogenesis and Cognitive Function. *Adv Nutr.* Nov 15;8(6):804-811.

[209] Fidaleo M, Cavallucci V, Pani G. (2017). Nutrients, neurogenesis and brain aging: From disease mechanisms to therapeutic opportunities. *Biochem Pharmacol.* Oct 1;141:63-76.

[210] Molteni R, Barnard RJ, Ying Z, Roberts CK, Gómez-Pinilla F. (2002). A high-fat, refined sugar diet reduces hippocampal brain-derived neurotrophic factor, neuronal plasticity, and learning. *Neuroscience.* 2002; 112(4):803-14.

[211] Tsai YC, Lin YC, Huang CC, Villaflores OB, Wu TY, et al. (2019). Hericium erinaceus Mycelium and Its Isolated Compound Erinacine A, Ameliorate High-Fat High-Sucrose Diet-Induced Metabolic Dysfunction and Spatial Learning Deficits in Aging Mice. *J Med Food.* May;22(5):469-478.

[212] Nam SM, Kim JW, Kwon HJ, Yoo DY, Jung HY, et al. (2017). Differential Effects of Low- and High-dose Zinc Supplementation on Synaptic Plasticity and Neurogenesis in the Hippocampus of Control and High-fat Diet-fed Mice. *Neurochem Res.* Nov;42(11):3149-3159.

[213] Brandhorst S, Choi IY, Wei M, Cheng CW, Sedrakyan S, et al. (2015). A Periodic Diet that Mimics Fasting Promotes Multi-system Regeneration, Enhanced Cognitive Performance, and Healthspan. *Cell Metab.* Jul 7;22(1):86-99.

[214] Yook JS, Rakwal R, Shibato J, Takahashi K, Koizumi H, et al. (2019). Leptin in hippocampus mediates benefits of mild exercise by an antioxidant on neurogenesis and memory. *Pro Natl Acad Sci U S A.* May 28;116(22):10966-10993.

[215] Bensalem J, Dudonne S, Gaudout D, Servant L, Calon F, et al. (2018). Polyphenol-rich extract from grape and blueberry attenuates cognitive decline and improves neuronal function in aged mice. *J Nutr Sci.* May 21;7:e19.

[216] Shukitt-Hale B, Bielinski DF, Lau FC, Willis LM, Carey AN, et al. (2015). The beneficial effects of berries on cognition, motor behavior and neuronal function in aging. *Br J Nutr.* Nov 28:114(10):1542-9.

[217] Devore EE, Kangs JH, Breteler MM, Grodstein FA. (2012). Dietary intakes of berries and flavonoids in relation to cognitive decline. *Neurology.* 72(1):135-43.

[218] Joseph JA, Shukitt-Hale B, Willis LM. (2009). Grape juice, berries, and walnuts affect brain aging and behavior. *J Med.* 139(9):1813S-7S.

[219] Tiwari SK, Agarwal S, Seth B, Yadav A, Nair S, et al. (2014). Curcumin-loaded nanoparticles potently induce adult neurogenesis and reverse cognitive deficits in Alzheimer's disease model via canonical Wnt/B-catenin pathway. *ACS Nano.* Jan 28;8(1):76-103.

[220] Ibid. Poulose. (2017). *Adv Nutr.*

[221] Shehzad A, Rehman G, Lee YS (2013). Curcumin in inflammatory diseases. *Biofactors.* Jan-Feb; 39(1):69-77.

[222] Kim GY, Kim KH, Lee SH, Yoon MS, Lee HJ, et al. (2005). Curcumin inhibits immunostimulatory function of dendritic cells: MAPKs and translocation of NF-kappa B as potential targets. *J Immunol.* Jun 15; 174(12):8116-24.

[223] Cheng J, Zhou ZW, Sheng HP, He LJ, Fan XW, et al. (2014). An evidence-based update on the pharmacological activities and possible molecular targets of Lycium barbarum polysaccharides. *Drug Des Devel Ther.* Dec 17;9:33-78.

[224] Po KK, Leung JW, Chan JN, Fung TK, Sanchez-Vidana DI, et al. (2017). Protective effect of Lycium Barbarum polysaccharides on dextromethorphan-induced mood impairment and neurogenesis suppression. *Brain Res Bull.* Sep;134:10-17.

[225] Ibid. Poulose. (2017).

[226] Calon F, Cole G. (2007). Neuroprotective action of omega-3 polyunsaturated fatty acids against neurodegenerative diseases: evidence from animal studies. *Prostaglandins Leukot Essent Fatty Acids.* Nov-Dec; 77(5-6):287-93.

[227] Ibid. Calon. (2007).

[228] Bousquet M, Calon F, Cicchetti F. (2011). Impact of ω-3 fatty acids in Parkinson's disease. *Ageing Res Rev.* Sep; 10(4):453-63.

[229] Ibid. Wysoczanski. (2016).

[230] Rathod R, Kale A, Joshi S. (2016). Novel insights into the effect of vitamin B12 and omega-3 fatty acids on brain function. *J Biomed Sci.* Jan 25;23:17.

[231] Alzheimer's Association. (2019). 2019 Alzheimer's disease facts and figures. Retrieved Aug 21 2019 from https://www.alz.org/media/Documents/alzheimers-facts-and-figures-2019-r.pdf.

[232] Ibid. Alzheimer's Association. (2019).

[233] Hong CH, Falvey C, Harris TB, Simonsick EM, Satterfield S, et al. (2013). Anemia and risk of dementia in older adults: findings from the Health ABC study. *Neurology.* Aug 6;81(6): 528-33.

[234] Biessels GJ, Staekenborg S, Brunner E, Brayne C, Scheltens P. (2006). Risk of dementia in diabetes mellitus: a system review. *Lancet Neurol.* Jan;5(1)64-74.

[235] Péneau S, Galan P, Jeandel C, Ferry M, Andreeva V, et al. (2011). Fruit and vegetable intake and cognitive function in the SU.VI.MAX 2 prospective study. *Am J Clin Nutr.* Nov; 94(5):1295-303.

[236] Ibid. Peneau. (2011).

[237] Mohajeri MH, Leuba G. (2009). Prevention of age-associated dementia. *Brain Res Bull.* Oct 28; 80(4-5):315-25

[238] Mohajeri MH, Troesch B, Weber P. (2015). Inadequate supply of vitamins and DHA in the elderly: implications for brain aging and Alzheimer-type dementia. *Nutrition.* Feb; 31(2):261-75

[239] Poulose SM, Miller MG, Scott T, Shukitt-Hale B. (2017). Nutritional Factors Affecting Adult Neurogenesis and Cognitive Function. *Adv Nutr.* Nov 15;8(6):804-811.

[240] Fidaleo M, Cavallucci V, Pani G. (2017). Nutrients, neurogenesis and brain aging: From disease mechanisms to therapeutic opportunities. *Biochem Pharmacol.* Oct 1;141:63-76.

[241] Loprinzi PD, Ponce P, Zou L, Li H. (2019). The Counteracting Effects of Exercise on High-Fat Diet-Induced Memory Impairment: A Systematic Review. *Brain Sci.* Jun 20:9(6):E145.

[242] Han TK, Leem YH, Kim HS. (2019). Treadmill exercise restores high fat diet-induced disturbance of hippocampal neurogenesis through B2-adrenergic receptor-dependent induction of thioredoxin-1 and .... *Brain Res.* Mar 15;1707:154-163.

[243] Kavoacevic A, Fenesi B, Paolucci E, Heisz JJ. (2019). The effects of aerobic exercise intensity on memory in older adults. *Appl Physiol Nutr Metab.* Oct 30.

[244] Haass C, Selkoe DJ. (2007). Soluble protein oligomers in neurodegeneration: lessons from the Alzheimer's amyloid beta-peptide. *Nat Rev Mol Cell Biol.* Feb; 8(2):101-12.

[245] Tanzi RE, Bertram L. (2005). Twenty years of the Alzheimer's disease amyloid hypothesis: a genetic perspective. *Cell.* Feb 25; 120(4):545-55.

[246] Kivipelto M, Ngandu T, Fratiglioni L, Viitanen M, Kåreholt I, et al. (2005). Obesity and vascular risk factors at midlife and the risk of dementia and Alzheimer disease. *Arch Neurol.* Oct; 62(10):1556-60.

[247] Whitmer RA, Sidney S, Selby J, Johnston SC, Yaffe K. (2005). Midlife cardiovascular risk factors and risk of dementia in late life. *Neurology.* Jan 25; 64(2):277-81.

[248] Shin LM, Rauch SL, Pitman RK. (2006). Amygdala, medial prefrontal cortex, and hippocampal function in PTSD. *Ann N Y Acad Sci.* Jul;1071:67-79.

[249] Lane CA, Barnes J, Nicholas JM. (2019). Associations Between Vascular Risk Across Adulthood and Brain Pathology in Late Life: Evidence from a British Birth Cohort. *JAMA Neurol.* Nov 4;1-9.

[250] Ibid. Lane. (2019). *JAMA Neurol.*

[251] Drzezga A, Becker JA, Van Dijk KR, Sreenivasan A, Talukdar T, et al. (2011). Neuronal dysfunction and disconnection of cortical hubs in non-demented subjects with elevated amyloid burden. *Brain.* Jun; 134(Pt 6):1635-46.

[252] Richardson K, Fox C, Maidment I, Steel N, Loke YK, et al. (2018). Anticholinergic drugs and risk of dementia: case-control study. *BMJ.* Apr 25;361:k1315.

[253] Greenwood CE, Winocur G. (2005). High-fat diets, insulin resistance and declining cognitive function. *Neurobiol Aging.* Dec; 26 Suppl 1():42-5

[254] Wu L, Sun D, He Y. (2017). Coffee intake and the incident risk of cognitive disorders: A dose-response meta-analysis of nine prospective cohort studies. *Clin Nutr.* 2017;36(3):730-6.

[255] Vaynman S, Ying Z, Wu A, Gomez-Pinilla F. (2006). Coupling energy metabolism with a mechanism to support brain-derived neurotrophic factor-mediated synaptic plasticity. *Neuroscience.* 139(4):1221-34.

[256] Wu A, Ying Z, Gomez-Pinilla F. (2004). The interplay between oxidative stress and brain-derived neurotrophic factor modulates the outcome of a saturated fat diet on synaptic plasticity and cognition. *Eur J Neurosci.* 19:1699–1707.

[257] Mattson MP. (2005). Energy intake, meal frequency, and health: a neurobiological perspective. *Annu Rev Nutr.* 2005; 25():237-60.

[258] Scheiermann C, Kunisaki Y, Frenette PS. (2013). Circadian control of the immune system. *Nat Rev Immunol.* Mar; 13(3):190-8.

[259] Hermida RC, Ayala DE, Smolensky MH, Mojón A, Fernández JR, et al. (2013). Chronotherapy improves blood pressure control and reduces vascular risk in CKD. *Nat Rev Nephrol.* Jun; 9(6):358-68.

[260] Levi F, Schibler U. (2007). Circadian rhythms: mechanisms and therapeutic implications. *Annu Rev Pharmacol Toxicol.* 2007;47():593-628.

[261] Sahar S, Sassone-Corsi P. (2009). Metabolism and cancer: the circadian clock connection. *Nat Rev Cancer.* Dec; 9(12):886-96.

[262] Coogan AN, Schutová B, Husung S, Furczyk K, Baune BT, et al. (2013). The circadian system in Alzheimer's disease: disturbances, mechanisms, and opportunities. *J Biol Psychiatry.* Sep 1; 74(5):333-9.

[263] Ibid. Coogan. (2013).

[264] Lupien SJ, McEwen BS, Gunnar MR, Heim C. (2009). Effects of stress throughout the lifespan on the brain, behavior and cognition *Nat Rev Neurosci.* Jun; 10(6):434-45.

[265] Lupien SJ, Lepage M. (2001). Stress, memory, and the hippocampus: can't live with it, can't live without it. Behav Brain Res. Dec 14; 127(1-2):137-58.

[266] Issa AM, Rowe W, Gauthier S, Meaney MJ. (1990). Hypothalamic-pituitary-adrenal activity in aged, cognitively impaired and cognitively unimpaired rats. *J Neurosci.* Oct; 10(10):3247-54.

[267] Gould E, Tanapat P. (1999). Stress and hippocampal neurogenesis. *Biol Psychiatry.* Dec 1; 46(11):1472-9

[268] Köhler S, Thomas AJ, Lloyd A, Barber R, Almeida OP, et al. (2010). White matter hyperintensities, cortisol levels, brain atrophy and continuing cognitive deficits in late-life depression. Br *J Psychiatry.* Feb; 196(2):143-9.

[269] Squire, L.R, Schacter DL. (2002). *The Neuropsychology of Memory*. Guilford Press.

[270] Borcel E, Pérez-Alvarez L, Herrero AI, Brionne T, Varea E, et al. (2008). Chronic stress in adulthood followed by intermittent stress impairs spatial memory and the survival of newborn hippocampal cells in aging animals: prevention by FGL, a peptide mimetic of neural cell adhesion molecule. *Behav Pharmacol*. Feb; 19(1):41-9.

[271] Wang C, Wang W, Dong H, Hou P, et al. (2008). Chronic mild stress impairs cognition in mice: from brain homeostasis to behavior. *Life Sci*. Apr 23; 82(17-18):934-42.

[272] Van der Kooij MA, Fantin M, Rejmak E, Grosse J, Zanoletti O, et al. (2014). Role for MMP-9 in stress-induced downregulation of nectin-3 in hippocampal CA1 and associated behavioural alterations. *Nat Comm*. 2014; 5: 4995.

[273] Branan N. (2007). Stress Kills Brain Cells Off. *Sci Am*. Jun-Jul.

[274] Kang HJ, Voleti B, Hajszan T, Rajkowska G, Stockmeier CA, et al. (2012). Decreased expression of synapse-related genes and loss of synapses in major depressive disorder. *Nat Med*. Sep;18(9):1413-7.

[275] Sanders R. (2014). New evidence that chronic stress predisposes brain to mental illness. Retrieved Sep 10 2019 from https://news.berkeley.edu/2014/02/11/chronic-stress-predisposes-brain-to-mental-illness/.

[276] Chetty S, Friedman AR, Taravosh-Lahn K, Kirby ED, Mirescu C, et al. (2014). Stress and glucocorticoids promote oligodendrogenesis in the adult hippocampus. *Mol Psychiatry*. Dec;19:1275–1283.

[277] Bergland C. (2014). Chronic Stress Can Damage Brain Structure and Connectivity. *Psy Today*. Feb 12, 2014.

[278] Song L, Che W, Min-Wei W, Murakami Y, Matsumoto K. (2006). Impairment of the spatial learning and memory induced by learned helplessness and chronic mild stress *Pharmacol Biochem Behav*. Feb; 83(2):186-93.

[279] López-Otín C, Blasco MA, Partridge L, Serrano M, Kroemer G. (2013). The hallmarks of aging. *Cell*. Jun 6; 153(6):1194-217.

[280] Rao AV, Balachandran B. (2002). Role of oxidative stress and antioxidants in neurodegenerative diseases. *Nutr Neurosci*. Oct; 5(5):291-309.

[281] Kayali R, Cakatay U, Akçay T, Altuğ T. (2006). Effect of alpha-lipoic acid supplementation on markers of protein oxidation in post-mitotic tissues of aging rat. *Cell Biochem Funct*. Jan-Feb; 24(1):79-85.

[282] La Fata G, Weber P, Mohajeri MH. (2014). Effects of Vitamin E on Cognitive Performance during Ageing and in Alzheimer's Disease. *Nutrients*. Dec; 6(12): 5453–5472.

[283] Trushina E, McMurray CT. (2007). Oxidative stress and mitochondrial dysfunction in neurodegenerative diseases. *Neuroscience*. Apr 14; 145(4):1233-48.

[284] Bennett IJ, Madden D. (2014). Disconnected aging: cerebral white matter integrity and age-related differences in cognition. *J Neuroscience*. Sep 12; 276():187-205.

[285] Miller E, Morel A, Saso L, Saluk. (2014). Isoprostanes and neuroprostanes as biomarkers of oxidative stress in neurodegenerative diseases. *J Oxid Med Cell Longev*. 2014:572491

[286] Ibid. Miller. (2014).

[287] Hernández-Avila M, Smith D, Meneses F, Sanin LH, Hu H. (1998). The influence of bone and blood lead on plasma lead levels in environmentally exposed adults. *Environ Health Perspect*. Aug; 106(8):473-7.

[288] Grosse SD, Matte TD, Schwartz J, Jackson RJ. (2002). Economic gains resulting from the reduction in children's exposure to lead in the United States. *Environ Health Perspect*. Jun; 110(6):563-9.

[289] Fewtrell LJ, Prüss-Ustün A, Landrigan P, Ayuso-Mateos JL. (2004). Estimating the global burden of disease of mild mental retardation and cardiovascular diseases from environmental lead exposure. Environ Res. Feb; 94(2):120-33.

[290] Wright RO, Tsaih SW, Schwartz J, Spiro A 3rd, McDonald K, et al. (2003). Lead exposure biomarkers and mini-mental status exam scores in older men. *Epidemiology*. Nov; 14(6):713-8.

[291] Weisskopf MG, Wright RO, Schwartz J, Spiro A 3rd, Sparrow D, et al. (2004). Cumulative lead exposure and prospective change in cognition among elderly men: the VA Normative Aging Study. *Am J Epidemiol*. Dec 15; 160(12):1184-93.

[292] Payton M, Riggs KM, Spiro A 3rd, Weiss ST, Hu H. (1998). Relations of bone and blood lead to cognitive function: the VA Normative Aging Study *Neurotoxicol Teratol*. Jan-Feb; 20(1):19-27.

[293] Dobbs MR. *Clinical Neurotoxicology*: Syndromes, Substances, Environments. Saunders; 2009

[294] Schwartz BS, Stewart WF, Bolla KI, Simon PD, Bandeen-Roche K, et al. (2000). Past adult lead exposure is associated with longitudinal decline in cognitive function. *Neurology*. Oct 24; 55(8):1144-50.

[295] Kamel F, Umbach DM, Hu H, Munsat TL, Shefner JM, et al. (2005). Lead exposure as a risk factor for amyotrophic lateral sclerosis. *Neurodegener Dis*. 2005; 2(3-4):195-201.

[296] Kamel F, Umbach DM, Lehman TA, Park LP, Munsat TL, et al. (2003). Amyotrophic lateral sclerosis, lead, and genetic susceptibility: polymorphisms in the delta-aminolevulinic acid dehydratase and vitamin D receptor genes. *Environ Health Perspect*. Aug; 111(10):1335-9.

[297] Weisskopf MG, Weuve J, Nie H, Saint-Hilaire MH, Sudarsky L, et al. (2010). Association of cumulative lead exposure with Parkinson's disease. *Environ Health Perspect.* Nov;118(11):1609-13.

[298] Calderon-Garciduenas L, Azzarelli B, Acuna H, Garcia R, Gambling TM, Osnaya N, et al. (2002). Air pollution and brain damage. *Toxicol Pathol.* 2002 May-Jun;30(3):373-89.

[299] Calderon-Garciduenas L, Reynoso-Robles R, Vargas-Martinez J, Gomez-Maqueo-Chew A, Parez-Guille B. (2016). Prefrontal white matter pathology in air pollution exposed Mexico City young urbanites and their potential impact on neurovascular unit dysfunction and the development of Alzheimer's disease. *Environ Res.* 2016 Apr;146:404-17.

[300] Calderon-Garciduenas L, Leray F, Heydarpour P, Torres-Jardon R, Reis J. (2016). Air pollution, a rising environmental risk factor for cognition, neuroinflammation and neurodegeneration: The clinical impact on children and beyond. *Rev Neurol (Paris).* 2016 Jan;172(1):69-80.

[301] Calderon-Garciduenas L, Reynoso-Robles R, Gonzalez-Maciel A. (2019). Combustion and friction-derived nanoparticles and industrial-sourced nanoparticles: The culprit of Alzheimer and Parkinson's diseases. *Environ Res.* 2019 Jul 5;176:108574.

[302] Bessis A, Béchade C, Bernard D, Roumier A. (2007). Microglial control of neuronal death and synaptic properties. *Glia.* Feb; 55(3):233-8.

[303] Calderó J, Brunet N, Ciutat D, Hereu M, Esquerda JE. (2009). Development of microglia in the chick embryo spinal cord: implications in the regulation of motoneuronal survival and death. *J Neurosci Res.* Aug 15; 87(11):2447-66.

[304] NIH. What Happens to the Brain in Alzheimer's Disease. Retrieved Aug 2 2019 from https://www.nia.nih.gov/health/what-happens-brain-alzheimers-disease.

[305] Cortright B. (2015). *The Neurogenesis Diet & Lifestyle.* Psyche Media.

[306] Ibid. NIH. What Happens to the Brain in Alzheimer's Disease.

[307] Solerte SB, Cravello L, Ferrari E, Fioravanti M. (2000). Overproduction of IFN-gamma and TNF-alpha from natural killer (NK) cells is associated with abnormal NK reactivity and cognitive derangement in Alzheimer's disease. *Ann N Y Acad Sci.* 917():331-40.

[308] Marsland AL, Petersen KL, Sathanoori R, Muldoon MF, Neumann SA, et al. (2006). Interleukin-6 covaries inversely with cognitive performance among middle-aged community volunteers. *Psychosom Med.* Nov-Dec; 68(6):895-903.

[309] Li S, Wang C, Wang W, Dong H, Hou P, et al. (2008). Chronic mild stress impairs cognition in mice: from brain homeostasis to behavior. *Life Sci.* Apr 23; 82(17-18):934-42.

[310] Zhou J, Yu JT, Wang HF, Meng XF, Tan CC, et al. (2015). Association between stroke and Alzheimer's disease: systematic review and meta-analysis. J Alzheimers Dis. 2015;43(2):479-89.

[311] Launer LJ. (2002). Demonstrating the case that AD is a vascular disease: epidemiologic evidence. *Ageing Res Rev.* Feb; 1(1):61-77.

[312] Stampfer MJ. (2006). Cardiovascular disease and Alzheimer's disease: common links. J *Intern Med.* Sep; 260(3):211-23

[313] Kin T, Yamano S, Sakurai R, Kajitani M, Okahashi Y, et al. (2007). Carotid atherosclerosis is associated with brain atrophy in Japanese elders. *Gerontology.* 53(1):1-6.

[314] Karayiannis C, Moran C, Sharman JE, Beare R, Quin SJ, et al. (2019). Blood Pressure, Aortic Stiffness, Hemodynamics, and Cognition in Twin Pairs Discordant for Type 2 Diabetes. *J Alzheimers Dis.* Aug 16. [Epub ahead of print.]

[315] Den Heijer T, Launer LJ, Prins ND, van Dijk EJ, Vermeer SE, et al. (2005). Association between blood pressure, white matter lesions, and atrophy of the medial temporal lobe. *Neurology.* Jan 25; 64(2):263-7.

[316] Seshadri S, Beiser A, Selhub J, Jacques PF, Rosenberg IH, et al. (2002). Plasma homocysteine as a risk factor for dementia and Alzheimer's disease. *N Engl J Med.* Feb 14; 346(7):476-83.

[317] Tata AM, Velluto L, D'Angelo C, Reale M. (2014). Cholinergic system dysfunction and neurodegenerative diseases: cause or effect? *CNS Neurol Disord Drug Targets.* 2014;13(7):1294-303.

[318] Lee YS, Jung WM, Jan H, Kim S, Chung SY, et al. (2017). The dynamic relationship between emotional and physical states: an observational study of personal health records. *Neuropsychiatr Dis Treat.* 2017; 13: 411–419.

[319] Rocca WA, Grossardt BR, Shuster LT, Stewart EA. (2012). Hysterectomy. Oophorectomy, estrogen, and risk of dementia. *Neurodegenerative Disease* 10: 175-178.

[320] Schilling MA. (2016). Unraveling Alzheimer's: Making Sense of the Relationship between Diabetes and Alzheimer's Disease. *J Alzheimers Dis.* 2016;51(4):961-77.

[321] Tups A, Benzler J, Sergi D, Ladyman SR, Williams LM. (2017). Central Regulation of Glucose Homeostasis. *Compr Physiol.* Mar 16;7(2):741-764.

[322] Sauer A. (2018). PET Scans Show Many Being Treated for Alzheimer's May Not Have Disease. Retrieved Jun 22 2020 from https://www.alzheimers.net/pet-scans-show-many-treated-for-alzheimers/.

[323] Bergmann C, Sano M. (2006). Cardiac risk factors and potential treatments in Alzheimer's disease. *Neurol Res.* Sep; 28(6):595-604.

[324] Ratey J, Loehr JE. (2011). The positive impact of physical activity on cognition during adulthood: A review of underlying mechanisms, evidence, and recommendations. *Rev Neurosci.* 22(2):171-85.

[325] Müller S, Preische O, Sohrabi HR, Gräber S, Jucker M, et al. (2018). Relationship between physical activity, cognition, and Alzheimer pathology in autosomal dominant Alzheimer's disease. *Alzheimers Dement*. Nov;14(11):1427-1437.

[326] Head D, Bugg JM, Goate AM, Fagan AM, Mintun MA, et al. (2012). Exercise engagement as a moderator of the effect of ApoE genotype on amyloid deposition. *Arch Neurol*. May;69(5):636-43.

[327] Fox KC, Nijeboer S, Dixon ML, Floman JL, Ellamil M, et al. (2014). Is meditation associated with altered brain structure? A systematic review and meta-analysis of morphometric neuroimaging in meditation practitioners. *Neurosci Biobehav Rev*. 2014 Jun; 43:48-73.

[328] Tang YY, Tang Y, Tang R, Lewis-Peacock JA. (2017). Brief Mental Training Reorganizes Large-Scale Brain Networks. *Front Syst Neurosci*. 2017; 11:6.

[329] Baer RA. (2003). Mindfulness training as a clinical intervention: A conceptual and empirical review. *Clinical Psychology: Science & Practice*. 2003;10:125–143.

[330] Kuyken W, Byford S, Taylor RS, Watkins E, Holden E, White K, Barrett B, Byng R, Evans A, Mullan E, Teasdale JDet al. (2008). Mindfulness-based cognitive therapy to prevent relapse in recurrent depression. J *Consult Clin Psychol*. 2008 Dec; 76(6):966-78.

[331] Carlson LE, Garland SN. (2005). Impact of mindfulness-based stress reduction (MBSR) on sleep, mood, stress, and fatigue symptoms in cancer outpatients. *Int J Behav Med*. 12(4):278-85.

[332] Ong JC, Shapiro SL, Manber R. (2009). Mindfulness meditation and cognitive behavioral therapy for insomnia: a naturalistic 12-month follow-up. *Explore* (NY). Jan-Feb; 5(1):30-6.

[333] Jha AP, Krompinger J, Baime MJ. (2007). Mindfulness training modified subsystems of attention. *Cogn Affect Behav Neurosci*. Jun; 7(2):109-19.

[334] Malinowski P, Moore AW, Mead BR, Gruber T. (2017). *Mindful Aging*: The Effects of Regular Brief Mindfulness Practice on Electrophysiological Markers of Cognitive and Affective Processing in Older Adults. *Mindfulness (N Y)*. 2017; 8(1):78-94.

[335] Yang L, Zhao Y, Wang Y, Liu L, Zhang X, et al. (2015). The Effects of Psychological Stress on Depression. *Urr Neuropharmacol*. 2015;13(4):494-504.

[336] Murphy MP, LeVine H. (2010). Alzheimer's Disease and the B-Amyloid Peptide. *J Alzheimers Dis*. Jan;19(1):311.

[337] Sosa-Ortiz AL, Acosta-Castillo I, Prince M. (2012). Epidemiology of dementias and Alzheimer's disease. *J Arch Med Res*. Nov; 43(8):600-8.

[338] James BD, Leurgans SE, Hebert LE, Scherr PA, Yaffe K. (2014). Contribution of Alzheimer disease to mortality in the United States. *Neurology*. Mar 25; 82(12):1045-50.

[339] Matthews KA, Xu W, Gaglioti AH, Holt JB, Croft JB, et al. (2019). Racial and ethnic estimates of Alzheimer's disease and related dementias in the United States (2015–2060) in adults aged≥ 65 years. *Alzheimers Dement*. Jan;15(1):17-24.

[340] Alzheimer's Association. Facts and Figures. Retrieved Jun 2 2019 from https://www.alz.org/alzheimers-dementia/facts-figures.

[341] Mohajeri MH, Troesch B, Weber P. (2015). Inadequate supply of vitamins and DHA in the elderly: implications for brain aging and Alzheimer-type dementia. *Nutrition*. Feb; 31(2):261-75.

[342] Gillette-Guyonnet S, Secher M, Vellas B. (2013). Nutrition and neurodegeneration: epidemiological evidence and challenges for future research. Br *J Clin Pharmacol*. Mar; 75(3):738-55.

[343] Bredesen DE. (2015). Metabolic profiling distinguishes three subtypes of Alzheimer's disease. *Aging (Albany NY)*, Aug;7(8):595-600.

[344] Ibid. Bredesen. (2015).

[345] Su B, Wang X, Nunomura A, Moreira PI, Lee HG, et al. (2008). Oxidative stress signaling in Alzheimer's Disease. *Curr Alzheimer Res*. Dec;5(6):525-32.

[346] Bredesen D. (2017). The End of Alzheimer's: The First Program to Reverse Cognitive Decline. New York, Avery.

[347] Ibid. Bredesen. (2017).

[348] Reitz C. (2012). Alzheimer's Disease and the Amyloid Cascade Hypothesis: A Critical Review. *Int J Alzheimers Dis*, 2012:369808.

[349] Ibid. Reitz. (2012).

[350] Huang Y, Mucke L. (2012). Alzheimer mechanisms and therapeutic strategies. *Cell*. Mar 16; 148(6):1204-22.

[351] Glenner GG. (1983). Alzheimer's disease. The commonest form of amyloidosis. *Arch Pathol Lab Med*. Jun; 107(6):281-2.

[352] Masters CL, Simms G, Weinman NA, Multhaup G, McDonald BL, et al. (1985). Amyloid plaque core protein in Alzheimer disease and Down syndrome. *Proc Natl Acad Sci U S A*. Jun; 82(12):4245-9.

[353] Ballatore C, Lee VM, Trojanowski JQ. (2007). Tau-mediated neurodegeneration in Alzheimer's disease and related disorders. *Nat Rev Neurosci*. Sep; 8(9):663-72.

[354] Haass C, Selkoe D. (2007). Soluble protein oligomers in neurodegeneration: lessons from the Alzheimer's amyloid beta-peptide. J *Nat Rev Mol* Cell Biol. Feb; 8(2):101-12.

[355] Tanzi RE, Bertram L. Twenty years of the Alzheimer's disease amyloid hypothesis: a genetic perspective. *Cell*. 2005 Feb 25; 120(4):545-55.

[356] Zempel H, Thies E, Mandelkow E, Mandelkow EM. (2010). Abeta oligomers cause localized Ca(2+) elevation, missorting of endogenous Tau into dendrites, Tau phosphorylation, and destruction of microtubules and spines. *J Neurosci.* Sep 8;30(36):11938-50.

[357] Holmes C, Boche D, Wilkinson D, Yadegarfar G, Hopkins V. (2008). Long-term effects of Abeta42 immunisation in Alzheimer's disease: follow-up of a randomised, placebo-controlled phase I trial. *Lancet.* Jul 19; 372(9634):216-23.

[358] Holtzman DM. (2008). Alzheimer's disease: Moving towards a vaccine. *Nature.* Jul 24; 454(7203):418-20.

[359] Iwata N, Tsubuki S, Takaki Y, Watanabe K, Sekiguchi M, et al. (2000). Identification of the major Abeta1-42-degrading catabolic pathway in brain parenchyma: suppression leads to biochemical and pathological deposition. *Nat Med.* 2000 Feb; 6(2):143-50.

[360] Huang SM, Mouri A, Kokubo H, Nakajima R, Suemoto T, et al. (2006). Neprilysin-sensitive synapse-associated amyloid-beta peptide oligomers impair neuronal plasticity and cognitive function. *J Biol Chem.* Jun 30;281(26):17941-51.

[361] Dacks P. (2016). What APOE means for your health. *Cognitive Vitality.* Retrieved May 22 2019 from https://www.alzdiscovery.org/cognitive-vitality/blog/what-apoe-means-for-your-health.

[362] Ibid. Dacks. (2016).

[363] Altmann A, Tian L, Henderson VW, Greicius MD. (2014). Sex Modifies the APOE-Related Risk of Developing Alzheimer's Disease. *Ann Neurol.* Apr; 75(4): 563–573.

[364] Corder EH, Saunders AM, Strittmatter WJ, Schmechel DE, Gaskell PC, et al. (1993). Gene dose of apolipoprotein E type 4 allele and the risk of Alzheimer's disease in late onset families. *Science.* Aug 13; 261(5123):921-3.

[365] Kim J, Basak JM, Holtzman DM. (2009). The role of apolipoprotein E in Alzheimer's disease. *Neuron.* Aug 13; 63(3):287-303.

[366] Bertram L, Tanzi RE. (2008). Thirty years of Alzheimer's disease genetics: the implications of systematic meta-analyses. *Nat Rev Neurosci.* Oct; 9(10):768-78.

[367] Carter DB. (2005). The interaction of amyloid-beta with ApoE. *Subcell Biochem.* 2005;38:255-72.

[368] Michaelson DM. (2014). APOE epsilon4: the most prevalent yet understudied risk factor for Alzheimer's disease. *Alzheimers Dement,* 10(6): p. 861-8.

[369] Ibid. Michaelson. (2014).

[370] Alzheimer's Society. Alzheimer's disease and genes. Retrieved Jun 10 2019 from https://www.alzheimers.org.uk/about-dementia/risk-factors-and-prevention/alzheimers-disease-and-genes.

[371] Bu G. (2009). Apolipoprotein E and its receptors in Alzheimer's disease: pathways, pathogenesis and therapy. *Nat Rev Neurosci.* May; 10(5):333-44.

[372] Mayo Clinic. Alzheimer's genes: Are You at Risk? Retrieved 5/22/19 from https://www.mayoclinic.org/diseases-conditions/alzheimers-disease/in-depth/alzheimers-genes/art-20046552.

[373] Ibid. Mayo Clinic. Alzheimer's Genes.

[374] NIH. (2019). CLU clusterin. Retrieved May 22 2019 from https://www.ncbi.nlm.nih.gov/gene/1191.

[375] NIH. (2019). CR1 complement C3b/C4b receptor 1. Retrieved May 22 2019 from https://www.ncbi.nlm.nih.gov/gene/1378.

[376] NIH. (2019). PICALM phosphatidylinositol binding clathrin assembly protein. Retrieved May 22 2019 from https://www.ncbi.nlm.nih.gov/gene/8301.

[377] NIH. (2019). PLD3 phospholipase D family member 3. Retreved May 22 2019 from https://www.ncbi.nlm.nih.gov/gene/23646.

[378] Gratuze M, Leyns CEG, Holtzman DM. (2018). New insights into the role of TREM2 in Alzheimer's disease. *Mol Neurodegenerl,* Dec 20;13(1):66.

[379] Yin RH, Yu JT, Tan L. (2015). The Role of AORL1 in Alzheimer's Disease. *Mol Neurobiol,* 2015:51(3):909-18.

[380] Mill J. (2011). Toward an integrated genetic and epigenetic approach to Alzheimer's disease. *Neurobiol Aging.* Jul; 32(7):1188-91.

[381] Mastroeni D, Grover A, Delvaux E, Whiteside C, Coleman PD, et al. (2011). Epigenetic mechanisms in Alzheimer's disease. *Neurobiol Aging.* Jul; 32(7):1161-80.

[382] Santos-Rebouças CB, Pimentel MM (2007). Implication of abnormal epigenetic patterns for human diseases. *Eur J Hum Genet.* Jan; 15(1):10-7.

[383] Calderon-Garciduenas L, Azzarelli B, Acuna H, Garcia R, Gambling TM, Osnaya N, et al. (2002). Air pollution and brain damage. *Toxicol Pathol.* 2002 May-Jun;30(3):373-89.

[384] Calderon-Garciduenas L, Reynoso-Robles R, Vargas-Martinez J, Gomez-Maqueo-Chew A, Parez-Guille B. (2016). Prefrontal white matter pathology in air pollution exposed Mexico City young urbanites and their potential impact on neurovascular unit dysfunction and the development of Alzheimer's disease. *Environ Res.* 2016 Apr;146:404-17.

[385] Calderon-Garciduenas L, Leray F, Heydarpour P, Torres-Jardon R, Reis J. (2016). Air pollution, a rising environmental risk factor for cognition, neuroinflammation and neurodegeneration: The clinical impact on children and beyond. *Rev Neurol (Paris).* 2016 Jan;172(1):69-80.

[386] Calderon-Garciduenas L, Reynoso-Robles R, Gonzalez-Maciel A. (2019). Combustion and friction-derived nanoparticles and industrial-sourced nanoparticles: The culprit of Alzheimer and Parkinson's diseases. *Environ Res.* 2019 Jul 5;176:108574.

[387] Chen JJ, Rosas HD, Salat DH. (2011). Age-associated reductions in cerebral blood flow are independent from regional atrophy. *Neuroimage.* Mar 15;55(2):468-78.

[388] Stampfer MJ. (2006). Cardiovascular disease and Alzheimer's disease: common links. *J Intern Med.* Sep; 260(3):211-23.

[389] Newman AB, Fitzpatrick AL, Lopez O, Jackson S, Lyketsos C, et al. (2005). Dementia and Alzheimer's disease incidence in relationship to cardiovascular disease in the Cardiovascular Health Study cohort. *J Am Geriatr Soc.* Jul; 53(7):1101-7.

[390] Bergmann C, Sano M. (2006). Cardiac risk factors and potential treatments in Alzheimer's disease. *Neurol Res.* Sep; 28(6):595-604.

[391] Ibid. Bredesen. (2015).

[392] Andreoulakis E, Hyphantis T, Kandylis D, Iacovides A. (2012). Depression in diabetes mellitus: a comprehensive review. *Hippokratia.* Jul;16(3):205-14.

[393] Huang C, Chung C, Leu H, et al. (2014). Diabetes mellitus and the risk of Alzheimer's disease: a nationwide population-based study. *PloS One.* 2014;9(1):e87095.

[394] Chew BH, Sherina MS, Hassan NH. (2015). Association of diabetes-related distress, depression, medication adherence, and health-related quality of life with glycated hemoglobin, blood pressure, and lipids in adult patients with type 2 diabetes: a cross-sectional study. *Ther Clin Risk Manag.* 2015;11:669-81

[395] K. Talbot. (2013). Brain insulin resistance in Alzheimer's disease and its potential treatment with a Mediterranean diet and GLP-1 analogues. *Psychiatric Times.* Aug 20:18-21.

[396] Ibid. Bredesen. (2015).

[397] Seshadri S, Beiser A, Selhub J, Jacques PF, Rosenberg IH, et al. (2002). Plasma homocysteine as a risk factor for dementia and Alzheimer's disease. *N Engl J Med.* Feb 14; 346(7):476-83.

[398] Pappolla MA, Bryant-Thomas TK, Herbert D, Pacheco J, Fabra Garcia M, et al. (2003). Mild hypercholesterolemia is an early risk factor for the development of Alzheimer amyloid pathology, *Neurology.* 2003 Jul 22; 61(2):199-205.

[399] Grimm MOW, Michaelson DM, Hartmann T. (2017). Omega-3 fatty acids, lipids, and apoE lipidation in Alzheimer's disease: a rationale for multi-nutrient dementia prevention. *J Lipid Res.* Nov;58(11):2083-2101.

[400] Michikawa M. (2006). Role of cholesterol in amyloid cascade: cholesterol-dependent modulation of tau phosphorylation and mitochondrial function. *Acta Neurol Scand Suppl.* 2006;185():21-6.

[401] Yaffe K, Barrett-Connor E, Lin F, Grady D. (2002). Serum lipoprotein levels, statin use, and cognitive function in older women. *Arch Neurol.* Mar; 59(3):378-84.

[402] Kivipelto M, Helkala EL, Laakso MP, Hänninen T, Hallikainen M, et al. (2002). Apolipoprotein E epsilon4 allele, elevated midlife total cholesterol level, and high midlife systolic blood pressure are independent risk factors for late-life Alzheimer disease. *Ann Intern Med.* Aug 6; 137(3):149-55.

[403] Jarvik GP, Wijsman EM, Kukull WA, Schellenberg GD, Yu C, et al. (1995). Interactions of apolipoprotein E genotype, total cholesterol level, age, and sex in prediction of Alzheimer's disease: a case-control study. *Neurology.* Jun; 45(6):1092-6.

[404] Loera-Valencia R, Goikolea J, Parrado-Fernandez C, Merino-Serrais P, Maioli S. (2019). Alterations in cholesterol metabolism as a risk factor for developing Alzheimer's disease: Potential novel targets for treatment. *J Steroid Biochem Mol Biol.* Jun;190:104-114.

[405] Jiang S, Li Y, Zhang C, Zhao Y, Bu G, et al. (2014). M1 muscarinic acetylecholine receptor in Alzheimer's disease. *Neurosci Bull.* Apr;30(2);295-307.

[406] Verma S, Kumar A, Tripathi T, Kumar A. (2018). Muscarinic and nicotinic acetylecholine receptor agonists: current scenario in Alzheimer's disease therapy. *J Pharm Pharmacol.* Aug;70(8):985-993.

[407] G. C. Román. (2005). Cholinergic dysfunction in vascular dementia. *Curr Psychiatry Rep. 7(1):18-26.*

[408] Wang J, Zhang HY, Tang XC. (2009). Cholinergic deficiency involved in vascular dementia: possible mechanism and strategy of treatment. *Acta Pharmacologica Sinica.* 30(7):879-88.

[409] Higgins JP, Flicker L. (2003). Lecithin for dementia and cognitive impairment. *Cochrane Database Syst Rev.* 2003;(3):CD001015.

[410] Velaquez R, Ferreria E, Winslow W, Dave N, Piras IS, et al. (2019). Maternal choline supplementation ameliorates Alzheimer's disease pathology by reducing brain homocysteine levels across multiple generations. *Mol Psychiatry.* Jan 8.

[411] Geula C, Mesulam MM. (1996). Systematic regional variations in the loss of cortical cholinergic fibers in Alzheimer's disease. *Cereb Cortex.* Mar-Apr; 6(2):165-77.

[412] Geula C, Mesulam MM. (1989). Cortical cholinergic fibers in aging and Alzheimer's disease: a morphometric study. *Neuroscience.* 1989; 33(3):469-81.

[413] Schliebs R, Arendt T. (2011). The cholinergic system in aging and neuronal degeneration. *Behav Brain Res.* 2011 Aug 10; 221(2):555-63.

[414] Shukla D, Mandal PK, Ersland L, Gruner ER, Tripathi M, et al. (2018). Multi-Center Study on Human Brain Glutathione Conformation using Magnetic Resonance Spectroscopy. *J Alzheimers Dis.* 2018;66(2):517-532.

[415] Sung HY, Choi EN, Ahn Jo S, Oh S, Ahn JH. (2011). Amyloid protein-mediated differential DNA methylation status regulates gene expression in Alzheimer's disease model cell line. *Biochem Biophys Res Commun.* Nov;414(4):700-5.

[416] Hodgson N, Trivedi M, Muratore C, Li S, Deth R. (2013). Soluble oligomers of amyloid-β cause changes in redox state, DNA methylation, and gene transcription by inhibiting EAAT3 mediated cysteine uptake. *J Alzheimers Dis.* (1):197-209.

[417] Chen KL, Wang SS, Yang YY, Yuan RY, Chen RM, et al. (2009). The epigenetic effects of amyloid-beta(1-40) on global DNA and neprilysin genes in murine cerebral endothelial cells. *Biochem Biophys Res Commun.* Jan 2; 378(1):57-61.

[418] Swerdlow RH, Burns JM, Khan SM. (2014). The Alzheimer's disease mitochondrial cascade hypothesis: progress and perspectives. *Biochim Biophys Acta.* Aug; 1842(8):1219-31.

[419] Picone P, Nuzzo D, Caruana L, Scafidi V, Di Carlo M. (2014). Mitochondrial dysfunction: different routes to Alzheimer's disease therapy. *Oxid Med Cell Longev.* 2014():780179.

[420] Scarpulla RC. (2008). Transcriptional paradigms in mammalian mitochondrial biogenesis and function. *Physiol Rev.* Apr; 88(2):611-38.

[421] Mosconi L, Brys M, Switalski R, Mistur R, Glodzik L, et al. (2007). Maternal family history of Alzheimer's disease predisposes to reduced brain glucose metabolism. *Proc Natl Acad Sci U S A.* Nov 27; 104(48):19067-72.

[422] Murray J, Tsui WH, Li Y, McHugh P, Williams S, et al. (2014). FDG and Amyloid PET in Cognitively Normal Individuals at Risk for Late-Onset Alzheimer's Disease. *Adv J Mol Imaging.* Apr; 4(2):15-26.

[423] Hirai K, Aliev G, Nunomura A, Fujioka H, Russell RL, et al. (2001). Mitochondrial abnormalities in Alzheimer's disease. *J Neurosci.* May 1; 21(9):3017-23.

[424] Moreira PI, Siedlak SL, Wang X, Santos MS, Oliveira CR, et al. (2007). Increased autophagic degradation of mitochondria in Alzheimer disease. *Autophagy.* Nov-Dec; 3(6):614-5.

[425] Wang X, Su B, Siedlak SL, Moreira PI, Fujioka H, et al. (2008). Amyloid-beta overproduction causes abnormal mitochondrial dynamics via differential modulation of mitochondrial fission/fusion proteins. *Proc Natl Acad Sci U S A.* Dec 9; 105(49):19318-23.

[426] Manczak M, Calkins MJ, Reddy PH. (2011). Impaired mitochondrial dynamics and abnormal interaction of amyloid beta with mitochondrial protein Drp1 in neurons from patients with Alzheimer's disease: implications for neuronal damage. *Hum Mol Genet.* Jul 1; 20(13):2495-509.

[427] Wang H, Lim PJ, Karbowski M, Monteiro MJ. (2009). Effects of overexpression of huntingtin proteins on mitochondrial integrity. *Hum Mol Genet.* Feb 15; 18(4):737-52.

[428] Keller JN, Pang Z, Geddes JW, Begley JG, Germeyer A, et al. (1997). Impairment of glucose and glutamate transport and induction of mitochondrial oxidative stress and dysfunction in synaptosomes by amyloid beta-peptide: role of the lipid peroxidation product 4-hydroxynonenal. *J Neurochem.* Jul; 69(1):273-84.

[429] Manczak M, Anekonda TS, Henson E, Park BS, et al. (2006). Mitochondria are a direct site of A beta accumulation in Alzheimer's disease neurons: implications for free radical generation and oxidative damage in disease progression. *Hum Mol Genet.* May 1; 15(9):1437-49.

[430] Mattson MP, Partin J, Begley JG. (1998). Amyloid beta-peptide induces apoptosis-related events in synapses and dendrites. *Brain Res.* Oct 5; 807(1-2):167-76.

[431] Reddy PH. (2008). Mitochondrial medicine for aging and neurodegenerative diseases. *Neuromolecular Med.* 10(4):291-315.

[432] Calkins MJ, Manczak M, Reddy PH. (2012). Mitochondria-Targeted Antioxidant SS31 Prevents Amyloid Beta-Induced Mitochondrial Abnormalities and Synaptic Degeneration in Alzheimer's Disease. *Pharmaceuticals (Basel).* 5(10):1103-19.

[433] Reddy PH, Tripathi R, Troung Q, Tirumala K, Reddy TP, et al. (2012). Abnormal mitochondrial dynamics and synaptic degeneration as early events in Alzheimer's disease: implications to mitochondria-targeted antioxidant therapeutics. *Biochim Biophys Acta.* May; 1822(5):639-49.

[434] Ryan MT, Hoogenraad NJ. (2007). Mitochondrial-nuclear communications. *Annu Rev Biochem.* 76():701-22.

[435] Liu X, Hajnóczky G. (2011). Altered fusion dynamics underlie unique morphological changes in mitochondria during hypoxia-reoxygenation stress. *Cell Death Differ.* Oct; 18(10):1561-72.

[436] Medeiros DM. (2008). Assessing mitochondria biogenesis. *Methods.* Dec; 46(4):288-94.

[437] Kim I, Rodriguez-Enriquez S, Lemasters JJ. (2007). Selective degradation of mitochondria by mitophagy. *Arch Biochem Biophys.* Jun 15; 462(2):245-53.

[438] Steiner JL, Murphy EA, McClellan JL, Carmichael MD, Davis JM. (2011). Exercise training increases mitochondrial biogenesis in the brain. *J Appl Physiol* (1985). Oct; 111(4):1066-71.

[439] Scherz-Shouval R, Elazar Z. (2011). Regulation of autophagy by ROS: physiology and pathology. *Trends Biochem Sci.* Jan; 36(1):30-8.

[440] Yamamoto A, Yue Z. (2014). Autography and its normal pathogenic states in the brain. *Annu Rev Neurosci.* 2014; 37:55-78.

441 Ariosa AR, Klionsky DJ. (2016). Autography core machinery: overcoming spatial barriers in neurons. *J Mol Med (Berl)*. 94:1217-1227.

442 Kulkami VV, Maday S. (2018). Compartment-specific dynamics and functions of autography in neurons. *Dev Neurobiol*. 78:298-310.

443 Kim M, Sandford E, Gatica D, Qiu Y, Liu X, et al. (2016). Mutation in ATG5 reduces autophagy and leads to ataxia with developmental delay. *Elife* 2016:5. e12245.

444 Maday S. (2016). Mechanisms of neuronal homeostasis: autophagy in the axon. *Brain Res*. 1649:143-150.

445 Frake RA, Ricketts T, Menzies FM, Rubinsztein DC. (2015). Autophagy and neurodegeneration. *J Clin Invest*. Jan;125(1)65-74.

446 De Vivo G, Gentile V. (2008). Transglutaminase-catalyzed post-translational modifications of proteins in the nervous system and their possible involvement in neurodegenerative diseases. *CNS Neurol Disord Drug Targets*. Oct;7(4):370-5.

447 Galasko D, Montine T. (2010). Biomarkers of oxidative damage and inflammation in Alzheimer's disease. *J Biomark Med*. Feb; 4(1):27-36.

448 Steele M, Stuchbury G, Münch G. (2007). The molecular basis of the prevention of Alzheimer's disease through healthy nutrition. *Exp Gerontol*. Jan-Feb; 42(1-2):28-36.

449 Bennett S, Grant MM, and Aldred S. (2009). Oxidative stress in vascular dementia and Alzheimer's disease: a common pathology. *J Alzheimer's Dis*. 2009;17(2):245-57.

450 Schwhab C, McGeer PL. (2008). Inflammatory aspects of Alzheimer disease and other neurodegenerative disorders. *J Alzheimers Dis*. May; 13(4):359-69

451 Bonda DJ, Wang X, Perry G, Nunomura A, Tabaton M, et al. (2010). Oxidative stress in Alzheimer disease: a possibility for prevention. *Neuropharmacology*. Sep-Oct; 59(4-5):290-4.

452 Ibid. Steele. (2007). *Exp Gerontol*.

453 Alzheimer's Association. (2017). Alzheimer's Disease Facts and Figures. Retrieved Jun 29 2019 from https://www.alzheimersanddementia.com/article/S1552-5260(17)30051-1/fulltext.

454 Ibid. Bonda. (2010). *Neuropharmacology*.

455 Chauhan V, Chauhan A. (2006). Oxidative stress in Alzheimer's disease. *Pathophysiology*. Aug; 13(3):195-208.

456 Gibson GE, Huang HM. (2002). Oxidative processes in the brain and non-neuronal tissues as biomarkers of Alzheimer's disease. *Front Biosci*. Apr 1; 7():d1007-15

457 Montine TJ, Neely MD, Quinn JF, Beal MF, Markesbery WR, et al. (2002). Lipid peroxidation in aging brain and Alzheimer's disease. *Free Radic Biol Med*. Sep 1; 33(5):620-6.

458 Arlt S, Beisiegel U, Kontush A. (2002). Lipid peroxidation in neurodegeneration: new insights into Alzheimer's disease. *Curr Opin Lipidol*. Jun; 13(3):289-94.

459 Lovell MA, Gabbita SP, Markesbery WR. (1999). Increased DNA oxidation and decreased levels of repair products in Alzheimer's disease ventricular CSF. *J Neurochem*. Feb; 72(2):771-6.

460 Harris ME, Hensley K, Butterfield DA, Leedle RA, Carney JM. (1995). Direct evidence of oxidative injury produced by the Alzheimer's beta-amyloid peptide (1-40) in cultured hippocampal neurons. *Exp Neurol*. Feb; 131(2):193-202

461 Sponne I, Fifre A, Drouet B, Klein C, Koziel V, et al. (2003). Apoptotic neuronal cell death induced by the non-fibrillar amyloid-beta peptide proceeds through an early reactive oxygen species-dependent cytoskeleton perturbation. *J Biol Chem*. Jan 31; 278(5):3437-45.

462 Stampfer MJ. (2006). Cardiovascular disease and Alzheimer's disease: common links. *J Intern Med*. 2006 Sep; 260(3):211-23.

463 Ozawa M, Shipley M, Kivimaki M, Singh-Manoux A. (2017). Dietary pattern, inflammation and cognitive decline: The Whilehall II prospective cohort study. *Clin Nutr*. Apr;36(2):506-512.

464 Venegas C, Kumar S, Franklin BS, Dierkes T, Brinkschulte R, et al. (2017). Microglia-derived ASC specks cross-seed amyloid-B in Alzheimer's disease. *Nature*, Dec 20:552(7685):355.

465 Di Benedetto S, Muller L, Wenger E, Duzel S, Pawelec G. (2017). Contribution of neuroinflammation and immunity to brain aging and the mitigating effects of physical and cognitive interventions. *Neurosci Biobehav Rev*. Apr;75:114-128.

466 Heneka MT, Carson MJ, El Khoury J, et al. (2015). Neuroinflammation in Alzheimer's Disease. *Lancet Neurol*. Apr;14(4):388-405.

467 Sperling RA, Aisen PS, Beckett LA, Bennett DA, Craft S, et al. (2011). Toward defining the preclinical stages of Alzheimer's disease: recommendations from the National Institute on Aging-Alzheimer's Association workgroups on diagnostic guidelines for Alzheimer's disease. *Alzheimers Dement*. May; 7(3):280-92.

468 Wirth M, Madison CM, Rabinovici GD, Oh H, Landau SM, et al. (2013). Alzheimer's disease neurodegenerative biomarkers are associated with decreased cognitive function but not β-amyloid in cognitively normal older individuals. *J Neurosci*. Mar 27; 33(13):5553-63.

469 Asgari N, Berg CT, Morch MT, Khorooshi R, Owens T. (2015). Cerebrospinal fluid aquaporin-4-immunoglobulin G disrupts blood brain barrier. *Ann Clin Transl Neurol*. Aug;2(8):857-863.

470 Abbot NJ. (2000). Inflammatory mediators and modulation of blood-brain permeability. *Cell Mol Neurobiol*. 2000 Apr;20(2):131-47.

471 Sofroniew MV. (2015). Astrocyte barriers to neurotoxic inflammation. *Nat Rev Neurosci*. May;16(5):249-263

[472] The potential role of aluminium in Alzheimer's disease. Campbell A *Nephrol Dial Transplant*. 2002; 17 Suppl 2():17-20.

[473] The role of metals in neurodegenerative processes: aluminum, manganese, and zinc. Zatta P, Lucchini R, van Rensburg SJ, Taylor A *Brain Res Bull*. 2003 Nov 15; 62(1):15-28

[474] Aluminium as a risk factor in Alzheimer's disease, with emphasis on drinking water. Flaten TP *Brain Res Bull*. 2001 May 15; 55(2):187-96.

[475] Aluminum and silica in drinking water and the risk of Alzheimer's disease or cognitive decline: findings from 15-year follow-up of the PAQUID cohort. Rondeau V, Jacqmin-Gadda H, Commenges D, Helmer C, Dartigues JF
Am J Epidemiol. 2009 Feb 15; 169(4):489-96.

[476] Wang Z, Wei X, Yang J, Suo J, Chen J, et al. (2016). Chronic exposure to aluminum and risk of Alzheimer's disease: a meta-analysis. *Neurosci Lett*. Jan 1;610:200-6.

[477] Colomina MT, Peris-Sampedro F. (2017). Aluminum and Alzheimer's Disease. *Adv Neurobiol*, 2017;18:183-197.

[478] Mutter J, Curth A, Naumann J, Deth R, Walach H. (2010). Does inorganic mercury play a role in Alzheimer's disease? A systematic review and an integrated molecular mechanism. *J Alzheimers Dis*. 2010;22(2):357-74.

[479] Chakraborty P. (2017). Mercury exposure and Alzheimer's disease in India - An imminent threat? *Sci Total Environ*. Jul 1;589:232-235.

[480] Sensi SL, Paoletti P, Bush AI, Sekler I. (2009). Zinc in the physiology and pathology of the CNS. *Nat Rev Neurosci*. Nov; 10(11):780-91.

[481] Hung YH, Bush AI, Cherny RA. (2010). Copper in the brain and Alzheimer's disease. *J Biol Inorg Chem*. Jan; 15(1):61-76.

[482] Wright RO, Baccarelli A. (2007). Metals and neurotoxicology. *J Nutr*. Dec; 137(12):2809-13.

[483] Strong MJ, Garruto RM, Joshi JG, Mundy WR, Shafer TJ. (1996). Can the mechanisms of aluminum neurotoxicity be integrated into a unified scheme? *J Toxicol Environ Health*. Aug 30; 48(6):599-613.

[484] Tyer CR, Allan AM. (2014). The effects of arsenic exposure on neurological and cognitive dysfunction in human and rodent studies: a review. *Curr Environ Health Rep*. Mar21;1:132-147.

[485] Basha MR, Wei W, Bakheet SA, Benitez N, Siddiqi HK, et al. (2005). The fetal basis of amyloidogenesis: exposure to lead and latent over-expression of amyloid precursor protein and beta-amyloid in the aging brain. *J Neurosci*. Jan 26;25(4):823-829.

[486] Silbergeld EK. (1992). Mechanisms of lead neurotoxicity, or looking beyond the lamppost. *FASEB J*. Oct; 6(13):3201-6.

[487] Bressler JP, Goldstein GW. (1991). Mechanisms of lead neurotoxicity. *Biochem Pharmacol*. Feb 15; 41(4):479-84.

[488] Cookman GR, King W, Regan CM. (1987). Chronic low-level lead exposure impairs embryonic to adult conversion of the neural cell adhesion molecule. *J Neurochem*. Aug; 49(2):399-403.

[489] Guilarte TR, Miceli RC, Altmann L, Weinsberg F, Winneke G, et al. (1993). Chronic prenatal and postnatal Pb2+ exposure increases [3H]MK801 binding sites in adult rat forebrain. *Eur J Pharmacol*. Oct 1; 248(3):273-5.

[490] Verity MA. Nervous system. In: Goyer RA, Klaassen CD, Waalkes MP, editors. *Metal Toxicology*. San Diego, Calif, USA: Academic Press; 1995. pp. 199–226

[491] US Department of Health and Human Services. (2007). Toxicological Profile For Lead. Washington, DC, USA.

[492] Kumar S, Jain S, Aggarwal CS, Ahuja GK. (1987). Encephalopathy due to inorganic lead exposure in an adult. *Jpn J Med*. May; 26(2):253-4.

[493] Khalil N, Morrow LA, Needleman H, Talbott EO, Wilson JW, et al. (2009). Association of cumulative lead and neurocognitive function in an occupational cohort. *Neuropsychology*. 2009 Jan; 23(1):10-9.

[494] Stewart WF, Schwartz BS. (2007). Effects of lead on the adult brain: a 15-year exploration. *Am J Ind Med*. Oct; 50(10):729-39.

[495] Ashok A, Rai NK, Tripathi S, Bandyopadhyay S. (2015). Exposure to As-Cd-, and Pb-mixture induces AB, amyloidogenic APP processing and cognitive impairments via oxidative stress-dependent neuroinflammation in young rats. *Toxicol Sci*. Jan;143(1):64-80.

[496] Fleming SM. (2017). Mechanisms of gene-environment interactions in Parkinson's disease. *Curr Environ Health Rep*. June;4(2):192-199.

[497] Narayan S, Liew Z, Bronstein JM, Ritz B. (2017). Occupational pesticide use and Parkinson's disease in the Parkinson Environmental Gene (PEG) study. *Environ Int*. Oct;107:266-273.

[498] Sabarwal A, Kumar K, Singh RP. (2018). Hazardous effects of chemical pesticides on human health-cancer and other associated disorders. *Environ Toxicol Pharmacol*. Oct;63:103-114.

[499] Gunnarsson LG, Bodin L. (2019). Occupational exposures and neurodegenerative diseases-a systematic literature review and meta-analyses. *Int J Environ Res Public Health*. Jan 26;16(3).

[500] Pohanka M. (2019). Diagnoses of pathological states based on acetylcholinesterase and butyrylcholinesterase. *Curr Med Chem*. Jan 30.

[501] Desai V, Kaler SG. (2008). Role of copper in human neurological disorders. *Am J Clin Nutr*. Sep; 88(3):855S-8S.

[502] Shaw CA, Tomljenovic L. (2013). Aluminum in the central nervous system (CNS): toxicity in humans and animals, vaccine adjuvants, and autoimmunity. *Immunol Res*. Jul; 56(2-3):304-16.

[503] Chen P, Chakraborty S, Peres TV, Bowman AB, Aschner M. (2015). Manganese-induced Neurotoxicity: From C. elegans to Humans. *Toxicol Res* (Camb). Mar 1; 4(2):191-202.

[504] Bredesen, D.E. (2016). Inhalational Alzheimer's disease: an unrecognized – and treatable – epidemic. *Aging* (Albany NY). 8: 304-313.

[505] Poole S, Singhrao SK, Kesavalu L, Curtis MA, Crean S. (2013). Determining the presence of periodontopathic virulence factors in short-term postmortem Alzheimer's disease brain tissue. *J Alzheimers Dis*. 36(4):665-677.

[506] Chen P, Stärkel P, Turner JR, Ho SB, Schnabl B. (2015). Dysbiosis-induced intestinal inflammation activates tumor necrosis factor receptor I and mediates alcoholic liver disease in mice *Hepatology*. Mar; 61(3):883-94.

[507] Yan AW, Fouts DE, Brandl J, Stärkel P, Torralba M, et al. (2011). Enteric dysbiosis associated with a mouse model of alcoholic liver disease. *Hepatology*. Jan; 53(1):96-105.

[508] Ibid. Chen. (2015).

[509] Adachi Y, Moore LE, Bradford BU, Gao W, Thurman RG. (1995). Antibiotics prevent liver injury in rats following long-term exposure to ethanol. *Gastroenterology*. 1995 Jan; 108(1):218-24.

[510] Engen PA, Kwasny M, Lau CK, Keshavarzian A. (2012). Colonic microbiome is altered in alcoholism. *Am J Physiol Gastrointest Liver Physiol*. May 1; 302(9):G966-78.

[511] Yan AW, Fouts DE, Brandl J, Stärkel P, Torralba M, et al. (2011). Enteric dysbiosis associated with a mouse model of alcoholic liver disease. *Hepatology*. Jan; 53(1):96-105.

[512] Mutlu EA, Gillevet PM, Rangwala H, Sikaroodi M, Naqvi A, et al. (2012). Colonic microbiome is altered in alcoholism. *Am J Physiol Gastrointest Liver Physiol*. 302(9):G966–78.10.1152/ajpgi.00380.2011

[513] Weller RO, Massey A, Newman TA, Hutchings M, Kuo YM, et al. (1998). Cerebral amyloid angiopathy: amyloid beta accumulates in putative interstitial fluid drainage pathways in Alzheimer's disease. *Am J Pathol*. 1998 Sep; 153(3):725-33.

[514] Nedergaard M. (2013). Neuroscience. Garbage truck of the brain. *Science*. Jun 28; 340(6140):1529-30.

[515] Carare RO, Hawkes CA, Jeffrey M, Kalaria RN, Weller RO. (2013). Review: cerebral amyloid angiopathy, prion angiopathy, CADASIL and the spectrum of protein elimination failure angiopathies (PEFA) in neurodegenerative disease with a focus on therapy. Neuropathol *Appl Neurobiol*. Oct; 39(6):593-611.

[516] Ibid. Nedergaard. (2013).

[517] Jessen NA, Munk AS, Lundgaard I, Nedergaard M. (2015). *Neurochem Res*. Dec;40(12):2583-99.

[518] Tarasoff-Conway JM, Carare RO, Osorio RS, Glodzik L, Butler T, et al. (2015). Clearance systems in the brain-implications for Alzheimer disease. *Nat Rev Neurol*. 2015 Aug; 11(8): 457–470.

[519] Potter R, Patterson BW, Elbert DL, Ovod V, Kasten T, et al. (2013). Increased in vivo amyloid-β42 production, exchange, and loss in presenilin mutation carriers. *Sci Transl Med*. Jun 12; 5(189):189ra77.

[520] Mawuenyega KG, Sigurdson W, Ovod V, Munsell L, Kasten T, et al. (2010). Decreased clearance of CNS beta-amyloid in Alzheimer's disease. *Science*. Dec 24; 330(6012):1774.

[521] Pasinetti GM, Wang J, Ho L, Zhao W, Dubner L. (2015). Roles of resveratrol and other grape-derived polyphenols in Alzheimer's disease prevention and treatment. *Biochim Biophys Acta*. Jun; 1852(6):1202-8.

[522] Atwood CS, Obrenovich ME, Liu T, Chan H, Perry G, et al. (2003). Amyloid-B: a chameleon walking in two worlds: a review of the trophic and toxic properties of amyloid-B. *Brain Research Reviews*. Sep;43(1):1-16.

[523] Plant LD, Bole JP, Smith IF, Peers C, Pearson HA. (2003). The production of amyloid beta peptide is a critical requirement for the viability of central neurons. *J Neurosci*. Jul 2;23(13):5531-5.

[524] Ozawa M, Shipley M, Kivimaki M, Singh-Manoux A. (2017). Dietary pattern, inflammation and cognitive decline: The Whilehall II prospective cohort study. *Clin Nutr*. Apr;36(2):506-512.

[525] Suzuki T. (2013). Regulation of intestinal epithelial permeability by tight junctions. *Cell Mol Life Sci*. Feb; 70(4):631-59.

[526] Barnard ND. (2014). Saturated and trans fats and dementia: a systematic review. *Neurobiol Aging*. Sep;35(2):S65-S73.

[527] Englehart MJ, Geerlings MI, Ruitenberg A, Van Swieten JC, Hofman A, et al. (2002). Diet and risk of dementia: Does fat matter? The Rotterdam Study. *Neurology*. Dec 24;59(12):1915-21.

[528] Sun Q, Ma J, Campos H, Hankinson SE, Rexrode KM, et al. (2007). A prospective Study of Trans Fatty Acids in Erythrocytes and Risk of Coronary Heart Disease. *Circulation*. 2007;115:1858-1865.

[529] Mazaffarian D, Pischon T, Hankinson SE, Rifai N, Joshipura K, et al. (2004). Dietary intake of trans fatty acids and system inflammation in women. *Am J Clin Nutr*. Apr;79(4):606-12.

[530] Barnard ND, Bush AI, Ceccarelli A, Cooper J, de Jager CA, et al. (2014). Dietary and lifestyle guidelines for the prevention of Alzheimer's disease. *Neurobiol Aging*. Sep;35 Suppl 2:S74-8.

[531] Farruggia MC, Small DM. (2019). Effects of adiposity and metabolic dysfunction on cognition: A review. *Physiol Behav*. Jun 11;208:112578.

[532] Feng Y, He D, Yo Z, Klionsky DJ: The machinery of macroautography. *Cell Res* 2014, 24:24-41.

[533] Weidberg H., Shvets E. Elazar Z. (2011). Biogenesis and cargo selectivity of autophagosomes. *Annu Rev Biochem* 80:125-156.

[534] Mizushima N. Yoshimori T, Ohsumi Y. (2011). The role of Atg proteins in autophagosome formation. *Annu Rev Cell Biol* 27:107-132.

[535] Sprecher KE, Koscik RL, Carlsson CM, Zetterberg H, Blennow K, et al. (2017). Poor sleep is associated with CSF biomarkers of amyloid pathology in cognitively normal adults. *Neurology.* Aug 1; 89(5): 445–453.

[536] Robb, A. (2018). *Why We Dream: The Transformative Power of Our Nightly Journey.* (p. 162). Boston, MA: Houghton Mifflin Harcourt.

[537] Xie L, Kang H, Xu Q, Chen MJ, Liao Y, et al. (2013). Sleep drives metabolite clearance from the adult brain. *Science.* Oct 18; 342(6156):373-7.

[538] Di Meco A, Joshi YB, Praticò D. (2014). Sleep deprivation impairs memory, tau metabolism, and synaptic integrity of a mouse model of Alzheimer's disease with plaques and tangles. *Neurobiol Aging.* Aug; 35(8):1813-20.

[539] Cantero JL, Hita-Yañez E, Moreno-Lopez B, Portillo F, et al. (2010). Tau protein role in sleep-wake cycle. *J Alzheimers Dis.* 21(2):411-21.

[540] Maret S, Faraguna U, Nelson AB, Cirelli C, Tononi G. (2011). Sleep and waking modulate spine turnover in the adolescent mouse cortex. *Nat Neurosci.* Oct 9; 14(11):1418-20.

[541] Faraut B, Boudjeltia KZ, Vanhamme L, Kerkhofs M. (2012). Immune, inflammatory and cardiovascular consequences of sleep restriction and recovery. *Sleep Med Rev.* 2012 Apr; 16(2):137-49.

[542] Potter R, Patterson BW, Elbert DL, Ovod V, Kasten T, et al. (2013). Increased in vivo amyloid-β42 production, exchange, and loss in presenilin mutation carriers. *Sci Transl Med.* Jun 12; 5(189):189ra77.

[543] Reiman EM, Quiroz YT, Fleisher AS, Chen K, Velez-Pardo C, et al. (2012). Brain imaging and fluid biomarker analysis in young adults at genetic risk for autosomal dominant Alzheimer's disease in the presenilin 1 E280A kindred: a case-control study. *Lancet Neurol.* Dec; 11(12):1048-56.

[544] Ibid. Potter. (2013).

[545] Ibid. Xie. (2013).

[546] Chen Q, Yoshida H, Schubert D, Maher P, Mallory M, et al. (2001). Presenilin Binding Protein Is Associated with Neurofibrillary Alterations in Alzheimer's Disease and Stimulates Tau Phosphorylation. *Am J Pathol.* Nov; 159(5): 1597–1602.

[547] Melao A. (2018). Obesity, Sedentary Behavior Not Linked to Parkinson's Disease Risk, Study Shows. *Parkinsons News Today.* May 25.

[548] Ellis T, Rochester L. (2018). Mobilizing Parkinson's Disease: The Future of Exercise. *J Parkinsons Dis.* 2018;8(Supple 1):S95-S100.

[549] Whitman H. (2017). Sedentary behavior raises Alzheimer's risk as much as genetic factors. *Med News Today.* Jan 15.

[550] Wheeler MJ, Dempsey PC, Grace MS, Ellis KA, Gardiner PA, et al. (2017). Sedentary behavior as a risk factor for cognitive decline? A focus on the influence of glycemic control in brain health. *Alzheimers Dement (NY).* Sep;3(3):291-300.

[551] Ibid. Heneka. (2015).

[552] Anderson KM, Olson KE, Estes KA, Flanagan K, Gendelman HE, et al. (2014). Dual destructive and protective roles of adaptive immunity in neurodegenerative disorders. *Transl Neurodegener.* Nov 13;3(1):25.

[553] Rabins PV (Reviewer). (2016). Alzheimer's Treatment Options: Benefits and Risks: Retreived Oct 2 2019 from https://www.healthcentral.com/article/alzheimers-treatment-options-benefits-and-risks.

[554] Bryan J. (2010). Donepezil – a major breakthrough in the treatment of Alzheimer's disease. *Pharmaceutical J.* Dec 17, 2010.

[555] Ibid. Rabins. (2016). Alzheimer's Treatment Options

[556] Ibid. Rabins. (2016).

[557] Ibid. Rabins. (2016).

[558] Bredesen DE. (2014). Reversal of cognitive decline: a novel therapeutic program. *Aging* (Albany NY). Sep; 6(9):707-17.

[559] Mutter J, Currh A, Naumann N, Deth R, Walach H. (2010). Does inorganic mercury play a role in Alzheimer's disease? A systemic review and an integrated molecular mechanism. *J Alz Dis.* 22: 357-374.

[560] Petersson SD, Philippou E. (2016). Mediterranean Diet, Cognitive Function, and Dementia: A Systematic Review of the Evidence. *Adv Nutr.* Sep 15;7(5):889-904.

[561] Safouris A, Tsiygoulis G, Sergentanis TN, Psaltopoulou T. (2015). Mediterranean Diet and Risk of Dementia. *Curr Alzheimer Res.* 2015;12(8):736-44.

[562] Roman GC, Jackson RE, Gadhia R, Roman AN, Reis J. (2019). Mediterranean diet: The role of long-chain omega-3 fatty acids in fish; polyphenols in fruits, vegetables, cereals, coffee, tea, cacao and wine; probiotics and vitamins in prevention of stroke, age-related cognitive decline, and Alzheimer disease. *Rev Neurol (Paris).* Sep 11:S0035-3787(19)30773-8.

[563] Mayo Clinic. Mediterranean diet: A heart-healthy eating plan. Retrieved Jun 20 2019 from http://www.mayoclinic.org/ healthylifestyle/nutrition-and-healthy-eating/in-depth/mediterranean-diet/art-20047801.

[564] Scarmeas N, Stern Y, Tang MX, Mayeux R, Luchsinger JA. (2006). Mediterranean diet and risk for Alzheimer's disease. *Ann Neurol.* Jun;59(6):912-21.

565 Lourida I, Soni M, Thompson-Coon J, Purandare N, Lang IA, et al. (2013). Mediterranean diet, cognitive function, and dementia: a systematic review. *J Epidemiology*. Jul;24(4):479-89.

566 Allès B, Samieri C, Féart C, Jutand MA, Laurin D, et al. (2012). Dietary patterns: a novel approach to examine the link between nutrition and cognitive function in older individuals. *Nutr Res Rev*. Dec; 25(2):207-22.

567 Rainey-Smith SR, Gu Y, Gardener SL, Doecke JD, Villemagne VL, et al. (2018). Mediterranean diet adherence and rate of cerebral AB-amyloid accumulation: Data from the Australian Imaging, Biomarkers and Lifestyle Study of Aging. *Transl Psychiatry*. Oct 30;8(1):238.

568 Hill E, Szoeke C, Dennerstein L, Campbell S, Clifton P. (2018). Adherence to the Mediterranean Diet is not related to Beta-Amyloid Deposition: Data from the Women's Healthy Aging Project. *J Prev Alzheimers Dis*. 5(2):137-141.

569 Vassilaki M, Aakre JA, Syrianen JA, Mielke MM, Geda YE, et al. (2018). Mediterranean Diet, Its Components, and Amyloid Imaging Biomarkers. *J Alzheimers Dis*. 64(1):281-290.

570 Berti V, Walters M, Sterling J, Quinn CG, Logue M, et al. (2018). Mediterranean diet and 3-year Alzheimer brain biomarker changes in middle-aged adults. *Neurology*. May 15;90(20):e1789-e1798.

571 Harnedo-Ortega R, Cerezo AB, de Pablos RM, Krisa S, Richard T, et al. (2018). Phenolic Compounds Characteristic of the Mediterranean Diet in Mitigating Microglia-Mediated Neuroinflammation. *Front Cell Neurosci*. Oct 23;12:273.

572 Peterson CM, Johannsen DL, Ravussin E. (2012). Skeletal muscle mitochondria and aging: a review. *J Aging Res*. 2012:194821.

573 Qiu X, Brown KV, Moran Y, Chen D. (2010). Sirtuin regulation in calorie restriction. *Biochim Biophys Acta*. Aug;1804(8):1576-83.

574 Sohal RS, Ku HH, Agarwal S, Forster MJ, Lal H. (1994). Oxidative damage, mitochondrial oxidant generation and antioxidant defenses during aging and in response to food restriction in the mouse. *Mech Ageing Dev*. May; 74(1-2):121-33.

575 Melov S, Hinerfeld D, Esposito L, Wallace DC. (1997). Multi-organ characterization of mitochondrial genomic rearrangements in ad libitum and caloric restricted mice show striking somatic mitochondrial DNA rearrangements with age. *Nucleic Acids Res*. Mar 1; 25(5):974-82.

576 Mattson MP. (2012). Energy intake and exercise as determinants of brain health and vulnerability to injury and disease. *Cell Metab*. Dec 5; 16(6):706-22.

577 Gillette-Guyonnet S, Secher M, Vellas B. (2013). Nutrition and neurodegeneration: epidemiological evidence and challenges for future research. *Br J Clin Pharmacol*. Mar;75(3):738-55.

578 Wikipedia. Metal Toxicity. Retrieved Dec 20 2019 from https://en.wikipedia.org/wiki/Metal_toxicity

579 Menshikova EV, Ritov VB, Fairfull L, Ferrell RE, Kelley DE, et al. (2006). Effects of exercise on mitochondrial content and function in aging human skeletal muscle. *J Gerontol* A *Biol Sci Med Sci*. Jun; 61(6):534-40.

580 Viña J, Gomez-Cabrera MC, Borras C, Froio T, Sanchis-Gomar F, et al. (2009). Mitochondrial biogenesis in exercise and in ageing. *Adv Drug Deliv Rev*. Nov 30; 61(14):1369-74.

581 Steiner JL, Murphy EA, McClellan JL, Carmichael MD, Davis JM. (2011). Exercise training increases mitochondrial biogenesis in the brain *J Appl Physiol* (1985). Oct; 111(4):1066-71.

582 Ibid. Bredesen. (2017). *The End of Alzheimer's*.

583 Dröge W, Schipper HM. (2007). Oxidative stress and aberrant signaling in aging and cognitive decline. *Aging Cell*. Jun; 6(3):361-70.

584 Mariani E, Polidori MC, Cherubini A, Mecocci P. (2005). Oxidative stress in brain aging, neurodegenerative and vascular diseases: an overview. *J Chromatogr B Analyt Technol Biomed Life Sci*. Nov 15; 827(1):65-75.

585 Niedzielska E, Smaga I, Gawlik M, Moniczewski A, Stankowicz P, et al. (2016). Oxidative Stress in Neurodegenerative Diseases. *Mol Neurobiol*. Aug; 53(6):4094-4125.

586 Suzuki M, Willcox DC, Rosenbaum MW, Willcox BJ. (2010). Oxidative stress and longevity in okinawa: an investigation of blood lipid peroxidation and tocopherol in okinawan centenarians. *Curr Gerontol Geriatr Res*. 2010; 2010:380460.

587 Tian J., Shi J., Zhang X., Wang Y. Herbal therapy: a new pathway for the treatment of Alzheimer's disease. *Alzheimers Res Ther*. 2010;2:30

588 Wang Z.Y., Liu J.G., Li H., Yang H.M. Pharmacological effects of active components of Chinese herbal medicine in the treatment of Alzheimer's disease: a review. *Am J Chin Med*. 2016;44(8):1525–1541

589 Yang W.T., Zheng X.W., Chen S., Shan C.S., Xu Q.Q., Zhu J.Z., Bao X.Y., Lin Y., Zheng G.Q., Wang Y. Chinese herbal medicine for Alzheimer's disease: clinical evidence and possible mechanism of neurogenesis. *Biochem Pharmacol*. 2017;141:143–155.

590 Pettigrew JW, Klunk WE, Panchalingam K, Kanfer JN, McClure RJ. (1995). Clinical and neurochemical effects of acetyle-L-carnitine in Alzheimer's disease. *Neurobiol Aging*. Jan-Feb;16(1):1-4.

591 Brooks JO, Yesavage JA, Carta A, Bravi D. (1998). Acetyl L-carnitine slows decline in younger patients with Alzheimer's disease: a reanalysis of a double-blind, placebo-controlled study using the trilinear approach. *Int Psychogeriatr*. Jun;10(2):193-203.

592 Zhou P, Chen Z, Zhao N, Liu D, Guo ZY, et al. (2011). Acetyl-L-carnitine attenuates homocysteine-induced Alzheimer-like histopathological and behavioral abnormalities. *Rejuvenation Res*. Dec;14(6):669-79.

[593] Malaguarnera M, Gargante MP, Cristaldi E, Colonna V, Messano M. et al. (2008) Acetyl L-carnitine (ALC) treatment in elderly patients with fatigue. *Arc Geron Geriatr.* Mar-Apr; 46(2):181-190.

[594] Jones LL, McDonald DA, Borum PR. (2010). Acylcarnitines: role in brain. *Prog Lipid Res.* Jan;49(1):61-75.

[595] Yin YY, Liu H, Cong XB, Liu Z, Wang Q, et al (2010). Acetyl-L-carnitine attenuates okadaic acid induced tau hyperphosphorylation and spatial memory impairment in rats. *J Alzheimers Dis.* 2010;19(2):735-46.

[596] Salvioli G, Neri M. (1994). L-acetylcarnitine treatment of mental decline in the elderly. *Drugs Exp Clin Res.* 1994;20(4):169-76.

[597] Ames BN, Liu J. (2004). Delaying the mitochondrial decay of aging with acetylcarnitine. *Ann N Y Acad Sci.* Nov;1033:108-16.

[598] Gavrilova SI, Kalyn IaB, Kolykhalov IV, Roshchina IF, Selezneva ND. (2011). [Acetyl-L-carnitine (carnicetine) in the treatment of early stages of Alzheimer's disease and vascular dementia]. *Zh Nevrol Psikhiatr Im S S Korsakova.* 2011;111(9):16-22.

[599] Sehgal N, Gupta A, Valli RK, Joshi SD, Mills JT, et al. (2012). Withania somnifera reverses Alzheimer's disease pathology by enhancing low-density lipoprotein receptor-related protein in liver. *Prac Natl Acad Sci U S A.* Feb 28;109(9):3510-5.

[600] Witter S, Witter R, Vilu R, Samoson A. (2018). Medical Plants and Nutraceuticals for Amyloid-B Fibrillation Inhibition. *J Alzheimers Dis Rep.* Dec 24;2(1):239-252.

[601] Kuboyama T, Tohda C, Komatsu K. (2014). Effects of Ashwagandha (Roots of Withania somnifera) on Neurodegenerative Diseases. *Biol Pharm Bull.* 2014;37(6):892-7.

[602] Jayaprakasam B, Padmanabhan K, Nair MG. (2010). Withanamides in Withania somnifera fruit protect PC-12 cells from beta-amyloid responsible for Alzheimer's disease. *Phytother Res.* Jun; 24(6):859-63.

[603] No author listed. (2004). Monograph. Withania somnifera. *Altern Med Rev.* Jun; 9(2):211-4

[604] Parihar MS, Hemnani T. (2003). Phenolic antioxidants attenuate hippocampal neuronal cell damage against kainic acid induced excitotoxicity. *J Biosci.* Feb;28(1):121-8.

[605] Uddin MS, Al Mamun A, Kabir MT, Jakaria M, Mathew B, et al. (2019). Nootropic and Anti-Alzheimer's Actions of Medicinal Plants: Molecular Insight into Therapeutic Potential to Alleviate Alzheimer's Neuropathology. *Mol Neurobiol.* Jul;56(7):4925-44.

[606] Ibid. Kyboyama. (2002). *Biol Pharm Bull.*

[607] Schliebs R, Liebmann A, Bhattacharya SK, et al. (1997). Systemic administration of defined extracts from Withania somnifera (Indian Ginseng) and Shilajit differentially affects cholinergic but not glutamatergic and GABAergic markers in rat brain. *Neurochem Int.* Feb;30(2):181-90.

[608] Wadhwa R, Konar A, Kaul SC. (2016). Nootropic potential of Ashwagandha leaves: Beyond traditional root extracts. *Neurochem Int.* May;95:109-18.

[609] Mattei R, Polotow TG, Vardaris CV, Guerra BA, Leite JR, et al. (2011). Astaxanthin limits fish oil-related oxidative insult in the anterior forebrain of Wistar rats: Putative anxiolytic effects? *Pharmacol Biochem Behav.* 2011;99:349-355.

[610] Che H, Li Q, Zhang T, Wang D, Yang L, et al. (2018). Effects of Astaxanthin and Docosahexaenoic-Acid Acylated Astaxanthin on Alzheimer's Disease in APP/PS1 Double-Transgenic Mice. *J Agric Food Chem.* May 16;66(19):4948-4957.

[611] Abdul Manap AS, Vijayabalan S, Madhavan P, Chia YY, et al. (2019). Bacopa monnieri, a Neuroprotective Lead in Alzheimer Disease: A Review on Its Properties, Mechanisms of Action, and Preclinical and Clinical Studies. *Drug Target Insights.* Jul 31;13:1177392819866412.

[612] Shinde P, Vidyasagar N, Dhulap S, Dhulap A, Hirwani R. (2015). Natural Products based P-glycoprotein Activators for Improved B-amyloid clearance in Alzheimer's Disease: An in silico Approach. *Cent Nerv Syst Agents Med Chem.* 2015;16(1):50-9.

[613] Uabundit N, Wattanathorn J, Mucimapura S, Ingkaninan K. (2010). Cognitive enhancement and neuroprotective effects of Bacopa monnieri in Alzheimer's disease model. *J Ethnopharmacol.* Jan 8;127(1):26-31.

[614] Limpeanchob N, Jaipan S, Rattanakaruna S, Phrompittayarat W, Ingkaninan K. (2008). Neuroprotective effect of Bacopa monnieri on beta-amyloid-induced cell death in primary cortical culture. *J Ethnopharmacol.* Oct 30; 120(1):112-7.

[615] Nemetcheck MD, Stierle AA, Stierle DB, Lurie DI. (2017). The Ayurvedic plant Bacopa monnieri inhibits inflammatory pathways in the brain. *J Ethnopharmacol.* Feb 2;199:92-100.

[616] Chaudhari KS, Tiwari NR, Tiwari NR, Sharma RS. (2017). Neurocognitive Effect of Nootropic Drug Brahmi (Bacopa monnieri) in Alzheimer's Disease. *Ann Neurosci.* May;24(2):111-122.

[617] Gasiorowski K, Lamer-Zarawska E, Leszek J, Parvathaneni K, Yendluri BB, et al. (2011). Flavones from root of Scutellaria baicalensis Georgi: Drugs of the future in neurodegeneration? *CNS Neurol Disord Drug Targets.* Mar;10:184-191.

[618] Sowndhararajan K, Deepa P, Kim M, Park SJ, Kim S. (2017). Baicalein as a potent neuroprotective agent: A review. *Biomed Pharmacother.* Nov;95:1021-1032.

[619] Li Y, Zhao J, Holscher C. (2017). Therapeutic Potential of Baicalein in Alzheimer's Disease and Parkinson's Disease. *CNS Drugs.* Aug:31(8):639-852.

[620] Zhou L, Tan S, Shan YL, Wang YG, Cai W, et al. (2016). Baicalein improves behavioral dysfunction induced by Alzheimer's disease in rats. *Neuropsychiatr Dis Treat.* Dec 9;12:3145-3152.

[621] Gu XH, Xu LJ, Liu ZQ, Wei B, Yang YJ, et al. (2016). The flavonoid baicalein rescues synaptic pasticity and memory deficits in a mouse model of Alzheimer's disease. *Behav Brain Res.* Sep 15;311:309-321.

[622] Wei D, Tang J, Bai W, Wang Y, Zhang Z. (2014). Ameliorative effects of baicalein on amyloid-B induced Alzheimer's disease rat model: a proteomics study. *Curr Alzheimer Res.* 2014;11(9):869-81.

[623] Chirumbolo S, Bjorklund G. (2016). Commentary: The Flavonoid Baicalein Rescues Synaptic Plasticity and Memory Deficits in a Mouse Model of Alzheimer's Disease. *Front Neurol.* Aug 29;7:141.

[624] Kelly E, Vyas P, Weber JT. (2017). Biochemical Properties and Neuroprotective Effects of Compounds in Various Species of Berries. *Molecules.* Dec 22;23(1):E26.

[625] Businaro R, Corsi M, Asprino R, Di Lorenzo C, Laskin D, et al. (2018). Modulation of Inflammation as a Way of Delaying Alzheimer's Disease Progression: The Diet's Role. *Curr Alzheimer Res.* Feb 22;15(4):33-380.

[626] Rashid K, Wachira FN, Nyabuga JN, Wanyonyi B, Murilla G, et al. (2014). Kenyan purple tea anthocyanins ability to cross the blood brain barrier and reinforce brain antioxidant capacity in mice. *Nutr Neurosci.* Ul;17(4):178-85.

[627] Tan L, Yang H, Pang W, Li H, Liu W, et al. (2017). Investigation on the Role of BDNF in the Benefits of Blueberry Extracts for the Improvement of Learning and Memory in Alzheimer's Disease Mouse Model. *J Alzheimers Dis.* 2017;56(2):629-640.

[628] Businaro R, Corsi M, Asprino R, Di Lorenzo C, Laskin D, et al. (2018). Modulation of Inflammation as a Way of Delaying Alzyeimer's Disease Progression: The Diet's Role. *Curr Alzheimer Res.* Feb 22;15(4):363-380.

[629] Bensalem J, Dudonne S, Gaudout D, Servant L, Calon F, et al. (2018). Polyphenol-rich extract from grape and blueberry attenuates cognitive decline and improves neuronal function in aged mice. *J Nutr Sci.* May 21;7:e19.

[630] Boespflug EL, Eliassen JC, Dudley JA, Shidler MD, Kalt W, et al. (2018). Enhaned neural activation with blueberry supplementation in mild cognitive impairment. *Nutr Neurosci.* May;2194):297-305.

[631] Blount PJ, Nguyen CD, McDeavitt JT. (2002). Clinical use of cholinomimetic agents: a review. *J Head Trauma Rehabil.* Aug; 17(4):314-21

[632] Gavrilova SI, Federova laB, Gantman, Kalyn laB, Kolykhalov IV. (2011). [Ceraxon (citicoline) in the treatment of the mild cognitive impairment syndrome.]. *Zh Nevrol Psikhiatr Im S S Korsakova.* 2011;111(12):16-20.

[633] Lee M, McGeer MG, McGeer PL. (2016). Quercetin, not caffeine, is a major neuroprotective component in coffee. *Neurobiol Aging.* Oct;46:113-23.

[634] Barranco Quintana J.L. et al. (2007) Alzheimer's disease and coffee: a quantitative review. *Neurol Res,* 29:91-5.

[635] Butt MS, Sultan MT. (2011). Coffee and its consumption: benefits and risks. *Crit Rev Food Sci Nutr.* Apr; 51(4):363-73.

[636] Tang M, Taghibiglou C. (2017). The Mechanisms of Action of Curcumin in Alzheimer's Disease. *J Alzheimers Dis.* 2017;58(4):1003-1016.

[637] Shehzad A, Rehman G, Lee YS (2013). Curcumin in inflammatory diseases. *Biofactors.* Jan-Feb; 39(1):69-77.

[638] Ibid. Shehzad. (2013).

[639] Kim GY, Kim KH, Lee SH, Yoon MS, Lee HJ, et al. (2005). Curcumin inhibits immunostimulatory function of dendritic cells: MAPKs and translocation of NF-kappa B as potential targets. *J Immunol.* Jun 15; 174(12):8116-24.

[640] Ibid. Shehzad. (2013).

[641] Yuan J, Liu W, Zhu H, Zhang X, Feng Y, et al. (2017). Curcumin attenuates blood-brain disruption after subarachnoid hemmorrhage in mice. J Surg Res. Jan;207:85-91.

[642] Polazzi E, Monti B. (2010). Microglia and neuroprotection: from in vitro studies to therapeutic applications. *Prog Neurobiol.* Nov; 92(3):293-315.

[643] Dong S, Zeng Q, Mitchell ES, Xiu J, Duan Y, et al. (2012). Curcumin enhances neuro genesis and cognition in aged rats: implications for transcriptional interactions related to growth and synaptic plasticity. *PloS One.* 7(2):e31211.

[644] Ng TP, Chiam PC, Lee T, Chua HC, Lim L, et al. (2006). Curry consumption and cognitive function in the elderly. *Am J Epidemiol.* Nov 1;164(9):898-906.

[645] Bigford GE, Del Rossi. (2014). Supplemental substances derived from foods as adjunctive therapeutic agents for treatment of neurodegenerative diseases and disorders. *G Adv Nutr.* Jul; 5(4):394-403.

[646] Mourtas S, Lazar AN, Markoutsa E, Duyckaerts C, Antimisiaris SG. (2014). Multifunctional nanoliposomes with curcumin-lipid derivative and brain targeting functionality with potential applications for Alzheimer disease. *Eur J Med Chem.* Jun 10;80():175-83.

[647] Serafini MM, Catanzaro M, Rosini M, Racchi M, Lanni C. (2017). Curcumin in Alzheimer's disease: Can we think to new strategies and perspectives for this molecule? *Pharmacol Res.* Oct;124:146-155.

[648] Shoba G, Joy D, Joseph T, Majeed M, Rajendran R, et al. (1998). Influence of piperine on the pharmacokinetics of curcumin in animals and human volunteers. *Planta Med.* May;64(4):353-6.

[649] Dyall SC. (2015). Long-chain omega-3 fatty acids and the brain: a reiview of the independent and shared effects of EPA, DPA, and DHA. *Front Aging Neurosci*. Apr 21;7:52.

[650] Grimm MOW, Michaelson DM, Hartmann T. (2017). Omega-3 fatty acids, lipids, and apoE lipidation in Alzheimer's disease: a rationale for multi-nutrient dementia prevention. *J Lipid Res*. Nov;58(11):2083-2101.

[651] Cardoso C, Afonso C, Bandarra N. (2016). Dietary DHA and health: cognitive function aging. *Nutr Res Rev*. Dec;29(2):281-94.

[652] Mohaibes RJ, Fiol-deRoque MA, Torres M, Ordinas M, Lopez DJ, et al. (2017). The hydroxylated form of docosahexaenoic acid (DHA-H) modifies the brain lipid composition in a model of Alzheimer's disease, improving behavioral motor function and survival. *Biochem Biophy Acta Biomembr*. Sep;1859(9 Pt B):1596-1603.

[653] Matsuoka Y, Nishi D, Tanima Y, Itakura M, et al. (2015). Serum pro-BDNF/BDNF as a treatment biomarker for respose to docosahexaenoic acid in traumatized people vulnerable to developing psychological distress. *Transl Psychiatry*. Jul 7;5:e596.

[654] Weiser MJ, Butt CM, Mohajeri MH. (2016). Docosahexaenoic Acid and Cognition throughout the Lifespan. *Nutrients*. Feb 17;8(2):99.

[655] Ibid. Grimm. (2017).

[656] Bakhtiari M, Panahi Y, Ameli J, Darvishi B. (2017). Protective effects of flavonoids against Alzheimer's disease-related neural dysfunctions. *Biomed Pharmacother*. Sep;93:218-229.

[657] Pandey KB, Rizvi SI. (2009). Plant polyphenols as dietary antioxidants in human health and disease. *Oxid Med Cell Longev*. Nov-Dec;2(5):270-278.

[658] Das S, Laskar MA, Sarker SD, Choudhury MD, Coudhury PR, et al. (2017). Prediction of Anti-Alzheimer's Activity of Flavonoids Targeting Acetylcholinesterase in silico. *Phytochem Anal*. Jul;28(4):324-331.

[659] Braidy N, Behzad S, Habtemariam S, Ahmed T, Daglia M, et al. (2017). Neuroprotective Effects of Citrus Fruit-Derived Flavonoids, Nobiletin and tangeretin in Alzheimer's and Parkinson's. *CNS Neurol Disord Drug Targets*. 2017;16(4):387-397.

[660] Wang J, Bi W, Cheng A, Freire D, Vempati P, et al. (2014). Targeting multiple pathogenic mechanisms with polyphenols for the treatment of Alzheimer's disease-experimental approach and therapeutic implications. *Front Aging Neurosci*. Mar 14;6:42.

[661] Steiner M, Li W. (2001). Aged garlic extract, a modulator of cardiovascular risk factors: a dose-finding study on the effects of AGE on platelet functions. J *Nutr*. Mar; 131(3s):980S-4S.

[662] Jeong YY, Park HJ, Cho YW, Kim EJ, Kim GT, et al. (2012). Aged red garlic extract reduces cigarette smoke extract-induced cell death in human bronchial smooth muscle cells by increasing intracellular glutathione levels. *Phytother Res*. Jan;26(1):18-25.

[663] Weiss N, Papatheodorou L, Morihara N, Hilge R, Ide N. (2013). Aged garlic extract restores nitric oxide bioavailability in cultured human endothelial cells even under conditions of homocysteine elevation. *J Ethnopharmacol*. Jan 9;145(1):162-7.

[664] Ishikawa H, Saeki T, Otani T, Suzuki T, Shimozuma K, et al. (2006). Aged garlic extract prevents a decline of NK cell number and activity in patients with advanced cancer. *J Nutr*. Mar;136(3 Suppl):816S-820S.

[665] Morioka N, Sze LL, Morton DL, Irie RF. (1993). A protein fraction from aged garlic extract enhances cytotoxicity and proliferation of human lymphocytes mediated by interleukin-2 and concanavalin A. *Cancer Immunol Immunother*. Oct;37(5):316-22.

[666] Thorajak P, Pannangrong W, Welbat JU, Chaijaroonkhanarak W, Sripanidkulchai K, et al. (2017). Effects of Aged Garlic Extract on Cholinergic, Glutamatergic and GABAergic Systems with Regard to Cognitive Impairment in Aβ-Induced Rats. *Nutrients*. Jul 1;9(7):E686.

[667] Nillert N, Pannangrong W, Weilbat JU, Chijaroonkhanarak W, Sripanidkulchai K, et al. (2017). Neuroprotective Effects of Aged Garlic Extract on Cognitive Dysfunction and Neuroinflammation Induced by β-Amyloid in Rats. *Nutrients*. Jan 3;9(1):E24.

[668] Cemil B, Gokce EC, Kahveci R, Gokce A, Aksoy N, et al. (2016). Aged Garlic Extract Attenuates Neuronal Injury in a Rat Model of Spinal Cord Ischemia/Reperfusion Injury. *J Med Food*. Jun;19(6):601-6.

[669] Griffin B, Selassie M, Gwebu ET. (2000). Effect of Aged Garlic Extract on the Cytotoxicity of Alzheimer β-Amyloid Peptide in Neuronal PC12 Cells. *Nutr Neurosci*. 2000;3(2):139-42.

[670] Ray B, Cauhan NB, Lahiri DK. (2011). The "aged garlic extract:" (AGE) and one of its active ingredients S-allyl-L-cysteine (SAC) as potential preventive and therapeutic agents for Alzheimer's disease (AD). *Curr Med Chem*. 2011;18(22):330-13.

[671] Jeong JH, Jeong HR, Jo YN, Kim HJ, Shin JH, et al. (2013). Ameliorating effects of aged garlic extracts against AB-induced neurotoxicity and cognitive impairment. *SMC Complement Altern Med*. Oct 18;13:268.

[672] Li F, Kim MR. (2019). Effect of Aged Garlic Ethyl Acetate Extract on Oxidative Stress and Cholinergic Function of Scopolamine-Induced Cognitive Impairment in Mice. *Prev Nutr Food Sci*. Jun;24(2):165-170.

[673] Ibid. Li. (2019).

[674] Nillert N, Pannangrong W, Welbat JU, Chaijaroonkhanarak W, Sripanidkulchai K, et al. (2017). Neuroprotective Effects of Aged Garlic Extract on Cognitive Dysfunction and Neuroinflammation Induced by B-Amyloid in Rats. *Nutrients*. Jan 3;9(1):E24.

[675] Azam F, Amer AM, Abulifa AR, Elzwawi MM. (2014). Ginger components as new leads for the design and development of novel multi-targeted anti-Alzheimer's drugs: a computational investigation. *Drug Des Devel Ther*. Oct 23;8:2045-59.

[676] Huh E, Lim S, Kim HG, Ha SK, Park HY, et al. (2018). Ginger fermented with Schizosaccharomyces pombe alleviates memory impairment via protecting hippocampal neuroal cells in amyloid beta(1-42) plaque injected mice. *Food Funct*. Jan 24;9(1):171-8.

[677] Lim S, Choi JG, Moon M, Kim HG, Lee W, et al. (2016). An Optimized Combination of Ginger and Peony Root Effectively Inhibits Amyloid-B Accumulation and Amyloid-B-Mediated Pathology in ABPP/PS1 Double-Transgenic Mice. *J Alzheimers Dis*. 2016;50(1):189-200.

[678] Zeng GF, Zhang ZY, Lu L, Xiao DQ, Zong SH, et al. (2013). Protective effects of ginger root extract on Alzheimer disease-induced behavioral dysfunction in rats. *Rejuvenation Res*. Apr;16(2):124-33.

[679] Mathew M, Subramanian S. (2014). In vitro evaluation of anti-Alzheimer effects of dry ginger (Zingiber officinale Roscoe) extract. *Indian J Exp Biol*. Jun;52(6):606-12.

[680] Cuya T, Baptista L, Celmar Costa Franca T. (2018). A molecular dynamics study of components of the ginger (Zingiber officinale) extract inside human acetylcholinesterase: implications for Alzheimer disease. *J Biomol Struct Dyn*. Nov;36(14):3843-3855.

[681] Tchantchou F, Lacor PN, Cao Z, Lao L, Hou Y, et al. (2009). Stimulation of neurogenesis and synaptogenesis bilobalide and quercetin via common final pathway in hippocampal neurons. *J Alz Dis*. 18(4):787-98.

[682] Yoo DY, Nam Y, Kim W, Yoo KY, Park J, et al. (2011). Effects of Gingko Biloba extract on promotion of neurogenesis in the hippocampal dentate gyrus in C57BL/6 mice. *J Vet Med Sci*. 73(1):71-6.

[683] Funakoshi H, Kanai M, Nakamura T. (2011). Modulation and alteration of anxiety-related behavior in tryptophan metabolism, promotion of neurogenesis and alteration of anxiety-related behavior n tryptophan 2,3-dioxygenase-deficient mice. *Intl J Tryptophan Res*. 4:7-18.

[684] Hou Y, Aboukhatwa MA, Lei DL, Manaye K, Khan I, et al. (2010). Antidepressant flavonols modulate BDNF and beta amyloid in neurons and hippocampus of double TgAD mice. *Neurophamarcology*. 58(6): 911-920.

[685] Surh Y. J. Molecular mechanisms of chemopreventive effects of selected dietary and medicinal phenolic substances. *Mutat Res*. 1999;428(1-2):305–27.

[686] Grzanna R, Phan P, Polotsky A, Lindmark L, Frondoza CG. (2004). Ginger extract inhibits beta-amyloid peptide-induced cytokine and chemokine expression in cultured THP-1 monocytes. *J Altern Complement Med*. Dec;10(6):1009-13.

[687] Young HY, Luo YL, Cheng HY, Hsieh WC, Liao JC, et al. (2005). Analgesic and anti-inflammatory activities of [6]-gingerol. J *Ethnopharmacol*. 2005;96(1-2):207–10.

[688] Minghetti P, Sosa S, Cilurzo F, Casiraghi A, Alberti E, et al. (2007). Evaluation of the topical anti-inflammatory activity of ginger dry extracts from solutions and plasters. *Planta Med*. Dec;73(15):1525–30

[689] Marcus D. M, Suarez-Almazor M. E. (2001). Is there a role for ginger in the treatment of osteoarthritis? *Arthritis Rheum*. 2001;44(11):2461–2

[690] Yang G, Wang Y, Sun J, Zhang K, Liu J. (2016). Ginkgo Biloba for Mild Cognitive Impairment and Alzheimer's Disease: A Systematic Review and Meta-Analysis of Randomized Controlled Trials. *Curr Top Med Chem*. 2016;16(5):520-8.

[691] Wightman EL. (2017). Potential benefits of phytochemicals against Alzheimer's disease. *Proc Nutr Soc*. May;76(2):106-112.

[692] Rege NN, Thatte UM, Dahanukar SA (1999). Adaptogenic properties of six rasayana herbs used in Ayurvedic medicine. *Phytother Res*. 1999;13:275–291

[693] Heo J.H., Lee S.T., Chu K., Oh M.J., Park H.J., Shim J.Y., Kim M. An open-label trial of Korean red ginseng as an adjuvant treatment for cognitive impairment in patients with Alzheimer's disease. *Eur J Neurol*. 2008;15:865–868

[694] Heo J.H., Lee S.T., Oh M.J., Park H.J., Shim J.Y., Chu K., Kim M. Improvement of cognitive deficit in Alzheimer's disease patients by long term treatment with Korean red ginseng. *J Ginseng Res*. 2011;35:457–461

[695] Lee S.T., Chu K., Sim J.Y., Heo J.H., Kim M. Panax ginseng enhances cognitive performance in Alzheimer disease. *Alzheimer Dis Assoc Disord*. 2008;22:222–226

[696] Hwang S.H., Shin E.J., Shin T.J., Lee B.H., Choi S.H., Kang J., Kim H.J., Kwon S.H., Jang C.G., Lee J.H. Gintonin, a ginseng-derived lysophosphatidic acid receptor ligand, attenuates Alzheimer's disease-related neuropathies: involvement of non-amyloidogenic processing. *J Alzheimer's Dis*. 2012;31:207–223

[697] Sohal RS, Orr WC. (2012). The redox stress hypothesis of aging. *Free Radic Biol Med*. Feb 1; 52(3):539-555.

[698] Ballatori N, Krance SM, Notenboom S, Shi S, Tieu K, et al. (2009). Glutathione dysregulation and the etiology and progression of human diseases. *Biol Chem*. Mar; 390(3):191-214.

[699] Rae CD, Williams SR. (2017). Glutathione in the human brain: Review of its roles and measurement by magnetic resonance spectroscopy. *Anal Biochem*. Jul 15;529:127-143.

[700] Mazzetti AP, Fiorile MC, Primavera A, Lo Bello M. (2015). Glutathione transferases and neurodegenerative diseases. *Neurochem Int*. Mar;82:10-8.

[701] Shukla D, Mandal PK, Ersland L, Gruner ER, Tripathi M, et al. (2018). Multi-Center Study on Human Brain Glutathione Conformation using Magnetic Resonance Spectroscopy. *J Alzheimers Dis*. 2018;66(2):517-532.

[702] Saharan S, Mandal PK. (2014). The emerging role of glutathione in Alzheimer's disease. *J Alzheimers Dis.* 2014;40(3):519-29.

[703] Mandal PK, Saharan S, Tripathi M, Murari G. (2015). Brain glutathione levels—a novel biomarker for mild cognitive impairment and Alzheimer's disease. *Biol Psychiatry.* Nov 15;78(10):702-10.

[704] Peter C, Braidy N, Zarka M, Welch J, Bridge W. (2015). Therapeutic approaches to modulating glutathione levels as a pharmacological strategy in Alzheimer's disease. *Curr Alzheimer Res.* 2015;12(4):298-313.

[705] Liu Y, Lukala TL, Musgrave IF, Williams DM, Dehle FC, et al. (2013). Gallic acid is the major component of grape seed extract that inhibits amyloid fibril formation. *Bioor Med Chem Lett.* Dec 1;23(23):6336-40.

[706] Ono K, Condron MM, Ho L, Wang J, Zhao W, et al. (2008). Effects of grape seed-derived polyphenols on amyloid beta protein self-assembly and cytoxicity. *J Biol Chem.* Nov 21;283(47):32176-87.

[707] Asha Devi S, Sagar Chandrasekar BK, Manjula KR, Ishii N. (2011). Grape seed proanthocyandin lowers brain oxidative stress in adult and middle-aged rats. *Exp Gerontol.* Nov;46(11):958-64.

[708] Wang J, Ho L, Zhao W, Ono K, Rosensweig C, et al. (2008). Grape-derived polyphenolics prevent Abeta oligomerization and attenuate cognitive deterioration in a mouse model of Alzheimer's disease. *J Neurosci.* Jun 18;28(25):6388-92.

[709] Ibid. Ono. (2008).

[710] Sarkaki A, Rafiereirad M, Hossini SE, Farbood Y, Motamedi F, et al. (2013). Improvement in Memory and Brain Long-term Potentiation Deficits Due to Permanent Hypoperfusion/Ischemia by Grape Seed Extract in Rats. *Iran J Basic Med Sci.* 2013 Sep;16(9):1004-10.

[711] Wang JY, Thomas P, Zhong JH, Bi FF, Kosaraju S, et al. (2009). Consumption of grape seed extract prevents amyloid-beta deposition and attenuates inflammation in brain of an Alzheimer's disease mouse. *Neurotox Res.* Jan;15(1):3-14.

[712] Nones J, E Spohr TC, Gomes FC. (2011). Hesperidin, a flavone glycoside, as mediator of neuronal survival. *Neurochem Res.* Oct; 36(10):1776-84.

[713] Nones J, Spohr TC, Gomes FC. (2012). Effects of the flavonoid hesperidin in cerebral cortical progenitors in vitro: indirect action through astrocytes. *Int J Dev Neurosci.* Jun; 30(4):303-13.

[714] Thenmozhi JA, Raja WTR, Manivasagam T, Janakiraman U, Essa MM. (2017). Hesperidin ameliorates cognitive dysfunction, oxidative stress, and apoptosis against aluminum chloride induced rat model of Alzheimer's disease. *Nutr Neurosci.* Jul;20(6):360-366.

[715] Chakraborty S, Bandyopadhyay J, Chakraborty S, Basu S. (2016). Multi-target screening mines hesperidin as a multi-potent inhibitor: Implication in Alzheimer's disease therapeutics. *Eur J Med Chem.* Oct 4;121:810-822.

[716] Bauer BA. Huperzine A: Can it treat Alzheimer's? Retrieved Oct 15 2019 from https://www.mayoclinic.org/diseases-conditions/alzheimers-disease/expert-answers/huperzine-a/faq-20058259

[717] Di Mascio P, Kaiser S, Sies H. (1989). Lycopene as the most efficient biological carotenoid singlet oxygen quencher. *Arch Biochem Biophys.* Nov 1; 274(2):532-8.

[718] Wang J, Li L, Wang Z, Cui Y, Tan X, et al. (2018). Supplementation of lycopene attenuates lipopolysaccharide-induced amyloidogenesis and cognitive impairments via mediating neuroinflammation and oxidative stress. *J Nutr Biochem.* Jun; 56():16-25.

[719] Liu CB, Wang R, Yi YF, Gao Z, Chen YZ. (2018). Lycopene mitigates B-amyloid induced inflammatory response and inhibits NF-kB signaling at the choroid plexus in early stages of Alzheimer's disease rats. *J Nutr Biochem.* Mar;53-66-71.

[720] Wang J, Wang Z, Li B, Qiang Y, Yuan T, et al. (2019). Lycopene attenuates western-diet-induced cognitive deficits via improving glycolipid metabolism dysfunction and inflammatory responses in gut-liver-brain axis. *Int J Obes* (Lond). Sep; 43(9):1735-1746.

[721] Chen D, Huang C, Chen Z. (2019). A review for the pharmacological effect of lycopene in central nervous system disorders. *Biomed Pharmacother.* Mar; 111():791-801.

[722] Veronese N, Zurlo A, Solmi M, Luchini C, Trevisan C, et al. (2016). Magnesium Status in Alzheimer's Disease: A Systematic Review. *Am J Alzheimers Dis Other Demen.* May;31(3):208-13.

[723] Zhu D, Su Y, Fu B, Xu H. (2018). Magnesium Reduces Blood-Brain Barrier Permeability and Regulates Amyloid-B Transcytosis. *Mol Neurobiol.* Sep;55(9):7118-7131.

[724] Wang YY, Zheng W, Ng CH, Ungvari GS, Wei W, et al. (2017). Meta-analysis of randomized, double-blind, placebo-controlled trials of melatonin in Alzheimer's disease. *Int J Geriatr Psychiatry.* Jan;32(1):50-57.

[725] Shukla M, Govitrapong P, Boontem P, Reiter RJ, Satayavivad J. (2017). Mechanisms of Melatonin in Alleviating Alzheimer's Disease. *Curr Neuropharmacol.* 2017;15(7):1010-1031.

[726] Lin L, Huang QX, Yang SS, Chu J, Wang JZ, et al. (2013). Melatonin in Alzheimer's disease. *Int J Mol Sci.* Jul 12;14(7):14575-93.

[727] Sulkaya S, Muggalla P, Sulkava R, Ollila HM, Peuralinna T, et al. (2018). Melatonin receptor type 1A gene linked to Alzheimer's disease in old age. *Sleep.* Jul;41(7):zsy103.

[728] Rahman MA, Abdullah N, Aminudin N. (2016). Interpretation of mushroom as a common therapeutic agent for Alzheimer's disease and cardiovascular diseases. *Crit Rev Biotechnol.* Dec;36(6):1131-1142.

729 Phan CW, David P, Naidu M, Wong KH, Sabaratnam V. (2015). Therapeutic potential of culinary-medicinal mushrooms for the management of neurodegenerative diseases: diversity, metabolite, and mechanism. *Crit Rev Biotechnol.* 2015;35(3):355-68.

730 Li IC, Lee LY, Tzeng TT, Chen WP, Chen YP, et al. (2018). Neurohealth Properties of Hericium eranceus Mycelia Enriched with Erinacines. *Behav Neurol.* May 21;2018:5802634.

731 Huang S, Mao J, Ding K, Zhou Y, Zeng X, et al. (2017). Polysaccharides from Ganoderma lucidum Promote Cognitive Function and Neural Progenitor Proliferation in Mouse Model of Alzheimer's Disease. *Stem Cell Reports.* Jan 10;8(1):84-94.

732 Baskaran A, Chua KH, Sabaratnam V, Ravishankar RM. (2017). Pleurotus giganteus (Berk. Karun & Hyde), the giant oyster mushroom inhibits NO production in PLS/H2O2 stimulated RAW 264.7 cells via STAT3 and COX-2 pathways. *BMC Complement Altern Med.* Jan 13;17(1):40.

733 Lee LY, Li IC, Chen WP, Tsai TY, Chen CC, et al. (2019). Thirteen-Week Oral Toxicity Evaluation of Erinacine A Enriched Lion's Medicinal Muchroom, Hericium erinaceus (Agaricomycetes), Mycelia in Spraque-Dawley Rats. In J Med Mushrooms. 2019;21(4):401-411.

734 Bhatt PC, Pathak S, Kumar V, Panda BP. (2018). Attenuation of neurobehavioral and neurochemical abnormalities in animal model of cognitive deficits of Alzheimer's disease by fermented soybean nanonutraceutical. *Inflammopharmacology.* Feb;26(1):105-118.

735 Almed HH, Nevein NF, Karima A, Hamza AH. (2013). Miracle enzymes serrapeptase and nattokinase mitigate neuroinflammation and apoptosis associated with Alzheimer's disease in experimental model. *WJPPS.* 2013;3:876-891.

736 Fadi NN, Ahmed HH, Booles HF, Sayed AH. (2013). Serrapeptase and nattokinase intervention for relieving Alzheimer's disease pathophysiology in rat model. *Hum Exp Toxicol.* Jul;32(7):721-35.

737 Bhatt PC, Verma A, Al-Abbasi FA, Anwar F, Kumar V, et al. (2017). Development of surface-engineered PLGA nanoparticulate-delivery system of Tet1-conjugated nattokinase enzyme for inhibition of AB40 plaques in Alzheimer's disease. *Int J Nanomedicine.* Dec 13;12:9849-8758.

738 Ibid. Bhatt. (2018).

739 Hsu RL, Lee KT, Wang JH, Lee LY, Chen RP. (2009). Amyloid-degrading ability of nattokinase from Bacillus subtilis natto. *J Agric Food Chem.* Jan 28;57(2):503-8.

740 Ibid. Bhatt. (2018).

741 Borji N, Moeini R, Memariani Z. (2018). Almond, hazelnut and walnut. Three nuts for neuroprotection in Alzheimer's disease: A neuropharmacological review of their bioactive constituents. *Pharmacol Res.* Mar;129:115-127.

742 Bahaeddin Z, Yans A, Khodagholi F, Hajimehdipoor H, Sahranavard S. (2017). Hazelnut and neuroprotection: Improved memory and hindered anxiety in response to intra-hippocampal AB injection. *Nutr Neurosci.* Jul;20(6):317-326.

743 Muthaiyah B, Essa MM, Lee M, Chauhan V, Kaur K, et al. (2014). Dietary supplementation of walnuts improves memory deficits and learning skills in transgenic mouse model of Alzheimer's disease. *J Alzheimers Dis.* 42(4):1397-405.

744 Barbaro B, Toietta G, Maggio R, Arciello M, Tarocchi M, et al. (2014). Effects of the olive-derived polyphenol oleuropein on human health. *In J Mol Sci.* Oct 14;15(10:18508-24.

745 More MI, Freitas U, Rutenberg D. (2014). Positive effects of soy lecithin-derived phosphatidylserine plus phosphatidic acid on memory, cognition, daily functioning, and mood in elderly patients with Alzheimer's disease and dementia. *Adv Ther.* Dec;31(12):1247-52.

746 Fünfgeld EW, Baggen M, Nedwidek P, Richstein B, Mistlberger G. (1989). Double-blind study with phosphatidylserine (PS) in parkinsonian patients with senile dementia of Alzheimer's type (SDAT). *Clin Biol Res.* 1989;317:1235-46.

747 Zhang YY, Yang LQ, Guo LM. (2015). Effect of phosphtidylersine on memory in patients and rats with Alzheimer's disease. *Genet Mol Res.* Aug 10;14(3):9325-33.

748 Kuboyama T, Hirotsu K, Arai T, Yamasaki H, Tohda C. (2017). Polygalae Radix Extract Prevents Axonal Degeneration and Memory Deficits in a Transgenic Mouse Model of Alzheimer's Disease. *Front Pharmacol.* Nov 14;8:805.

749 Cao C, Xiao J, Liu M, Ge Z, Huang R, et al. (2018). Active components, derived from Kai-xin-san, a herbal formula, increase the expressions of neurotrophic factor NGF and BDNF on mouse astrocyte primary cultures via cAMP-dependent signaling pathway. *J Ethnopharmacol.* Oct 5;224:554-562.

750 Castillo S. (2015). Pomegranate Health Benefits: The Fruit Helps Protect Against Plaque, Hunger, and Certain Cancers. *Medical Daily.* Jun 26, 2015.

751 Hartman RE, Shah A, Fagan AM, Schwetye KE, Parsadanian M, et al. (2006) Pomegranate juice decreases amyloid load and improves behavior in a mouse model of Alzheimer's disease. *Neurobiol Dis* 24: 506-515.

752 Yuan T, Ma H, Liu W, Niesen DB, Shah N, et al. (2016). Pomegranate's Neuroprotective Effects against Alzheimer's Disease are Mediated by Urolithins, Its Ellagitannin-Gut Microbial Derived Metabolites. *ACS Chem Neurosci.* Jan20;7(1):26-33.

753 Khan MM, Kempuraj D, Thangavel R, Zaheer A. (2013). Protection of MPTP-induced neuroinflammation and neurodegeneration by Pycnogenol. *Neurochem Int.* Mar;62(4):379-88.

[754] Simpson T, Kure C, Stough C. (2019). Assessing the Efficacy and Mechanisms of Pycnogenol® on Cognitive Aging From In Vitro Animal and Human Studies. *Front Pharmacol.* Jul 3;10:694.

[755] Sawmiller D, Li S, Mori T, Habib A, Rongo D, et al. (2017). Beneficial effects of a pyrroloquinolinequinone-containing dietary formulation on motor deficiency, cognitive decline and mitochondrial dysfunction in a mouse model of Alzheimer's disease. *Heliyon.* Apr 4;3(4):e00279.

[756] Hynd MR, Scott HL, Dodd PR. (2004). Glutamate-mediated excitotoxicity and neurodegeneration in Alzheimer's disease. *Neurochem Int.* Oct;45(5):583-95.

[757] Silva B, Oliveira PJ, Dias A, Malva JO. (2008). Quercetin, kaempferol and biapigenin from Hypericum perforatum are neuroprotective against excitotoxic insults. *Neurotox Res.* May-Jun;13(3-4):265-79.

[758] Yang EJ, Kim GS, Kim JA, Song KS. (2013). Protective effects of onion-derived quercetin on glutamate-mediated hippocampal neuronal cell death. *Pharmacogn Mag.* Oct;9(36):302-8.

[759] Dong XX, Wang Y, Qin ZH. (2009). Molecular mechanisms of excitotoxicity and their relevance to pathogenesis of neurodegenerative diseases. *Acta Pharmacologica Sinica.* Apr;30(4):379-87.

[760] Moussa C, Hebron M, Huang X, Ahn J, Rissman RA, et al. (2017). Resveratrol regulates neuro-inflammation and induces adaptive immunity in Alzheimer's disease. *JNeuroinflammation.* Jan 3;14:1.

[761] Turner RS, Thomas RG, Craft S, van Dyck CH, Mintzer J, et al. (2015). A randomized, double-blind, placebo-controlled trial of resveratrol for Alzheimer disease. Neurology. Oct 20;85:1383–1391.

[762] Georgetown University Medical Center. (2016, July 27). Resveratrol appears to restore blood-brain barrier integrity in Alzheimer's disease. ScienceDaily. Retrieved January 6, 2021 from www.sciencedaily.com/releases/2016/07/160727140041.htm.

[763] Marambaud P, Zhao H, Davies P. (2005). Resveratrol promotes clearance of Alzheimer's disease amyloid beta peptides. *J Biol Chem.* Nov 11;280(45):37377-82.

[764] Savaskan E, Olivieri G, Meier F, Seifritz E, Wirz-Justis A, et al. (2003). Red wine ingredient resveratrol protects from beta-amyloid neurotoxicity. *Gerontology.* Nov-Dec;49(6):380-3.

[765] Lee JE Song J, Cheon SY, Jung W, Lee WT. (2014). Resveratrol induces the expression of interleukin-10 and brain-derived neurotrophic factor in BV2 microglia under hypoxia. *Int J Mol Sci.* 2014 Sep 2; 15(9):15512-29.

[766] Sawda C, Moussa C, Turner RS. (2017). Resveratrol for Alzheimer's disease. *Ann N Y Acad Sci.* Sep;1403(1):142-9.

[767] Ibid. Sawda. (2017).

[768] Ahmed T, Javed S, Javed S, Tariq A, Samec D, et al. (2017). Resveratrol and Alzheimer's Disease: Mechanistic Insights. *Mol Neurobiol.* May;54(4):2622-2635.

[769] Kou X, Chen N. (2017). Resveratrol as a Natural Autophagy Regulator for Prevention and Treatment of Alzheimer's Disease. *Nutrients.* Aug 24;9(9):E927.

[770] Ibid. Wightman. (2017).

[771] Lopresti AL. (2017). Salvia (Sage):A Review of its Potential Cognitive-Enhancing and Protective Effects. *Drgus R D.*, Mar;17(1):53-64.

[772] Zhang XZ, Qian SS, Zhang YJ, Wang RQ. (2016). Salvia miltiorrhiza: A source for anti-Alzheimer's disease drugs. *Pharm Biol.* 2016;54(1):18-24.

[773] Park SE, Sapkota K, Choi JH, Kim MK, Him YH, et al. (2014). Rutin from Dendropanax morbifera Leveille protects human dopaminergic cells against rotenone induced cell injury through inhibiting JNK and p38 MAPK signaling. *Neurochemical Res.* Apr;39(4):707-18.

[774] Magalingam KB, Radhakrishnan A, Haleagrahara N. (2013). Rutin, a bioflavonoid antioxidant protects rat pheochromocytoma (PC-12) cells against 6-hydroxydopamine (6-OHDA)-induced neurotoxicity. *Int J Mol Med.* Jul;23(1):235-40.

[775] Wang YB, Ge ZM, Kang WQ, Lian ZX, Yao J, Zhou CY. (2015). Rutin alleviates diabetic cardiomyopathy in a rat model of type 2 diabetes. *Exp Ther Med.* Feb;9(2):451-455.

[776] Ibid. Park. (2014). *Neurochemical Res.*

[777] Yu XL, Li YN, Zhang H, Su YJ, Zhou WW, et al. (2015). Rutin inhibits amylin-induced neurocytotoxicity and oxidative stress. *Food Funct.* Oct;6(10):3296-306.

[778] Enogieru AB, Haylett W, Hiss DC, Bardien S, Ekpo OE. (2018). Rutin as a Potent Antioxidant: Implications for Neurodegenerative Disorders. *Oxid Med Cell Longev.* Jun 27;2018:6241017.

[779] Hablemariam S. (2016). Rutin as a Natural Therapy for Alzheimer's Disease: Insights into its Mechanisms of Action. *Curr Med Chem.* 2016;23(9):860-73.

[780] Akhondzadeh S, Shafiee Sabet M, Harichian MH, Togha M, Cheraghmakani H, et al. (2010). A 22-week, multicenter, randomized, double-blind controlled trial of Crocus sativus in the treatment of mild-to-moderate Alzheimer's disease. *Psychopharmacology (Berl).* Jan;207(4):637-43.

[781] Hatziagapiou K, Kakouri E, Lambrou GI, Bethanis K, Tarantilis PA. (2019). Antioxidant Properties of Crocus Sativus L. and Its Constituents and Relevance to Neurodegenerative Diseases; Focus on Alzheimer's and Parkinson's Disease. *Curr Neuropharmacol.* 2019;17(4):377-402.

[782] Chen C, Xia s, He J, Lu G, Xie Z, et al. (2019). Roles of taurine in cognitive function of physiology, pathology, and toxication. *Life Sci.* Aug 15;231:116584.

[783] Jang H, Lee S, Choi SL, Kim HY, Baek S, Kim Y. (2017). Taurine Directly Binds to Oligomeric Amyloid-B and Recovers Cognitive Deficits in Alzheimer Model Mice. *Adv Exp Med Biol.* 2017;975 Pt 1:233-241.

[784] Wakabayashi C, Numakawa T, Ninomiya M, Chiba S, Kunugi H. (2012). Behavioral and molecular evidence for psychotropic effects in L-theanine. *Psychopharmacology* (Berl). Feb; 219(4):1099-109.

[785] Tamano H, Fukura K, Suzuki M, Sakamoto K, Yokogoshi H, et al. (2014). Advantageous effect of theanine intake on cognition. *Nutr Neurosci.* Nov; 17(6):279-83.

[786] Kakuda T, Nozawa A, Sugimoto A, Niino H. (2002). Inhibition by theanine of binding of [3H]AMPA, [3H]kainate, and [3H]MDL 105,519 to glutamate receptors. *Biosci Biotechnol Biochem.* Dec; 66(12):2683-6.

[787] Kakuda T. (2011). Neuroprotective effects of theanine and preventive effects on cognitive dysfunction. *Pharmacol Res.* Aug;64(2):162-8.

[788] Di X, Yan J, Zhao Y, Zhang J, Shi Z, et al. (2010). L-theanine protects the APP (Swedish mutation) transgenic SH-SY5Y cell against glutamate-induced excitotoxicity via inhibition of the NMDA receptor pathway. *Neuroscience.* Jul 14; 168(3):778-86.

[789] Hidese S, Ogawa S, Ota M, Ishida I, Yasukawa Z, et al. Effects of l-theanine administration on stress-related symptoms and cognitive functions in healthy adults: A randomized controlled trial. Nutrients. 2019;11(10):2362.

[790] Park S, Kim DS, Kang S, Kim HJ. (2018). The combination of luteolin and l-theanine improved Alzheimer disease-like symptoms by potentiating hippocampal insulin signaling and decreasing neuroinflammation and norepinephrine degradation in amyloid-B-infused rats. *Nutr Res.* Dec;60:116-131.

[791] Zhu G, Yang S, Xie Z, Wan X. (2018). Synaptic modification by L-theanine, a natural constituent in green tea, rescues the impairment of hippocampal long-term potentiation and memory in AD mice. *Neuropharmacology.* Aug;138:331-340.

[792] Ali AA, Ahmed HI, Khaleel SA, Abu-Elfotuh K. (2019). Vinpocetine mitigates aluminum-induced cognitive impairment in socially isolated rats. *Physiol Behav.* Sep 1;208:112571.

[793] Ali AA, Abo El-Ella DM, El-Emam SZ, Shahat AS, El-Sayed RM. (2019). Physical & mental activities enhance the neuroprotective effect of inpocetine & coenzyme Q10 combination against Alzheimer & bone remodeling in rats. *Life Sci.* Jul 15;229:21-35.

[794] Heckman PR, Wouters C, Prickaerts J. (2015). Phosphodiesterase inhibitors as a target for cognition enhancement in aging and Alzheimer's disease: a translational overview. *Curr Pharm Des.* 2015;21(3):317-31.

[795] Landel V, Annweiler C, Millet P, Morelio M, Feron F. (2016). Vitamin D, Cognition and Alzheimer's Disease: The Therapeutic Benefit is in the D-tails. *J Alzheimers Dis.* May 11;53(2):419-44.

[796] Lakey-Beitia J, Doens D, Jagadeesh Kumar D, Murillo E, Fernandez PL, et al. (2017). Anti-amyloid aggregation activity of novel carotenoids: implications for Alzheimer's drug discovery. *Clin Interv Aging.* May 15;12:815-822.

[797] Min JY, Min KB. (2014). Serum lycopene, lutein and zeaxanthin, and the risk of Alzheimer's disease mortality in older adults. *Dement Geriatr Cogn Disord.* 2014;37(3-4):246-56.

[798] Hammond BR Jr, Miller LS, Bello MO, Lindbergh CA, et al. (2017). Effects of Lutein/Zeaxanthin Supplementation on the Cognitive Function of Community Dwelling Older Adults: A Randomized, Double-Masked, Placebo-Controlled Trial. *Front Aging Neurosci.* 2017; 9: 254.

[799] *J Alzheimers Dis.* 2015;44(4):1157-69. doi: 10.3233/JAD-142265. The impact of supplemental macular carotenoids in Alzheimer's disease: a randomized clinical trial. Nolan JM1, Loskutova E1, Howard A2, Mulcahy R3, Moran R1, Stack J1, Bolger M3, Coen RF4, Dennison J1, Akuffo KO1, Owens N1, Power R1, Thurnham D5, Beatty S1.

[800] De Lau LM, Breteler MM. (2006). Epidemiology of Parkinson's disease. *Lancet Neuro.* 5;6:525–535, 2006.

[801] Malek N, Grosset DG. (2015). Medication adherence in patients with Parkinson's disease. *CNS Drugs.* 29:47-53.

[802] Ding H, Huang Z, Chen M, Wang C, Chen X, et al. (2016). Identification of a panel of five serum miRNAs as a biomarker for Parkinson's disease. *Parkinsonism Relat Disord.* 2016;22:68-73.

[803] Kessler II. (1972). Epidemiologic studies of Parkinson's disease: II. A hospital-based survey. *Am J Epidemiol.* Apr;95(4):308-18.

[804] Schoenberg BS, Osuntokun BO, Adeuja AOG, et al. (1985). Comparison of the prevalence of Parkinson's disease in the biracial population of Copiah County, Mississippi. *Neur.* 35:841-845.

[805] Poewe W, (2006). The natural history of Parkinson's disease. *J Neurol.* 253;7(supp): 2–6.

[806] Sita G, Hrelia P, Tarozzi A, Morroni F. (2016). Isothiocyanates are promising compounds against oxidative stress, neuroinflammation and cell death that may benefit neurodegeneration in Parkinson's Disease. *Int J Mol Sci.* 2016;17(9).

[807] Bernheimer H, Birkmayer W, Hornykiewicz O, Jellinger K, Seitelberg F. (1973). Brain dopamine and the syndromes of Parkinson and Huntington. *J Neurol Sci.* 1973 Dec;20(4):415-55.

[808] Muller LMTM, Bohnen NI. (2013). Cholinergic Dysfunction in Parkinson's Disease. *Curr Neurol Neurosci Rep*. Sep;13(9):377.

[809] Braak H, Del Tredici K, Rüb U, de Vos RA, Jansen Steur EN, et al. (2003). Staging of brain pathology related to sporadic Parkinson's disease. *Neurobiol Aging*. Mar-Apr; 24(2):197-211.

[810] Conway KA, Lee SJ, Rochet JC, Ding TT, Williamson RE, et al. (2000). Acceleration of oligomerization, not fibrillization, is a shared property of both alpha-synuclein mutations linked to early-onset Parkinson's disease: implications for pathogenesis and therapy. *Proc Natl Acad Sci USA*. Jan 18;97(2):571-6.

[811] Bohnen NI, Kaufer DI, Ivanco LS, Lopresti B, Koeppe RA, et al. (2003). Cortical cholinergic function is more severely affected in parkinsonian dementia than in Alzheimer disease: an in vivo positron emission tomographic study. *Arch Neurol*. Dec; 60(12):1745-8.

[812] Bohnen NI, Muller MLTM. (2018). Imaging in Movement Disorders: Imaging Methodology and Applications in Parkinson's Disease. *Internal R Neurobio*. 141:131-172.

[813] Genetics Home Reference. PRKN gene. Retrieved Jun 27 2019 from https://ghr.nlm.nih.gov/gene/PRKN.

[814] Li JQ, Tan L, Yu JT. (2014). The role of the LRRK2 gene in Parkinsonism. *Mol Neurodegener*. 9:47.

[815] Calderon-Garciduenas L, Azzarelli B, Acuna H, Garcia R, Gambling TM, Osnaya N, et al. (2002). Air pollution and brain damage. *Toxicol Pathol*. 2002 May-Jun;30(3):373-89.

[816] Calderon-Garciduenas L, Reynoso-Robles R, Vargas-Martinez J, Gomez-Maqueo-Chew A, Parez-Guille B. (2016). Prefrontal white matter pathology in air pollution exposed Mexico City young urbanites and their potential impact on neurovascular unit dysfunction and the development of Alzheimer's disease. *Environ Res*. 2016 Apr;146:404-17.

[817] Calderon-Garciduenas L, Leray F, Heydarpour P, Torres-Jardon R, Reis J. (2016). Air pollution, a rising environmental risk factor for cognition, neuroinflammation and neurodegeneration: The clinical impact on children and beyond. *Rev Neurol (Paris)*. 2016 Jan;172(1):69-80.

[818] Calderon-Garciduenas L, Reynoso-Robles R, Gonzalez-Maciel A. (2019). Combustion and friction-derived nanoparticl es and industrial-sourced nanoparticles: The culprit of Alzheimer and Parkinson's diseases. *Environ Res*. 2019 Jul 5;176:108574.

[819] Tata AM, Velluto L, D'Angelo C, Reale M. (2014). Cholinergic system dysfunction and neurodegenerative diseases: cause or effect? *CNS Neurol Disord Drug Targets*. 13(7):1294-303.

[820] Andreoulakis E, Hyphantis T, Kandylis D, Lacovides A. (2012). Depression in diabetes mellitus: a comprehensive review. *Hippokratia*. Jul;16(3):205-14.

[821] Huang C, Chung C, Leu H, Lin LY, Chiu CC, et al. (2014). Diabetes mellitus and the risk of Alzheimer's disease: a nationwide population-based study. *PloS One*. Jan 29;9(1):e87095.

[822] Chew BH, Sherina MS, Hassan NH. (2015). Association of diabetes-related distress, depression, medication adherence, and health-related quality of life with glycated hemoglobin, blood pressure, and lipids in adult patients with type 2 diabetes: a cross-sectional study. *Ther Clin Risk Manag*. 2015;11:669-81

[823] Tinkhauser G, Pogosyan A, Little S, Beudel M, Herz DM, et al. (2017). The modular effect of adaptive deep brain stimulation on beta bursts in Parkinson's disease. *Brain*. Apr; 140(4): 1053–1067.

[824] Rocha EM, De Miranda B, Sanders LH. (2018). Alpha-synuclein: Pathology, mitochondrial dysfunction and neuroinflammation in Parkinson's disase. *Neurobiol Dis*. Jan;109(Pt B):249-257.

[825] Ibid. Schapira. (2013).

[826] Ibid. Schapira. (2013).

[827] Yamamoto A, Yue Z. (2014). Autography and its normal pathogenic states in the brain. *Annu Rev Neurosci*. 37:55-78.

[828] Ariosa AR Klionsky DJ. (2016). Autography core machinery: overcoming spatial barriers in neurons. *J Mol Med* (Berl). 94: 1217-1227.

[829] Kulkami VV, Maday S (2018). Compartment-specific dynamics and functions of autography in neurons. *Dev Neurobiol*. 78:298-310.

[830] Cushman M, Johnson BS, King OD, Gitler AD, Shorter J. (2010). Prionlike disorders: blurring the divide between transmissibility and infectivity. *J Cell Sci*, 123:1191-1201.

[831] Nagatsu T. (2002). Amine-related neurotoxins in Parkinson's disease: past, present, and future. *Neurotoxicol Teratol*. Sep-Oct;24(5):565-9.

[832] De Vivo G, Gentile V. (2008). Transglutaminase-catalyzed post-translational modifications of proteins in the nervous system and their possible involvement in neurodegenerative diseases. *CNS Neurol Disord Drug Targets*. 2008 Oct;7(4):370-5.

[833] Jin X, Liu MY, Zhang DF, Gao H. Wei MJ. (2018). Elevated circulating magnesium levels in patients with Parkinson's disease: a meta-analysis. *Neurospychiatr Dis Treat*. Nov 19;14:3159-3158.

[834] Endo R. Saito T, Asada A, Kawahara H, Ohshima T, Hisanaga SI. (2009). Commitment of 1-methyl-4-phenylpyrinidinium ion-induced neuronal cell deathby proteasome-mediated degradation of p35 cyclin-dependent kinase 5 activator. *J Biol Chem*. 284;38:26029–26039.

[835] Hirsch EC, Jenner P, Przedborski S. (2013). Pathogenesis of Parkinson's disease. *Mov Disord*. Jan;28(1):24-30.

[836] Schrag M, Mueller C, Zabel M, Crofton A, Kirsch WM, Ghribi O, et al. Oxidative stress in blood in Alzheimer's disease and mild cognitive impairment: a meta-analysis. *Neurobiol Dis*. 2013;59:100–110.

837 Sita G, Hrelia P, Tarozzi A, Morroni F. (2016). Isothiocyanates are promising compounds against oxidative stress, neuroinflammation and cell death that may benefit neurodegeneration in Parkinson's Disease. *Int J Mol Sci*. 2016;17(9).

838 Peterson LJ, Flood PM. (2012) Oxidative stress and microglial cells in Parkinson's disease. *Mediators Inflamm*. 2012:401264.

839 Belaidi AA, Bush AI. (2016). Iron neurochemistry in Alzheimer's disease and Parkinson's disease: targets for therapeutics. *J Neurochem*. Oct;139 Suppl 1:179-197.

840 Schapira AH, Olanow CW. (2004). Neuroprotection in Parkinson disease: mysteries, myths, and misconceptions. *JAMA*. Jan 21; 291(3):358-64.

841 Boyko AA, Troyanova NI, Kovalenko EI, Sapozhnikov AM. (2017). Similarity and Differences in Inflammation-Related Characteristics of the Peripheral Immune System of Patients with Parkinson's and Alzheimer's Diseases. *Int J Mol Sci*. Dec 6;18(12).

842 De Virgilio A, Greco A, Fabbrini G, Inghilleri M, Rizzo MI, et al. (2016). Parkinson's disease: Autoimmunity and neuroinflammation. *Autoimmun Rev*. Oct;15(10):1005-11.

843 Desai V, Kaler SG. (2008). Role of copper in human neurological disorders. *Am J Clin Nutr*. Sep; 88(3):855S-8S.

844 Shaw CA, Tomljenovic L. (2013). Aluminum in the central nervous system (CNS): toxicity in humans and animals, vaccine adjuvants, and autoimmunity. *Immunol Res*. Jul; 56(2-3):304-16.

845 Chen P, Chakraborty S, Peres TV, Bowman AB, Aschner M. (2015). Manganese-induced Neurotoxicity: From C. elegans to Humans. *Toxicol Res (Camb)*. Mar 1; 4(2):191-202.

846 Kamel F, Umbach DM, Hu H, Munsat TL, Shefner JM. (2005). Lead exposure as a risk factor for amyotrophic lateral sclerosis. *Neurodegener Dis*. 2(3-4):195-201.

847 Kamel F, Umbach DM, Lehman TA, Park LP, Munsat TL, et al. (2003). Amyotrophic lateral sclerosis, lead, and genetic susceptibility: polymorphisms in the delta-aminolevulinic acid dehydratase and vitamin D receptor genes. *Health Perspect*. Aug; 111(10):1335-9.

848 Weisskopf MG, Weuve J, Nie H, Saint-Hillaire MH, Sudarsky L, et al. (2010). Association of Cumulative Lead Exposure with Parkinson's Disease. *Environ Health Perspect*. Nov;118(11):1609-13.

849 Mischley LK, Lau RC, Bennett RD. (2017). Role of Diet and Nutritional Supplements in Parkinson's Disease Progression. *Oxid Med Cell Longev*. 2017: 6405278.

850 Chen H, Zhang SM, Hernán MA, Willett WC, Ascherio A. (2002). Diet and Parkinson's disease: a potential role of dairy products in men. *Ann Neurol*. Dec; 52(6):793-801.

851 Kyrozis A, Ghika A, Stathopoulos P, Vassilopoulos D, Trichopoulos D, et al. (2013). Dietary and lifestyle variables in relation to incidence of Parkinson's disease in Greece. *J Epidemiol*. Jan; 28(1):67-77.

852 Chen H, O'Reilly E, McCullough ML, Rodriguez C, Schwarzschild MA, Calle EE, et al. (2007). Consumption of dairy products and risk of Parkinson's disease. *Am J Epidemiol*. May 1; 165(9):998-1006.

853 Ibid. Chen. (2002).

854 Park M, Ross GW, Petrovitch H, White LR, Masaki KH, et al. (2005). Consumption of milk and calcium in midlife and the future risk of Parkinson disease. *Neurology*. Mar 22; 64(6):1047-51.

855 Kyrozis A, Ghika A, Stathopoulos P, Vassilopoulos D, Trichopoulos D, et al. (2013). Dietary and lifestyle variables in relation to incidence of Parkinson's disease in Greece. *Eur J Epidemiol*. Jan; 28(1):67-77.

856 Le Corre L, Besnard P, Chagnon MC. (2015). BPA, an energy balance disruptor. *Crit Rev Food Sci Nutr*. 55(6):769-77.

857 Campdelacreu J. (2014). Parkinson disease and Alzheimer disease: environmental risk factors. *Neurologia*. Nov-Dec; 29(9):541-9.

858 Bonaz BL, Bernstein CN. (2013). Brain-gut interactions in inflammatory bowel disease. *Gastroenterology*. Jan; 144(1):36-49.

859 Dinan TG, Cryan JF. (2013). Melancholic microbes: a link between gut microbiota and depression? *Neurogastroenterol Motil*. Sep; 25(9):713-9.

860 Hsiao EY, McBride SW, Hsien S, Sharon G, Hyde ER, et al. (2013). Microbiota modulate behavioral and physiological abnormalities associated with neurodevelopmental disorders. *Cell*. Dec 19; 155(7):1451-63.

861 Borre YE, O'Keeffe GW, Clarke G, Stanton C, Dinan TG, et al. (2014). Microbiota and neurodevelopmental windows: implications for brain disorders. *Trends Mol Med*. Sep; 20(9):509-18.

862 Choi HK, Liu S, Curhan G. (2005). Intake of purine-rich foods, protein, and dairy products and relationship to serum levels of uric acid: the Third National Health and Nutrition Examination Survey. *Arthritis Rheum*. Jan; 52(1):283-9.

863 Weisskopf MG, O'Reilly E, Chen H, Schwarzschild MA, Ascherio A. (2007). Plasma urate and risk of Parkinson's disease. *Am J Epidemiol*. Sep 1; 166(5):561-7.

864 Schlesinger I, Schlesinger N. (2008). Uric acid in Parkinson's disease *Mov Disord*. Sep 15; 23(12):1653-7.

865 Andreadou E, Nikolaou C, Gournaras F, Rentzos M, Boufidou F, et al. (2009). Serum uric acid levels in patients with Parkinson's disease: their relationship to treatment and disease duration. *Clin Neurol Neurosurg*. 2009 Nov; 111(9):724-8.

[866] Shen C, Guo Y, Luo W, Lin C, Ding M. (2013). Serum urate and the risk of Parkinson's disease: results from a meta-analysis *Can J Neurol Sci*. Jan; 40(1):73-9.

[867] Ibid. Schlesinger. (2008).

[868] Ibid. Shen. (2013).

[869] O'Reilly EJ, Gao X, Weisskopf MG, Chen H, Schwarzschild MA, et al. (2010). Plasma urate and Parkinson's disease in women. *Am J Epidemiol*. Sep 15; 172(6):666-70.

[870] Ragonese P, Salemi G, Morgante L, Aridon P, Epifanio A, et al. (2003). A case-control study on cigarette, alcohol, and coffee consumption preceding Parkinson's disease. *Neuroepidemiology*. Sep-Oct; 22(5):297-304.

[871] Liu R, Guo X, Park Y, Wang J, Huang X, et al. (2013). Alcohol Consumption, Types of Alcohol, and Parkinson's Disease. *PLoS One*. 8(6):e66452.

[872] Eriksson AK, Lofving S, Callaghan RC, Allebeck P. (2013). Alcohol use disorders and risk of Parkinson's disease: findings from a Swedish national cohort study 1972-2008. *BMC Neurol*. Dec 5;13:190.

[873] Malik VS, Schulze MB, Hu FB. (2006). Intake of sugar-sweetened beverages and weight gain: a systematic review. *Am J Clin Nutr*. Aug; 84(2):274-88.

[874] Maher TJ, Wurtman R. (1987). Possible neurologic effects of aspartame, a widely used food additive. *J Environ Health Perspect*. Nov; 75():53-7.

[875] Rycerz K, Jaworska-Adamu JE. (2013). Effects of aspartame metabolites on astrocytes and neurons. *Folia Neuropathol*. 51(1):10-7.

[876] Plotegher N, Bubacco L. (2016). Lysines, Achilles' heel in alpha-synuclein conversion to a deadly neuronal endotoxin. *Ageing Res Rev*. Mar; 26():62-71.

[877] Shamoto-Nagai M, Maruyama W, Hashizume Y, Yoshida M, Osawa T, et al. (2007). In parkinsonian substantia nigra, alpha-synuclein is modified by acrolein, a lipid-peroxidation product, and accumulates in the dopamine neurons with inhibition of proteasome activity. *J Neural Transm* (Vienna). 114(12):1559-67.

[878] Stolzenberg E, Berry D, Yang, Lee EY, Kroemer A, et al. (2017). A Role for Neuronal Alpha-Synuclein in Gastrointestinal Immunity. *J Innate Immun*. 9(5):456-463.

[879] Robb, A. (2018). *Why We Dream: The Transformative Power of Our Nightly Journey*. (p. 162). Boston, MA: Houghton Mifflin Harcourt.

[880] Stefani A, Hogl B. (2019). Sleep in Parkinson's Disease. *Neuropsychopharmacology*. Jun 24.

[881] Gardner RC, Byers AL, Barnes DE, Li Y, Boscardin J, et al. (2018). Mild TBI and risk of Parkinson disease: Chronic Effects of Neurotrauma Consortium Study. *Neurology*. May 15;90(20):e1771-e1779.

[882] Wikipedia. Signs and Symptoms of Parkinson's Disease. Retrieved Dec 29 2019 from https://en.m.wikipedia.org/wiki/Signs_and_symptoms_of_Parkinson%27s_disease.

[883] Ahlskog JE, Muenter MD. (2001). Frequency of levodopa-related dyskinesias and motor fluctuations as estimated from the cumulative literature. *Mov Disord*. May; 16(3):448-58.

[884] Miyawaki E, Lyons K, Pahwa R, Tröster AI, Hubble J, et al. (1997). Motor complications of chronic levodopa therapy in Parkinson's disease. *Clin Neuropharmacol*. Dec; 20(6):523-30.

[885] O'Sullivan SS, Evans AH, Lees AJ. (2009). Dopamine dysregulation syndrome: an overview of its epidemiology, mechanisms and management. *CNS Drugs*. 2009;23(2):157-70.

[886] Warren N, O'Gorman C, Lehn A, Siskind D. (2017). Dopamine dysregulation syndrome in Parkinson's disease: a systemic review of published cases. *J Neurol Neurosurg Psychiatry*. Dec;88(12):1060-1064.

[887] Kakish J, Allen KJH, Harkness TA, Krol ES, Lee JS. (2016). Novel Dimer Compounds That Bind a-synuclean Can Rescue Cell Growth in a Yeast Model Overexpressing a-Synuclein. *ACS Chem Neurosci*, Sep 12;7(12):1671-1680.

[888] Maher P. (2017). Protective effects of fisetin and berry flavonoids in Parkinson's disease. *Food Funct*. Sep 20;8(9):3033-3042.

[889] Dauncey MJ, Bicknell R. (1999). Nutrition and neurodevelopment: mechanisms of developmental dysfunction and disease in later life. *J Nutr Res Rev*. Dec; 12(2):231-53.

[890] Dauncey M. (2012). Recent advances in nutrition, genes and brain health. *J Proc Nutr Soc*. Nov; 71(4):581-91.

[891] Gao X, Chen H, Fung TT, Logroscino G, Schwarzschild MA, et al. (2007). Prospective study of dietary pattern and risk of Parkinson disease. *Am J Clin Nutr*. Nov; 86(5):1486-94.

[892] Okubo H, Miyake Y, Sasaki S, Murakami K, Tanaka K, et al. (2012). Dietary patterns and risk of Parkinson's disease: a case-control study in Japan. *Eur J Neurol*. May; 19(5):681-8.

[893] Liu RH. (2003). Health benefits of fruit and vegetables are from additive and synergistic combinations of phytochemicals. *Am J Clin Nutr*. Sep; 78(3 Suppl):517S-520S.

[894] Miyake Y, Fukushima W, Tanaka K, Sasaki S, Kiyohara C, et al. (2011). Dietary intake of antioxidant vitamins and risk of Parkinson's disease: a case-control study in Japan. *Eur J Neurol*. Jan; 18(1):106-13.

[895] Gao X, Cassidy A, Schwarzschild MA, Rimm EB, Ascherio A. (2012). Habitual intake of dietary flavonoids and risk of Parkinson disease. *Neurology*. Apr 10; 78(15):1138-45.

[896] Hu G, Bidel S, Jousilahti P, Antikainen R, Tuomilehto J. (2007). Coffee and tea consumption and the risk of Parkinson's disease. *Mov Disord*. Nov 15; 22(15):2242-8.

[897] Alcalay RN, Gu Y, Mejia-Santana H, Cote L, Marder KS, et al. (2012). The association between Mediterranean diet adherence and Parkinson's disease. *Mov Disord*. May; 27(6):771-4.

[898] Ibid. Alcalay. (2012).

[899] Wlodarek D. (2019). Role of Ketogenic Diets in Neurodegenerative Diseases (Alzheimer's Disease and Parkinson's Disease). *Nutrients*. Jan;11(1):169.

[900] Neth MJ, Mintz A, Whitlow C, Jung Y, Solingapuram SK, et al. (2019). Modified ketogenic diet is associated with improved cerebrospinal fluid biomarker profile, cerebral perfusion, and cerebral ketone body uptake in older adults at risk for Alzheimer's disease: a pilot study. *Neurobiol Aging*. Sep 26;S0197-4580.

[901] WebMD. Eating Right with Parkinson's Disease. Retrieved Jun 10 2019 from https://www.webmd.com/parkinsons-disease/guide/eating-right-parkinsons#1.

[902] Zhang H, Jia H, Liu J, Ao N, Yan B, et al. (2010). Combined R-alpha-lipoic acid and acetyl-L-carnitine exerts efficient preventative effects in a cellular model of Parkinson's disease. *J Cell Mol Med*. Jan;14(1-2):215-25.

[903] Phillipson OT. (2014). Management of the aging risk factor for Parkinson's disease. *Neurobiol Aging*. Apr;35(4):847-57.

[904] Monti DA, Zabrecky G, Kremens D, Liang TW, Wintering NA, et al. (2016). N-Acetyl Cysteine May Support Dopamine Neurons in Parkinson's Disease: Preliminary Clinical and Cell Line Data. *PLoS One*. 11(6):e0157602.

[905] Afshin-Majd S, Bashiri K, Kiasalari Z, Baluchnejadmojarad T, Sedaghat R, et al. (2017). Acetyl-l-carnitine protects nigrostriatal pathway in 6-hydroxydopamine-induced model of Parkinson's disease in the rat. *Biomed Pharmacother*. May;89:1-9.

[906] Li YH, He Q, Yu JZ, Liu CY, Feng L, et al. (2015). Lipoic acid protects dopaminergic neurons in LPS-induced Parkinson's disease model. *Metab Brain Dis*. Oct;30(5):1217-26.

[907] Zhao H, Zhao X, Liu L, Zhang H, Xuan M, et al. (2017). Neurochemical effects of the R form of a-lipoic acid and its neuroprotective mechanism in cellular models of Parkinson's disease. *Int J Biochem Cell Biol*. Jun;87:86-94.

[908] Zhou B, Wen M, Lin X, Chen YH, Gou Y, et al. (2018). Alpha Lipoamide Ameliorates Motor Deficits and Mitochondrial Dynamics in the Parkinson's Disease Model Induced by 6-hydroxydopamine. *Neurotox Res*. May;33(4):7590767.

[909] Srivastav S, Fatima M, Mondal AC. (2017). Important medicinal herbs in Parkinson's disease pharmacotherapy. *Biomed Pharmacother*. Aug;92:856-863.

[910] Ahmad M, Saleem S, Ahmad AS, Ansari MA, Yousuf S, et al. (2005). Neuroprotective effects of Withania somnifera on 6-hydroxydopamine induced Parkinsonism in rats. *Hum Exp Toxicol*. Mar; 24(3):137-47.

[911] Kyboyama T, Tohda C, Zhao J, Nakamura, N, Hattori M, Komatsu K. (2002). Axon- or dendrite-predominant outgrowth induced by constituents from Ashwagandha. *Neuroreport* Oct. 7; 13(14): 1715-20.

[912] Kuboyama T, Tohda C, Komatsu K. (2005). Neuritic regeneration and synaptic reconstruction induced by withanolide A. *Br J Pharmacol*. Apr; 144(7):961-71

[913] Tohda C, Kuboyama T, Komatsu K. (2000). Dendrite extension by methanol extract of Ashwagandha (roots of Withania somnifera) in SK-N-SH cells. *Neuroreport*. Jun 26; 11(9):1981-5.

[914] Ibid. Kyboyama. (2002).

[915] Ibid. Kuboyama. (2005).

[916] Ibid. Kyboyama. (2002).

[917] Schliebs R, Liebmann A, Bhattacharya SK, Kumar A, Ghosal S, Bigl V. (1997). Systemic administration of defined extracts from Withania somnifera (Indian Ginseng) and Shilajit differentially affects cholinergic but not glutamatergic and GABAergic markers in rat brain. *Neurochem Int*. Feb;30(2):181-90.

[918] Dar NJ, Hamid A, Ahmad M. (2015). Pharmacologic overview of Withania somnifera, the Indian Ginseng. *Cell Mol Life Sci*. Dec;72(23):4445-60.

[919] Galasso C, Orefice I, Pellone P, Cirino P, Miele R, et al. (2018). On the Neuroprotective Role of Astaxanthin: New Perspectives? *Mar Drugs*. Jul 27;16(8):E247.

[920] Grimmig B, Daly L, Subbarayan M, Hudson C, Williamson R, et al. (2017). Astaxanthin is neuroprotective in an aged mouse model of Parkinson's disease. *Oncotarget*. Dec 28;9(12):10388-10401.

[921] Grimmig B, Morganti J, Nash K, Bickford PC. (2016). Immunomodulators as Therapeutic Agents in Mitigating the Progression of Parkinson's Disease. *Brain Sci.* Sep 23;6(4):E41.

[922] Ye Q, Zhang K, Huang B, Zhu Y, Chen X. (2013). Astaxanthin suppresses MPP(+)-induced oxidative damage in PC12 cells through a Sp1/NR1 signaling pathway. *Mar Drugs.* Mar 28;11(4):1019-34.

[923] Lee DH, Kim CS, Lee YJ. (2011). Astaxanthin protects against MPTP/MPP+-induced mitochondria dysfunction and ROS production in vivo and in vitro. *Food Chem Toxicol.* Jan;49(1):271-80.

[924] Fakhri S, Aneva IY, Farzaei MH, Sobarzo-Sanchez E. (2019). The Neuroprotective Effects of Astaxanthin: Therapeutic Targets and Clinic Perspective. *Molecules.* Jul 20;24(14):E2640.

[925] Jadiya P, Khan A, Sammi SR, Kaur S, Mir SS, et al. (2011). Anti-Parkinsonian effects of Bacopa monnieri: insights from transgenic and pharmacological Caenorhabditis elegans models of Parkinson's disease. *Biochem Biophys Res Commun.* Oct 7;413(4):605-10.

[926] Singh B, Pandey S, Yadav SK, Verma R, Singh SP, et al. (2017). Role of ethanolic extract of Bacopa monnieri against 1-methyl-4-phenyl-1,2,3,6-tetrahydropyridine (MPTP) induced mice model via inhibition of apoptotic pathways of dopaminergic neurons. *Brain Res Bull.* Oct;135:120-128.

[927] Ibid. Jadiya. (2011). Biochem Biophy Res Commun.

[928] Gasiorowski K, Lamer-Zarawska E, Leszek J, Parvathaneni K, Yendluri BB, et al. (2011). Flavones from root of Scutellaria baicalensis Georgi: Drugs of the future in neurodegeneration? *CNS Neurol Disord Drug Targets.* Mar;10:184-191.

[929] Li Y, Zhao J, Holscher C. (2017). Therapeutic Potential of Baicalein in Alzheimer's Disease and Parkinson's Disease. *CNS Drugs.* Aug;31(8):639-852.

[930] Zhang X, Du L, Zhang W, Yang Y, Zhou Q, et al. (2017). Therapeutic effects of baicalein on rotenone-induced Parkinson's disease through protecting mitochondrial function and biogenesis. *Sci Rep.* Aug 30;7(1):9968.

[931] Kuang L, Cao X, Lu Z. (2017). Baicalein Protects against Rotenone-Induced Neurotoxicity through Induction of Autophagy. *Biol Parm Bull.* Sep 1;40(9):1537-1543.

[932] Dinda B, Dinda S, DasSharma S, Banik R, Chakraborty A, et al. (2017). Therapeutic potentials of baicalein and its aglycone, baicalein against inflammatory disorders. *Eur J Med Chem.* May 5;131:68-80.

[933] Chen M, Lai L, Li X, Zhang X, He X, et al. (2016). Baicalein attenuates neurological deficits and preserves blood-brain barrier integrity in a rat model of intracerebral hemorrhage. *Neurochem Res.* Nov;41:3095-3102.

[934] Lu JH, Ardah MT, Durairajan SS, Liu LF, Xie LX, et al. (2011). Baicalein inhibits formation of alpha-synuclein oligomers within living cells and prevents aβ peptide fibrillation and oligomerisation. *Chembiochem.* Mar 7;12:615-624.

[935] Jiang M, Porat-Shliom Y, Pei Z, Cheng Y, Xiang L, et al. (2010). Baicalein reduces E46K alpha-synuclein aggregation in vitro and protects cells against E46K alpha-synuclein toxicity in cell models of familiar parkinsonism. *J Neurochem.* Jul;114:419-429

[936] Zhu M, Rajamani S, Kaylor J, Han S, Zhou F, et al. (2004). The flavonoid baicalein inhibits fibrillation of alpha-synuclein and disaggregates existing fibrils. *J Bio Chem.* June 25;279:26846-26857

[937] Yu X, He G, Du G. (2012). [Neuroprotective effect of baicalein in patients with Parkinson's disease]. *Zhongguo Zhong Yao Za Zhi.* Feb;37(4):421-5.

[938] Strathearn KE, Yousef GG, Grace MH, Roy SL, Tambe, MA, et al. (2014). Neuroprotective effects of anthocyanin-and proanthocyanidin-rich extracts in cellular models of Parkinson's disease. *Brain Res.* Mar 25;1555:60-77.

[939] Gao X, Cassidy A, Schwarzschild MA, Rimm EB, Ascherio A. (2012). Habitual intake of dietary flavonoids and risk of Parkinson disease. *Neurology.* Apr 10; 78(15):1138-45.

[940] Blount PJ, Nguyen CD, McDeavitt JT. (2002). Clinical use of cholinomimetic agents: a review. *J Head Trauma Rehabil.* Aug; 17(4):314-21

[941] Saver JL. (2008). Citicoline: update on a promising and widely available agent for neuroprotection and neurorepair. *Rev Neurol Dis.* Fall;5(4):167-77.

[942] McDaniel MA, Maier SF, Einstein GO. (2003). Brain-specific nutrients: a memory cure? *Nutrition.* Nov-Dec; 19(11-12):957-75.

[943] Abad-Santos F, Novalbos-Reina J, Gallego-Sandín S, García AG. (2002). [Treatment of mild cognitive impairment: value of citicoline]. *Rev Neurol.* Oct 1-15; 35(7):675-82.

[944] Kashkin VA, Shekunova EV, Mararova MN, Makarov VG. (2017). [A study of combination treatment with nacom (levodopa + carbodope) and citocoline in the model of Parkinson disease in rats]. *Zh Nevrol Psikhiatr Im S S Korsakova.* 2017;117(7):59-63.

[945] Secades JJ, Lorenzo JL. (2006). Citicoline: pharmacological and clinical review, 2006 update. *Methods Find Exp Clin Pharmacol.* Sep;28 Supple B:1-56.

[946] Shehzad A, Rehman G, Lee YS (2013). Curcumin in inflammatory diseases. *Biofactors.* Jan-Feb; 39(1):69-77.

[947] Kim GY, Kim KH, Lee SH, Yoon MS, Lee HJ, et al. (2005). Curcumin inhibits immunostimulatory function of dendritic cells: MAPKs and translocation of NF-kappa B as potential targets. *J Immunol.* Jun 15; 174(12):8116-24.

[948] Bigford GE, Del Rossi. (2014). Supplemental substances derived from foods as adjunctive therapeutic agents for treatment of neuro-degenerative diseases and disorders. *G Adv Nutr*. Jul; 5(4):394-403.

[949] Siddique YH, Naz F, Jyoti S. (2014). Effect of curcumin on lifespan, activity pattern, oxidative stress, and apoptosis in the brains of transgenic Drosophila model of Parkinson's disease. *Biomed Res Int*. 2014; 2014():606928.

[950] Qu Z, Mossine VV, Cui J, Sun GY, Gu Z. (2016). Protective Effects of AGE and Its Components on Neuroinflammation and Neurodegeneration. *Neuromolecular Med*. Sep;18(3):474-82.

[951] Rojas P, Serrano-Garcia N, Medina-Campos ON, Pedraza-Chaverri J, Maldonado PD, et al. (2011). S-Allylcysteine, a garlic compound, protects against oxidative stress in 1-methyl-4-phenylpyridinium-induced parkinsonism in mice. *J Nutr Biochem*. Oct:22(10):937-44.

[952] Ibid. Rojas. (2011).

[953] Maher P. (2017). Protective effects of fisetin and other berry flavonoids in Parkinson's disease. *Food Funct*. Sep 20;8(9):3033-3042.

[954] Sagara Y, Vanhnasy J, Maher P. (2004). Induction of PC12 cell differentiation by flavonoids is dependent upon extracellular signal-regulated kinase activation. *J Neurochem*. Sep; 90(5):1144-55.

[955] Maher P, Akaishi T, Abe K. (2006). Flavonoid fisetin promotes ERK-dependent long-term potentiation and enhances memory. *Proc Natl Acad Sci U S A*. Oct 31; 103(44):16568-73.

[956] Ibid. Sagara. (2004).

[957] Ishige K, Schubert D, Sagara Y. (2001). Flavonoids protect neuronal cells from oxidative stress by three distinct mechanisms. *Free Radic Biol Med*. Feb 15; 30(4):433-46.

[958] Nabavi SF, Braidy N, Hablemariam S, Sureda A, Manayi A, et al. (2016). Neuroprotective Effects of Fisetin in Alzheimer's and Parkinson's Diseases: From Chemistry to Medicine. *Curr Top Med Chem*. 16(17):1910-5.

[959] Simon A, Darcsi A, Kery A, Riethmuller E. (2019). Blood-brain barrier permeability study of ginger constituents. *J Pharm Biomed Anal*. Aug 19;177:112820.

[960] Park G, Kim HG, Ju MS, Ha SK, Park Y, et al. (2013). 6-Shogaol, an active compound of ginger, protects dopaminergic neurons in Parkinson's disease models via anti-neuroinflammation. *Acta Pharmacol Sin*. Sep;34(9):1131-9.

[961] Huh E, Choi JG, Noh D, Yoo HS, Ryu J, et al. (2018). Ginger and 6-shogaol protect intestinal tight junction and enteric dopaminergic neurons against 1-methyl-4-phenyl 1,2,3,6-tetrahydropyridine in mice. *Nutr Neurosci*. Sep 19:1-10.

[962] Xing X, Liu F, Xiao J, So KF. (2016). Neuro-protective Mechanisms of Lycium barbarum. *Neuromolecular Med*. Sep;18(3):253-63.

[963] Cheng J, Zhou ZW, Sheng HP, He LJ, Fan XW, et al. (2014). An evidence-based update on the pharmacological activities as possible molecular targets of Lycium barbarum polysaccharides. *Drug Des Devl Ther*. Dec 17;9:33-78.

[964] Amro MS, Teoh SL, Norzana AG, Srijit D. (2018). The potential role of herbal products in the treatment of Parkinson's disease. *Clin Ter*. Jan-Feb;169(1):e23-e33.

[965] Srivastav S, Fatima M, Mondal AC. (2017) Important medicinal herbs in Parkinson's disease pharmacotherapy. *Biomed Pharmacother*. Aug;92:856-863.

[966] Banjari I, Marcek T, Tomic S, Waisundara VY. (2018). Forestalling the Epidemics of Parkinson's Disease Through Plant-Based Remedies. *Font Nutr*. Oct 30;5:95.

[967] Zhang C, Zang Y, Song Q, Li H, Hu L, Zhao W, et al. (2019). The efficacy of a "cocktail therapy" on Parkinson's disease with dementia. *Neuropsychiatr Dis Treat*. Jun 24;15:1639-1647.

[968] Huang X, Li N, Pu Y, Zhang T, Wang B. (2019). Neuroprotective Effects of Ginseng Phytochemicals: Recent Perspectives. *Molecules*. Aug;24(16):E2939.

[969] Gonzalez-Burgos E, Fernandex-Moriano C, Gomez-Serranillos MP. (2015). Potential neuroprotective activity of Ginseng I Parkinson's disease: a review. *J Neuroimmune Parmacol*. Mar;10(1):14-29.

[970] Kim D, Jeon H, Ryu S, Koo S, Ha KT, et al. (2016). Proteomic Analysis of the Effect of Korean Red Ginseng in the Striatum of a Parkinson's Disease Mouse Model. *PLoS One*. Oct 27;11(10:e0164906.

[971] Ardah MT, Paleologou KE, Lv G, Menon SA, Abul Khair SB, et al. (2015). Ginsenoside Rb1 inhibits fibrillation and toxicity of alpha-synuclein and disaggregates preformed fibrils. *Neurobiol Dis*. Feb; 74():89-101

[972] Radad K, Gille G, Moldzio R, Saito H, Ishige K, et al. (2004). Ginsenosides Rb1 and Rg1 effects on survival and neurite growth of MPP+-affected mesencephalic dopaminergic cells. *J Neural Transm (Vienna)*. 2004 Jan; 111(1):37-45.

[973] Ibid. Huang. (2019).

[974] Sohal RS, Orr WC. (2012). The redox stress hypothesis of aging. *Free Radic Biol Med*. Feb 1; 52(3):539-555.

[975] Zeevalk GD, Razmpour R, Bernard LP. (2008). Glutathione and Parkinson's disease: is this the elephant in the room? *Biomed Pharmacother*. Apr-May; 62(4):236-49.

976 Monti DA, Zabrecky G, Kremens D, Liang TW, Wintering NA, et al. (2016). N-Acetyl Cysteine May Support Dopamine Neurons in Parkinson's Disease: Preliminary Clinical and Cell Line Data. *PLoS One.* 2016; 11(6):e0157602.

977 Sarkaki A, Eidypour Z, Motamedi F, Keramati K, Farbood Y. (2012). Motor disturbances and thalamic electrical power of frequency bands' improve by grape seed extract in animal model of Parkinson's disease. *Avicenna J Phytomed.* Fal;2(4):222-32.

978 Strathearn KE, Yousef CG, Grace MH, Roy SL, Tambe MA, et al. (2014). Neuroprotective effects of anthocyanin- and proanthocyanidin-rich extracts in cellular models of Parkinson's disease. *Brain Res.* Mar 25;1155:60-77.

979 Ben Youssef S, Brisson G, Doucet-Beaupre H, Castonguay AM, Gora C, et al. (2019). Neuroprotective benefits of grape seed and skin extract in a mouse model of Parkinson's disease. *Nutr Neurosci.* May 25:1-15.

980 Nataraj J, Manivasagam T, Thenmozhi AJ, Essa MM. (2016). Lutein protects dopaminergic neurons against MPTP-induced apoptotic death and motor dysfunction by ameliorating mitochondrial disruption and oxidative stress. *Nutr Neurosci.* Jul;19(6):237-46.

981 Bovier ER, Renzi LM, Hammond BR Jr. (2014). A double-blind, placebo-controlled study on the effects of lutein and zeaxanthin on neural processing speed and efficiency. *PLoS One.* 2014; 9(9):e108178 .

982 Takeda A, Nyssen OP, Syed A, Jansen E, Bueno-de-Mesquita B, et al. (2014). Vitamin A and carotenoids and the risk of Parkinson's disease: a systematic review and meta-analysis. *Neuroepidemiology.* 2014;42(1):25-38.

983 Agarwal P, Wang Y, Buchman AS, Holland TM, Bennett D, et al. (2020). Dietary Antioxidants Associated with Slower Progression of Parkinsonian Signs in Older Adults. *Nutr Neurosci.* May 22;1-8.

984 Suzuki K, Miyamoto M, Miyamoto T, Iwanami M, Hirata K. (2011). Sleep disturbances associated with Parkinson's disease. *Parkinsons Dis.* 2011():219056.

985 St Louis EK, Boeve AR, Boeve BF. (2017). REM Sleep Behavior Disorder in Parkinson's Disease and Other Synucleinopathies. *Mov Disord.* May;32(5):645-658.

986 Mack JM, Schamne MG, Sampaio TB, Pértile RA, Fernandes PA, et al. (2016). Melatoninergic system in Parkinson's disease: from neuroprotection to the management of motor and nonmotor symptoms. *Oxid Med Cell Longev.* 2016:3472032.

987 Ibid. Mack. (2016).

988 Patil RR, Gholave AR, Jadhav JP, Yadav SR, Bapat VA. (2015). Mucuna sanjappae Aitawade et Yadav: A new species of Mucuna with promising yield of anti-Parkinson's drug l-DOPA. *Genet Resour Crop Evol.* 2015;62(1):155–162.

989 Manyam BV, Dhanasekaran M, Hare TA. (2004). Neuroprotective effects of the antiparkinson drug Mucuna pruriens. *Phytother Res.* 2004;18(9):706–712.

990 Hussian G, Manyam BV. (1997). Mucuna pruriens proves more effective than l-DOPA in Parkinson's disease animal model. *Phytother Res.* 1997;11(6):419–423.

991 Katzenschlager R, Evans A, Manson A, Patsalos PN, Ratnaraj N, et al. (2004). Mucuna pruriens in Parkinson's disease: A double blind clinical and pharmacological study. *J Neurol Neurosurg Psychiatry.* Dec;75(12):1672–1677.

992 Kim HG, Ju MS, Shim JS, Kim MC, Lee SH, et al. (2010). Mulberry fruit protects dopaminergic neurons in toxin-induced Parkinson's disease models. *Brit J Nutr.* Jul;104(1):8-16.

993 Kim AJ, Park S. (2006). Mulberry extract supplements ameliorate the inflammation-related hematological parameters in carrageenan-induced arthritic rats. *J Med Food.* Fall;9(3)431–435.

994 Fahimi Z, Jahromy MH. (2018). Effects of blackberry (Morus nigra) fruit juice on levodopa-induced dyskinesia in a mice model of Parkinson's disease. *J Exp Pharmacol. 2018;10():29-35.*

995 Rahman MA, Abdullah N, Aminudin N. (2016). Interpretation of mushroom as a common therapeutic agent for Alzheimer's disease and cardiovascular diseases. *Crit Rev Biotechnol.* Dec;36(6):1131-1142.

996 Lee LY, Li IC, Chen WP, Tsai TY, Chen CC, et al. (2019). Thirteen-Week Oral Toxicity Evaluation of Erinacine A Enriched Lion's Mane Medicinal Muchroom, Hericium erinaceus (Agaricomycetes), Mycelia in Spraque-Dawley Rats. In *J Med Mushrooms.* 2019;21(4):401-411.

997 Pribis P, Shukitt-Hale B. (2014). Cognition: the new frontier for nuts and berries. *Am J Clin Nutr.* Jul;100 Suppl 1:347S-52S.

998 Vinson JA, Cai Y. (2012). Nuts, especially walnuts have both antioxidant quantity and efficacy and exhibit significant potential health benefits. *Food Funct.* 2012 Feb;3(2):134-40.

999 Essa MM, Subash S, Dhanalakshmi C, Manivasagam T, A-Adawi S, et al. (2015). Dietary Supplementation of Walnut Partially Reverses 1-Methyl-4-phenyl-1,2,3,5-tetrahydrophyridine Induced Neurodegeneration in a Mouse Model of Parkinson's Disease. *Neurochem Res.* Jun;40(6):1283-93.

1000 Choi JG, Park G, Kim HG, Oh DS, Kim H, et al. (2016). In Vitro and in Vivo Neuroprotective Effects of Walnut (Juglandis Semen) in Models of Parkinson's Disease. *Int J Mol Sci.* Jan 15;17(1):E108.

1001 Mohammad-Beigi H, Allakbari F, Sahin C, Lomax C, Tawfike A, et al. (2019). Oleuropein derivatives from olive fruit extracts reduce a-sunuclein fibrillation and oligomer toxicity. *J Biol Chem.* Mar 15;294(11):4215-4232.

[1002] Bousquet M, Calon F, Cicchetti F. (2011). Impact of ω-3 fatty acids in Parkinson's disease. *Ageing Res Rev.* Sep; 10(4):453-63.

[1003] Calon F, Cole G. (2007). Neuroprotective action of omega-3 polyunsaturated fatty acids against neurodegenerative diseases: evidence from animal studies. *Prostaglandins Leukot Essent Fatty Acids.* Nov-Dec; 77(5-6):287-93.

[1004] Ibid. Calon. (2007).

[1005] da Silva TM, Munhoz RP, Alvarez C, Naliwaiko K, Kiss A, et al. (2008). Depression in Parkinson's disease: a double-blind, randomized, placebo-controlled pilot study of omega-3 fatty-acid supplementation. *J Affect Disord.* Dec; 111(2-3):351-9.

[1006] Wysoczański T, Sokoła-Wysoczańska E, Pękala J, Lochyński S, Czyż K, et al. (2016). Omega-3 Fatty Acids and their Role in Central Nervous System - A Review. *Curr Med Chem.* 2016;23(8):816-31.

[1007] Ibid. Wysoczanski. (2016).

[1008] Rathod R, Kale A, Joshi S. (2016). Novel insights into the effect of vitamin B12 and omega-3 fatty acids on brain function. *J Biomed Sci.* Jan 25;23:17.

[1009] Taghizadeh M, Tamtaji OR, Dadgostar E, Daneshvar KR, Bahmani F, et al. (2017). The effects of omega-3 fatty acids and vitamin E co-supplementation on clinical and metabolic status in patients with Parkinson's disease: A randomized, double-blind, placebo-controlled trial. *Neurochem Int.* Sep;108:183-189.

[1010] Valadas JS, Esposito G, Vandekerkhove D, Miskiewicz K, Deaulmerie L, et al. (2018). ER Lipid Defects in Neuropeptidergic Neurons Impair Sleep Patterns in Parkinson's Disease. *Neuron.* Jun 27;98(6):1155-1169.

[1011] Fünfgeld EW, Baggen M, Nedwidek P, Richstein B, Mistlberger G. (1989). Double-blind study with phosphatidylserine (PS) in parkinsonian patients with senile dementia of Alzheimer's type (SDAT). *Clin Biol Res.* 1989;317:1235-46.

[1012] Choi JG, Kim HG, Kim MC, Yang WM, Huh Y, et al. (2011). Polygalae radix inhibits toxin-induced neuronal death in the Parkinson's disease models. *J Ethnopharmacol.* Mar 24;134(2):414-21.

[1013] Wu AG, Wong VK, Xu SW, Chan WK, Ng CL, et al. (2013). Onjisaponin B derived from Radix Polygalae enhances autophagy and accelerates the degradation of mutan a-synuclein and huntingtin in PC-12 cells. *In J Mol Sci.* Nov 15;14(11):22618-41.

[1014] Lin CM, Lin RD, Chen ST. (2010). Neurocytoprotective effects of the bioactive constituents of Pueraria thomsonii in 6-hydroxydopamine (6-OHDA)-treated nerve growth factor (NGF)-differentiated PC12 cells. *Phytochemistry.* 2010;71:2147-56.

[1015] Gong P, Deng F, Zhang W, Ji J, Liu J, et al. (2017). Tectorigenin attenuates the MPP+ -induced SH-SY5Y cell damage indicating a potential beneficial role in Parkinson's disease by oxidative stress inhibition.

[1016] Khan MM, Kempuraj D, Thangavel R, Zaheer A. (2013). Protection of MPTP-induced neuroinflammation and neurodegeneration by Pycnogenol. *Neurochem Int.* Mar;62(4):379-88.

[1017] Zhang Q, Chen S, Yu S, Qin J, Zhang J, et al. (2016). Neuroprotective effects of pyrroloquinoline quinone against rotenone injury in primary cultured midbrain neurons and in a rat model of Parkinson's disease. *Neuropharmacology.* Sep;108:238-51.

[1018] Kobayashi M, Kim J, Kobayashi N, Han S, Nakamura C, et al. (2006). Pyrroloquinoline quinone (PQQ) prevents fibril formation of alpha-synuclein. *Biochem Biophys Res Commun.* Oct 27;349(3):1139-44.

[1019] Elumalai P, Lakshmi S. (2016). Role of Quercetin Benefits in Neurodegeneration. *Adv Neurobiol.* 2016;12:229-45.

[1020] Bournival J, Plouffe M, Renaud J, Provencher C, Martinoli MG. (2012). Quercetin and sesamin protect dopaminergic cells from MPP+-induced neuroinflammation in a microglial (N9)-neuronal (PC12) coculture system. *Oxid Med Cell Longev.* 2012;2012:921941

[1021] Wenk GL, McGann-Gramling K, Hauss-Wegrzyniak B, Ronchetti D, Maucci R, et al. (2004). Attenuation of chronic neuroinflammation by a nitric oxide-releasing derivative of the antioxidant ferulic acid. *J Neurochem.* Apr;89(2):484-93.

[1022] El-Horany HE, El-Latif RN, ElBatsh MM, Emam MN. (2016). Ameliorative Effect of Quercetin on Neurochemical and Behavioral Deficits in Rotenone Rat Model of Parkinson's Disease: Modulating Autophagy (Quercetin on Experimental Parkinson's Disease). *J Biochem Mol Toxicol.* Jul;30(7):360-9.

[1023] Lee M, McGeer MG, McGeer PL. (2016). Quercetin, not caffeine, is a major neuroprotective component in coffee. *Neurobiol Aging.* Oct;46:113-23.

[1024] Ren B, Zhang YX, Zhou HX, Sun FW, Zhang ZF, et al. (2015). Tanshione IIA prevents the loss of nigrostriatal dopaminergic neurons by inhibiting NADPH oxidase and iNOS in the MPTP model of Parkinson's disease. *J Neurol Sci.* Jan 15;348(1-2):142-152.

[1025] Wang S, Jing H, Yang H, Liu Z, Guo H, et al. (2015). Tanshione I selectively suppresses pro-inflammatory genes expression in activated microglia and prevents nigrostriatal dopaminergic neurodegeneration in a mouse model of Parkinson's disease. *J Ethnopharmacol.* Apr 22;164:247-55.

[1026] Xia D, Sui R, Zhang Z. (2019). Administration of resveratrol improved Parkinson's disease-like phenotype by suppressing apoptosis of neurons via modulating the MALAT1/miR-129/SNCA signaling pathway. *J Cell Biochem.* Apr;120(4):4942-4951.

[1027] Morgan LA, Grundmann O. (2017). Preclinical and Potential Applications of Common Western Herbal Supplements as Complementary Treatment in Parkinson's Disease. *J Diet Suppl.* Jul 4;14(4):453-466.

[1028] Zhuang W, Yue L, Dang X, Chen F, Gong Y, et al. (2019). Rosenroot (Rhodiola): Potential Applications in Aging-related diseases. *Aging Dis.* Feb 1;10(1):134–146.

[1029] Jacob R, Nalini G, Chidambaranathan N. (2013). Neuroprotective effect of Rhodiola rosea Linn against MPTP induced cognitive impairment and oxidative stress. *Ann Neurosci.* Apr;20(2): 47–51.

[1030] Wang S, He H, Chen L, Zhang W, Zhang X, et al. (2015). Protective effects of salidroside in the MPTP/MPP(+)-induced model of Parkinson's disease through ROS-NO-related mitochondrion pathway. *Mol Neurobiol.* Apr;51(2):718-28.

[1031] Meininger V, Flamier A, Phan T, Ferris O, Uzan A, et al. (1982). [L- Methionine treatment of Parkinson's disease: preliminary results]. [Article in French]. *Rev Neurol* (Paris). 1982;138(4):297-303.

[1032] Methinonine Sulfoxide Reductase A CMRSA and Parkinson's Disease Pathogenesis. Funded Study. Retrieved Jun 28 2019 from https://www.michaeljfox.org/foundation/grant-detail.php?grant_id=88.

[1033] Hatziagapiou K, Kakouri E, Lambrou GI, Bethanis K, Tarantilis PA. (2019). Antioxidant Properties of Crocus Sativus L. and Its Constituents and Relevance to Neurodegenerative Diseases; Focus on Alzheimer's and Parkinson's Disease. *Curr Neuropharmacol.* 2019;17(4):377-402.

[1034] Perry TL, Bratty PJ, Hansen S, Kennedy J, Urquhart N, et al. (1975). Hereditary mental depression and Parkinsonism with taurine deficiency. *Arch Neurol.* Feb;32(2):108-13.

[1035] Zhang L, Yuan Y, Tong Q, Jiang S, Xu Q, et al. (2016). Reduced plasma taurine level in Parkinson's disease: association with motor severity and levodopa treatment. *Int J Neurosci.* 2016;126(7):630-6.

[1036] Ibid. Zhang. (2016).

[1037] Hou L, Che Y, Sun F, Wang Q. (2018). Taurine protects noradrenergic locus coeruleus neurons in a mouse Parkinson's disease model by inhibiting microglial M1 polarization. *Amino Acids.* May;50(5):547-556.

[1038] Chan DK, Woo J, Ho SC, Pang CP, Law LK, et al. (1998). Genetic and environmental risk factors for Parkinson's disease in a Chinese population. *J Neurol Neurosurg Psychiatry.* Nov;65(5):781-4.

[1039] Checkoway H, Powers K, Smith-Weller T, Franklin GM, Longstreth WT Jr, et al. (2002). Parkinson's disease risks associated with cigarette smoking, alcohol consumption, and caffeine intake. *Am J Epidemiol.* Apr 15; 155(8):732-8.

[1040] Hu G, Bidel S, Jousilahti P, Antikainen R, Tuomilehto J. (2007). Coffee and tea consumption and the risk of Parkinson's disease. *Mov Disord.* Nov 15; 22(15):2242-8.

[1041] Kandinov B, Giladi N, Korczyn AD. (2009). Smoking and tea consumption delay onset of Parkinson's disease. *Parkinsonism Relat Disord.* Jan; 15(1):41-6.

[1042] Kuriyama S, Hozawa A, Ohmori K, Shimazu T, Matsui T, et al. (2006). Green tea consumption and cognitive function: a cross-sectional study from the Tsurugaya Project 1. *Am J Clin Nutr.* Feb; 83(2):355-61.

[1043] Noguchi-Shinohara M, Yuki S, Dohmoto C, Ikeda Y, Samuraki M, et al. (2014). Consumption of green tea, but not black tea or coffee, is associated with reduced risk of cognitive decline. *PLoS ONE.* 2014;9:e96013.

[1044] Anandhan A, Tamilselvam K, Radhiga T, Rao S, Essa MM, et al. (2012). Theaflavin, a black tea polyphenol, protects nigral dopaminergic neurons against chronic MPTP/probenecid induced Parkinson's disease. *Brain Res.* Jan 18;1433:104- 13.

[1045] Anandhan A, Essa MM, Manivasagam T. (2013). Therapeutic Attenuation of Neuroinflammation and Apoptosis by Black Tea Theaflavin in Chronic MPTP/Probenecid Model of Parkinson's Disease. *Neurotox Res* 2013;23:166-73.

[1046] Levites Y, Weinreb O, Maor G, Youdim MBH, Mandel S. (2001). Green tea polyphenol (_)-epigallocatechin-3-gallate prevents N-methyl-4phenyl-1,2,3,6- tetrahydropyridine-induced dopaminergic neurodegeneration. *J Neurochem.* 78:1073–82.

[1047] Deleu D, Northway MG, Hanssens Y. (2002). Clinical pharmacokinetic and pharmacodynamic properties of drugs used in the treatment of Parkinson's disease. *Clin Pharmacokinet.* 41:261–309.

[1048] Satoh T, Nakatsuka D, Watanabe Y, Nagatal, Kikuchi H, et al. (2000). Neuroprotection by MAPK/ERK kinase inhibition with U0126 against oxidative stress in a mouse neuronal cell line and rat primary cultured cortical neurons. *Neurosci Lett.* 288:163–6.

[1049] Levites Y, Youdim MBH, Maor G, Mandel S. (2002). Attenuation of 6-hydroxydopamine (6-OHDA)-induced nuclear factor-kappaB (NFkappaB) activation and cell death by tea extracts in neuronal cultures. *Biochem Pharmacol.* 2002;63:21–9.

[1050] Guo Q, Zhao B, Li M, Shen S, Xin W. (1996). Studies on protective mechanisms of four components of green tea polyphenols against lipid peroxidation in synaptosomes. *Biochim Biophys Acta.* 1996;1304:210-22.

[1051] Salazar J, Mena N, Núñez MT. (2006). Iron dyshomeostasis in Parkinson's disease. *J Neural Transm Suppl.* 2006;(71):205-13.

[1052] Daubner SC, Le T, Wang S. (2011). Tyrsoine hydroxylase and regulation of dopamine synthesis. *Arch Biochem Biophys.* 2011;508:1-12.

[1053] Ping Z, Xiaomu W, Xufang X, Liang S. (2019). Vinpocetine regulates levels of circulating TLRs in Parkinson's disease patients. *Neurol Sci.* Jan;40(1):113-120.

[1054] Sharma S, Desmukh R. (2015). Vinpocetine attenuates MPTP-induced motor deficit and biochemical abnormalities in Wistar rats. *Neuroscience.* Feb 12;286:393-403.

[1055] Ishola IO, Akinyede AA, Aduluwa TP, Micah C. (2018). Novel action of vinpocetine in the prevention of paraquat-induced parkinsonism in mice: involvement of oxidative stress and neuroinflammation. *Metab Brain Dis.* Oct;33(5):1493-1500.

[1056] Zaitone SA, Abo-Elmatty DM, Elshazly SM. (2012). Piracetam and vinpocetine ameliorate rotenone-induced Parkinsonism in rats. *Indian J Pharmacol.* Nov-Dec;44(6):774-9.

[1057] Ibid. Kim. (2017).

[1058] De Jager CA, Ouihaj A, Jacoby R, Refsum H, Smith AD. (2012). Cognitive and clinical outcomes of homocysteine-lowering B-vitamin treatment in mild cognitive impairment: a randomized controlled trial. *Int J Geriatr Psychiatry.* 2012 Jun;27(6):592-600.

[1059] Shen L. (2015). Associations between B Vitamins and Parkinson's Disease. *Nutrients.* Aug 27;7(9):7197-208.

[1060] Smith AD, Smith SM, de Jager CA, Whitbread P, Johnston C, et al. (2010). Homocysteine-lowering by B vitamins slows the rate of accelerated brain atrophy in mild cognitive impairment: a randomized controlled trial. *PLoS One.* 2010 Sep 8;5(9):e12244.

[1061] Kinsella LJ, Riley DE. Nutritional deficiencies and syndromes associated with alcoholism. In: Goetz CG, Pappert EJ, editors. Textbook of Clinical Neurology. Philadelphia: *W.B. Saunders Company;* 1999. pp. 803–806

[1062] Luong KV, Nguyen LT. (2013). The beneficial role of thiamine in Parkinson disease. *CNS Neurosci Ther.* Jul;19(7):461-8.

[1063] Murakami K, Miyake Y, Sasaki S, Tanaka K, Fukushima W, et al. (2010). Dietary intake of folate, vitamin B6, vitamin B12 and riboflavin and risk of Parkinson's disease: a case-control study in Japan. *Br J Nutr.* Sep; 104(5):757-64.

[1064] Loens S, Chorbadzhieva E, Kleinmann A, Dressler D, Schrader C. (2017). Effects of levodopa/carbidopa intestinal gel versus oral levodopa/carbidopa on B vitamin levels and neuropathy. *Brain Behav.* Apr 7;7(5):e00698.

[1065] De Lau LM, Koudstaal PJ, Witteman JC, Hofman A, Breteler MM. (2006). Dietary folate, vitamin B12, and vitamin B6 and the risk of Parkinson disease. *Neurology.* Jul 25;67(2):315-8.

[1066] Shen L. (2015). Associations between B Vitamins and Parkinson's Disease. *Nutrients.* Aug 27;7(9):7197-208.

[1067] Wu XY, Lu L. (2012). Vitamin B6 deficiency, genome instability and cancer. *Asian Pac J Cancer Prev.* 2012;13(11):5333-8.

[1068] Corrada MM, Kawas CH, Hallfrisch J, Muller D, Brookmeyer R. (2005). Reduced risk of Alzheimer's disease with high folate intake: the Baltimore Longitudinal Study of Aging. *Alzheimers Dement.* Jul; 1(1):11-8.

[1069] Fioravanti M, Ferrario E, Massaia M, Cappa G, Rivolta G, et al. (1998). Low folate levels in the cognitive decline of elderly patients and the efficacy of folate as a treatment for improving memory deficits. *Arch Gerontol Geriatr.* Jan-Feb; 26(1):1-13.

[1070] Ramos MI, Allen LH, Mungas DM, Jagust WJ, Haan MN, et al. (2005). Low folate status is associated with impaired cognitive function and dementia in the Sacramento Area Latino Study on Aging. *Am J Clin Nutr.* Dec; 82(6):1346-52.

[1071] Nilsson K, Gustafson L, Hultberg B. (2001). Improvement of cognitive functions after cobalamin/folate supplementation in elderly patients with dementia and elevated plasma homocysteine. *Int J Geriatr Psychiatry.* Jun; 16(6):609-14.

[1072] Durga J, van Boxtel MP, Schouten EG, Kok FJ, Jolles J, et al. (2007). Effect of 3-year folic acid supplementation on cognitive function in older adults in the FACIT trial: a randomized, double blind, controlled trial. *Lancet.* Jan 20; 369(9557):208-16.

[1073] Connelly PJ, Prentice NP, Cousland G, Bonham J. (2008). A randomised double-blind placebo-controled trial of folic acid supplementation of cholinesterase inhibitors in Alzheimer's disease. *Int J Geriatr Psychiatry.* Feb;23(2):155-60.

[1074] Morris MS, Jacques PF, Rosenberg IH, Selhub J. (2002). Elevated serum methylmalonic acid concentrations are common among elderly Americans. *J Nutr.* Sep; 132(9):2799-803.

[1075] Reynolds EH. (2002). Folic acid, ageing, depression, and dementia. *BMJ.* Jun 22; 324(7352):1512-5.

[1076] Miller AL. (2008). The methylation, neurotransmitter, and antioxidant connections between folate and depression. *Alt Med Rev.* Sept;12(3):216-26.

[1077] Clarke R, Smith AD, Jobst KA, Refsum H, Sutton L, Ueland PM. (1998). Folate, Vitamin B12, Vitamin B12, and serum total homocysteine levels in confirmed Alzheimer's disease. *Arch Neurol.* Nov;55(11):1449-55.

[1078] Quadri P, Fragiacomo C, Pezzati R, Zanda E, Forloni G, et al. (2004). Homocysteine, folate, and Vitamin B-12 in mild cognitive impairment, Alzheimer's disease, and vascular dementia. *Am J Clin Nutr.* Jul;80(1):114-22.

[1079] Ibid. Ramos. (2005).

[1080] Quinlivan EP, McPartlin J, McNulty H, Ward M, Strain JJ, et al. (2002). Importance of both folic acid and vitamin B12 in reduction of vascular disease. *Lancet.* Jan 19;359(9302):227-8.

[1081] Sato Y, Kikuyama M, Oizumi K. (1997). High prevalence of vitamin D deficiency and reduced bone mass in Parkinson's disease. *Neurology.* Nov; 49(5):1273-8.

[1082] Wang JY, Wu JN, Cherng TL, Hoffer BJ, Chen HH, et al. (2001). Vitamin D(3) attenuates 6-hydroxydopamine-induced neurotoxicity in rats. *Brain Res.* Jun 15; 904(1):67-75.

[1083] Smith MP, Fletcher-Turner A, Yurek DM, Cass WA. (2006). Calcitriol protection against dopamine loss induced by intracerebroventricular administration of 6-hydroxydopamine. *Neurochem Res.* Apr; 31(4):533-9.

[1084] Holick MF. (2007). Vitamin D deficiency. *N Engl J Med*. Jul 19; 357(3):266-81.

[1085] Fulgoni VL 3rd, Keast DR, Bailey RL, Dwyer J. (2011). Foods, fortificants, and supplements: Where do Americans get their nutrients? *J Nutr*. Oct; 141(10):1847-54.

[1086] Morris MC, Evans DA, Bienias JL, Tangney CC, Wilson RS. (2002). Vitamin E and cognitive decline in older persons. *Arch Neurol*. Jul; 59(7):1125-32.

[1087] Burton GW, Traber MG. (1990). Vitamin E: antioxidant activity, biokinetics, and bioavailability. *Annu Rev Nutr*. 1990;10():357-82.

[1088] Ibid. Morris. (2002).

[1089] Schrag M, Mueller C, Zabel M, Crofton A, Kirsch WM, et al. (2013). Oxidative stress in blood in Alzheimer's disease and mild cognitive impairment: a meta-analysis. *Neurobiol Dis*. Nov; 59():100-10.

[1090] Kang JH, Cook N, Manson J, Buring JE, Grodstein F. (2006). A randomized trial of vitamin E supplementation and cognitive function in women. *Arch Intern Med*. Dec 11-25; 166(22):2462-8.

[1091] Jiménez-Jiménez FJ, de Bustos F, Molina JA, Benito-León J, Tallón-Barranco A, et al. (1997). Cerebrospinal fluid levels of alpha-tocopherol (vitamin E) in Alzheimer's disease. *J Neural Transm* (Vienna). 104(6-7):703-10.

[1092] Prakash A, Bharti K, Majeed AB. (2015). Zinc: indications in brain disorders. *Fundam Clin Pharmacol*. Apr;29(2):131-49.

[1093] Ibid. Prakash. (2015).

[1094] Frederickson CJ, Koh JY, Bush A. (2005). The neurobiology of zinc in health and disease. *Nat Rev Neurosci*. Jun; 6(6):449-62.

[1095] Bremner JD. (2006). Traumatic stress: effects on the brain. *Dialogues Clin Neurosci*. Dec;8(4):445-461.

[1096] Kontos AP, Van Cott AC, Roberts J, Pan JW, Kelly MB, et al. (2017). Clinical and Magnetic Resonance Spectroscopic Imaging Findings in Veterans with Blast Mild Traumatic Brain Injury and Post-Traumatic Stress Disorder. *Mil Med*. Mar;182(S1):99-104.

[1097] Ibid. Bremner. (2006). Dialogues Clin Neurosci.

[1098] Newcomb B. (2018). How your brain records the memory of a stressful experience. Retrieved Sep 25 2019 from https://news.usc.edu/136280/in-a-stressful-situation-this-part-of-the-brain-helps-you-turn-that-experience-into-a-vivid-memory/.

[1099] Schwarz LA, Luo L. (2015). Organization of the locus coeruleus-norepinephrine system. *Curr Biol*. Nov 2;25(21):R1051-R1056.

[1100] Clewett DV, Huang R, Valasco R, Lee TH, Mather M. (2018). Locus Coeruleus Activity Strengthens Prioritized Memories Under Arousal. *J Neurosci*. Feb7;38(6):1558-1574.

[1101] Lambert HK, McLaughlin KA. (2019). Impaired Hippocampus-Dependent Associative Learning as a Mechanism Underlying PTSD: a Meta-Analysis. *Neurosci Biobehav Rev*. Sep 20:S0149-763(19)30138-1.

[1102] Ibid. Bremner. (2006). *Dialogues Clin Neurosci*.

[1103] Ibid. Bremner. (2006).

[1104] Ahmed-Leitao F, Spies G, van den Heuvel L, Seedat S. (2016). Hippocampal and amygdala volumes in adults with posttraumatic stress disorder secondary to childhood abuse or maltreatment: A systematic review. *Psychiatry Red Neuroimaging*. Oct30;256:33-43.

[1105] Starcevic A, Postic S, Radojicic Z, Starcevic B, Milovanovic S, et al. (2014). Volumetric analysis of amygdala, hippocampus, and prefrontal cortex in therapy-naïve PTSD participants. *Biomed Res Int*. 2014:968495.

[1106] Sublette ME, Galfalvy HC, Oquendo MA, Bart CP, Schneck N, et al. (2016). Relationship of recent stress to amygdala volume in depression and healthy adults. *J Affect Disord*. Oct;203:136-142.

[1107] Gray JD, Rubin TG, Hunter RG, McEwen BS. (2014). Hippocampal gene expression changes underlying stress sensitization and recovery. *Mol Psychiatry*. Nov;19(11):1171-8.

[1108] Xie H, Claycomb EM, Elhai JD, Wall JT, Tamburrino MB, et al. (2018). Relationship of Hippocampal Volumes and Posttraumatic Stress Disorder Symptoms Over Early Posttrauma Periods. *Biol Psychiatry Cogn Neurosci Neuroiming*. Nov;3(11):968-975.

[1109] Kempuraj D, Selvakumar GP, Thangavel R, Ahmed ME, Zaheer S, et al. (2017). Mast Cell Activation in Brain Injury, Stress, and Post-traumatic Stress Disorder and Alzheimer's Disease Pathogenesis. *Front Neurosci*. Dec 12;11:703.

[1110] Felger JC. (2018). Imaging the Role of Inflammation in Mood and Anxiety-related Disorders. *Curr Neuropharmacol*. 15(5):533-558.

[1111] Sherin JE, Nemeroff CB. (2011). Post-traumatic stress disorder: the neurobiological impact of psychological trauma. *Dialogues Clin Neurosci*. Sep;13(3):263-278.

[1112] Ibid. Sherin. (2011). *Dialogues Clin Neurosci*.

[1113] Ibid. Sherin. (2011).

[1114] Danniowski U, Stuhrmann A, Beutelmann V, Zwanger P, Lenzen T, et al. (2012). Limbic scars: long-term consequences of childhood maltreatment revealed by functional and structural magnetic resonance imaging. *Biol Psychiatry*. Feb 15;71(4):286-93.

[1115] Olff M. (2017). Sex and gender differences in post-traumatic stress disorder: an update. *Psychotraumatology in Greece: Abstracts of the First Greek Psychotraumatology Conference*. Jul 27:13351204.

[1116] Ibid. Olff. (2017).

[1117] Tull M. (2019). Causes and Risk Factors of PTSD. Retrieved Sep 27 2019 from https://www.verywellmind.com/ptsd-causes-and-risk-factors-2797397.

[1118] Van der Merwe C, Jahanshad N, Cheung JW, Mufford M, Groenewold NA, et al. (2019). Concordance of genetic variation that increases risk for anxiety disorders and posttraumatic stress disorders and that influence their underlying neurocicuitry. *J Affect Disord.* Feb 15;245:885-896.

[1119] Mukherjee, S. (2016). *The Gene.* (p. 459). New York, Simon & Shuster, Inc.

[1120] Duncan LE, Ratanatharathorn A, Aiello AE, et al. (20180. Largest GWAS of PTSD (N=20 070) yields genetic overlap with schizophrenia and sex differences in heritability. *Mol Psychiatry.* 2018;23(3):666-673.

[1121] Zohar J, Yahalom H, Kozlovsky N, Cwikel-Hamzany S, Matar MA, et al. (2011). High dose hydrocortisone immediately after trauma may alter trajectory of PTSD: interplay between clinical and animal studies. *Eur Neuropsychopharmacol.* Nov; 21(11):796-809.

[1122] Schelling G, Roozendaal B, De Quervain DJ. (2004). Can posttraumatic stress disorder be prevented with glucocorticoids? Ann *N Y Acad Sci.* Dec; 1032():158-66.

[1123] Alzoubi KH, Al Hilo AS, Al-Balas QA, El-Salem K, El-Elimat T, et al. (2019). Withania somnifera root powder protects against post-traumatic stress disorder-induced memory impairment. *Mol Biol Rep.* Jun 19.

[1124] Sarris J, McIntyre E, Carnfield DA. (2013). Plant-based medicines for anxiety disorders, part 2: a review of clinical studies with supporting preclinical evidence. *CNS Drugs.* Apr;27(4):301-19.

[1125] Ibid. Sarris. (2013).

[1126] Ibid. Sarris. (2013).

[1127] Ebenezer PJ, Wilson CB, Wilson LD, Nair AR, J F. (2016). The Anti-Inflammatory Effects of Blueberries in an Animal Model of Post-Traumatic Stress Disorder (PTSD). *PloS One.* Sep 7;11(9):e0160923.

[1128] Lee B, Lee H. (2018). System Administration of Curcumin Affect Anxiety-Related Behaviors in a Rat Model of Posttraumatic Stress Disorder via Activation of Serotonergic Systems. *Evid Based Complement Alternat Med.* Jun 19:218:9041309.

[1129] Lopresti AL. (2017). Curcumin for neuropsychiatric disorders: a review of in vitro, animal and human studies. *J Psychopharmacol.* Mar;31(3):287-302.

[1130] Kaufmann FN, Gazal M, Bastos CR, Kaster MP, Ghisleni G. (2016). Curcumin in depressive disorders: An overview of potential mechanisms, preclinical and clinical findings. *Eur J Pharmacol.* Aug 5;784:192-8.

[1131] Monsey MS, Gerhard DM, Boyle LM, Briones MA, Seligsohn M, et al. (2015). A diet enriched with curcumin impairs newly acquired and reactivated fear memories. *Neuropsychopharmacology.* Mar 13;40(5):1278-88.

[1132] De Vries GJ, Mocking R, Lok A, Assies J, Schene A, et al. (2016). Fatty acid concentrations in patients with posttraumatic stress disorder compared to healthy controls. *J Affect Disord.* Nov 15;205:351-359.

[1133] Matsuoka YJ, Hamazaki K, Nishi D, Hamazaki T. (2016). Change in blood levels of eicosapentaenoic acid and posttraumatic stress symptom: A secondary analysis of data from a placebo-controlled trial of omega3 supplements. *J Affect Disord.* Nov 15;205:289-291.

[1134] Nasir M, Bloch MH. (2019). Trim the fat: the role of omega-3 fatty acids in psychopharmacology. *Ther Adv Psychopharmacol.* Aug 27;9:20451253.

[1135] Matsuoka Y, Nishi D, Tanima Y, Itakura M, Kojima A, et al. (2015). Serum pro-BDNF/BDNF as a treatment biomarker for response to docosahexaenoic acid in traumatized people vulnerable to developing psychological distress: a randomized controlled trial. *Transl Psychiatry.* Jul 7;5:e596.

[1136] Lee B, Sur B, Cho SG, Yeom M, Shim I, et al. (2016). Ginsenoside Rb1 rescues anxiety-like responses in a rat model of post-traumatic stress disorder. *J Nat Med.* Apr;70(2):133-44.

[1137] Lee B, Shim I, Lee H, Habm DH. (2018). Effects of Epigallocatechin Gallate on Behavioral and Cognitive Impairments, Hypothalamic-Pituitary-Adrenal Axis Dysfunctions and Alterations in Hippocampal BDNF Expression Under Single Prolonged Stress. *J Med Food.* Oct;21(10):979-989.

[1138] Ibid. Sarris. (2013).

[1139] Lai S, Shi L, Jiang Z, Lin Z. (2019). Glycyrrhizin treatment ameliorates posttraumatic stress disorder-like behaviors and restores circadian oscillation of intracranial serotonin. *Clin Exp Pharmacol Physiol.* Sept 8.

[1140] Ibid. Sarris. (2013).

[1141] Garcia-Keller C, Smiley C, Monforton C, Melton S, Kalivas PW, et al. (2019). N-Acetylecystein treatment during acute stress prevents stress-induced augmentation of addictive drug use and relapse. *Addict Biol.* Jul 7:e12798.

[1142] Coulter ID. (2014). The response of an expert panel to Nutritional armor for the warfighter: can omega-3 fatty acids enhance stress resilience, wellness, and military performance? *Mil Med.* Nov;179(11 Suppl):192-8.

[1143] Ibid. Sarris. (2013).

[1144] Zhang ZS, Qui ZK, He JL, Liu X, Chen JS, et al. (2017). Resveratrol ameliorated the behavioral deficits in a mouse model of post-traumatic stress disorder. *Pharmacol Biochem Behav.* Oct;161:68-76.

[1145] Li G, Wang G, Shi J, Xie X, Fei N, et al. (2018). Trans-Resveratrol ameliorates anxiety-like behaviors and fear memory deficits in a rat model of post-traumatic stress disorder. *Neuropharmacology.* May 1;133:181-188.

[1146] Ibid. Sarris. (2013).

[1147] De Souza Cp, Gambeta E, Stern CAJ, Zanoveli JM. (2019). Posttraumatic stress disorder-type behaviors in streptozotocin-induced diabetic rats can be prevents by prolonged treatment with vitamin E. *Behav Brain Res.* Feb;359:749-754.

[1148] Gaal L, Molnar P. (1990). Effect of vinpocetine on noradrenergic neurons in rat locus coeruleus. *Eur J Pharmacol.* Oct 23;187(3):537-9.

[1149] Alzheimer's Association. Chronic Traumatic Encephalopathy. Retrieved Oct 1 2019 from https://www.alz.org/alzheimers-dementia/what-is-dementia/related_conditions/chronic-traumatic-encephalopathy-(cte).

[1150] Gaetz M. (2017). The multi-factorial origins of Chronic Traumatic Encephalopathy (CTE) symptomology in post-career atheletes: The athlete post-career adjustment (AP-CA) model. Med *Hypotheses.* May;102:130-143.

[1151] Mez J, Daneshvar DH, Kierman PT, Abdolmohammadi B, Alvarez VE, et al. (2017). Clinicopathological Evaluation of Chronic Traumatic Encephalopathy in Players of American Football. *JAMA.* Jul 25;318(4):360-370.

[1152] Stone P. (2014). First Soccer and Rugby Players Diagnosed With CTE. Neurologic Rehabilitation Institute at Brookhaven Hospital. Retrieved Oct 1 2019 from https://traumaticbraininjury.net/2014/03/18/first-soccer-and-rugby-players-diagnosed-with-c.

[1153] Lee EB, Kinch K, Johnson VE, Trojanowski JQ, Smith DH, et al. (2019). Chronic traumatic encephalopathy is a common co-morbidty, but less frequent primary dementia in former soccer and rugby players. *Acta Neuropathol.* Sep;138(3):389-399.

[1154] Panchal H, Sollman N, Pasternak O, Alosco ML, Kinzel P, et al. (2018). Neuro-Metabolite Changes in a Single Season of Unniversity Ice Hockey Using Magnetic Resonance Spectroscopy. *Front Neurol.* Aug 20;9:616.

[1155] Montenigro PH, Corp DT, Stein TD, Cantu RC, Stern RA. (2015). Chronic traumatic encephalopathy: historical origins and current perspective. *Annu Rev Clin Psychol.* 2015;11:309-30.

[1156] Lim LJH, Ho RCM, Ho CSH. (2019). Dangers of Mixed Martial Arts in the Development of Chronic Traumatic Encephalopathy. *Int J Environ Res Public Health.* Jan 17;16(2).

[1157] Daneshvar DH, Nowinski CJ, McKee AC, Cantu RC. (2011). The epidemiology of sport-related concussion. *Clin Sports Med.* 30 (1): 1–17.

[1158] Agoston DV. (2017). Modeling the Long-Term Consequences of Repeated Blast-Induced Mild Traumatic Brain Injuries. *J Neurotrauma.* Sep;34(S1):S44-S52.

[1159] McKee AC, Robinson ME. (2014). Military-related traumatic brain injury and neurodegeneration. *Alzheimers Dement.* Jun;10(3 Suppl):S242-53.

[1160] Omalu B, Hammers JL, Bailes J, Hamilton RL, Kamboh MI, et al. (2011). Chronic traumatic encephalopathy in an Iragi war veteran with posttraumatic stress disorder who committed suicide. *Neurosurg Focus.* Nov;31(5):E3.

[1161] Gardner R, Yaffe K. (2015). Epidemiology of mild traumatic brain injury & neurodegenerative disease. *Mol Cell Neurosci.* May;66(B):75-80.

[1162] Katsumoto A, Takeuchi H, Tanaka F. (2019). Tau Pathology in Chronic Traumatic Encephalopathy and Alzheimer's Disease: Similarities and Differences. *Front Neurol.* Sep 10;10:980.

[1163] Mufson EJ, Perez SE, Nadeem M, Mahady L, Kanaan NM, et al. (2016). Progression of tau pathology within cholinergic nucleus basalis neurons in chronic traumatic encephalopathy: A chronic effects of neurotrauma consortium study. *Brain Inj.* 2016;30(12):1399-1413.

[1164] Hirad AA, Bazarian JJ, Merchant-Borna K, Garcea FE, Heilbronner S, et al. (2019). *Sci Adv.* Aug 7;5(8):eaau3460.

[1165] Zhang H, Zhang Z, Wang Z, Zhen Y, Yu J, et al. (2018). Research on the changes in balance motion behavior and learning, as well as memory abilities of rats with multiple cerebral concussion-induced chronic traumatic encephalopathy and the underlying mechanism. *Exp Ther Med.* Sep;16(3):2295-2302.

[1166] Ibid. Panchal. (2018). *Front Neurol.*

[1167] Alosco ML, Tripodis Y, Rowland B, Chua AS, Liao H, et al. (2019). A magnetic resonance spectroscopy investigation in symptomatic former NFL players. *Brain Imaging Behav.* Mar 8.

[1168] Paslakis G, Traber F, Roberz J, Block W, Jessen F. (2014). N-acetyl-aspartate (NAA) as a correlate of pharmacological treatment in psychiatrict disorders: a systematic review. *Eur Neuropsychopharmacol.* Oct;24(10):1659-75.

[1169] Ibid. Panchal. (2018). *Front Neurol.*

[1170] Ibid. Alosco. (2019).

[1171] NIH. Glutathione synthetase deficiency. Retrieved Oct 2 2019 from https://rarediseases.info.nih.gov/diseases/10047/glutathione-synthetase-deficiency.

[1172] Alosco ML, Koerte IK, Tripodis Y, Mariani M, Chua AS, et al. (2018). White matter signal abnormalities in former National Football League players. *Alzheimers Dement (Amst).* 2018:10:56-65.

[1173] Ibid. Gaetz. (2017). *Med Hypotheses.*

[1174] Ibid. Gaetz. (2017). *Med Hypotheses.*

[1175] Ibid. Katsumoto. (2019). *Front Neurol.*

[1176] Ibid. Gaetz. (2017).

[1177] Asken BM, Sullan MJ, Snyder AR, Houck ZM, Bryant VE, et al. (2016). Factors Influencing Clinical Correlates of Chronic Encephalopathy (CTE): a Review. *Neuropsychol Rev.* Dec;26(4):340-363.

[1178] Zetterberg H, Blennow K. (2018). Chronic traumatic encephalopathy: fluid biomarkers. *Handb Clin Neurol.* 2018;158:323-333.

[1179] Shinoda J, Nagamine Y, Kobayashi S, Odaki M, Oka N, et al. (2019). Multidisciplinary attentive treatment for patients with chronic disorders of consciousness following severe traumatic brain injury in the NASVA of Japan. *Brain Inj.* Sep 17:1-11.

[1180] Steinberg L. (2018). Helmet Rule Change: NFL's Next Step Toward Player Safety. *Forbes.* Aug 14, 2018.

[1181] France24. NFL concussions show sharp drop after rule changes. Retrieved Oct 1 2019 from https://www.france24.com/en/20190124-nfl-concussions-show-sharp-drop-after-rule-changes.

[1182] Bakala B. (2018). House Committee Passes Tackle Football Ban for Illinoisans Under Age 12. Retrieved Oct 1 2019 from https://www.illinoispolicy.org/house-committee-passes-tackle-football-ban-for-illinoisans-under-age-12/.

[1183] Fainaru-Wada M, Steele M. (2018). Debate over youth tackle football an extension of country's polarized politics. Retrieved Oct 1 2019 from https://www.espn.com/espn/otl/story/_/id/24773919/efforts-ban-youth-tackle-football-five-states-draw-comparisons-nanny-state-grass-roots-politics.

[1184] Coulter ID. (2014). The response of an expert panel to Nutritional armor for the warfighter: can omega-3 fatty acids enhance stress resilience, wellness, and military performance? *Mil Med.* Nov;179(11 Suppl):192-8.

[1185] Alzoubi KH, Al Hilo AS, Al-Balas QA, El-Salem K, El-Elimat T, et al. (2019). Withania somnifera root powder protects against post-traumatic stress disorder-induced memory impairment. *Mol Biol Rep.* Jun 19.

[1186] Sarris J, McIntyre E, Carnfield DA. (2013). Plant-based medicines for anxiety disorders, part 2: a review of clinical studies with supporting preclinical evidence. *CNS Drugs.* Apr;27(4):301-19.

[1187] Grimmig B, Daly L, Subbarayan M, Hudson C, Williamson R, et al. (2017). Astaxanthin is neuroprotective in an aged mouse model of Parkinson's disease. *Oncotarget.* Dec 28;9(12):10388-10401.

[1188] Grimmig B, Morganti J, Nash K, Bickford PC. (2016). Immunomodulators as Therapeutic Agents in Mitigating the Progression of Parkinson's Disease. *Brain Sci.* Sep 23;6(4):E41.

[1189] Ye Q, Zhang K, Huang B, Zhu Y, Chen X. (2013). Astaxanthin suppresses MPP(+)-induced oxidative damage in PC12 cells through a Sp1/NR1 signaling pathway. *Mar Drugs.* Mar 28;11(4):1019-34.

[1190] Lee DH, Kim CS, Lee YJ. (2011). Astaxanthin protects against MPTP/MPP+-induced mitochondria dysfunction and ROS production in vivo and in vitro. *Food Chem Toxicol.* Jan;49(1):271-80.

[1191] Fakhri S, Aneva IY, Farzaei MH, Sobarzo-Sanchez E. (2019). The Neuroprotective Effects of Astaxanthin: Therapeutic Targets and Clinic Perspective. *Molecules.* Jul 20;24(14):E2640.

[1192] Dinda B, Dinda S, DasSharma S, Banik R, Chakraborty A, et al. (2017). Therapeutic potentials of baicalein and its aglycone, baicalein against inflammatory disorders. *Eur J Med Chem.* May 5;131:68-80.

[1193] Chen M, Lai L, Li X, Zhang X, He X, et al. (2016). Baicalein attenuates neurological deficits and preserves blood-brain barrier integrity in a rat model of intracerebral hemorrhage. *Neurochem Res.* Nov;41:3095-3102.

[1194] Lu JH, Ardah MT, Durairajan SS, Liu LF, Xie LX, et al. (2011). Baicalein inhibits formation of alpha-synuclein oligomers within living cells and prevents aβ peptide fibrillation and oligomerisation. *Chembiochem.* Mar 7;12:615-624.

[1195] Jiang M, Porat-Shliom Y, Pei Z, Cheng Y, Xiang L, et al. (2010). Baicalein reduces E46K alpha-synuclein aggregation in vitro and protects cells against E46K alpha-synuclein toxicity in cell models of familiar parkinsonism. *J Neurochem.* Jul;114:419-429

[1196] Zhu M, Rajamani S, Kaylor J, Han S, Zhou F, et al. (2004). The flavonoid baicalein inhibits fibrillation of alpha-synuclein and disaggregates existing fibrils. *J Bio Chem.* June 25;279:26846-26857

[1197] Yu X, He G, Du G. (2012). [Neuroprotective effect of baicalein in patients with Parkinson's disease]. *Zhongguo Zhong Yao Za Zhi.* Feb;37(4):421-5.

[1198] Ibid. Sarris. (2013). *CNS Drugs.*

[1199] Ebenezer PJ, Wilson CB, Wilson LD, Nair AR, J F. (2016). The Anti-Inflammatory Effects of Blueberries in an Animal Model of Post-Traumatic Stress Disorder (PTSD). *PloS One.* Sep 7;11(9):e0160923.

[1200] Lee B, Lee H. (2018). System Administration of Curcumin Affect Anxiety-Related Behaviors in a Rat Model of Posttraumatic Stress Disorder via Activation of Serotonergic Systems. *Evid Based Complement Alternat Med.* Jun 19:218:9041309.

[1201] Lopresti AL. (2017). Curcumin for neuropsychiatric disorders: a review of in vitro, animal and human studies. *J Psychopharmacol.* Mar;31(3):287-302.

[1202] Kaufmann FN, Gazal M, Bastos CR, Kaster MP, Ghisleni G. (2016). Curcumin in depressive disorders: An overview of potential mechanisms, preclinical and clinical findings. *Eur J Pharmacol.* Aug 5;784:192-8.

[1203] Monsey MS, Gerhard DM, Boyle LM, Briones MA, Seligsohn M, et al. (2015). A diet enriched with curcumin impairs newly acquired and reactivated fear memories. *Neuropsychopharmacology.* Mar 13;40(5):1278-88.

[1204] De Vries GJ, Mocking R, Lok A, Assies J, Schene A, et al. (2016). Fatty acid concentrations in patients with posttraumatic stress disorder compared to healthy controls. *J Affect Disord.* Nov 15;205:351-359.

[1205] Matsuoka YJ, Hamazaki K, Nishi D, Hamazaki T. (2016). Change in blood levels of eicosapentaenoic acid and posttraumatic stress symptom: A secondary analysis of data from a placebo-controlled trial of omega3 supplements. *J Affect Disord.* Nov 15;205:289-291.

[1206] Nasir M, Bloch MH. (2019). Trim the fat: the role of omega-3 fatty acids in psychopharmacology. *Ther Adv Psychopharmacol.* Aug 27;9:20451253.

[1207] Matsuoka Y, Nishi D, Tanima Y, Itakura M, Kojima A, et al. (2015). Serum pro-BDNF/BDNF as a treatment biomarker for response to docosahexaenoic acid in traumatized people vulnerable to developing psychological distress: a randomized controlled trial. *Transl Psychiatry.* Jul 7;5:e596.

[1208] Lee B, Sur B, Cho SG, Yeom M, Shim I, et al. (2016). Ginsenoside Rb1 rescues anxiety-like responses in a rat model of post-traumatic stress disorder. *J Nat Med.* Apr;70(2):133-44.

[1209] Sohal RS, Orr WC. (2012). The redox stress hypothesis of aging. *Free Radic Biol Med.* Feb 1; 52(3):539-555.

[1210] Zeevalk GD, Razmpour R, Bernard LP. (2008). Glutathione and Parkinson's disease: is this the elephant in the room? *Biomed Pharmacother.* Apr-May; 62(4):236-49.

[1211] Ibid. Sarris. (2013). *CNS Drugs.*

[1212] Ibid. Sarris. (2013).

[1213] Garcia-Keller C, Smiley C, Monforton C, Melton S, Kalivas PW, et al. (2019). N-Acetylecystein treatment during acute stress prevents stress-induced augmentation of addictive drug use and relapse. *Addict Biol.* Jul 7:e12798.

[1214] Coulter ID. (2014). The response of an expert panel to Nutritional armor for the warfighter: can omega-3 fatty acids enhance stress resilience, wellness, and military performance? *Mil Med.* Nov;179(11 Suppl):192-8.

[1215] Zhang P, Ye Y, Qian Y, Yin B, Zhao J, et al. (2017). The Effect of Pyrroloquinoline Quinone on Apoptosis and Autophagy in Traumatic Brain Injury. *CNS Neurol Disord Drug Targets.* 2017;16(6):724-736.

[1216] Ibid. Sarris. (2013). *CNS Drugs.*

[1217] Ibid. Sarris. (2013).

[1218] De Souza Cp, Gambeta E, Stern CAJ, Zanoveli JM. (2019). Posttraumatic stress disorder-type behaviors in streptozotocin-induced diabetic rats can be prevents by prolonged treatment with vitamin E. *Behav Brain Res.* Feb;359:749-754.

[1219] Ross AJ, Medow MS, Rowe PC, Stewart JM. (2013). What is brain fog? An evaluation of the symptom in postural tachycardia syndrome. *Clin Auton Res.* Dec;23(6):305-11.

[1220] Martin S, Chen K, Harris N, Vera-Llonch M, Krasner A. (2019). Development of a Patient-Reported Outcome Measuring Chronic Hypoparathyroidism. *Adv Ther.* Jun 10.

[1221] Fukuda K, Straus SE, Hickie I, Sharpe MC, Dobbins JG. (1994). Chronic fatigue syndrome: a comprehensive approach to its definition and study. *Komaroff A Ann Intern Med.* Dec 15; 121(12):953-9.

[1222] Theocharides TC, Stewart JM, Hatziagelaki E, Kolaitis G. (2015). Brain "fog," inflammation and obesity: key aspects of neuropsychiatric disorders improved by luteolin. *Font Neurosci.* Jul3;9:225.

[1223] Yalland GW. (2017). Gluten-induced cognitive impairment ("brain fog") in coeliac disease. *J Gastroenterol Hepatol.* Mar;32 Suppl 1:90-93.

[1224] Deans M. (2015). Heavy Metal: Iron and the Brain. *Psychology Today.* Nov 29.

[1225] Kovalchuk A, Kolb B. (2017). Chemo brain: From discerning mechanisms to lifting the brain fog-An aging connection. *Cell Cycle.* Jul 19;16(15):1345-49.

[1226] Schmidt S. (2019). Brain Fog: Does Air Pollution Make Us Less Productive? Environ Health Perspect. May;127(5):52011.

[1227] Calderon-Garciduenas L, Azzarelli B, Acuna H, Garcia R, Gambling TM, Osnaya N, et al. (2002). Air pollution and brain damage. Toxicol Pathol. 2002 May-Jun;30(3):373-89.

[1228] Calderon-Garciduenas L, Reynoso-Robles R, Vargas-Martinez J, Gomez-Maqueo-Chew A, Parez-Guille B. (2016). Prefrontal white matter pathology in air pollution exposed Mexico City young urbanites and their potential impact on neurovascular unit dysfunction and the development of Alzheimer's disease. *Environ Res.* 2016 Apr;146:404-17.

1229 Calderon-Garciduenas L, Leray F, Heydarpour P, Torres-Jardon R, Reis J. (2016). Air pollution, a rising environmental risk factor for cognition, neuroinflammation and neurodegeneration: The clinical impact on children and beyond. *Rev Neurol (Paris)*. 2016 Jan;172(1):69-80.

1230Calderon-Garciduenas L, Reynoso-Robles R, Gonzalez-Maciel A. (2019). Combustion and friction-derived nanoparticles and industrial-sourced nanoparticles: The culprit of Alzheimer and Parkinson's diseases. *Environ Res*. 2019 Jul 5;176:108574.

1231 Kim KM, Zameleeva AI, Lee YW, Ahmed MR, Kim E. (2018). Characterization of Brain Dysfunction Induced by Bacterial Lipopeptides that Alter Neuronal Activity and Network in Rodent Brains. *J Neurosci*. Dec 12;38(50):10672-10691.

1232 Eaneff S, Wang V, Hanger M, Levy M, Mealy MA, et al. (2017). Patient perspectives on neuromyelitis optica spectrum disorders: Data from the PatientsLikeMe online community. *Mult Scler Relat Disord*. Oct;17:116-122.

1233 Manzo C, Martinez-Suarez E, Kechida M, Isetta M, Serra-Mestres J. (2019). Cognitive Function in Primary Sjogren's Syndrome: A Systematic Review. *Brain Sci*. Apr 15;9(4):E85.

1234 Stoykovich S, Gibas K. (2019). APOEe4, the door to insulin-resistant dyslipidemia and brain fog? A case study. *Alzheimers Dement iAmst)*. Mar 14;11:264-269.

1235 Colucci L, Bosco M, Ziello AR, Rea R, Amenta F, et al. (2012). Effectiveness of nootropic drugs with cholinergic activity in treatment of cognitive deficit: a review. *J Exp Pharmacol*. 2012;4:163-172.

1236 Rebello CJ, Keller JN, Liu AG, Johnson WD, Greenway FL. (2015). Pilot feasibility and safety study examining the effect of medium chain triglyceride supplementation in subjects with mild cognitive impairment: A randomized controlled trial. *BBA Clin*. Jan 16;3:123-5.

1237 Onore C, Careaga M, Ashwood P. (2012). The role of immune dysfunction in the pathophysiology of autism. *Brain Behav Immun*. Mar; 26(3):383-92.

1238 Theoharides TC, Zhang B. (2011). Neuro-inflammation, blood-brain barrier, seizures and autism. *J Neuroinflammation*. Nov 30; 8():168.

1239 Najjar S, Pearlman DM, Alper K, Najjar A, Devinsky O. (2013). Neuroinflammation and psychiatric illness. *J Neuroinflammation*. Apr 1; 10():43.

1240 Zhao Q, Peng C, Wu X, Chen Y, Wang C, et al. (2014). Maternal sleep deprivation inhibits hippocampal neurogenesis associated with inflammatory response in young offspring rats. *Neurobiol Dis*. 2014 Aug; 68():57-65.

1241 Heneka MT, Carson MJ, El Ehoury J, Landreth GE, Brosseron F, et al. (2015). Neuroinflammation in Alzheimer's disease. *Lancet Neurol*. Apr;14(4):388-405.

1242 Réus GZ, Fries GR, Stertz L, Badawy M, Passos IC, et al. (2015). The role of inflammation and microglial activation in the pathophysiology of psychiatric disorders. *J Neuroscience*. Aug 6; 300():141-54.

1243 Steiner N, Balez R, Karunaweera N, Lind JM, et al. (2016). Neuroprotection of Neuro2a cells and the cytokine suppressive and anti-inflammatory mode of action of resveratrol in activated RAW264.7 macrophages and C8-B4 microglia. *Neurochem Int*. May; 95():46-54.

1244 Perry VH. (2004). The influence of systemin inflammation on inflammation in the brain: implications for chronic neurodegenerative disease. *Brain Behav Immun*. Sept;1. 8(5):407-13.

1245 Perry VH. (2010). Contribution of systemic inflammation to chronic neurodegeneration. *Acta Neuropathol*. Sep;120(3):277-86

1246 Miyake S, Yamamura T. (2009). Ghrelin: friend or foe for neuroinflammation. *Discov Med*. Aug;8(41):64-7.

1247 Schrepf A, Kaplan CM, Ichesco E, Larkin T, Harte SE, et al. (2018). A multi-modal MRI study of the central response to inflammation in rheumatoid arthritis. *Nat Commun*. Jun 8;9(1):2243.

1248 Sin SY, Katz P, Wallhagen M, Julian L. (2012). Cognitive impairment in persons with rheumatoid arthritis. *Arthritis Care Res* , (Hoboken). Aug; 64(8): 1144–1150.

1249 Calderon-Garciduenas L, Azzarelli B, Acuna H, Garcia R, Gambling TM, Osnaya N, et al. (2002). Air pollution and brain damage. *Toxicol Pathol*. 2002 May-Jun;30(3):373-89.

1250 Calderon-Garciduenas L, Reynoso-Robles R, Vargas-Martinez J, Gomez-Maqueo-Chew A, Parez-Guille B. (2016). Prefrontal white matter pathology in air pollution exposed Mexico City young urbanites and their potential impact on neurovascular unit dysfunction and the development of Alzheimer's disease. *Environ Res*. 2016 Apr;146:404-17.

1251 Calderon-Garciduenas L, Leray F, Heydarpour P, Torres-Jardon R, Reis J. (2016). Air pollution, a rising environmental risk factor for cognition, neuroinflammation and neurodegeneration: The clinical impact on children and beyond. *Rev Neurol (Paris)*. 2016 Jan;172(1):69-80.

1252Calderon-Garciduenas L, Reynoso-Robles R, Gonzalez-Maciel A. (2019). Combustion and friction-derived nanoparticles and industrial-sourced nanoparticles: The culprit of Alzheimer and Parkinson's diseases. *Environ Res*. 2019 Jul 5;176:108574.

1253 Li Y, Li M, Zuo L, Shi Q, Qin W, et al. (2018). Compromised Blood-Brain Barrier Integrity is Associated with Total Magnetic Resonance Imaging Burden of Cerebral Small Vessel Disease. *Front Neurol*. Apr 6;9:221.

1254 McGeer PL, Schulzer M, McGeer EG. (1996). Arthritis and anti-inflammatory agents as possible protective factors for Alzheimer's disease: a review of 17 epidemiologic studies. *Neurology*. Aug; 47(2):425-32.

[1255] Shen Y, Kapfhammer D, Minella AM, Kim JE, Won SJ, et al. (2017). Bioenergetic state regulates innate inflammatory responses through the transcriptional co-repressor CtBP. *Nat Commun.* 2017;8(624).

[1256] Beilharz JE, Maniam J, Morris MJ. (2015). Diet-Induced Cognitive Deficits: The Role of Fat and Sugar, Potential Mechanisms and Nutritional Interventions. *Nutrients.* Aug 12;7(8):6719-38.

[1257] Volek JS, Fernandez ML, Feinman RD, Phinney SD. (2008). Dietary carbohydrate restriction induces a unique metabolic state positively affecting atherogenic dyslipidemia, fatty acid partitioning, and metabolic syndrome. *Prog Lipid Res.* Sep;47(5):307-18.

[1258] Roberts RO, Roberts LA, Geda YE, Cha RH, Pankratz VS, et al. (2012). Relative intake of macronutrients impacts risk of mild cognitive impairment or dementia. *J Alzheimers Dis.* 2012;32(2):329-39.

[1259] Obrenovich MEM. (2018). Leaky Gut, Leaky Brain? *Microorganisms.* 2018 Oct 18;6(4):E107.

[1260] Wikipedia. Intestinal mucosal barrier. Retrieved Oct 17 2019 from https://en.wikipedia.org/wiki/Intestinal_mucosal_barrier.

[1261] Ibid. Obrenovich. (2018).

[1262] Wikipedia. Gastrointestinal tract. Retrieved Oct 19 2019 from https://en.wikipedia.org/wiki/Gastrointestinal_tract.

[1263] Hill JM, Clement C, Pogue AI, Bhattacharjee S, Zhao Y, et al. (2014). Pathogenic microbes, the microbiome, and Alzheimer's disease (AD). *Front Aging Neurosci.* 6():127.

[1264] Foster JA, Neufeld KAM. (2013). Gut-brain axis: how the microbiome influences anxiety and depression. *Trends Neurosci.* May;36(5):305-12.

[1265] Turnbaugh PJ, Ley RE, Hamady M, Fraser-Liggett CM, Knight R, et al. (2007). The human microbiome project. *Nature.* Oct 18; 449(7164):804-10.

[1266] Clemente JC, Ursell LK, Parfrey LW, Knight R. (2012). The impact of the gut microbiota on human health: an integrative view. *Cell.* Mar 16; 148(6):1258-70.

[1267] Human Microbiome Project Consortium. (2012). Structure, function and diversity of the healthy human microbiome. *Nature.* Jun 13; 486(7402):207-14.

[1268] Raes J, Arumugam M, Burgdorf KS, et al. (2010). A human gut microbial gene catalogue established by metagenomic sequencing. *Nature.* 2010 Mar 4; 464(7285):59-65.

[1269] Grenham S, Clarke G, Cryan JF, Dinan TG. (2011). Brain-gut-microbe communication in health and disease. *Front Physiol.* 2011; 2():94.

[1270] Wade PR, Cowen T. Neurodegeneration: a key factor in the ageing gut. *Neurogastroenterol Motil.* 2004 Apr;16 Suppl 1:19-23

[1271] Wang Y, Kondo T, Suzukamo Y, Oouchidaa Y, Izumi S. (2010). Vagal nerve regulation is essential for the increase in gastric motility in response to mild exercise. *Tohoku J Exp Med.* 222(2):155-62.

[1272] Zhu X, Han Y, Du J, Liu R, Jin K, et al. (2017). Microbiota-gut-brain axis and the central nervous system. *Oncotarget.* Aug 8;8(32):53829-53838.

[1273] Alkasir R, Li J, Li X, Jin M, Zhu B. (2017). Human gut microbiota: the links with dementia development. *Protein Cell.* Feb;8(2):90-102.

[1274] Viswanathan VK, Koutsouris A, Lukic S, Pilkinton M, Simonovic I, et al. (2004). Comparative analysis of EspF from enteropathogenic and enterohemorrhagic Escherichia coli in alteration of epithelial barrier function. *Infect Immun.* 2004 Jun; 72(6):3218-27.

[1275] Wilmore DW, Smith RJ, O'Dwyer ST, Jacobs DO, Ziegler TR, et al. (1998). The gut: a central organ after surgical stress. *Surgery.* 1988 Nov; 104(5):917-23.

[1276] Welsh FK, Farmery SM, MacLennan K, Sheridan MB, Barclay GR, et al. (1998). Gut barrier function in malnourished patients. *Gut.* Mar; 42(3):396-401.

[1277] Rupani B, Caputo FJ, Watkins AC, Vega D, Magnotti LJ, et al. (2007). Relationship between disruption of the unstirred mucus layer and intestinal restitution in loss of gut barrier function after trauma hemorrhagic shock. *Surgery.* Apr; 141(4):481-9.

[1278] Carneiro-Filho BA, Lima IP, Araujo DH, Cavalcante MC, Carvalho GH, et al. (2004). Intestinal barrier function and secretion in methotrexate-induced rat intestinal mucositis. *Dig Dis Sci.* Jan; 49(1):65-72.

[1279] Illig KA, Ryan CK, Hardy DJ, Rhodes J, Locke W, et al. (1992). Total parenteral nutrition-induced changes in gut mucosal function: atrophy alone is not the issue. *Surgery.* Oct; 112(4):631-7.

[1280] Yoshida S, Matsui M, Shirouzu Y, Fujita H, Yamana H, et al. (1998). Effects of glutamine supplements and radiochemotherapy on systemic immune and gut barrier function in patients with advanced esophageal cancer. *An Surg.* Apr; 227(4):485-91.

[1281] Ferrier L, Mazelin L, Cenac N, Desreumaux P, Janin A, et al. (2003). Stress-induced disruption of colonic epithelial barrier: role of interferon-gamma and myosin light chain kinase in mice. *Gastroenterology.* Sep; 125(3):795-804.

[1282] Fasano A. (2011). Zonulin and its regulation of intestinal barrier function: the biological door to inflammation, autoimmunity, and cancer. *Physiol Rev.* Jan; 91(1):151-75.

[1283] Gammon C. (2009). Weed-Whacking Herbicide Proves Deadly to Human Cells. Retrieved Oct 22 2019 from https://www.scientificamerican.com/article/weed-whacking-herbicide-p/.

[1284] Samsel A, Seneff S. (2013). Glyphosate's suppression of cytochrome P450 enzymes and amino acid biosynthesis by the gut microbiome: Pathways to modern diseases. *Entropy.* 2013;15:1416–1463.

[1285] Flint HJ, Duncan SH, Louis P. (2017). The impact of nutrition on intestinal bacterial communities. *Curr Opin Microbiol.* Aug; 38():59-65.

[1286] Bansal V, Constantini T, Ryu SY, Peterson C, Loomis W, et al. (2010). Stimulating the central nervous system to prevent intestinal dysfunction after traumatic brain injury. *J Trauma.* May;68(5):1059-64.

[1287] Hollander D. (1999). Intestinal permeability, leaky gut, and intestinal disorders. *Curr Gastroenterol Rep.* Oct;(5):410-6.

[1288] Axe J. (2015). 5 Signs You're Suffering From Candida Overgrowth – and What You Can Do About It. US News Health. Dec 23.

[1289] Galland L. (1983). Nutrition and Candidiasis. Yeast-Human Interaction Symposium, Birmingham Alabama Dec 10.

[1290] Gamaletsou MN, Rammaert B, Bueno MA, Sipsas NV, Moriyama B, et al. (2016). Candida Arthritis: Analysis of 112 Pediatric and Adult Cases. *Open Forum Infect Dis.* Jan;3(1):ofv207.

[1291] McDonell K. (2017). 7 Symptoms of Candida Overgrowth (Plus How to Get Rid of It). Healthline. Aug 24.

[1292] Centers for Disease Control and Prevention. (no date). Invasive candidiasis. Retrieved Aug 21 2020 from https://www.cdc.gov/fungal/diseases/candidiasis/invasive/index.html.

[1293] Zhang JR, Tuomanen E. (1999). Molecular and cellular mechanisms for microbial entry into the CNS. *J Neuroviol.* Dec;5(6):581-603.

[1294] Antinori S, Milazzo L, Sallima S, Galli M, Corbellino M. (2016). Candidemia and invasive candidiasis in adults: A narrative review. *Eur J Intern Med.* Oct;34:21-28.

[1295] Barchiesi F, Orsetti E, Mazzanti S, Trave F, Salvi A, et al. (2017). Candidemia in the elderly: What does it change? PLoS One. May 11;12(5):e0176576.

[1296] Parker JC, McCloskey JJ, Lee RS. (1981). Human cerebral candidosis—a postmortem evaluation of 19 patients. *Hum Pathol.* Jan;12(1):23-8.

[1297] Wu Y, Du S, Johnson JL, Tung HY, Landers CT, et al. (2019). Microglia and amyloid precursor protein coordinate control of transient Candida cerebritis with memory deficits. *Nat Commun.* Jan 4;10(1):58.

[1298] Lone SA, Ahmad A. (2019). Candida auris-the growing menace to global health. Mycoses. Aug;62(8):620-637.

[1299] Maes M, Kubera M, Leunis JC. (2008). The gut-brain barrier in major depression: intestinal mucosal dysfunction with an increased translocation of LPS from gram negative enterobacteria (leaky gut) plays a role in the inflammatory pathophysiology of depression. *Neuro Endocrinol Lett.* Feb; 29(1):117-24.

[1300] Purohit V, Bode JC, Bode C, Brenner DA, et al. (2008). Alcohol, intestinal bacterial growth, intestinal permeability to endotoxin, and medical consequences: summary of a symposium. *Alcohol.* Aug:42(5):349-61.

[1301] Hawkes CH, Del Tredici K, Braak H. (2007). Parkinson's disease: a dual-hit hypothesis. *Neuropathol Appl Neurobiol.* Dec; 33(6):599-614.

[1302] Hill JM, Lukiw WJ. (2015). Microbial-generated amyloids and Alzheimer's disease (AD). *Front Aging Neurosci.* 2015;7():9.

[1303] Hill JM, Clement C, Pogue AI, Bhattacharjee S, Zhao Y, et al. (2014). Pathogenic microbes, the microbiome, and Alzheimer's disease (AD). *Jn Front Aging Neurosci.* 2014 6():127.

[1304] Ibid. Hill. (2014).

[1305] Dignass AU. (2001). Mechanisms and modulation of intestinal epithelial repair. *Inflamm Bowel Dis.* Feb; 7(1):68-77.

[1306] Duggan C, Gannon J, Walker WA. (2002). Protective nutrients and functional foods for the gastrointestinal tract. *Am J Clin Nutr.* May; 75(5):789-808.

[1307] Bansal V, Constantini T, Kroll L, Peterson C, Loomis W, et al. (2009). Traumatic brain injury and intestinal dysfunction: uncovering the neuro-enteric axis. *J Neurotrauma.* Aug:26(8):1353-9.

[1308] Bonaz BL, Bernstein CN. (2013). Brain-gut interactions in inflammatory bowel disease. *Gastroenterology.* Jan; 144(1):36-49.

[1309] Engelborghs S, De Brabander M, De Crée J, D'Hooge R, Geerts H, et al. (1999). Unchanged levels of interleukins, neopterin, interferon-gamma and tumor necrosis factor-alpha in cerebrospinal fluid of patients with dementia of the Alzheimer type. *Neurochem Int.* Jun; 34(6):523-30.

[1310] Yaffe K, Lindquist K, Penninx BW, Simonsick EM, Pahor M, et al. (2003). Inflammatory markers and cognition in well-functioning African-American and white elders. *Neurology.* Jul 8; 61(1):76-80.

[1311] Harris TB, Benjamin EJ, Au R, Kiel DP, Wolf PA, et al. (2007). Inflammatory markers and the risk of Alzheimer's disease: the Framingham Study. *Neurolgy.* May 29; 68(22):1902-8.

[1312] Zuliani G, Ranzini M, Guerra G, Rossi L, Munari MR, et al. (2007). Plasma cytokines profile in older subjects with late onset Alzheimer's disease or vascular dementia. *J Psychiatr Res.* Oct; 41(8):686-93.

[1313] Aisen PS, Davis KL. (1994). Inflammatory mechanisms in Alzheimer's disease: implications for therapy. *Am J Psychiatry.* Aug; 151(8):1105-13.

[1314] Nagpal R, Neth BJ, Wang S, Craft S, Yadav H. (2019). Modified Mediterrean-ketogenic diet modulates gut microbiome and short-chain fatty acids in association with Alzheimer's disease markers in subjects with mild cognitive impairment. *EBioMedicine.* Sep;47:529-542.

[1315] Dinan TG, Cryan JF. (2013). Melancholic microbes: a link between gut microbiota and depression? *Neurogastroenterol Motil.* Sep; 25(9):713-9.

[1316] Hsiao EY, McBride SW, Hsien S, Sharon G, Hyde ER, et al. (2013). Microbiota modulate behavioral and physiological abnormalities associated with neurodevelopmental disorders. *Cell.* Dec 19; 155(7):1451-63.

[1317] Borre YE, O'Keeffe GW, Clarke G, Stanton C, Dinan TG, et al. (2014). Microbiota and neurodevelopmental windows: implications for brain disorders. *Trends Mol Med.* Sep; 20(9):509-18.

[1318] Hazen SL, Smith JD. (2012). An antiatherosclerotic signaling cascade involving intestinal microbiota, microRNA-10b, and ABCA1/ABCG1-mediated reverse cholesterol transport. *Circ Res.* Sep 28; 111(8):948-50.

[1319] Davson H, Segal MB. (1996). Physiology of the CSF and Blood-Brain Barriers. Boca Raton: *CRC Press;* 1996.

[1320] Biesmans S, Bouwknecht JA, Ver Donck L, Langlois X, Acton PD, et al. (2015). Peripheral Administration of Tumor Necrosis Factor-Alpha Induces Neuroinflammation and Sickness but Not Depressive-Like Behavior in Mice. *Biomed Res Int.* 2015():716920.

[1321] Gądek-Michalska A, Tadeusz J, Rachwalska P, Bugajski J. (2013). Cytokines, prostaglandins and nitric oxide in the regulation of stress-response systems. *Pharmacol Rep.* 65(6):1655-62.

[1322] Lopez-Ramirez MA, Wu D, Pryce G, Simpson JE, Reijerkerk A, et al. (2014). MicroRNA-155 negatively affects blood-brain barrier function during neuroinflammation. *FASEB J.* Jun;28(6):2551-65.

[1323] Block ML, Hong JS. (2005). Microglia and inflammation-mediated neurodegeneration: multiple triggers with a common mechanism. Prog Neurobiol. Jun;76(2):77-98.

[1324] Carabotti M, Scirocco A, Maselli MA, Severi C. (2015). The gut-brain axis: interactions between enteric microbiota, central and enteric nervous systems. *Ann Gastroenterol.* Apr-Jun; 28(2):203-209.

[1325] Mayer EA, Padua D, Tillisch K. (2014). Altered brain-gut axis in autism: comorbidity or causative mechanisms? *Bioessays.* Oct; 36(10):933-9.

[1326] Dinan TG, Stanton C, Cryan JF. (2013). Psychobiotics: a novel class of psychotropic. *Biol Psychiatry.* Nov 15; 74(10):720-6.

[1327] Ibid. Nagpal (2019).

[1328] Hamer HM, Jonkers D, Venema K, Vanhoutvin S, Troost FJ, et al. (2008). Review article: the role of butyrate on colonic function. *Aliment Pharmacol Ther.* Jan 15;27(2):104-19.

[1329] Selhub EM, Logan AC, Bested AC. (2014). Fermented foods, microbiota, and mental health: ancient practice meets nutritional psychiatry. *J Physiol Anthropol.* Jan 15; 33():2.

[1330] Lamprecht M, Bogner S, Schippinger G, Steinbauer K, et al. (2012).Probiotic supplementation affects markers of intestinal barrier, oxidation, and inflammation in trained men; a randomized, double-blinded, placebo-controlled trial. *J Int Soc Sports Nutr* 9(1):45.

[1331] Markowiak P, Slizewska K. (2017). Effects of Probiotics, Prebiotics, and Synbiotics on Human Health. *Nutrients.* Sep;9(9):1021.

[1332] Rao RK, Samak G. (2013). Protection and Restitution of Gut Barrier by Probiotics: Nutritional and Clinical Implications. *Curr Nutr Food Sci.* May 1; 9(2): 99–107.

[1333] Ibid. Rao. (2013).

[1334] Smith CJ, Emge JR, Berzins K, Lung L, Khamishon R, et al. (2014). Probiotics normalize the gut-brain-microbiota axis in immunodeficient mice. *Am J Physiol Gastrointest Liver Physiol.* Oct 15; 307(8):G793-802.

[1335] Ait-Belgnaoui A, Durand H, Cartier C, Chaumaz G, Eutamene H, et al. (2012). Prevention of gut leakiness by a probiotic treatment leads to attenuated HPA response to an acute psychological stress in rats. *Psychoneuroendocrinology.* Nov; 37(11):1885-95.

[1336] Benton D, Williams C, Brown A. (2007). Impact of consuming a milk drink containing a probiotic on mood and cognition. *Eur J Clin Nutr.* Mar; 61(3):355-61.

[1337] Messaoudi M, Lalonde R, Violle N, Javelot H, Desor D, et al. (2011). Assessment of psychotropic-like properties of a probiotic formulation (Lactobacillus helveticus R0052 and Bifidobacterium longum R0175) in rats and human subjects. *Br J Nutr.* Mar; 105(5):755-64.

[1338] Steenbergen L, Sellaro R, van Hemert S, Bosch JA, Colzato LS. (2015). A randomized controlled trial to test the effect of multispecies probiotics on cognitive reactivity to sad mood. *Brain Behav Immun.* Aug; 48():258-64.

[1339] Schmidt K, Cowen PJ, Harmer CJ, Tzortzis G, Errington S, et al. (2015). Prebiotic intake reduces the waking cortisol response and alters emotional bias in healthy volunteers. *Psychopharmacology (Berl).* May; 232(10):1793-801.

[1340] Ibid. Markowiak. (2017).

[1341] De Vrese M, Schrezenmeir J. (2008). Probiotics, prebiotics, and synbiotics. *Adv Biochem Eng Biotechnol.* 111:1-66.

[1342] Konturek PC, Brzozowski T, Konturek SJ. (2011). Stress and the gut: pathophysiology, clinical consequences, diagnostic approach and treatment options. *J Physiol Pharmacol.* Dec;62(60:591-9.

[1343] Suarez K, Mayer C, Ehlert U, Nater UM. (2010). Psychological Stress and Self-Reported Functional Gastrointestinal Disorders. *J Nerv Ment Dis.* March;198(3):226-9.

1344 Kiecolt-Glaser JK, Derry HM, Fagundes CP. (2015). Inflammation: depression fans the flames and feasts on the heat. *Am J Psychiatry.* Nov 1;172(11):1075-91.

1345 Lamprecht M, Frauwallner A. (2012). Exercise, intestinal barrier dysfunction and probiotic supplementation. *Med Sport Sci.* 59:47-56.

1346 Karper WB. (2011). Intestinal permeability, moderate exercise, and older adult health. *Holist Nurs Pract.* Jan-Feb;25(1):45-8.

1347 Marks IN. (1988). Site-protective agents. *Baillieres Clin Gastroenterol.* Jul;2(3):609-20.

1348 Marks IN, Boyd E. (1985). Mucosal protective agents in the long-term management of gastric ulcer. *Med J Aust.* 1985 Feb 4;142(3):S23-5.

1349 Rees WD, Rhodes J, Wright JE, Stamford LF, Bennett A. Effect of deglycyrrhizinated liquorice on gastic mucosal damage by aspirin. Scand *J Gastroenterol.* 1979;14(5):605-7.

1350 Sharma V, Agrawal RC. (2013). Glycyrrhiza glabra – A Plant for the Future. *Min J Pharmaceu Med Sci.* Jul-Sep;2(3).

1351 (2018). 12 Best Supplements for Leaky Gut Syndrome. Retrieved Oct 2 2019 from https://blog.thryveinside.com/12-best-supplements-for-leaky-gut-syndrome/.

1352 Van Ampting MT, Schonewille AJ, Vink C, Brummer RJ, van der Meer R, et al. (2009). Intestinal barrier function in response to abundant or depleted mucosal glutathione in Salmonella-infected rats. *MBC Physiol.* Apr 17; 9:6.

1353 Van der Hulst RR, van Kreel BK, von Meyenfeldt MF, Brummer RJ, Arends JW, et al. (1993). Glutamine and the preservation of gut integrity. *Lancet.* May 29;341(8857):1363-5.

1354 Rao R, Samak G. (2012). Role of Glutamine in Protection of Intestinal Epithelial Tight Junctions. *J Epithel Biol Pharmacol.* Jan;5(Suppl 1-M7):47-54.

1355 Amasheh M, Andres S, Amasheh S, Fromm M, Schulzke JD. (2009). Barrier effects of nutritional factors. *Ann N Y Acad Sci.* May;1165:267-73.

1356 Coeffier M, Claeysenns S, Lecleire S, Leblond J, Coquard A, et al. (2008). Combined interal infusion of glutamine, carbohydrates, and antioxidant modulates gut protein metabolism in humans. *Am J Clinic Nutr.* Nov;88(5):1284-90.

1357 Engels G. (2007). Marshmallow. *Herbal Gram.* 2007;75:1–5.

1358 Yamada HT, Nagai JC, Cyong Y, et al. (1985). Relationship between chemical structure and anti-complementary activity of plant polysaccharides. *Carbohydr Res.* 1(1):28–31.

1359 Deters A, Zippel J, Hellenbrand N, Pappai D, Possemeyer C, et al. (2010). Aqueous extracts and polysaccharides from Marshmallow roots (Althea officinalis L.): cellular internalization and stimulation of cell physiology of human epithelial cells in vitro. *J. Ethnopharmacol.* Jan. 8;127(1):62-9.

1360 Iauk L, Lo Bue AM, Milazzo I, Rapisarda A, Blandino G. (2003). Antibacterial activity of medicinal plant extracts against periodontopathic bacteria. *Phytother Res.* Jun;17(6):599-604.

1361 Zaghlool SS, Shehata BA, Abo-Seif AA, Abd El-Latif HA. (2015). Protective effects of ginger and marshmallow extracts on indomethacin-induced peptic ulcer in rats. *J Nat Sci Biol Med.* Jul-Dec; 6(2): 421–428.

1362 Kim YH, Kim DH, Lim H, Baek DY, Shin HK, et al. (2009). The anti-inflammatory effects of methylsulfonylmethane on lipopolysaccharide-induced inflammatory responses in murine macrophages. Kim JK *Biol Pharm Bull.* Apr; 32(4):651-6.

1363 Ibid. Kim. (2009).

1364 Ahn H, Kim J, Lee MJ, Kim YJ, Cho YW, et al. (2015). Methylsulfonylmethane inhibits NLRP3 inflammasome activation. *Cytokine.* Feb; 71(2):223-31.

1365 Oshima Y, Amiel D, Theodosakis J. (2007). The effect of distilled methylsulfonylmethane (msm) on human chondrocytes in vitro. *Osteoarthr. Cartil.* 2007;15:C123.

1366 Parcell S. (2017). Sulfur in human nutrition and applications in medicine. *Altern Med Rev.* Feb;7(1):22-24.

1367 Butawan M, Benjamin RL, Bloomer RJ. (2017). Methylsulfonylmethane: Applications and Safety of a Novel Dietary Supplement. *Nutrients.* Mar;9(3):290.

1368 Bak YK, Lampe JW, Sung MK. (2014). Effects of dietary supplementation of glucosamine sulfate on intestinal inflammation in a mouse model of experimental colitis. *J Gastroenterol Hepatol.* May;29(5):957-63.

1369 Li Q, Zhang Q, Wang M, Zhao S, Xu G, et al. (2008). n-3 polyunsaturated fatty acids prevent disruption of epithelial barrier function induced by proinflammatory cytokines. *J Mol Immunol.* Mar; 45(5):1356-65.

1370 Mani V, Hollis JH, Gabler NK. (2013). Dietary oil composition differentially modulates intestinal endotoxin transport and postprandial endotoxemia. *Nutr Metab (Lond).* Jan 10; 10(1):6.

1371 Costantini L, Molinari R, Farinon B, Merendino N. (2017). . Impact of Omega-3 Fatty Acids on the Gut Microbiota. *Int J Mol Sci.* Dec 7;18(12): E2645.

1372 Suzuki T, Hara H. (2011). Role of flavonoids in intestinal tight junction regulation. *J Nutr Biochem.* May;22(5):401-408.

[1373] Suzuki T, Hara H. (2009). Quercetin Enhances Intestinal Barrier Function through the Assembly of Zonnula Occludens-2, Occludin, and Claudin-1 and the Expression of Claudin-4 in Caco-2 Cells *J Nutr Biochem. May 1;139(5):965-974.*

[1374] Santos J, Yang PC, Soderholm JD, Benjamin M, Perdue MH. (2001). Role of mast cells in chronic stress induced colonic epithelial barrier dysfunction in the rat. *Gut.* May;48(5):630-6.

[1375] Pearce FL, Befus AD, Bienenstock J. (1984). Mucosal mast cells. III. Effect of quercetin and other flavonoids on antigen-induced histamine seceation from rate intestinal mast cells. *J Allergy Clin Immunol.* Jun;73(6):819-23.

[1376] WebMD. Slippery Elm. Retrieved Oct 22 from https://www.webmd.com/vitamins/ai/ingredientmono-978/slippery-elm.

[1377] Ibid. WebMD. Slippery Elm.

[1378] Joo YE. (2014). Natural Product-Derived Drugs for the Treatment of Inflammatory Bowel Diseases. *Intestinal Res.* Apr;12(2):103-109.

[1379] Chen P, Soares AM, Lima AAM, Gamble MV, Schorling JB, et al. (2003). Association of Vitamin A and Zinc Status with Altered Intestinal Permeability: Analyses of Cohort Data from Northeastern Brazil. *J Health Pop Nutr.* Dec;21(4):309-15.

[1380] Sturniolo GC, Di Leo V, Ferronato A, D'Odorico A, D'Inca R. (2001). Zinc supplementation tightens "leaky gut" in Crohn's disease. *Inflamm Bowel Dis.* May;7(2):94-8.

[1381] Shelton RM. (1991). Aloe vera. Its chemical and therapeutic properties. *Int J Dermatol.* Oct; 30(10):679-83.

[1382] Hamman JH. (2008). Composition and applications of Aloe vera leaf gel. *Molecules.* Aug 8; 13(8):1599-616.

[1383] Fawole OA, Amoo SO, Ndhlala AR, Light ME, Finnie JF, et al. (2010). Anti-inflammatory, anticholinesterase, antioxidant and phytochemical properties of medicinal plants used for pain-related ailments in South Africa. *J Ethnopharmacol.* Feb 3;127(2):235-41.

[1384] Rosca-Casian O, Parvu M, Vlase L, Tamas M. (2007). Antifungal activity of Aloe vera leaves. *Fitoterapia.* Apr;78(3):219-22

[1385] Lamm S, Sheng Y, Pero RW. (2001). Persistent response to pneumococcal vaccine in individuals supplemented with a novel water soluble extract of Uncaria tomentosa, C-Med-100. *Phytomedicine.* Jul;8(4):267-74.

[1386] WebMD. Cat's Claw. Retrieved Oct 22 2019 from ://www.webmd.com/vitamins/ai/ingredientmono-395/cats-claw

[1387] Rocha BS, Gago B, Barbosa RM. (2009). Dietary polyphenols generate nitric oxide from nitrite in the stomach and induce smooth muscle relaxation. *Laranjinha J Toxicology.* Nov 9; 265(1-2):41-8.

[1388] Bernardes I, Felipe Rodrigues MP, Bacelli GK, Munin E, Alves LP, et al. (2012). Aloe vera extract reduces both growth and germ tube formation by Candida albicans. *Mycoses.* May;55(3):257-61.

[1389] Cataldi V, Di Bartolomeo S, Di Campli E, Nostro A, Cellini L, et al. (2015). . In vitro activity of Aloe vera inner gel against microorganisms grown in planktonic and sessile phases. *Int J Immunopathol Pharmacol.* Dec;28(4):595-602.

[1390] Kosalec I, Pepeljnjak S, Kustrak D. *(2005).* Antifungal activity of fluid extract and essential oil from anise fruits (Pimpinella anisum L., Apiaceae). *Acta Pharm.* Dec;55(4):377-85.

[1391] Swamy MK, Akhtar MS, Sinniah UR. (2016). Antimicrobial Properties of Plant Essential Oils against Human Pathogens and Their Mode of Action: An Updated Review. *Evid Based Complement Alternat Med.* 2016: 3012462.

[1392] Stampar F., Solar A., Hudina M., Veberic R., and Colaric M. (2006). Traditional walnut liqueur - cocktail of phenolics. *Food Chem.* 95:627–631.

[1393] Vinson J. A., and Cai Y. X. ()2012. Nuts, especially walnuts, have both antioxidant quantity and efficacy and exhibit significant potential health benefits. *Food Funct.* 3:134–140.

[1394] Oliveira I., Sousa A., Ferreira I., Bento A., Estevinho L., and Pereira J. A. (2008). Total phenols, antioxidant potential and antimicrobial activity of walnut (Juglans regia L.) green husks. *Food Chem. Toxicol.* 46:2326–2331.

[1395] Fernandez-Agullo A., Pereira E., Freire M. S., Valentao P., Andrade P. B., Gonzalez-Alvarez J., et al. 2013. Influence of solvent on the antioxidant and antimicrobial properties of walnut (Juglans regia L.) green husk extracts. *Ind. Crops Prod.* 42:126–132.

[1396] Wang X., Zhao M. M., Su G. W., Cai M. S., Zhou C. M., Huang J. Y., et al. 2015. The antioxidant activities and the xanthine oxidase inhibition effects of walnut (Juglans regia L.) fruit, stem and leaf. *Int. J. Food Sci. Technol.* 50:233–239.

[1397] Noumi E, Snoussi M, Hajlaoui H, Valentin E, Bakhrouf A. (2010). Antifungal properties of Salvadora persica and Juglans regia L. extracts against oral Candida strains. *Eur J Clin Microbiol Infect Dis.* Jan;29(1):81-8.

[1398] Clark AM, Jurgens TM, Hufford CD. (1990). Antimicrobial activity of juglone. *Phytother Res.* Feb. 1990.

[1399] Ogbolu DO, Oni AA, Daini OA, Oloko AP. (2007). In vitro antimicrobial properties of coconut oil on Candida species in Ibadan, Nigeria. *J Med Food.* Jun;10(2):384-7.

[1400] Omura Y, O'Young B, Jones M, Pallos A, Duvvi H, et al. (2011). Caprylic acid in the effective treatment of intractable medical problems of frequent urination, incontinence, chronic upper respiratory infection, root canalled tooth infection, ALS, etc., caused by asbestos & mixed infections of Candida albicans, Helicobacter pylori & cytomegalovirus with or without other microorganisms & mercury. *Acupunct Electrother Res.* 2011;36(1-2):19-64.

[1401] Rath CC, Mohapatra S. (2015). Susceptibility characterisation of Candida spp. to four essential oils. *Indian J Med Microbiol.* Feb;33 Suppl:93-6.

[1402] Naeini A, Naderi NJ, Shokri H. (2013). Analysis and in vitro anti-Candida antifungal activity of Cuminum cyminum and Salvadora persica herbs extracts against pathogenic Candida strains. *J Mycol Med.* Mar;24(1):13-8.

[1403] Irkin R, Korukluoglu M. (2009). Growth inhibition of pathogenic bacteria and some yeasts by selected essential oils and survival of L. monocytogenes and C. albicans in apple-carrot juice. *Foodborne Pathog Dis.* Apr;6(3):387-94.

[1404] Chan JY, Yuen AC, Chan RY, Chan SW. (2013). A review of the cardiovascular benefits and antioxidant properties of allicin. *Phytother Res.* May; 27(5):637-46.

[1405] Lemar KM, Turner MP, Lloyd D. (2002). Garlic (Allium sativum) as an anti-Candida agent: a comparison of the efficacy of fresh garlic and freeze-dried extracts. *J Appl Microbiol.* 93(3):398-405.

[1406] Ankri S, Mirelman D. (1999). Antimicrobial properties of allicin from garlic. *Microbes Infect.* Feb;1(2):125-9.

[1407] Ibid. Lemar. (2002).

[1408] WebMD. Calendula. Retrieved Oct 10 2019 from https://www.webmd.com/vitamins/ai/ingredientmono-235/calendula.

[1409] Preethi KC, Kuttan G, Kuttan R. (2009). Anti-inflammatory of flower extract of Calendula officinalis Linn and its possible mechanism of action. *Indian J Exp Biol.* Feb;47(2):113-20.

[1410] Bashir S, Gilani AH. (2008). Studies on the antioxidant and analgesic activities of Aztec marigold (Tagetes erecta) flowers. *Phytother Res.* Dec;22(12):1692-4.

[1411] Wang M, Tsao R, Zhang S, Dong Z, Yang R, et al. (2006). Antioxidant activity, mutagenicity/anti-mutagenicity, and clastogenicity/anti-clastogenicity of lutein from marigold flowers. *Food Chem Toxicol.* Sep;44(9):1522-9.

[1412] Bona E, Cantamessa S, Pavan M, Novello G, Massa N, et al. (2016). Sensitivity of Candida albicans to essential oils: are they an alternative to antifungal agents? *J Appl Microbiol.* Dec;121(6):1530-1545.

[1413] Pozzatti P1, Scheid LA, Spader TB, Atayde ML, Santurio JM, et al. (2008). In vitro activity of essential oils extracted from plants used as spices against fluconazole-resistant and fluconazole-susceptible Candida spp. *Can J Microbiol.* Nov;54(11):950-6. doi: 10.1139/w08-097.

[1414] Elchinger PH, Delattre C, Faure S, Roy O, Badel S, et al. (2014). Effect of proteases against biofilms of Staphylococcus aureus and Staphylococcus epidermidis. *Lett Appl Microbiol.* Nov;59(5):507-13.

[1415] Mitrofanova O, Mardanova A, Evtugyn V, Bogomolnaya L, Sharipova M. (2017). Effects of Bacillus Serine Proteases on the Bacterial Biofilms. *Biomed Res Int.* 2017: 8525912.

[1416] Jin X, Ruiz Beguerie J, Sze DM, Chan GC. (2012). Ganoderma lucidum (Reishi mushroom) for cancer treatment. *Cochrane Database Syst Rev.* Jun 13;(6):CD007731.

[1417] Goel RK, Banerjee RS, Acharya SB. (1990). Antiulcerogenic and antinflammatory studies with shilajit. *J Ethnopharmacol.* Apr;29(1):95-103.

[1418] Wachtel-Galor S, Yuen J, Buswell J, Benzie IFF. (2011). Chapter 9. Ganoderma lucidum (Lingzhi or Reishi) A Medicinal Mushroom. *Herbal Medicine: Biomolecular and Clinical Aspects. 2nd edition.* CRC Press.

[1419] Bhardwaj A, Gupta P, Kumar N, Mishra J, Kumar A, et al. (2017). Lingzhi or Reishi Medicinal Mushroom, Ganoderma lucidum (Agaricomycetes), Inhibits Candida Biofilms: A Metabolomic Approach. *Int J Med Mushrooms.* 2017;19(8):685-696.

[1420] WebMD. Pau D'Arco. Retrieved Oct 22 2019 from https://www.webmd.com/vitamins/ai/ingredientmono-647/pau-darco.

[1421] Neelofar K, Shreaz S, Rimple B, Muralidhar S, Nikhat M, et al. (2011). Curcumin as a promising anticandidal of clinical interest. *Can J Microbiol.* Mar;57(3):204-10.

[1422] Moghadamtousi SZ, Kadir HA, Hassandarvish P, Tajik H, Abubakar S, et al. (2014). Review on Antibacterial, Antiviral, and Antifungal Activity of Curcumin. *Biomed Res Int.* 2014: 186864.

[1423] Ekamed AP, Brisibe EA. (2010). Effects of ethanol extract of Artemisia annua L. against monogenean parasites of Heterobranchus longifilis. *Parasitol Res.* Apr;106(5):1135-9.

[1424] Tagboto S, Townson S. (2001). Antiparasitic properties of medicinal plants and other naturally occurring products. *Adv Parasitol.* 2001;50:199-295.

[1425] Ahameetthunisa AR, Hopper W. (2010). Antibacterial activity of Artemesia nilagirica leaf extracts against clinical and phytopathogenic bacteria. *BMC Complement Altern Med.* Jan 29;10:6.

[1426] Cha JD, Jeong MR, Jeong SI, Moon SE, Kim MY, et al. (2005). Chemical composition and antimicrobial activity of the essential oils Artemisa scoparia and A. capillaris. *Planta Med.* Fec;71(2):186-90.

[1427] Li W, Mo W, Shen D, Sun L, Wang J, et al. (2005). Yeast model uncovers dual roles of mitochondria in action of artemisinin. *PLoS Genet.* Sep; 1(3): e36.

[1428] De Cremer K, Lanckacker E, Cools TL, Bax M, De Brucker K, et al. (2015). Artemisinins, New Miconazole Potentiators Resulting in Increased Activity against Candida albicans biofilms. *Antimicrob Agents Chemother.* Jan;59(1):421-6.

[1429] Hadjivassiliou M, Williamson CA, Woodroofe N. (2004). The immunology of gluten sensitivity: beyond the gut. *Trends Immunol.* Nov; 25(11):578-82.

[1430] Fasano A, Catassi C. (2001). Current approaches to diagnosis and treatment of celiac disease: an evolving spectrum. *Gastroenterology.* Feb; 120(3):636-51.

[1431] Hadjivassiliou M, Grünewald RA, Davies-Jones GA. (2002). Gluten sensitivity as a neurological illness. *J Neurol Neurosurg Psychiatry.* May; 72(5):560-3.

[1432] Cebolla A, Moreno ML, Coto L, Sousa C. (2018). Gluten Immunogenic Peptides as Standard for the Evaluation of Potential Harmful Prolamin Content in Food and Human Specimen. *Nutrients.* Dec;10(12):1927.

[1433] Shan L, Molberg Ø, Parrot I, Hausch F, Filiz F, et al. (2002). Structural basis for gluten intolerance in celiac sprue. *Science.* Sep 27; 297(5590):2275-9.

[1434] Zimmer KP, Fischer I, Mothes T, Weissen-Plenz G, Schmitz M, et al. (2010). Endocytotic segregation of gliadin peptide 31-49 in enterocytes. *Gut.* Mar; 59(3):300-10.

[1435] Thomas H, Beck K, Adamcryk M, Aeschlimann P, Langley M, et al. (2011). Transglutaminase 6: a protein associated with central nervous system development and motor function. *Amino Acids.* Oct. 8.

[1436] Stamnaes J, Dorum S, Fleckenstein B, Aeschlimann D, Sollid LM. (2010). Gluten T cell epitope targeting by TG3 an TG6; implications for dermatitis herpetiformis and gluten ataxia. *Amino Acids.* Nov;39(5):1183-91.

[1437] Kristjansson G, Venge P, Hallgren R. (2007). Mucosal reactivity to cow's milk protein in coeliac disease. *Clin Exp Immunol.* Mar;147(3):449-55.

[1438] Briani C, Zara G, Alaedini A, Grassivaro F, Ruggero S, et al. (2008). Neurological complications of celiac disease and autoimmune mechanisms: a prospective study. *J Neuroimmunol.* Mar; 195(1-2):171-5.

[1439] Hadjivassiliou M, Grünewald RA, Chattopadhyay AK, Davies-Jones GA, Gibson A, et al. (1998). Clinical, radiological, neurophysiological, and neuropathological characteristics of gluten ataxia. *Lancet.* Nov 14; 352(9140):1582-5.

[1440] Hu WT, Murray JA, Greenaway MC, Parisi JE, Josephs KA. (2006). Cognitive Impairment and Celiac Disease. *Arch Neurol.* 2006;63(10):1440-1446.

[1441] Borhani Haghighi A, Ansari N, Mokhtari M, Geramizadeh B, Lankarani KB. (2007). Multiple sclerosis and gluten sensitivity. *Clin Neurol Neurosurg.* Oct:109(8):651-3.

[1442] Konishi T. (2004). Dementia due to celiac disease. [in Japanese]. *Nihon Rinsho.* Jan;62 Suppl:450-5.

[1443] Greengard P, Valtorta F, Czernik AJ, Benfenati F. (1993). Synaptic vesicle phosphoproteins and regulation of synaptic function. *Science.* Feb 5; 259(5096):780-5.

[1444] Kao HT, Porton B, Hilfiker S, Stefani G, Pieribone VA, et al. (1999). Molecular evolution of the synapsin gene family. *Exp Zool.* Dec 15; 285(4):360-77.

[1445] Alaedini A, Okamoto H, Briani C, Wollenberg K, Shill HA, et al. (2007). Immune cross-reactivity in celiac disease: anti-gliadin antibodies bind to neuronal synapsin I. *J Immunol.* May 15:178(10):6590-5.

[1446] Hadjivassiliou M, Boscolo S, Davies-Jones GA, Grunewald RA, Not T, et al. (2002). The humoral response in the pathogenesis of gluten ataxia. *Neurology.* Apr 23:58(8):1221-6.

[1447] Hadjivassiliou M. (2012). Immune-mediated acquired ataxias. *Handb Clin Neurol.* 2012;103:189-99.

[1448] Hemmings WA. (1978). The entry into the brain of large molecules derived from dietary protein. *Proc R Soc Lond B Biol Sci.* 1978 Feb;200(1139):175-92.

[1449] Visser J, Rozing J, Sapone A, Lammers K, Fasano A. (2009). Tight junctions, intestinal permeability, and autoimmunity: celiac disease and type 1 diabetes paradigms. *Ann N Y Acad Sci.* May;1165:195-205.

[1450] Woodroofe N, Wood N, Davies-Jones A. (2003). Gluten ataxia in perspective: epidemiology, genetic susceptibility and clinical characteristics., *Brain.* Mar; 126(Pt 3):685-91.

[1451] Hadjivassiliou M, Grünewald R, Sharrack B, Sanders D, Lobo A, et al. (2001). Brain white-matter lesions in celiac disease: a prospective study of 75 diet-treated patients. *Pediatrics.* Aug; 108(2):E21.

[1452] Hadjivassiliou M, Rao DG, Wharton SB, Sanders DS, Grünewald RA, et al. (2010). Sensory ganglionopathy due to gluten sensitivity. *Neurology.* Sep 14; 75(11):1003-8.

[1453] Hadjivassiliou M, Chattopadhyay AK, Grünewald RA, Jarratt JA, Kandler RH, et al. (2007). Myopathy associated with gluten sensitivity. *Muscle Nerve.* Apr; 35(4):443-50.

[1454] Ibid. Hadjivassiliou. (2002).

[1455] Gabrielli M, Cremonini F, Fiore G, Addolorato G, Padalino C, et al. (2003). Association between migraine and Celiac disease: results from a preliminary case-control and therapeutic study. *Am J Gastroenterol.* Mar; 98(3):625-9.

[1456] Poloni N, Vender S, Bolla E, Bortolaso P, Costantini C, et al. (2009). Gluten encephalopathy with psychiatric onset: case report. *Clin Pract Epidemiol Ment Health.* Jun 26; 5():16.

[1457] Jackson JR, Eaton WW, Cascella NG, Fasano A, Kelly DL. (2012). Neurologic and psychiatric manifestations of celiac disease and gluten sensitivity. *Psychiatr Q.* Mar; 83(1): 91–102.

[1458] Daulatzai MA. (2015). Non-celiac gluten sensitivity triggers gut dysbiosis, neuroinflammation, gut-brain axis dysfunction, and vulnerability for dementia. *CNS Neurol Disord Drug Targets.* 2015;14(1):110-31.

[1459] Ibid. Daulatzai. (2015).

[1460] Nadal I, Donat E, Ribes-Koninckx C, Calabuig M, Sanz Y. (2007). Sulfate-reducing bacterial counts were also elevated. Imbalance in the composition of the duodenal microbiota of children with coeliac disease. *J Med Microbiol.* Dec; 56(Pt 12):1669-74.

[1461] Collado MC, Calabuig M, Sanz Y. (2007). Differences between the fecal microbiota of coeliac infants and healthy controls. *Curr Issues Intest Microbiol.* Mar; 8(1):9-14.

[1462] Sanz Y, De Pama G, Laparra M. (2011). Unraveling the ties between celiac disease and intestinal microbiota. *Int Rev Immunol.* Aug; 30(4):207-18.

[1463] Di Cagno R, De Angelis M, De Pasquale I, Ndagijimana M, Vernocchi P, et al. (2011). Duodenal and faecal microbiota of celiac children: molecular, phenotype and metabolome characterization. *Microbiol.* Oct 4; 11():219.

[1464] Ibid. Collado. (2007).

[1465] Ibid. Di Cagno. (2011).

[1466] Hallert C, Grant C, Grehn S, Grännö C, Hultén S, et al. (2002). Evidence of poor vitamin status in coeliac patients on a gluten-free diet for 10 years. Aliment *Pharmacol Ther.* Jul; 16(7):1333-9.

[1467] Saibeni S, Lecchi A, Meucci G, Cattaneo M, Tagliabue L, et al. (2005). Prevalence of hyperhomocysteinemia in adult gluten-sensitive enteropathy at diagnosis: role of B12, folate, and genetics. *Clin Gastroenterol Hepatol.* Jun; 3(6):574-80.

[1468] Dickey W, Ward M, Whittle CR, Kelly MT, Pentieva K, et al. (2008). Homocysteine and related B-vitamin status in coeliac disease: Effects of gluten exclusion and histological recovery. *J Gastroenterol.* 2008;43(6):682-8.

[1469] Dahele A, Ghosh S. (2001). Vitamin B12 deficiency in untreated celiac disease. Am *J Gastroenterol.* Mar;96(3):745-50.

[1470] Refsum H, Yajnik CS, Gadkari M, Schneede J, Vollset SE, et al. (2001). Hyperhomocysteinemia and elevated methylmalonic acid indicate a high prevalence of cobalamin deficiency in Asian Indians. *Am J Clin Nutr.* Aug;74(2):233-41.

[1471] Hadithi M, Mulder CJ, Stam F, Azizi J, Crusius JB, et al. (2009). Effect of B vitamin supplementation on plasma homocysteine levels in celiac disease. *World J Gastroenterol.* Feb 28; 15(8):955-60.

[1472] Halfdanarson TR, Litzow MR, Murray JA. (2007). Hematologic manifestations of celiac disease. *Blood.* Jan 15; 109(2):412-21.

[1473] Bottaro G, Cataldo F, Rotolo N, Spina M, Corazza GR. (1999). The clinical pattern of subclinical/silent celiac disease: an analysis on 1026 consecutive cases. *Am J Gastroenterol.* Mar; 94(3):691-6.

[1474] Hershko C, Patz J. (2008). Ironing out the mechanism of anemia in celiac disease. *Haematologica.* Dec;93(12):1761-5.

[1475] Turnbull J, Powell A, Guimond S. (2001). Heparan sulfate: decoding a dynamic multifunctional cell regulator. *Trends Cell Biol.* Feb; 11(2):75-82.

[1476] Murch SH. (1995). Sulphation of proteoglycans and intestinal function. *J Gastroenterol Hepatol.* Mar-Apr;10(2):210-2.

[1477] Murch SH, MacDonald TT, Walker-Smith JA, Levin M, Lionetti P, et al. (1993). Disruption of sulphated glycosaminoglycans in intestinal inflammation. *Lancet.* Mar 20;341(8847):711-4.

[1478] Ibid. Collado. (2007).

[1479] Nadal I, Donat E, Ribes-Koninckx C, Calabuig M, Sanz Y. (2007). Imbalance in the composition of the duodenal microbiota of children with coeliac disease. *J Med Microbiol.* Dec; 56(Pt 12):1669-74.

[1480] Hinks LJ, Inwards KD, Lloyd B, Clayton BE. (1984). Body content of selenium in coeliac disease. *Br Med J (Clin Res Ed).* Jun 23; 288(6434):1862-3.

[1481] Rayman MP. (2000). The importance of selenium to human health. *Lancet.* Jul 15; 356(9225):233-41.

[1482] Chanoine JP, Nève J, Wu S, Vanderpas J, Bourdoux P. (2001). Selenium decreases thyroglobulin concentrations but does not affect the increased thyroxine-to-triiodothyronine ratio in children with congenital hypothyroidism. *J Clin Endocrinol Metab.* Mar; 86(3):1160-3.

[1483] Schuppan D, Zimmer KP. (2013). The diagnosis and treatment of celiac disease. *Dtsch Arztebl Intv.* Dec 6;110(49):835-46.

[1484] Schuppan D, Junker Y, Barisani D. (2009). Celiac disease: from pathogenesis to novel therapies. *Gastroenterology.* Dec; 137(6):1912-33.

[1485] Collin P, Kaukinen K, Välimäki M, Salmi J (2002). Endocrinological disorders and celiac disease. *Endocr Rev.* Aug; 23(4):464-83.

[1486] Valentino R, Savastano S, Maglio M, Paparo F, Ferrara F, et al. (2002). Markers of potential coeliac disease in patients with Hashimoto's thyroiditis. *Eur J Endocrinol.* Apr; 146(4):479-83.

[1487] Ibid. Valentino. (2002).

[1488] Iglesias P, Díez JJ. (2009). Thyroid dysfunction and kidney disease. *Eur J Endocrinol.* Apr; 160(4):503-15.

[1489] NIH. Dermatitis Herpetiformis. Retrieved Oct 25 2019 from https://www.niddk.nih.gov/health-information/digestive-diseases/dermatitis-herpetiformis/health-care-professionals.

[1490] Salmi TT, Hervonen K, Kurppa K, Collin P, Kaukinen K, et al. (2015). Celiac disease evolving into dermatitis herpetiformis in patient adhering to normal or gluten-free diet. *Scan J Gastroenterol.* Apr;50(4):387-92.

[1491] Rubio-Tapia A, Murray JA. (2010). Classification and Management of Refractory Celiac Disease. *Gut.* Apr;59(4):547-557.

[1492] Dewar DH, Donnelly SC, McLaughlin SD, Johnson MW, Ellis HJ, et al. (2012). Celiac disease: Management of persistent symptoms in patients on a gluten-free diet. *World J Gastroenterol.* Mar 28;18(12):1346-1356.

[1493] Ross-Smith P, Jenner FA. Diet (gluten) and schizophrenia. *J Hum Nutr.* 1980 Apr;34(2):107-12

[1494] Telega G, Bennet TR, Werlin S. (2008). Emerging new clinical patterns in the presentation of celiac disease. *Arch Pediatr Adolesc Med.* Feb; 162(2):164-8.

[1495] Husby S, Koletzko S, Korponay-Szabó IR, Mearin ML, Phillips A, et al. (2012). European Society for Pediatric Gastroenterology, Hepatology, and Nutrition guidelines for the diagnosis of coeliac disease. *J Pediatr Gastroenterol Nutr.* Jan; 54(1):136-60.

[1496] Ludvigsson JF, Leffler DA, Bai JC, Biagi F, Fasano A, et al. (2013) The Oslo definitions for coeliac disease and related terms. *Gut.* Jan; 62(1):43-52.

[1497] Zimmer KP. (2001). Klinische Bedeutung nichtklassischer Zöliakieformen. *Dt Ärztebl.* 2001;98:A 3285–A 3292.

[1498] Ibid. Schuppan. (2013).

[1499] Fine KD, Meyer RL, Lee EL. (1997). The prevalence and causes of chronic diarrhea in patients with celiac sprue treated with a gluten-free diet. *Gastroenterology.* Jun;112(6):1830-8.

[1500] Zipser RD, Patel S, Yahya KZ, Baisch DW, Monarch E. (2003). Presentations of adult celiac disease in a nationwide patient support group. *Dig Dis Sci.* Apr;48(4):761-4.

[1501] Ibid. Dewar. (2012).

[1502] Van Hees NJ, Van der Does W, Giltay EJ. (2013). Coeliac disease, diet adherence and depressive symptoms. *J Psychosom Res.* Feb;74(2):155-60.

[1503] Ibid. Schuppan. (2013).

[1504] Mayo Clinic. Celiac Disease. Retrieved Oct 25 2019 from https://www.mayoclinic.org/diseases-conditions/celiac-disease/diagnosis-treatment/drc-20352225.

[1505] Ibid. Mayo Clinic. Celiac Disease.

[1506] BeyondCeliac. Endoscopic Biopsy. Retrieved Oct 25 2019 from https://www.beyondceliac.org/celiac-disease/diagnostic-endoscopy/.

[1507] Carretero C, Sidhu R. (2018). Mistakes in capsule endoscopy and how o avoid them. Retrieved Oct 25 2019 from https://www.ueg.eu/education/latest-news/article/article/mistakes.

[1508] Pruimboom L, de Punder K. (2015). The opiod effects of gluten exorphins: asymptomatic disease. *J Health Popul Nutr.* Nov 24;33:24.

[1509] Dohan FC. (1980). Hypothesis: genes and neuroactive peptides from food as cause of schizophrenia. *Adv Biochem Psychopharmacol.* 198;22:535-48.

[1510] Hashimoto S, Hagino A. (1989). Wheat germ agglutinin, concanavalin A, and lens culinalis agglutinan block the inhibitory effect of nerve growth factor on cell-fee phosphorylation of Nsp10 in PC12h cells. *Cell Struct Funct.* Feb;14(1):87-93

[1511] Smecuol E, Hwang HJ, Sugai E, Corso L, Cherñavsky AC, et al. (2013). Exploratory, randomized, double-blind, placebo-controlled study on the effects of Bifidobacterium infantis natren life start strain super strain in active celiac disease. *J Clin Gastroenterol.* Feb; 47(2):139-47.

[1512] Whorwell PJ, Altringer L, Morel J, Bond Y, Charbonneau D, et al. (2006). Efficacy of an encapsulated probiotic Bifidobacterium infantis 35624 in women with irritable bowel syndrome. *Am J Gastroenterol.* Jul; 101(7):1581-90.

[1513] Medina M, De Palma G, Ribes-Koninckx C, Calabuig M, Sanz Y. (2008). Bifidobacterium strains suppress in vitro the pro-inflammatory milieu triggered by the large intestinal microbiota of coeliac patients. *J Inflamm (Lond).* Nov 3; 5():19.

[1514] Lindfors K, Blomqvist T, Juuti-Uusitalo K, Stenman S, Venäläinen J, et al. (2008). Live probiotic Bifidobacterium lactis bacteria inhibit the toxic effects induced by wheat gliadin in epithelial cell culture. *Clin Exp Immunol.* Jun; 152(3):552-8.

[1515] Kresser C. (2017). Is Gluten Killing Your Brain? Retrieved Oct 25 2019 https://kresserinstitute.com/gluten-killing-brain/.

[1516] Daulatzai MA. (2015). Non-celiac gluten sensitivity triggers gut dysbiosis, neuroinflammation, gut-brain axis dysfunction, and vulnerability for dementia. *CNS Neurol Disord Drug Targets.* 14(1):110-31.

[1517] Pohanka M. (2012). Alpha 7 Nicotinic Acetylcholine Receptor is a Target in Pharmacology and Toxicology. *Int J Mol Sci.* 13(2):2219-2238.

[1518] Ibid. Daulatzai. (2015).

[1519] Islami F, Ren JS, Taylor PR, Kamangar F. (2009). Pickled vegetables and the risk of oesophageal cancer: a meta-analysis. *Br J Cancer.* Nov 3; 101(9):1641-7.

[1520] Schroeder FA, Lin CL, Crusio WE, Akbarian S. (2007). Antidepressant-like effects of the histone deacetylase inhibitor, sodium butyrate, in the mouse. *Biol Psychiatry*. Jul 1; 62(1):55-64.

[1521] Tiruppathi c, Miyamoto Y, Ganapathy V, Leibach FH. Genetic evidence for role of DPP IV in intestinal hydrolysis and assimilation of prolyl peptides. *Am J Physiol*. 1993;265:G81-9

[1522] Kozakova H, Stepankva R, Kolinska J, et al. Brush border enzyme activities in the small intestine after long-term gliadin feeding in animal models of human celiac disease. *Folia Microbiol(Phraha)*. 1998;43(5):497-500.

[1523] Ruiz PA, Haller D. Functional diversity of flavonoids in the inhibition of the proinflammatory NF-kappa B, IRF, and Akt signaling pathways in murine and epithelial cells. *J Nutr*. 2006;136(3):664-71

[1524] Peng IW, Kuo SM. Flavonoid structure affects the inhibition of lipid peroxidation in Caco-2 intestinal cells at physiological concentrations. *J Nutr*. 2003;133(7):2184-7

[1525] De Stefano d, Maiuri MC, Simeon v, et al. Lycopene, Quercetin and tyrosol prevent macrophage activation induced by gliadin and IFN-gamma. *Eur J Pharmacol*. 2007; 566(1-3)_:192-9

[1526] Simons Al, Renouf M, Hendrich S, Murphy PA. Human gut microbial degradation of flavonoids: structure-function relationships. *J Agric Food Chem*. 2005:53(10:4258-63

[1527] Panes J, Gerritsen Me, Anderson DC, et al. Apigenin inhibits tumor necrosis factor-induces intercellular adhesion molecule-1 upregulation in vivo. *Microcirculation*. 1996;3(3):279-86

[1528] Kim JS, Jobin c. The flavonoid luteolin prevents lipopolysaccharide-induced NF-kappa B signaling and gene expression by blocking IkappaB kinase activity in intestinal epithelial cells an bone-marrow derived dendritic cells. *Immunology*. 2005;115(3):375-87

[1529] Ashokkumst p, Sudhandiran G. Protective role of luteolin on the status of lipid peroxidation and aPharntioxidant defense against azoxymethane-induced experimental colon carcinogenesis. *Biomed Pharmacother*. 2008;62(9):590-7

[1530] Manju V, Nalini N. Protective role of luteolin in 1,2-dimethylhydrazine induced experimental colon carcinogenesis. *Call Biochem Funct*. 2007;25(2):189-94

[1531] Francis H, Stevenson R. (2013). The longer-term impacts of Western diet on human cognition and the brain. *Appetite*. Apr;63(1):119-128.

[1532] Kanoski SE, Davidson TL. (2011). Western diet consumption and cognitive impairment: Links to hippocampal dysfunction and obesity. *Physiol Behav*. Apr 18;103(1):59-68.

[1533] Pearson KE, Wadley VG, McClure LA, Shikany JM, Unverzagt FW, et al. (2016). Dietary patterns are associated with cognitive function in the REasons for Geographic and Racial Differences in Stroke (REGARDS) cohort. *J Nutr Sci*. Sep 28;5:e38.

[1534] Ozawa M, Shipley M, Kivimaki M, Singh-Manoux A, Brunner EJ. (2017). Dietary pattern, inflammation and cognitive decline: The Whitehall II prospective cohort study. *Clin Nutr*. Apr;36(2):506-512.

[1535] Berti V, Murray J, Davies M, Spector N, Tsui WH, et al. (2015). Nutrient patterns and brain biomarkers of Alzheimer's disease in cognitively normal individuals. *J Nutr Health Aging*. Apr;19(4)413-23.

[1536] Solfrizzi V, Panza F, Capurso A. (2003). The role of diet in cognitive decline. *J Neural Transm (Vienna)*. Jan;110(1):95-110.

[1537] Zalecka A, Bugel S, Paoletti F, Kahl J, Bonanno A. (2014). The influence of organic production on food quality - research findings, gaps and future challenges. *J Sci Food Agric*. Oct;94;(13):2600-4.

[1538] Ibid. Zalecka. (2014).

[1539] Mitchell, A.E., Hong, Y.J., Barrett, D.M., Bryant, D.E., Denison, R.F., et al. (2007). Ten-Year Comparison of the Influence of Organic and Conventional Crop Management Practices on the Content of Flavonoids in Tomatoes. *J Agric Food Chem*, Jul 25;55(15):6154-9.

[1540] Vinha AF, Barreira SV, Costa AS, Alves RC, Oliveira MB. (2014). Organic versus conventional tomatoes: influence on physicochemical parameters, bioactive compounds and sensorial attributes. *Food Chem Toxicol*. May;67:139-44.

[1541] Hallmann, E., Lipowski, J., Marszalek, K., Rembialkowska, E. (2013). The seasonal variation in bioactive compounds content in juice from organic and non-organic tomatoes. *Plant Foods Hum Nutr,* Jun;68(2):171-6.

[1542] Palupi, E., Jayanegara, A., Ploeger, A., Kahl, J. (2012). Comparison of nutritional quality between conventional and organic dairy products: a meta-analysis. *J Sci Food Agric,* Nov;92(14):2774-81.

[1543] Ibid. Palupi. (2012).

[1544] Crinnon, W.J. (2010). Organic foods contain higher levels of certain nutrients, lower levels of pesticides, and may provide health benefits for the consumer. *Altern Med Rev,* Apr;15(1):4-12.

[1545] Reganold, J.P., Wachter, J.M. (2016). Organic agriculture in the twenty-first century. *Nat Plants,* Feb 3;2:15221.

[1546] Strasser, C., Cavoski, I., Di Cagno, R., Kahl, J., Kesse-Guyot, E., et al. (2015). How the Organic Food System Supports Sustainable Diets and Translates These into Practice. *Front Nutr,* Jun 29;2:19.

[1547] Clark, W.F., Sontrop, J.M., Huang, S.H., Moist, L., Bouby, N. et al. (2016). Hydration and Chronic Kidney Disease Progression: A Critical Review of the Evidence. *Am J Nephrol*, 43(4):281-92.

[1548] Saint SE, Renzi-Hammond LM, Khan NA, Hillman CH, Frick JF, et all. (2018). The Macular Carotenoids are Associated with Cognition in Preadolescent Children. *Nutrients.* Feb 10;10(2):E193.

[1549] Ramirez C, Lightfield K, Zuniga K. (2019). Macular Carotenoids and Cognitive Function in a Young Adult Population (FS04-07-19). *Curr Dev Nutr.* Jun 13;3(Suppl 1):nzz052.FS05-07-19.

[1550] Ceravolo SA, Hammond BR, Oliver W, Clementz B, Miller LS, et al. (2019). Dietary Carotenoids Lutein and Zeaxanthin Change Brain Activation in Older Adult Participants: A Randomized, Double-Masked, Placebo-Controlled Trial. *Mol Nutr Food Res.* Apr 5:e1801051.

[1551] Power R, Prado-Cabrero A, Mulcahy R, Howard A, Nolan JM. (2019). The Role of Nutrition for the Aging Population: Implications of Cognition and Alzheimer's Disease. *Ann Rev Food Sci Technol.* Mar 25;10:619-639.

[1552] Elkaim Y. Food Combining Rules: The Complete Guide. Retrieved from https://yurielkaim.com/food-combining-rules.

[1553] Fortune NC, Harville EW, Guralnik JM, Gustat J, Chen W, et al. (2019). Dietary intake and cognitive function: evidence from the Bogalusa Heart Study. *Am J Clin Nutr.* Jun 1;109(6):1656-1663.

[1554] Ibid. Ozawa. (2017).

[1555] Bechthold A, Boeing H, Schwedhelm C, Hoffmann G, Knuppel S, et al. (2017). Food groups and risk of coronary heart disease, stroke and heart failure: A systematic review and dose-response meta-analysis of prospective studies. *Crit Rev Food Sci Nutr.* Oct 17:0.

[1556] Mazza E, Fava A, Ferro Y, Moraca M, Rotundo S, et al. (2017). Impact of legumes and plant proteins consumption on cognitive performances in the elderly. *J Transl Med.* May 22;15(1):109.

[1557] Lin HC, Peng CH, Huang CN, Chiou JY. (2018). Soy-Based Foods are Negatively Associated with Cognitive Decline in Taiwan's Elderly. *J Nutr Sci Vitaminol (Tokyo).* 2018;64(5):335-339.

[1558] https://pubmed.ncbi.nlm.nih.gov/19774556/

[1559] Rajaram S, Valls-Pedret C, Cofan M, Sabate J, Serra-Mir M, et al. (2017). The Walnuts and Healthy Aging Study (WAHA): Protocol for a Nutritional Intervention Trial with Walnuts on Brain Aging. *Front Aging Neurosci.* Jan 10;8:333.

[1560] Esselun C, Dilberger B, Silaidos C, Eckert G. (2019). A Walnut-enriched Diet and Physical Activity Enhanced Cognitive and Motor Function in Aged Mice (P14-010-19). *Curr Dev Nutr.* Jun 13;3(Suppl 1):nzz052.P14-010-19.

[1561] Ren D, Zhao F, Liu C, Wang J, Guo Y, et al. (2018). Antioxidant hydrolyzed peptides from Manchuian walnut (Juglans mandshurica Maxim.) attenuate scopolamine-induced memory impairment in mice. *J Sci Food Agric.* Oct;98(13):5142-5152.

[1562] Batool Z, Sadir S, Liaqut L, Tabassum S, Madiha S, et al. (2016). Repeated administration of almonds increases brain acetylcholine levels and enhances memory function in healthy rats while attenuates memory deficits in animal model of amnesia. *Brain Res Bull.* Jan;120:63-74.

[1563] Dhillon J, Tan SY, Mattes RD. (2017). Effects of almond consumption on the post-lunch dip and long-term cognitive function in energy-restricted overweight and obese adults. *Br J Nutr.* Feb;117(3):395-402.

[1564] Morgan, W.A., Clayshulte, B.J. (2000). Pecans lower low-density lipoprotein cholesterol in people with normal lipid levels. *J Am Diet Assoc,* Mar;100(3):312-8.

[1565] Pacifico S, Piccolella S, Marciano S, Galasso S, Nocera P, et al. (2014). LC-MS/MS profiling of a mastic leaf phenol enriched extract and its effects on H2O2 and AB(25-35) oxidative injury in SK-B-NE©-2 cells. *J Agric Food Chem.* Dec 10;62(49):11957-66.

[1566] Hogervorst E, Sadjimim T, Yesufu A, Kreager P, Rahardjo TB. (2008). High tofu intake is associated with worse memory in elderly Indonesian men and women. *Dement Geriatr Cogn Disord.* 2008;26(1):50-7.

[1567] Xu X, Xiao S, Rahardjo TB, Hogervorst E. (2015). Tofu intake is associated with poor cognitive performance among community-dwelling elderly in China. *J Alzheimers Dis.* 2015;43(2):669-75.

[1568] Hogervorst E, Kassam S, Kridawati A, Soni M, Xin X, et al. (2017). Nutrition research in cognitive impairment/dementia with a focus on soya and folate. *Proc Nutr Soc.* Nov;76(4):437-442.

[1569] Ibid. Lin. (2018).

[1570] Gleason CE, Fischer BL, Dowling NM, Setchell KD, Atwood CS, et al. (2015). Cognitive Effects of Soy Isoflavones in Patients with Alzheimer's Disease. *J Alzheimers Dis.* 2015;47(4):1009-19.

[1571] Ibid. Gleason. (2015). *J Alzheimers Dis.*

[1572] Ruitenberg A, Kalmijn S, de Ridder MA, Redekop WK, van Harskamp F, et al. (2001). Prognosis of Alzheimer's disease: the Rotterdam Study. *Neuroepidemiology.* Aug; 20(3):188-95.

[1573] Barberger-Gateau P, Letenneur L, Deschamps V, Pérès K, Dartigues JF, et al. (2002). Fish, meat, and risk of dementia: cohort study. *BMJ.* Oct 26; 325(7370):932-3.

[1574] Morris MC, Evans DA, Bienias JL, Tangney CC, Bennett DA, et al. (2003). Dietary fats and the risk of incident Alzheimer disease. *Arch Neurol.* Feb; 60(2):194-200.

[1575] Knochel C, Voss M, Gruter F, Alves GS, Matura S, et al. (2017). Omega-3 Fatty Acids: Repurposing Opportunities for Cognitive and Biobehavioral Disturbances in MCI and Dementia. *Curr Alzheimer Res.* 2017;14(3):240-254.

[1576] Cooper RE, Tye C, Kuntsi J, Vassos F, Asherson P. (2015). Omega-3 polyunsaturated fatty acid supplementation and cognition: A systematic review and meta-analysis. *J Psychopharmacol.* Jul;29(7):753-63.

[1577] Kuszewski JC, Wong RHX, How PRC. (2017). Effects of Long-Chain Omega-3 Polyunsaturated Fatty Acis on Endothelial Vasodilator Function and Cognition-Are They Interrelated? *Nutrients.* May 12;9(5).

[1578] Pottala JV, Yaffe K, Robinson JG, Espeland MA, Wallace R, et al. (2014). Higher RBC EPA + DHA corresponds with larger total brain and hippocampal volumes. *Neurology.* Feb 4;82(5): 435-42.

[1579] Ruitenberg A, Kalmijn S, de Ridder MA, Redekop WK, van Harskamp F, et al. (2001). Prognosis of Alzheimer's disease: the Rotterdam Study. *Neuroepidemiology.* Aug; 20(3):188-95.

[1580] Ibid. Barberger-Gateau. (2002). *BMJ.*

[1581] Ibid. Morris (2003). *Arch Neurol.*

[1582] Hashimoto M, Hossain S, Shimada T, Sugioka K, Yamasaki H, et al. (2002). Docosahexaenoic acid provides protection from impairment of learning ability in Alzheimer's disease model rats. *J Neurochem.* Jun; 81(5):1084-91.

[1583] Hashimoto M, Tanabe Y, Fujii Y, Kikuta T, Shibata H, et al. (2005). Chronic administration of docosahexaenoic acid ameliorates the impairment of spatial cognition learning ability in amyloid beta-infused rats. *J Nutr.* Mar; 135(3):549-55.

[1584] Lim GP, Calon F, Morihara T, Yang F, Teter B, et al. (2005). A diet enriched with the omega-3 fatty acid docosahexaenoic acid reduces amyloid burden in an aged Alzheimer mouse model. *J Neurosci.* Mar 23; 25(12):3032-40.

[1585] Jansson P, Kay B. (2018). Aldehydes Identified in Commercially Available Omega-3 Supplements via 1H NMR spectroscopy. *Nutrition 60*, October 2018

[1586] Mason RP, Sherratt SCR. (2017). Omega-3 fatty acid fish oil dietary supplements contain saturated fats and oxidized lipds that may interfer with their intended biological benefits. *Biochem Biophys Res Comm.* Jan;483(1):425-429.

[1587] Calder PC. (2015). Marine omega-3 fatty acids and inflammatory processes: Effects, mechanisms and clinical relevance. *Biochim Biophys Acta.* Apr;1851(4):469-84.

[1588] Hooijmans CR, Pasker-de Jong PC, de Vries RB, Ritskes-Hoitinga M. The effects of long-term omega-3 fatty acid supplementation on cognition and Alzheimer's pathology in animal models of Alzheimer's disease: a systematic review and meta-analysis. *J Alzheimers Dis.* 2012;28(1):191-209.

[1589] Martin B, Mattson MP, Maudsley S. (2006). Caloric restriction and intermittent fasting: two potential diets for successful brain again. *Aging Res Rev.* Aug;5(3):332-53.

[1590] Roth GS, Lane MA, Ingram DK, Mattison JA, Elahi D, et al. (2002). Biomarkers of caloric restriction may predict longevity in humans. *Science.* Aug 2;297(5582):811.

[1591] Csiszar A, Labinskyy N, Jimenez R, Pinto JT, Ballabh P, et al. (2009). Anti-oxidative and anti-inflammatory vasoprotective effects of caloric restriction in aging: role of circulating factors and SIRT1. *Mech Aging Dev.* Aug;130(8):518-27.

[1592] Faris MA, Kacimi S, Al-Kurd RA, Fararjeh MA, Bustanji YK, et al. (2012). Intermittent fasting during Ramadan attenuates proinflammatory cytokines and immune cells in healthy subjects. *Nutr Res.* Dec;32(12):947-55.

[1593] Bhutani S, Klempel MC, Berger RA, Varady KA. (2010). Improvements in coronary heart disease risk indicators by alternate-day fasting involve adipose tissue modulations. *Obesity* (Silver Spring). Nov;18(11):2152-9.

[1594] Li L, Wang Z, Zuo Z. (2013). Chronic intermittent fasting improves cognitive functions and brain structures in mice. *PLoS One.* 2013 Jun 3;8(6):e66069.

[1595] Lee J, Duan W, Long JM, Ingram DK, Mattson MP. (2000). Dietary restriction increases the number of newly generated neural cells, and induces BDNF expression, in the detate gyrus of rats. *J Mol Neurosci.* Oct;15(2):99-108.

[1596] Tajes M, Gutierrez-Cuesta J, Folch J, Ortuno-Sahagun D, Verdaguer E, et al. (2010). Neuroprotective role of intermittent fasting in senescence-accelerated mice P8 (SAMP8). *Exp Gerontol.* 2010 Sep;45(9):702-10.

[1597] Halagappa VK, Guo Z, Pearson M, Matsuoka Y, Cutler RG, et al. (2007). Intermittent fasting and caloric restriction ameliorate age-related behavioral deficits in the triple-transgenic mouse model of Alzheimer's disease. *Neurobiol Dis.* 2007 Apr;26(1):212-20.

[1598] Duan W, Mattson MP. (1999). Dietary restriction and 2-deoxyglucose administration improves behavioral outcome and reduce degeneration of dopaminergetic neurons in models of Parkinson's disease. *J Neurosci Res.* 1999 Jul 15;57(2):195-206.

[1599] Szalay, J. (2015). Inflammation: Causes, Symptoms & Anti-Inflammatory Diet. *LiveScience.* Retrieved from https://www.livescience.com/52344-inflammation.html.

[1600] Kamat PK, Kalani A, Rai S, Swarnkar S, Tota S, et al. (2016). Mechanism of Oxidative Stress and Synapse Dysfunction in the Pathogenesis of Alzheimer's Disease: Understanding the Therapeutics Strategies. *Mol Neurobiol.* Jan;53(1):648-661.

[1601] Tonnies E, Trushina E. (2017). Oxidative Stress, Synaptic Dysfunction, and Alzheimer's Disease. *J Alzheimers Dis.* 2017;57(4):1105-1121.

[1602] Ganguly G, Chakrabarti S, Chatterjee U, Saso L. (2017). Proteinopathy, oxidative stress and mitochondrial dysfunction: cross talk in

Alzheimer's disease and Parkinson's disease. *Drug Des Devel Ther.* Mar 16;11:797-810.

[1603] Pena KB, Ramos CO, Soares NP, da Silva PF, Bandeira AC, et al. (2016). The administration of a high refined carbohydrate diet promoted and increase in pulmonary inflammation and oxidative stress in mice exposed to cigarette smoke. *Int J Chron Obstruct Pulmon Dis.* Dec 15;11:3207-3217.

[1604] Taylor MK, Sullivan DK, Swerdlow RH, Vidoni ED, Morris JK, et al. (2017). A high-glycemic diet is associated with cerebral amyloid burden in cognitively normal older adults. *Am J Clin Nutr.* Dec;106(6):1463-1470.

[1605] Lara HH, Alanis-Garza EJ, Estrada Puente MF, Mureyko LL, Alarcon Torres DA, et al. (2015). [Nutritional approaches to modulate oxidative stress that induce Alzheimer's disease. Nutritional approaches to prevent Alzheimer's disease.] [article in Spanish]. *Gac Med Mex.* Mar-Apr;151(2):245-51.

[1606] Phillppou E, Constantinou M. (2014). The influence of glycemic index on cognitive functioning: a systematic review of the evidence. *Adv Nutr.* Mar 1;5(2):119-30.

[1607] de Munter, JS, Hu FB, Spiegelman D, Franz M, van Dam RM. (2007). Whole grain, bran, and germ intake and risk of type 2 diabetes: a prospective cohort study and systematic review. *PLoS Med*, 4:e261.

[1608] Li W, Huang E, Gao S. (2017). Type 1 Diabetes Mellitus and Cognitive Impairments: A Systematic Review. *J Alzheimer's Dis.* 57(1):29-36.

[1609] Beulens JW, de Bruijne LM, Stolk RP, Peeters PH, Bots ML, et al. (2007). High dietary glycemic load and glycemic index increase risk of cardiovascular disease among middle-aged women: a population-based follow-up study. *J Am Coll Cardiol*, 50:14-21.

[1610] Halton TL, Willett WC, Liu S, Manson JE, Albert CM, et al. (2006). Low-carbohydrate-diet score and the risk of coronary heart disease in women. *N Engl J Med*, 355:1991-2002.

[1611] Anderson JW, Randles KM, Kendall CW, Jenkins DJ. (2004). Carbohydrate and fiber recommendations for individuals with diabetes: a quantitative assessment and meta-analysis of the evidence. *J Am Coll Nutr*, 23:5-17

[1612] Ebbeling CB, Leidig MM, Feldman HA, Lovesky MM, Ludwig DS. (2007). Effects of a low-glycemic load vs low-fat diet in obese young adults: a randomized trial. *JAMA*, 297:2092-102.

[1613] Maki KC, Rains TM, Kaden VN, Raneri KR, Davidson MH. (2007). Effects of a reduced-glycemic-load diet on body weight, body composition, and cardiovascular disease risk markers in overweight and obese adults. *Am J Clin Nutr*, 85:724-34.

[1614] WebMD. How to Use the Glycemic Index. Retrieved May 30 2018 from https://www.webmd.com/diabetes/guide/glycemic-index-good-versus-bad-carbs#1

[1615] Buyken, A.E., Goletzke, J., Joslowski, G., Felbick, A., Cheng, G., et al. (2014). Association between carbohydrate quality and inflammatory markers: systematic review of observational and interventional studies. *Am J Clin Nutr*, 99(4): 2014;813-33.

[1616] Ibid. WebMD. How to Use the Glycemic Index.

[1617] Bozzetto L, Alderisio A, Giorgini M, Barone F, Giacco A, et al. (2016). Extra-Virgin Olive Oil Reduces Glycemic Response to a High-Glycemic Index Meal in Patients with Type 1 Diabetes: A Randomized Controlled Trial., *Diabetes Care.* Apr;39(4):518-24.

[1618] Howarth C, Gleeson P, Attwell D. (2013). Updated energy budgets for neural computation in the neocortex and cerebellum. *J Cereb Blood Flow Metab.* Jul; 32(7):1222-32.

[1619] Dienel GA. (2012). Fueling and imaging brain activation. *ASN Neuro.* Jul 20; 4(5):e00093.

[1620] Ishibashi K, Sakurai K, Shimoji K, Takumaru AM, Ishii K. (2018). Altered functional connectivity of the default mode network by glucose loading in young, healthy participants.

[1621] Walsh EI, Shaw M, Sachdev P, Anstey KJ, Cherbuin N. (2018). Brain atrophy in aging: Estimating effects of blood glucose levels vs. other type 2 diabetes effects. *Diabetes Metab.* Feb;44(1):80-83.

[1622] Croteau E, Castellano CA, Fortier M, Bocti C, Fulop T, et al. (2018). A cross-sectional comparison of brain glucose and ketone metabolism in cognitively healthy older adults, mild cognitive impairment and early Alzheimer's disease. *Exp Gerontol.* Jul 1;107:18-26.

[1623] Edwards S. (2019). Sugar and the Brain. Retrieved Jun 18 2019 from https://neuro.hms.harvard.edu/harvard-mahoney-neuroscience-institute/brain-newsletter/and-brain-series/sugar-and-brain.

[1624] Crane PK, Walker R, Hubbard RA, Li G, Nathan DM, et al. (2013). Glucose levels and risk of dementia. *N Engl J Med.* Aug 8;369(6):540-548.

[1625] An Y, Varma VR, Varma S, Casanova R, Dammer E, et al. (2018). Evidence for brain glucose dysregulation in Alzheimer's disease. Mar;14(3):318-329.

[1626] An Y, Varma VR, Varma S, Casanova R, Dammer E, et al. (2018). Evidence for brain glucose dysregulation in Alzheimer's disease. *Alzheimers Dement.* Mar;14(3):318-329.

[1627] Doheny K. (2012). Americans Sweet on Sugar: Time to Regulate? WebMD. Retrieved from https://www.webmd.com/diet/news/20120201/americans-sweet-on-sugar-time-to-regulate#1

[1628] Leung CW, Laraia BA, Needham BL, Rehkopf DH, Adler NE, et al. (2014). Soda and cell aging: associations between sugar-sweetened beverage consumption an leukocyte telomere length in healthy adults from the National Health and Nutrition Examination Surveys. *Am J*

Public Health. Dec;104(12):2425-31.

[1629] Ashwell M. (2015). Stevia, Nature's Zero-Calorie Sustainable Sweetner: A New Player in the Fight Against Obesity. *Nutr Today.* May; 50(3):129–134.

[1630] Pass MP, Himali JJ, Beiser AS, Aparicio HJ, Satizabal CL, et al. (2017). Sugar- and Artificially Sweetened Beverages and the Risks of Incident Stroke and Dementia: A Prospective Cohort Study. *Stroke.* May;48(5):1139–1146.

[1631] Gorelick PB, Scuteri A, Black SE, Decarli C, Greenberg SM, et al. (2011). Vascular contributions to cognitive impairment and dementia: a statement for healthcare professionals from the american heart association/american stroke association. *Stroke.* Sep; 42(9):2672-713.

[1632] Romano M, Diomede L, Guiso G, Caccia S, Perego C, et al. (1990). Plasma and brain kenetics of large neutral amino acids and striatum monoamines in rats given aspartame. *Food Chem Toxicol.* May;28(5):317-321.

[1633] Pepino MY. (2015). Metabois effects of non-nutritive sweeteners. *Physio Behav.* Dec 1;152(Pt B):450-5.

[1634] Christian B, McConnaughey K, Bethea E, Brantley S, Coffey A , et al. (2004). Chronic aspartame affects T-maze performance, brain cholinergic receptors and Na+,K+-ATPase in rats *Pharmacol Biochem Behav.* May;78(1):121-127.

[1635] Chattopadhyay S, Raychaudhuri U, Chakraborty R. (2014). Artificial sweeteners-a review. *J Food Sci Technol.* Apr;51(4):611-621.

[1636] Qurrat-ul-Ain, Khan SA. (2015). Artificial sweeteners: safe or unsafe? *J Pak Med Assoc.* Feb;65(2):225-227.

[1637] Fernstrom JD. (2015). Non-nutritive sweeteners and obesity. *Annu Rev Food Sci Technol.* 2015;6:119-136.

[1638] Roberts JR. (2015). The paradox of artificial sweeteners in managing obesity. *Curr Gastroenterol Rep.* Jan;17(1):423.

[1639] Schiffman SS, Rother KI. (2013). Sucralose, a synthetic organochlorine sweetener: overview of biological issues *J Toxicol Environ Health B Crit Rev.* 2013;16(7):399-451

[1640] Studzinski CM, Li F, Bruce-Keller AJ, Fernandez-Kim SO, Zhang L, et al. (2009). Effects of short-term Western diet on cerebral oxidative stress and diabetes related factors in APP x PS1 knock-in mice. *J Neurochem.* Feb;108(4):860-6.

[1641] Ramassamy C, Belkacémi A. (2011). Nutrition and Alzheimer's disease: is there any connection? *Curr Alzheimer Res.* Aug; 8(5):443-4.

[1642] Ibid. Morris. (2003). *Arch Neurol.*

[1643] George AJ, Holsinger RM, McLean CA, Laughton KM, Beyreuther K, et al. (2004). APP intracellular domain is increased and soluble Abeta is reduced with diet-induced hypercholesterolemia in a transgenic mouse model of Alzheimer disease. *Neurobiol Dis.* Jun;16(1):124-32.

[1644] Ho L, Qin W, Pompl PN, Xiang Z, Wang J, et al. (2004). Diet-induced insulin resistance promotes amyloidosis in a transgenic mouse model of Alzheimer's disease. *FASEB J.* May;18(7):902-4.

[1645] Greenwood CE, Winocur G. (2005). High-fat diets, insulin resistance and declining cognitive function. *Neurobiol Aging.* Dec; 26 Sup1():42-5.

[1646] Molteni R, Barnard RJ, Ying Z, Roberts CK, Gómez-Pinilla F. (2002). A high-fat, refined sugar diet reduces hippocampal brain-derived neurotrophic factor, neuronal plasticity, and learning. *Neuroscience.* 2002;112(4):803-14.

[1647] Ibid. George. (2004). *Neurobiol Dis.*

[1648] Ibid. Ho. (2004). *FASEB J.*

[1649] Levin-Allerhand JA, Lominska CE, Smith JD. (2002). Increased amyloid- levels in APPSWE transgenic mice treated chronically with a physiological high-fat high-cholesterol diet. *J Nutr Health Aging.* 2002;6(5):315-9.

[1650] Shie FS, Jin LW, Cook DG, Leverenz JB, LeBoeuf RC. (2002). Diet-induced hypercholesterolemia enhances brain A beta accumulation in transgenic mice. *Neuroreport.* Mar 25;13(4):455-9.

[1651] Ibid. George. (2004).

[1652] Ibid. Ho. (2004).

[1653] Mozaffarian D., Katan MB, Ascherio A., Stampfer MJ, Willett WC. (2006). Trans fatty acids and cardiovascular disease. *N Engl J Med.* Apr 13;354(15):1601-13.

[1654] Cahill LE, Pan A, Chiuve SE, Sun Q Willett WC., et al. (2014). Fried-food consumption and risk of type 2 diabetes and coronary artery disease: a prospective study in 2 cohorts of US women and men. *Am J Clin Nutr,* Aug;100(2):667-675.

[1655] Association of Food and Drug Officials. Food Color Additives Banned in the USA. Retrieved from http://importedfoods.afdo.org/food-color-additives-banned-in-the-usa.html.

[1656] Seattle Organic Restaurants. Top 10 foods, additives and preservatives that are banned in many countries except US. Retrieved from http://www.seattleorganicrestaurants.com/vegan-whole-food/foods-banned-in-other-countries-but-we-eat-in-us.php.

[1657] Bjarnadottir A. (2015). How to Read Food Labels Without Being Tricked. Healthline Newsletter. Retrieved from https://www.healthline.com/nutrition/how-to-read-food-labels#section3.

[1658] WebMD. Food Additives: What's Hiding in Your Food? (2017). Retrieved from https://www.webmd.com/news/breaking-news/food-additives/food-additives-infographic.

[1659] Stefanatos R, Sanz A. (2018). The role of mitochondrial ROS in the aging brain. *FEBS Lett.* Mar;592(5):743-758.

[1660] Johnson RJ, Nakagawa T, Sanchez-Lozada LG, Shafiu M, Sundaram S, et al. (2013). Sugar, uric acid, and the etiology of diabetes and obesity. *Diabetes*. Oct;62(10):3307-15.

[1661] Ibid. WebMD. Food Additives.

[1662] Hyman M. (2011). *5 Reasons High Fructose Corn Syrup Will Kill You*. Retrieved from http://drhyman.com/blog/2011/05/13/5-reasons-high-fructose-corn-syrup-will-kill-you/.

[1663] Legeza B, Marcolongo P, Gamberucci A, Varga V, Banhegyi G. (2017). Fructose, Glucocorticoids and Adipose Tissue: Implications for the Metabolic Syndrome. *Nutrients*. Apr. 26;9(5).

[1664] Noble EE, Hsu TM, Liang J, Kanoski SE. (2017). Early-life sugar consumption has long-term negative effects on memory function in male rats. *Nutr Neurosci*. Sept 25:1-11.

[1665] Ibid. WebMD. Food Additives.

[1666] Ritz E, Hahn K, Ketteler M, Kuhlmann MK, et al. (2012). Phosphate Additives in Food—A Health Risk. *Dtsch Arztebl Int*. Jan;109(4):49–55.

[1667] Thiamine. Wikipedia. Retrieved from https://en.wikipedia.org/wiki/Thiamine.

[1668] Gibson GE, Hirsch JA, Fonzetti P, Jordan BD, Cirio RT, et al. (2016). Vitamin B1 (thiamine) and dementia. *Ann NY Acad Sci*. Mar;1367(1):21-30.

[1669] Ibid. WebMD. Food Additives.

[1670] Ibid. WebMD. Food Additives.

[1671] Driscoll I, Shumaker SA, Snively BM, Margolis KL, Manson JE, et al. (2016). Relationships Between Caffeine Intake and Risk for Probable Dementia or Global Cognitive Impairment: The Women's Health Initiative Memory Study. *J Gerontol A Biol Sci Med Sci*. Dec;71(12):1596-1602.

[1672] Lee M, McGeer EG, McGeer PL. (2016). Quercetin, not caffeine, is a major neuroprotective component in coffee. *Neurobiol Aging*. Oct;46:113-23.

[1673] Gokcen BB, Sanlier N. (2017). Coffee Consumption and Disease Correlations. *Crit Rev Food Sci Nutr*. Aug 30:1-13.

[1674] Pasquale LR, Wiggs JL, Willett WC, Kang JH. (2012). The Relationship between Caffeine and Coffee Consumption and Exfoliation Glaucoma or Glaucoma Suspect: A Prospective Study in Two Cohorts. *Invest Ophthalmol Vis Sci*. Sept 21;53(10):6427-6433.

[1675] Kromhout MA, Rius Ottenheim N, Giltay E, Numan ME, Achterberg WP. (2019). Caffeine and neuropsychiatric symptoms in patients with dementia: A systematic review. *Exp Gerontol*. Jul 15;122-85-91.

[1676] Brooks PJ, Zakhari S. (2013). Moderate alcohol consumption and breast cancer in women: from epidemiology to mechanisms and interventions. *Alcohol Clin Exp Res*. Jan;37(1):23-30.

[1677] Freeman D. (2018). 12 Health Risks of Chronic Heavy Drinking. Retrieved April 18 2018 from https://www.webmd.com/mental-health/addiction/features/12-health-risks-of-chronic-heavy-drinking#1

[1678] Xu W, Wang H, Wan Y, Tan C, Li J, et al. (2017). Alcohol consumption and dementia risk: a dose-response meta-analysis of prospective studies. *Eur J Epidemiol*. Jan;32(1):31-42.

[1679] Morris MC, Tangney CC, Wang Y, Sacks FM, Barnes LL, et al. (2015). MIND diet slows cognitive decline with aging. *Alzheimers Dement*. Sep;11(9):1015-22.

[1680] Adjibade M, Assmann KE, Julia C, Galan P, Hercberg S, et al. (2019). Prospective association between adherence to the MIND diet and subjective memory complaints in the French NutriNet-Sante cohort. *J Neurol*. Apr;266(4):942-952.

[1681] Berendsen AM, Kang JH, Fedkens EJM, de Grout CPGM, Grodstein F, et al. (2018). Association of Long-Term Adherence to the MIND Diet with Cognitive Function and Cognitive Decline in American Women. *J Nutr Health Aging*. 22(2:222-229.

[1682] Van den Brink AC, Brouwer-Brolsma EM, Berendsen AAM, van de Rest O. (2019). The Mediterranean, Dietary Approaches to Stop Hypertension (DASH), and Mediterranean-DASH Intervention for Neurodegenerative Delay (MIND) Diets Are Associated with Less Cognitive Decline and a Lower Risk of Alzheimer's Disease-A Review. *Adv Nutr*. Jun 18. [Epub ahead of print].

[1683] Morric MC, Tangney CC, Wang Y, Sacks FM, Bennett DA, et al. (2015). MIND diet associated with reduced incidence of Alzheimer's disease. *Alzheimers Dement*. Sep;11(9):1007-14.

[1684] Koch M, Jensen MK. (2016). Association of the MIND diet with cognition and risk of Alzheimer's disease. *Curr Opin Lipidol*. Jun;27(3):303-4.

[1685] Agarwal P, Wang Y, Buchman AS, Holland TM, Bennett DA, et al. (2018). MIND Diet Associated with Reduced Incidence and Delay of Progression of Parkinsonism in Old Age. *J Nutr Health Aging*. 2018;22(10):1211-1215.

[1686] Ibid. Morris. (2015).

[1687] Dominguez LJ, Barbagallo M, Godos J, Garcia MM, Martinez-Gonzalez MA. (2019). Dietary Patterns and Cognitive Decline: key features for prevention. *Curr Pharm Des*. Jul 22. [Epub ahead of print].

[1688] Makhlouf S, Messelmani M, Zaouali J, Mrissa R. (2018). Cognitive impairment in celiac disease and non-celiac gluten sensitivity: review of literature on the main cognitive impairments, the imaging and the effect of gluten free diet. *Acta Neurol Belg.* Mar;118(1):21-27.

[1689] Greenfield, B. (2018). The Hidden Dangers of a Low Carbohydrate Diet. BenGreenfieldFitness. Retrieved from https://bengreenfieldfitness.com/article/low-carb-ketogenic-diet-articles/the-hidden-dangers-of-a-low-carbohydrate-diet/.

[1690] WebMD. (2019). High-Protein, Low-Carb Diets Explained. Retrieved from https://www.webmd.com/diet/guide/high-protein-low-carbohydrate-diets.

[1691] Brandt J, Buchholz A, Henry-Barron B, Vizthum D, Avramopoulos D, et al. (2019). Preliminary Report on the Feasibility and Efficacy of the Atkins Diet for Treatment of Mild Cognitive Impairment and Early Alzheimer's disease. *J Alzheimers Dis.* 68(3):959-981.

[1692] D'Adamo P. (2019). Blood Type and Your Health. Retrieved from http://www.dadamo.com/txt/index.pl?1001.

[1693] D'Adamo P. (2015). Inflammation and the Blood Type Diet. Personalized Living. Retrieved from http://northamericanpharmacal.com/living/2015/08/inflammation-and-the-blood-type-diet.

[1694] Cusack L, De Buck E, Compernolle V, Vandekerckhove P. (2013). Blood type diets lack supporting evidence: a systematic review. *Am J Clin Nutr*, Jul:98(1):99-104.

[1695] Shmerling RH. (2017). Diet not working? Maybe it's not your type. *Harvard Health Publishing.* May 7, 2017.

[1696] Wang J, Garcia-Bailo B, Nielsen DE, El-Sohemy A. (2014). ABO Genotype, 'Blood-Type' Diet and Cardiometabolic Risk Factors. *PLoS One*, 9(1): e84749.

[1697] Alexander KS, Zakai NA, Gillet S, McClure LA, Wadley V, et al. (2014). ABO Blood Type, Factor VIII, and Incident Cognitive Impairment in the REGARDS cohort. *Neurology.* Sep 30;83(14):1271-1276.

[1698] Ibid. Alexander. (2014).

[1699] Pan JW, de Graaf RA, Petersen KF, Shulman GI, Hetherington HP, et al. (2002). [2,4-13 C2]-beta-Hydroxybutyrate metabolism in human brain Ketone bodies readily cross the blood–brain barrier. *J Cereb Blood Flow Metab.* Jul; 22(7):890-8.

[1700] Pierre K, Pellerin L. (2005). Monocarboxylate transporters in the central nervous system: distribution, regulation and function J Neurochem. Jul; 94(1):1-14.

[1701] Cunnane SC, Musa K, Ryan MA, Whiting S, Fraser DD. (2002). Potential role of polyunsaturates in seizure protection achieved with the ketogenic diet. *Prostaglandins Leukot Essent Fatty Acids.* Aug-Sep; 67(2-3):131-5.

[1702] Henderson ST. (2004). High carbohydrate diets and Alzheimer's disease. *Med Hypotheses.* 2004;62(5):689-700.

[1703] Kashiwaya Y, Takeshima T, Mori N, Nakashima K, Clarke K, et al. (2000). D-beta-hydroxybutyrate protects neurons in models of Alzheimer's and Parkinson's disease. *Proc Natl Acad Sci* U S A. May 9;97(10):5440-4.

[1704] Ziegler DR, Ribeiro LC, Hagenn M, Siqueira IR, Araújo E, et al. (2003). Ketogenic diet increases glutathione peroxidase activity in rat hippocampus. *Neurochem Res.* Dec; 28(12):1793-7.

[1705] Yudkoff M, Daikhin Y, Nissim I, Lazarow A, Nissim I. (2001). Ketogenic diet, amino acid metabolism, and seizure control. *J Neurosci Res.* Dec 1;66(5):931-40.

[1706] Veech RL (2004). The therapeutic implications of ketone bodies: the effects of ketone bodies in pathological conditions: ketosis, ketogenic diet, redox states, insulin resistance, and mitochondrial metabolism. *Prostaglandins Leukot Essent Fatty Acids.* Mar; 70(3):309-19.

[1707] Young KW, Greenwood CE, van Reekum R, Binns MA. (2005). A randomized, crossover trial of high-carbohydrate foods in nursing home residents with Alzheimer's disease: associations among intervention response, body mass index, and behavioral and cognitive function. *J Gerontol A Biol Sci Med Sci.* Aug;60(8):1039-45.

[1708] Sullivan PG, Rippy NA, Dorenbos K, Concepcion RC, Agarwal AK, et al. (2004). The ketogenic diet increases mitochondrial uncoupling protein levels and activity., *Ann Neurol.* Apr;55(4):576-80.

[1709] Noh HS, Kim YS, Lee HP, Chung KM, Kim DW, et al. (2003). The protective effect of a ketogenic diet on kainic acid-induced hippocampal cell death in the male ICR mice. *Epilepsy Res.* Feb;53(1-2):119-28.

[1710] Stamp LK, James MJ, Cleland LG. (2005). Diet and rheumatoid arthritis: a review of the literature. *Semin Arthritis Rheum.* Oct; 35(2):77-94.

[1711] Cullingford TE. (2004). The ketogenic diet; fatty acids, fatty acid-activated receptors and neurological disorders. *Prostaglandins Leukot Essent Fatty Acids.* Mar;70(3):253-64.

[1712] Jockers D. What is Your Metabolic Type? Retrieved Jun 18 2019 from http://drjockers.com/what-is-your-metabolic-type/.

[1713] Ibid. Jockers. (2019).

[1714] Wong C. (2017). The Metabolic Typing Diet. Verywell. Retrieved Jun 18 2019 from https://www.verywell.com/the-metabolic-typing-diet-89876.

[1715] Healthline Newsletter. Metabolic Diet Review: Fact or Fiction? Retrieved Jun 18 2019 from https://www.healthline.com/health/metabolic-diet-review-fact-or-fiction#changing-your-metabolism2.

[1716] Hosking DE, Eramudugolia R, Cherbuin N, Anstey KJ. (2019). MIND not Mediterranean diet related to 12-year incidence of cognitive impairment in an Australian longitudinal cohort study. *Alzheimers Dement.* Apr;15(4):581-589.

[1717] Gotsis E, Anagnostis P, Mariolis A, Vlachou A, Katsiki N, et al. (2015). Health benefits of the Mediterranean Diet: an update of research over the last 5 years. *Angiology.* Apr;66(4):304-18.

[1718] Bach-Faig A, Berry EM, Lairon D, Reguant J, Trichopoulou A, et al. (2011). Mediterranean diet pyramid today. Science and cultural updates. *Public Health Nutr.* Dec;14(12A):2274-84.

[1719] Ibid. Bach-Faig. (2011).

[1720] Petersson SD, Philippou E. (2016). Mediterranean Diet, Cognitive Function, and Dementia: A Systematic Review of the Evidence. *Adv Nutr.* Sep 15;7(5):889-904.

[1721] Safouris A, Tsiygoulis G, Sergentanis TN, Psaltopoulou T. (2015). Mediterranean Diet and Risk of Dementia. *Curr Alzheimer Res.* 2015;12(8):736-44.

[1722] Roman GC, Jackson RE, Gadhia R, Roman AN, Reis J. (2019). Mediterranean diet: The role of long-chain omega-3 fatty acids in fish; polyphenols in fruits, vegetables, cereals, coffee, tea, cacao and wine; probiotics and vitamins in prevention of stroke, age-related cognitive decline, and Alzheimer disease. *Rev Neurol (Paris).* Sep 11:S0035-3787(19)30773-8.

[1723] Mayo Clinic. Mediterranean diet: A heart-healthy eating plan. Retrieved Jun 20 2019 from http://www.mayoclinic.org/ healthylife-style/nutrition-and-healthy-eating/in-depth/mediterranean-diet/art-20047801.

[1724] Scarmeas N, Stern Y, Tang MX, Mayeux R, Luchsinger JA. (2006). Mediterranean diet and risk for Alzheimer's disease. *Ann Neurol.* Jun;59(6):912-21.

[1725] Lourida I, Soni M, Thompson-Coon J, Purandare N, Lang IA, et al. (2013). Mediterranean diet, cognitive function, and dementia: a systematic review. *J Epidemiology.* Jul;24(4):479-89.

[1726] Ibid. Agarwal. (2018).

[1727] Tangney CC. (2019). Diet to beat the odds of prodomal Parkinson's disease? *Mov Disord.* Jan;34(1):2-3.

[1728] Maraki MI, Yannakoulia M, Stamelou M, Stefanis L, Xiromerisious G, et al. (2019). Mediterranean diet adherence is related to reduced probability of prodromal Parkinson's disease. *Mov Disord.* Jan;34(1):48-57.

[1729] Keys A, Menotti A, Karvonen MJ, Aravanis C, Blackburn H, et al. (1986). The diet and 15-year death rate in the seven countries study. *Am J Epidemiol.* Dec;124(6):903-15.

[1730] Merle BM, Silver RE, Rosner B, Seddon JM. (2015). Adherence to a Mediterranean diet, genetic susceptibility, and progression to advanced macular degeneration: a prospective cohort study. *Am J Clin Nutr,* Nov;102(5):1196-206.

[1731] Hogg RE, Woodside JV, McGrath A, Young IS, Vioque JL. (2017). Mediterranean Diet Score and Its Association with Age-Related Macular Degeneration: The European Eye Study. *Ophthalmology,* Jan;124(1):82-89.

[1732] Ibid. Allès. (2012). *Nutr Res Rev.*

[1733] Rainey-Smith SR, Gu Y, Gardener SL, Doecke JD, Villemagne VL, et al. (2018). Mediterranean diet adherence and rate of cerebral AB-amyloid accumulation: Data from the Australian Imaging, Biomarkers and Lifestyle Study of Aging. *Transl Psychiatry.* Oct 30;8(1):238.

[1734] Hill E, Szoeke C, Dennerstein L, Campbell S, Clifton P. (2018). Adherence to the Mediterranean Diet is not related to Beta-Amyloid Deposition: Data from the Women's Healthy Aging Project. *J Prev Alzheimers Dis.* 5(2):137-141.

[1735] Vassilaki M, Aakre JA, Syrianen JA, Mielke MM, Geda YE, et al. (2018). Mediterranean Diet, Its Components, and Amyloid Imaging Biomarkers. *J Alzheimers Dis.* 64(1):281-290.

[1736] Berti V, Walters M, Sterling J, Quinn CG, Logue M, et al. (2018). Mediterranean diet and 3-year Alzheimer brain biomarker changes in middle-aged adults. *Neurology.* May 15;90(20):e1789-e1798.

[1737] Harnedo-Ortega R, Cerezo AB, de Pablos RM, Krisa S, Richard T, et al. (2018). Phenolic Compounds Characteristic of the Mediterranean Diet in Mitigating Microglia-Mediated Neuroinflammation. *Front Cell Neurosci.* Oct 23;12:273.

[1738] Redford, G.D. (2014). Ready to Ditch Your Low-Fat Diet? Not So Fast. AARP Newsletter. Retrieved Jun 22 2019 from https://www.aarp.org/health/healthy-living/info-2014/dean-ornish-low-fat-diet.html.

[1739] Berkeley Wellness. (2015). Ornish: Still Best for Heart Health? Retrieved Jun 22 2019 from http://www.berkeleywellness.com/healthy-eating/diet-weight-loss/article/ornish-still-ultimate-diet.

[1740] Mayo Clinic. Paleo diet: What is it and why is it so popular? Retrieved Jun 22 2019 from https://www.mayoclinic.org/healthy-life-style/nutrition-and-healthy-eating/in-depth/paleo-diet/art-20111182.

[1741] Keehan N. (2016). Paleo and Ketogenic Diets on the Brain. Retrieved Oct 15 2019 from https://www.alzdiscovery.org/cognitive-vital-ity/blog/paleo-and-keto-on-the-brain.

[1742] UC Davis Health. (2015). Is the paleo diet safe? Retrieved Jun 22 2019 from http://www.ucdmc.ucdavis.edu/ welcome/features/2014-2015/06/20150603_paleo-diet.html.

1743 Race B, Williams K, Orru CD, Hughson AG, Lubke L, Chesbro. (2018). Lack of transmission of chronic wasting disease to cynomogus macaques. *J Virol.* 92:300550-18.

1744 Illinois Department of Public Health. Tularemia. *HealthBeat*. Retrieved Jun 22 2019 from http://www.idph.state.il.us/public/hb/hbtu-lare.htm.

1745 Nordqvist C. (2014). What is the South Beach diet? Medical News Today. Retrieved Jun 24 2019 from https://www.medicalnewstoday.com/articles/7380.php.

1746 Ibid. Nordqvist. (2014).

1747 Nordqvist C. (2017). Vegan diet: Health benefits, risks, and meals tips. MedicalNewsToday. Retrieved Jun 24 2019 from https://www.medicalnewstoday.com/articles/149636.php

1748 Nordqvist C. (2017). Nine most popular diets rated by experts 2017. Retrieved Jun 24 2019 from http://www.medicalnewstoday.com/articles/5847.php#raw_food_diet.

1749 Howes MJ, Houghton PF. (2012). Ethnobotanical treatment strategies against Alzheimer's disease. *Curr Alzheimer Res.* Jan;9(1):67-85.

1750 Casadesus G, Shukitt-Hale B, Joseph JA. (2002). Qualitative versus quantitative caloric intake: are they equivalent paths to successful aging? *Neurobiol Aging.* Sep-Oct;23(5):747-69.

1751 Subash S, Essa MM, Al-Adawi S, Memon MA, Manivasagam T, et al. (2014). Neuroprotective effects of berry fruits on neurodegenerative diseases. *Neural Regen Res.* Aug 15;9(16):1557-1566.

1752 Kelly E, Vyas P, Weber J. (2017). Biochemical Properties and Neuroprotective Effects of Compounds in Various Species of Berries. *Molecules.* Dec 22;23(1):E26.

1753 Solleiro-Villavicencio H, Rivas-Arancibia S. (2018). Effect of Chronic Oxidative Stress on Neuroinflammatory Response Mediated by CD4+T Cells in Neurodegenerative Diseases. *Front Cell Neurosci.* Apr 27;12:114.

1754 Kempuraj D, Thangavel R, Natteru PA, Selvakumar GP, Saeed D, et al. (2016). Neuroinflammation Induces Neurodegeneration. *J Neurol Neurosurg Spine.* 2016;1(1):pii:1003.

1755 Almeida S, Alves MG, Sousa M, Oliveira PE, Silva BM. (2016). Are Polyphenols Strong Dietary Agents Against Neurotoxicity and Neurodegeneration? *Neurotox Res.* Oct;30(3):345-66.

1756 Molino S, Dossena M, Buonocore D, Ferrari F, Venturini L, et al. (2016). *Life Sci.* Sep 15; 161():69-77.

1757 Schaffer S, Asseburg H, Kuntz S, Muller WE, Eckert GP. (2012). *Mol Neurobiol.* Aug; 46(1):161-78.

1758 Bruno RM, Ghiadoni L. (2018). Polyphenols, Antioxidants and the Sympathetic Nervous System. *Curr Pharm Des.* 24(2):130-139.

1759 Arulselvan P, Fard MT, Tan WS, Gothai S, Fakurazi S, et al. (2016). Role of Antioxidants and Natural Products in Inflammation. *Oxid Med Cell Longev.* 2016:5276130.

1760 Molino S, Dossena M, Buonocore D, Ferrai F, Venturini L, et al. (2016). Polyphenols in dementia: From molecular basis to clinical trials. *Life Sci.* Sep 15;161:69-77.

1761 Desai A. (2016). Dietary Polyphenols as Potential Remedy for Dementia. *Adv Neurobiol.* 2016:12:41-56.

1762 Flanagan E, Muller M, Hornberger M, Vauzour D. (2018). Impact of Flavonoids on Cellular and Molecular Mechanisms Underlying Age-Related Cognitive Decline and Neurodegeneration. *Curr Nutr Res.* Jun;7(2):49-57.

1763 Savaskan E, Olivieri G, Meier F, Seifritz E, Wirz-Justice A, et al. (2003). Red wine ingredient resveratrol protects from beta-amyloid neurotoxicity. *Gerontology.* Nov-Dec;49(6):380-3.

1764 Braidy N, Behzad S, Hablemariam S, Ahmed T, Daglia M, et al. (2017). Neuroprotective Effects of Citrus Fruit-Derived Flavonoids Nobiletin and Tangeretin in Alzheimer's and Parkinson's Diseases. *CNS Neurol Disord Drug Targets.* 2017;16(4):387-397.

1765 Pandey KB, Rizvi SI. (2009). Plant polyphenols as dietary antioxidants in human health and disease. *Oxid Med Cell Longev.* Nov-Dec;2(5):270-8.

1766 Sokolov AN, Pavlova MA, Klosterhalfen S, Enck P. (2013). Chocolate and the brain: neurobiological impact of cocoa flavanols on cognition and behavior. *Neurosci Biobehav Rev.* Dec;37(10 Pt 2):2445-53.

1767 Bhullar KS, Rupasinghe HP. (2013). Polyphenols: multipotent therapeutic agents in neurodegenerative diseases. *Oxid Med Cell Longev.* 2013():891748.

1768 Orhan IE, Daglia M, Nabavi SF, Loizzo MR, Sobarzo-Sanchez E, et al. (2015). Flavonoids and dementia: an update. *Curr Med Chem.* 22(8):1004-15.

1769 Lange KW, Li S. (2018). Resveratrol, pterostilbene, and dementia. *Biofactors.* Jan;44(1):83-90.

1770 Grassi D, Ferri C, Desideri G. (2016). Brain Protection and Cognitive Function: Cocoa Flavones as Nutraceuticals. *Curr Pharm Des.* 22(2):145-51.

1771 Airoldi C, La Feria B, D Orazio G, Ciaramelli C, Palmioli A. (2018). Flavonoids in the Treatment of Alzheimer's and Other Neurodegenerative Diseases. *Curr Med Chem.* 25(27):3228-3246.

[1772] Ibid. Flanagan. (2018). *Curr Nutr Res.*

[1773] Scholey A, Owen L. (2013). Effects of chocolate on cognitive function and mood: a systematic review. *Nutr Rev.* Oct;71(10):665-81.

[1774] Field DT, Williams CM, Butler LT. (2011). Consumption of cocoa flavanols results in an acute improvement in visual and cognitive functions. *Physiol Behav.* 2011 Jun 1;103(3-4):255-60.

[1775] Goel A, Dignijaya, Garg A, Kumar A. (2016). Effect of Capparis spinosa Linn. Extract on lipopolysaccharide-induced cognitive impairment in rats. *Indian J Exp Biol.* Feb;54(2):126-32.

[1776] Szwajgier D, Baranowska-Wojcik E, Borowiec K. (2018). Phenolic Acids Exert Anticholinesterase and Cognition-Improving Effects. *Curr Alzheimer Res.* 15(6):531-543.

[1777] Moore K, Hughes CF, Ward M, Hoey L, McNulty H. (2018). Diet, nutrition and the aging brain: current evidence and directions. *Proc Nutr Soc.* May;77(2):152-163.

[1778] Hablemariam S. (2018). Molecular Pharmacology of Rosmarinic and Salvianolic Acids: Potential Seeds for Alzheimer's and Vascular Dementia. *Int J Mol Sci.* Feb 3;19(2):E458.

[1779] Szwajgier D, Borowiec K, Pustelniak K. (2017). The Neuroprotective Effects of Phenolic Acids: Molecular Mechanism of Action. *Nutrients.* May 10;9(5):E477.

[1780] Ibid. Lange. (2018). *Biofactors.*

[1781] Sawda C, Moussa C, Turner RS. (2017). Resveratrol for Alzheimer's disease. *Ann N Y Acad Sci.* Sep;1403(1):142-149.

[1782] Gomes BAQ, Silva JPB, Romeiro CFR, Dos Santos SM, Rodrigues CA, et al. (2018). Neuroprotective Mechanisms of Resveratrol in Alzheimer's Disease: Role of SIRT1. *Oxid Med Cell Longev.* Oct 30;2018:8152373.

[1783] Wei M, Liu Z, Liu Y, Li S, Hu M, et al. (2019). Urinary and plasmatic metabolomics strategy to explore the holistic mechanism of lignans in S. chinesis in treating Alzheimer's disease using UPLC-Q-TOF-MS. *Food Funct.* Sep 1;10(9):5656-5668.

[1784] Wei M, Liu Y, Pi Z, Li S, Hu M, et al. (2019). Systematically Characterize the Anti-Alzheimer's Disease Mechanisms of Lignans from S. chinensis based on In-Vivo Ingredient Analysis and Target-Network Pharmacology Strategy by UHPLC-Q-TOF-MS. *Molecules.* Mar 27;24(7):E1203.

[1785] Giuliano C, Siani F, Mus L, Ghezzi C, Cerri S, Pacchetti B, et al. (2019). Neuroprotective effects of lignan 7-hydroxymatairesinol (HMR/lignan) in a rodent model of Parkinson's disease. *Nutrition.* Apr 25;69:110494.

[1786] Almario RU, Karakas SE. (2013). Lignan content of the flaxseed influences its biological effects in healthy men and women. *J Am Coll Nutr.* 32(3):194-9.

[1787] Loera-Valencia R, Goikolea J, Prrado-Fernandez C, Merino-Serrais P, Maioli S. (2019). Alterations in cholesterol metabolism as a risk factor for developming Alzheimer's disease: Potential novel targets for treatment. *J Steroid Biochem Mol Biol.* Jun;190:104-114.

[1788] Kostova I, Bhatia S, Grigorov P, Balkansky S, Pramar VS, et al. (2011). Coumarins as antioxidants. *Curr Med Chem.* 2011;18:3929–395.

[1789] Shahidi F, Yeo JD. (2018). Bioactivities of Phenolics by Focusing on Suppression of Chronic Diseases: A Review. *Int J Mol Sci.* Jun;19(6):1573.

[1790] Anand P, Singh B, Singh N. (2012). A review on coumarins as acetylcholinesterase inhibitors for Alzheimer's disease. *Bioorgan Med Chem.* 2012;20:1175–1180.

[1791] Castillo J, Benavente-Garcia O, Lorente J, Alcaraz M, Redondo A, et al. (2000). Antioxidant activity and radioprotective effects against chromosomal damage induced in vivo by X-rays of flavan-3-ols (procyanidins) from grape seeds (Vitis Vinifera): Comparative study versus other phenolic and organic compounds. *J Agric Food Chem.* 2000;48:1738–1745.

[1792] Ibid. Shahidi. (2018). *Int J Mol Sci.*

[1793] MedlinePlus. Amino Acids. Retrieved Nov 15 2019 from https://medlineplus.gov/ency/article/002222.htm.

[1794] Banos G, Daniel PM, Moorhouse SR, Pratt OE. (1975). The requirements of the brain for some amino acids. *J Physiol.* Apr;246(3):539-48.

[1795] Fernstrom JD. (1994). Dietary amino acids and brain function. *J Am Diet Assoc.* Jan;94(1):71-7

[1796] Knochel C, Voss M, Gruter F, Alves GS, Matura S, et al. (2017). Omega-3 Fatty Acids: Repurposing Opportunities for Cognitive and Biobehavioral Disturbances in MCI and Dementia. *Curr Alzheimer Res.* 2017;14(3):240-254.

[1797] Calder PC. (2015). Marine omega-3 fatty acids and inflammatory processes: Effects, mechanisms and clinical relevance. *Biochim Biophys Acta.* Apr;1851(4):469-84.

[1798] Kerksick C, Willoughby D. (2005). The Antioxidant role of glutathione and N-acetyl-cysteine supplements and exercise-induced oxidative stress. *J Int Soc Sports Nutr.* 2005;2:38–44.

[1799] Smeland OB, Meisingset TW, Borges K, Sonnewald U. (2012). Chronic acetyl-L-carnitine alters brain energy metabolism and increases noradrenaline and serotonin content in healthy mice. *Neurochem Int.* Jul;61(1):100-7.

[1800] Malaguarnera M, Cammalleri L, Gargante MP et al. (2007) L-Carnitine treatment reduces severity of physical and mental fatigue and increases cognitive functions in centenarians: a randomized and controlled clinical trial. *Am J Clin Nutr.* 86;1738-1744.

[1801] Malaguarnera M, Gargante MP, Cristaldi E et al. (2008) Acetyl L-carnitine (ALC) treatment in elderly patients with fatigue. *Arc Geron Geriartrics.* 46;181-190.

[1802] Jones LL, McDonald DA, Borum PR. (2010). Acylcarnitines: role in brain. *Prog Lip Res.* 49;61-75.

[1803] Gavrilova SI, Kalyn IaB, Kolykhalov IV, Roshchina IF, Selezneva ND. (2011). [Acetyl-L-carnitine (carnicetine) in the treatment of early stages of Alzheimer's disease and vascular dementia]. *Zh Nevrol Psikhiatr Im S S Korsakova.* 2011;111(9):16-22.

[1804] Kobayashi S, Iwamoto M, Kon K, Waki H, Ando S, et al. (2010). Acetyl-L-carnitine improves aged brain function. *Geriatr Gerontol Int.* Jul;10 Suppl 1:S99-106.

[1805] Zhou P, Chen Z, Zhao N, Liu D, Guo ZY, et al. (2011). Acetyl-L-carnitine attenuates homocysteine-induced Alzheimer-like histopathological and behavioral abnormalities. *Rejuvenation Res.* Dec;14(6):669-679.

[1806] Yin YY, Liu H, Cong XB, Liu Z, Wang Q, et al. (2010). Acetyl-L-carnitine attenuates okadaic acid induced tau hyperphosphorylation and spatial memory impairment in rats. *J Alzheimers Dis.* 2010;19(2):735-46.

[1807] Salvioli G, Neri M. (1994). L-acetylcarnitine treatment of mental decline in the elderly. *Drugs Exp Clin Res.* 20(4):169-76.

[1808] Ames BN, Liu J. (2004). Delaying the mitochondrial decay of aging with acetylcarnitine. *Ann N Y Acad Sci.* Nov;1033:108-16.

[1809] Brooks JO, Yesavage JA, Carta A, Bravi D. (1998). Acetyl l-carnitine slows decline in younger patients with Alzheimer's disease: a reanalysis of a double-blind, placebo-controlled study using the trilinear .... *Int Psychogeriatr.* Jun;10(2):193-203.

[1810] Atkuri KR, Mantovani JJ, Herzenberg LA, Herzenberg LA. (2007). N-Acetylecysteine—a safe antidote for cysteine/glutathione deficiency. *Curr Opin Pharmacol.* Aug;7(4):355-9.

[1811] Ibid. Kerksick. (2005).

[1812] Banaclocha M. (2001). Therpautic potential of N-acetylcysteine in age-related mitochondrial neurogenerative diseases. *Med Hypothesis.* Apr;56(4):472-77.

[1813] Alavi Naini SM, Soussi-Yanicostas N. (2015). Tau Hyperphosphorylation and Oxidative Stress, a Critical Vicious Circle in Neurodegenerative Tauopathies? *Oxid Med Cell Longev.* 2015:151979.

[1814] Moreira P, et al. (2007). Lipoic acid and N-acetyl cysteine decrease mitochondrial-related oxidative stress in Alzheimer disease patient fibroblasts. *J Alz Dis.* 2007;12(2):195-206.

[1815] Joy T, Rae MS, Madhyastha S. (2018). N-Acetyl Cystein Supplement Minimize Tau Expression and Neuronal Loss in Animal Model of Alzheimer's Disease. *Brain Sci.* Oct; 8(10): 185.

[1816] Atkuri KR, Mantovani JJ, Herzenberg LA, Herzenberg LA. (2007). N-Acetylecysteine—a safe antidote for cysteine/glutathione deficiency. *Curr Opin Pharmacol.* Aug;7(4):355-9.

[1817] Farr SA, Poon HF, Dogrukol-Ak D, Drake J, Banks WA, et al. (2003). The antioxidants alpha-lipoic acid and N-acetylcysteine reverse memory impairment and brain oxidative stress in aged SAMP8 mice. *J Neurochem.* Mar;84(5):1173-83.

[1818] Manda K, Ueno M, Moritake T, Anzai K. (2007). Radiation-induced cognitive dysfunction and cerebellar oxidative stress in mice: protective effect of alpha-lipoic acid. *Behav. Brain Res.* 2007;177()7–14.

[1819] Mahboob A, Farhat SM, Iqbal G, Babar MM, Zaidi NU, et al. (2016). Alpha-lipoic acid-mediated activation of muscarinic receptors improves hippocampus- and amygdala-dependent memory. *Brain Res Bull.* 2016 Apr; 22():19-28.

[1820] Hiller S, DeKroon R, Hamlett ED, Xu L, Osorio C, et al. (2016). Alpha-lipoic acid supplementation protects enzymes from damage by nitrosative and oxidative stress. *Biochim Biophys Acta.* Jan;1860(1 Pt A):36-45.

[1821] Zhang YH, Wang DW, Xu SF, Zhang S, Fan YG, et al. (2018). A-Lipoic acid improves abnormal behavior by mitigation of oxidative stress, inflammation, ferroptosis, and tauopathy in P301S Tau transgenic mice. *Redox Biol.* Apr;14:535-548.

[1822] Shay KP, Moreau RF, Smith EJ, Smith AR, Hagen TM. (2009). Alpha-lipoic acid as a dietary supplement: molecular mechanisms and therapeutic potential. *Biochim Biophys Acta.* Oct;1790(10):1149-60.

[1823] Packer L, Tritschler HJ, Wessel K. (1997). Neuroprotection by the metabolic antioxidant alpha-lipoic acid. *Free Radic Biol Med.* 1997;22(1-2):359-78.

[1824] The effects and mechanisms of mitochondrial nutrient alpha-lipoic acid on improving age-associated mitochondrial and cognitive dysfunction: an overview. Liu J *Neurochem Res.* 2008 Jan; 33(1):194-203.

[1825] Hager K, Kenklies M, McAfoose J, Engel J, Münch G. (2007). Alpha-lipoic acid as a new treatment option for Alzheimer's disease--a 48 months follow-up analysis. *J Neural Transm Suppl.* 2007;(72):189-93.

[1826] Hager K, Marahrens A, Kenklies M, Riederer P, Münch G. (2001). Alpha-lipoic acid as a new treatment option for Alzheimer [corrected] type dementia. *Arch Gerontol Geriatr.* Jun;32(3):275-82.

[1827] Ibid. Moreira. (2007). *J Alz Dis.*

[1828] Kidd PM. (2005). Neurodegeneration from mitochondrial insufficiency: nutrients, stem cells, growth factors, and prospects for brain rebuilding using integrative management. *Altern Med Rev.* Dec;10(4):268-93.

[1829] Zhang H, Jia H, Liu J, Ao N, Yan B, et al. (2010). Combined R-alpha-lipoic acid and acetyl-L-carnitine exerts efficient preventative effects in a cellular model of Parkinson's disease. *J Cell Mol Med*. Jan;14(1-2):215-25.

[1830] Zuo L, Motherwell MS. (2013). The impact of reactive oxygen species and genetic mitochondrial mutations in Parkinson's disease. *Gene*. Dec 10;532(1):18-23.

[1831] Cui X, Zuo P, Zhang Q, Li X, Hu Y, et al. (2006). Chronic systemic D-galactose exposure induces memory loss, neurodegeneration, and oxidative damage in mice: protective effects of R-alpha-lipoic acid. *J Neurosci Res*. Aug 15; 84(3):647-54.

[1832] Khanna S, Atalay M, Laaksonen DE, Gul M, Roy S, et al. (1999). Alpha-lipoic acid supplementation: tissue glutathione homeostasis at rest and after exercise. *J Appl Physiol (1985)*. Apr;86(4):1191-6.

[1833] Hultberg M, Hultberg B. (2006). The effect of different antioxidants on glutathione turnover in human cell lines and their interaction with hydrogen peroxide. *Chem Biol Interact*. Nov 7;163(3):192-8.

[1834] Ibid. Hager. (2001). *Arch Gerontol Geriatr*.

[1835] Ibid. Hager. (2007). *J Neural Transm Suppl*.

[1836] Quinn JF, Bussiere JR, Hammond RS, Montine TJ, Henson E, et al. (2007). Chronic dietary alpha-lipoic acid reduces deficits in hippocampal memory of aged Tg2576 mice. *Neurobiol Aging*. Feb;28(2):213-25.

[1837] Farr SA, Price TO, Banks WA, Ercal N, Morley JE. (2012). Effect of alpha-lipoic acid on memory, oxidation, and lifespan in SAMP8 mice. *J Alzheimers Dis*. 2012;32(2):447-55.

[1838] Holmquist L, Stuchbury G, Berbaum K, Muscat S, Young S, et al. (2007). Lipoic acid as a novel treatment for Alzheimer's disease and related dementias. *Pharmacol Ther*. Jan;113(1):154-64.

[1839] Shinto L, Quinn J, Montine T, Dodge HH, Woodward W, et al. (2014). A randomized placebo-controlled pilot trial of omega-3 fatty acids and alpha lipoic acid in Alzheimer's disease. *J Alzheimers Dis*. 2014;38(1):111-20.

[1840] Blondeau N, Nguemeni C, Debruyne DN, Piens M, Wu X, et al. (2009). Subchronic alpha-linolenic acid treatment enhances brain plasticity and exerts an antidepressant effect: a versatile potential therapy for stroke. *Neuropsychopharmacology*. Nov;34(12):2548-59.

[1841] Valls-Pedret C, Sala-Vila A, Serra-Mir M, Corella D, de la Torre R, et al. (2015). Mediterranean Diet and Age-Related Cognitive Decline: A Randomized Clinical Trial. *JAMA Intern Med*. Jul;175(7):1094-1103.

[1842] Yadav SS, Singh MK, Singh PK, Kumar V. (2017). Traditional knowledge to clinical trials: A review on therapeutic actions of Emblica officinalis. *Biomed Pharmacother*. Sep;93:1291-1302.

[1843] Mani V, Parle M. (2007). Memory enhancing activity of Anwala churna (Emblica officinalis Gaertn.): An Ayurvedic preparation. *Phys Behav*. Jun;91(1):46-54.

[1844] Mathew M, Subramanian S. (2014). In vitro screening for anti-cholinesterase and antioxidant activity of methanolic extracts of ayurvedic medicinal plants used for cognitive disorders. *PLoS One*. Jan 23;9(1):486804.

[1845] Golechha M, Bhatia J, Arya DS. (2012). Studies on effects of Emblica officinalis (Amla) on oxidative stress and cholinergic function in scopolamine induced amnesia in mice. *J Environ Biol*. Jan;33(1):95-100.

[1846] Liu R, Zhang T, Yang H, Lan X, Ying J, et al. (2011). The flavonoid apigenin protects brain neurovascular coupling against amyloid-B25-35-induced toxicity in mice. *J Alzheimers Dis*. 2011;24(1):85-100.

[1847] Balez R, Steiner N, Engel M, Munez SS, Lum JS, et al. (2016). Neuroprotective effects of apigenin against inflammation, neuronal excitability and apoptosis in an induced pluripotent stem cell model of Alzheimer's disease *Sci Rep*. 2016;6:31450.

[1848] Saksena AK, Singh SP, Dixit KS, Singh N, Seth K, et al. (1993). Effect of Withania somnifera and Panax ginseng on dopaminergic receptors in rat brain during stress. *Planta Med*. 55(1):95.

[1849] Singh N. 1988. Effect of Withania somnifera and Panax ginseng on dopaminergic receptors in rat brain during stress; in *XXXVIth An Con Med Plant Res* (Freiburg). (p 28).

[1850] Singh N, Misra N. (1993). Experimental methods tools for assessment of anti-stress activity in medicinal plants. *J Biomed Res*. 1993;12(182):124–127.

[1851] Bhattacharya A, Ghosal S, Bhattacharya SK. (2001). Anti-oxidant effect of Withania somnifera glycowithanolides in chronic footshock stress-induced perturbations of oxidative free radical scavenging enzymes and lipid peroxidation in rat frontal cortex and striatum. *J Ethnopharmacol*. Jan;74(1):1-6.

[1852] Mishra LC, Singh BB, Dagenais S. (2000). Scientific basis for the therapeutic use of Withania somnifera (ashwagandha): a review. *Altern Med Rev*. Aug;5(4):334-46.

[1853] Russo A, Izzo AA, Cardile V, Borrelli F, Vanella A. (2001). Indian medicinal plants as antiradicals and DNA cleavage protectors. *Phytomedicine*. Mar; 8(2):125-32.

[1854] Nemetcheck MD, Stierle AA, Stierle DB, Lurie DI. (2017). The Ayurvedic plant Bacopa monnieri inhibits inflammatory pathways in the brain. *J Ethnopharmacol*. Feb 2;199:92-100.

1855 Jayaprakasam B, Padmanabhan K, Nair MG. (2010). Withanamides in Withania somnifera fruit protect PC-12 cells from beta-amyloid responsible for Alzheimer's disease *Phytother Res.* Jun;24(6):859-63

1856 Monograph. Withania somnifera. *Altern Med Rev.* 2004 Jun; 9(2):211-4.

1857 Parihar MS, Hemnani T. (2003). Phenolic antioxidants attenuate hippocampal neuronal cell damage against kainic acid induced excitotoxicity. *J Biosci.* Feb; 28(1):121-8.

1858 Sandhir R., Sood A. (2017). Neuroprotective Potential of Withania somnifera (Ashwagandha) in Neurological Conditions. In: Kaul S., Wadhwa R., editors. Cham, Germany: *Springer International Publishing.* pp. 373–387.

1859 Kyboyama T, Tohda C, Zhao J, Nakamura, N, Hattori M, et al. (2002). Axon- or dendrite-predominant outgrowth induced by constituents from Ashwagandha. *Neuroreport.* Oct. 7;13(14): 1715-20.

1860 Kuboyama T, Tohda C, Komatsu K. (2005). Neuritic regeneration and synaptic reconstruction induced by withanolide A. *Br J Pharmacol.* Apr;144(7):961-71.

1861 Tohda C, Kuboyama T, Komatsu K. (2000). Dendrite extension by methanol extract of Ashwagandha (roots of Withania somnifera) in SK-N-SH cells. *Neuroreport.* Jun 26;11(9):1981-5.

1862 Ibid. Kyboyama. (2002).

1863 Ibid. Kuboyama. (2005).

1864 Andrade C, Aswath A, Chaturvedi SK, Srinivasa M, Raguram R. (2000). A double-blind, placebo-controlled evaluation of the anxiolytic efficacy of an ethanolic extract of withania somnifera. *Indian J Psychiatry.* Jul;42(3):295-301.

1865 Ibid. Sandhir. (2017).

1866 Choudhary D, Bhattacharyya S, Bose S. (2017). Efficacy and Safety of Ashwagandha (Withania somnifera (L.) Dunal) Root Extract in Improving Memory and Cognitive Functions. *J Diet Suppl.* 2017;14(6):599-612.

1867 Tohda C, Kuboyama T, Komatsu K. (2005). Search for natural products related to regeneration of the neuronal network. *Neurosignals.* 2005;14(1-2):34-45.

1868 McPhee GM, Downey LA, Noble A, Stough C. (2016). Cognitive training and Bacopa monnieri: Evidence for a combined intervention to alleviate age associated cognitive decline.

1869 Sehgal N, Gupta A, Valli RK, Joshi SD, Mills JT, et al. (2012). Withania somnifera reverses Alzheimer's disease pathology by enhancing low-density lipoprotein receptor-related protein in liver. *Proc Natl Acad Sci U S A.* Feb 28;109:3510-3515

1870 Ibid. Kuboyama. (2005).

1871 Ibid. Kuboyama. (2002).

1872 Schliebs R, Liebmann A, Bhattacharya SK, Kumar A, Ghosal S, et al. (1997). Systemic administration of defined extracts from Withania somnifera (Indian Ginseng) and Shilajit differentially affects cholinergic but not glutamatergic and GABAergic markers in rat brain. *Neurochem Int.* 1997 Feb; 30(2):181-90.

1873 Ibid. Schliebs. (1997). *Neurochem Int.*

1874 Ibid. Jayaprakasam. (2010). *Phytother Res.*

1875 Kumar S, Harris RJ, Seal CJ, Okello EJ. (2012). An aqueous extract of Withania somnifera root inhibits amyloid β fibril formation in vitro. *Phytother Res.* Jan;26(1):113-7.

1876 Dhuley JN. (1998). Effect of ashwagandha on lipid peroxidation in stress-induced animals. *J Ethnopharmacol.* 1998 Mar; 60(2):173-8. 4

1877 Ibid. Monograph. Withania somnifera. (2004).

1878 Parihar MS, Hemnani TJ. (2003). Phenolic antioxidants attenuate hippocampal neuronal cell damage against kainic acid induced excitotoxicity. *Biosci.* Feb;28(1):121-8.

1879 Ibid. Monograph. Withania somnifera. (2004).

1880 Andrade C, Aswath A, Chaturvedi SK, Srinivasa M, Raguram R. (2000). A double-blind, placebo-controlled evaluation of the anxiolytic efficacy ff of an ethanolic extract of withania somnifera. *Indian J Psychiatry.* Jul;42(3):295-301.

1881 Pingali U, Pilli R, Fatima N. (2014). Effect of standardized aqueous extract of Withania somnifera on tests of cognitive and psychomotor performance in healthy human participants. *Pharmacognosy Res.* Jan;6(1):12-8.

1882 Auddy B, Hazra J, Mitra A, Abedon B, Ghosal S. (2008). A standardized Withania somnifera extract significantly reduces stress-related parameters in chronically stressed humans: a double-blind randomized, placebo-controlled study. *J Am Nutra Assoc.* 2008;11:50–56.

1883 Wadhwa R, Konar A, Kaul SC. (2016). Nootropic potential of Ashwagandha leaves: Beyond traditional root extracts. *Neurochem Int.* May;95:109-18.

1884 Galasso C, Orefice I, Pellone P, Cirino P, Miele R, et al. (2018). On the Neuroprotective Role of Astaxanthin: New Perspectives? *Mar Drugs.* Jul 27;16(8):E247.

[1885] Ambati RR, Phang SM, Ravi S, Aswathanarayana RG. (2014). Astaxanthin: sources, extraction, stability, biological activities and its commercial applications--a review. *Mar Drugs.* Jan 7; 12(1):128-52.

[1886] Balietti M, Giannubilo SR, Giorgetti B, Solazzi M, Turi A, et al. (2016). The effect of astaxanthin on the aging rat brain: gender-related differences in modulating inflammation. *J Sci Food Agric.* 2016;96:615–618.

[1887] Choi SK, Park YS, Choi DK, Chang HI. (2008). Effects of astaxanthin on the production of NO and the expression of COX-2 and iNOS in LPS-stimulated BV2 microglial cells. *J Microbiol Biotechnol.* Dec;18(12):1990-6.

[1888] Koutsilieri E, Scheller C, Tribl F, Riederer P. (2002). Degeneration of neuronal cells due to oxidative stress--microglial contribution. *Parkinsonism Relat Disord.* Sep;8(6):401-6.

[1889] Ibid. Galasso. (2018).

[1890] Liu X, Shibata T, Hisaka S, Osawa T. (2009). Astaxanthin inhibits reactive oxygen species-mediated cellular toxicity in dopaminergic SH-SY5Y cells via mitochondria-targeted protective mechanism. *Brain Res.* Feb 13;1254():18-27.

[1891] Ibid. Liu. (2009).

[1892] Lu Y, Xie T, He XX, Mao ZF, Jia LJ. (2015). Astaxanthin rescues neuron loss and attenuates oxidative stress induced by amygdala kindling in adult rat hippocampus. *Neurosci Lett.* 2015;597:49–53.

[1893] Park JS, Mathison BD, Hayek MG, Zhang J, Reinhart GA, et al. (2013). Astaxanthin modulates age-associated mitochondrial dysfunction in healthy dogs. *J Anim Sci.* Jan; 91(1):268-75.

[1894] Yook JS, Okamoto M, Rakwal R, Shibato J, Lee MC, et al. (2016). Astaxanthin supplementation enhances adult hippocampal neurogenesis and spatial memory in mice. *Mol Nutr Food Res.* Mar;60(3):589–599.

[1895] Li Z, Dong X, Liu H, Chen X, Shi H, et al. (2013). Astaxanthin protects ARPE-19 cells from oxidative stress via upregulation of Nrf2-regulated phase II enzymes through activation of PI3K/Akt. *Mol Vis.* 2013;19():1656-66.

[1896] Wibrand K, Berge K, Messaoudi M, Duffaud A, Panja D, et al. (2013). Enhanced cognitive function and antidepressant-like effects after krill oil supplementation in rats. *Lipids Health Dis.* Jan 25;12():6.

[1897] Wu W, Wang X, Xiang Q, Meng X, Peng Y. (2014). Astaxanthin alleviates brain aging in rats by attenuating oxidative stress and increasing BDNF levels. *Food Funct.* 2014;5:158–166.

[1898] Kim YH, Koh HK, Kim DS. (2010). Down-regulation of IL-6 production by astaxanthin via ERK-, MSK-, and NF-κB-mediated signals in activated microglia. *Int Immunopharmacol.* Dec; 10(12):1560-72.

[1899] Grimmig B, Kim SH, Nash K, Bickford PC, Douglas Shytie R. (2017). Neuroprotective mechanisms of astaxanthin: a potential therapeutic role in preserving cognitive function in age and neurodegeneration. *Geroscience.* Feb;39(1):19-32.

[1900] Katagiri M, Satoh A, Tsuji S, Shirasawa T. (2012). Effects of astaxanthin-rich Haematococcus pluvialis extract on cognitive function: a randomised, double-blind, placebo-controlled study. *J Clin Biochem Nutr.* Sep; 51(2):102-7.

[1901] Chang CH, Chen CY, Chiou JY, Peng RY, Peng CH. (2010). Astaxanthin secured apoptotic death of PC12 cells induced by beta-amyloid peptide 25-35: its molecular action targets. *J Med Food.* Jun;13(3):548-56.

[1902] Wang HQ, Sun XB, Xu YX, Zhao H, Zhu QY, et al. (2010). Astaxanthin upregulates heme oxygenase-1 expression through ERK1/2 pathway and its protective effect against beta-amyloid-induced cytotoxicity in SH-SY5Y cells. *Brain Res.* Nov 11; 1360():159-67.

[1903] Kim JH, Choi W, Lee JH, Jeon SJ, Choi YH, et al. (2009). Astaxanthin inhibits H2O2-mediated apoptotic cell death in mouse neural progenitor cells via modulation of P38 and MEK signaling pathways. *J Microbiol Biotechnol.* Nov;19(11):1355-63.

[1904] Mahmassani HA, Avendano EE, Raman G, Johnson EJ. (2018). Avocado consumption and risk factors for heart disease: a systematic review and meta-analysis. *Am J Clin Nutr.* April 1; 107(4): 523-536.

[1905] Ameer K. (2016). Avocado as a Major Dietary Source of Antioxidants and Its Preventative Role in Neurodegenerative Diseases. *Adv Neurobiol.* 12:237-54.

[1906] Dreher ML, Davenport AJ. (2013). Hass avocado composition and potential health effects. *Crit Rev Food Sci Nutr.* 2013;53(7):738-50.

[1907] Russo A, Borrelli F. (2005). Bacopa monniera, a reputed nootropic plant: an overview. *Phytomedicine.* Dec;12(4):305–317.

[1908] Singh HK, Srimal RC, Srivastava AK, Garg NK, Dhawan BN. (1990). Neuropsychopharmacological effects of bacosides A and B. in *Proc 4th Conf Neurobiol Learning Memory.* Irvine, CA, USA; pp. 17–20.

[1909] Prabhakar S, Saraf MK, Pandhi P, Anand A. (2008). Bacopa monniera exerts antiamnesic effect on diazepam-induced anterograde amnesia in mice. *Psychopharmacology.* Sep;200(1):27–37.

[1910] Sudharani D, Krishna KL, Deval K, Safia AK, Priya (2011). Pharmacological profiles of Bacopa monnieri: a review. *Intl J Pharm.* 1(1):15-23.

[1911] Stough C, Downey LA, Lloyd J, Silber B, Redman S, et al. (2008). Examining the nootropic effects of a special extract of Bacopa monniera on human cognitive functioning: 90 day double-blind placebo-controlled randomized trial. *Phytother Res.* Dec; 22(12):1629-34.

[1912] Meena H, Pandey HK, Pandey P, Arya MC, Ahmed Z. (2012). Evaluation of antioxidant activity of two important memory enhancing medicinal plants Baccopa monnieri and Centella asiatica. *Indian J Pharmacol.* Jan;44(1):114–117.

[1913] Chowdhuri DK, Parmar D, Kakkar P, Shukla R, Seth PK, et al. (2002). Antistress effects of bacosides of Bacopa monnieri: modulation of Hsp70 expression, superoxide dismutase and cytochrome P450 activity in rat brain. *Phytother Res.* 2002 Nov; 16(7):639-45.

[1914] Limpeanchob N, Jaipan S, Rattanakaruna S, Phrompittayarat W, Ingkaninan K. (2008). Neuroprotective effect of Bacopa monnieri on beta-amyloid-induced cell death in primary cortical culture. *J Ethnopharmacol.* Oct 30; 120(1):112-7.

[1915] Bhattacharya SK, Bhattacharya A, Kumar A, Ghosal S. (2000). Antioxidant activity of Bacopa monniera in rat frontal cortex, striatum and hippocampus. *Phytother Res.* May;14(3):174-9.

[1916] Ramakrishnan S., Sumathi T. (2007). Hepatoprotective activity of Bacopa monniera on D-galactosamine induced hepatotoxicity in rats. 2007;13(3):195–198.

[1917] Stough C, Downey LA, Lloyd J, Silber B, Redman S, et al. (2008). Examining the nootropic effects of a special extract of bacopa monniera on human cognitive functioning: 90 day double-blind placebo-controlled randomized trial. *Phytother Res.* Dec;22(12):1629-34.

[1918] Stough C, Lloyd J, Clarke J, Downey LA, Hutchison CW, et al. (2001). The chronic effects of an extract of Bacopa monniera on cognitive function in healthy human subjects. *Psychopharmacology* (Berl). Aug; 156(4):481-4.

[1919] Singh HK, Dhawan BN. (1982). Effect of Bacopa monniera Linn. (brahmi) extract on avoidance responses in rat. *J Ethnopharmacol.* ar; 5(2):205-14.

[1920] Chen M, Lai L, Li X, Zhang X, He X, et al. (2016). Baicalein attenuates neurological deficits and preserves blood-brain barrier integrity in a rat model of intracerebral hemorrhage. *Neurochem Res.* Nov;41:3095-3102.

[1921] Dinda B, Dinda S, DasSharma S, Banik R, Chakraborty A, et al. (2017). Therapeutic potentials of baicalein and its aglycone, baicalein against inflammatory disorders. *Eur J Med Chem.* May 5;131:68-80.

[1922] Viji V, Shobha B, Kavitha SK, Ratheesh M, Kripa K, et al. (2010). Betulinic acid isolated from Bacopa monniera (L.) Wettst suppresses lipopolysaccharide stimulated interleukin-6 production through modulation of nuclear factor-κB in peripheral blood mononuclear cells. *Int Immunopharmacol.* Aug;10(8):843-9.

[1923] Viji V, Kavitha SK, Helen A. (2010). Bacopa monniera (L.) Wettst inhibits type II collagen-induced arthritis in rats. *Phytother Res.* Sep;24(9):1377-83.

[1924] Gohil KJ, Patel JJ. (2010). A review on Bacopa monniera: current research and future prospects. *Internat J Green Pharm.* 4(1):1-9.

[1925] Khan R, Krishnakumar K, Paulose CS. (2008). Decreased glutamate receptor binding and NMDA R1 gene expression in hippocampus of pilocarpine-induced epileptic rats: neuroprotective role of Bacopa monnieri extract. *Epilepsy Behav.* 12(1)54-60.

[1926] Chronic effects of Brahmi (Bacopa monnieri) on human memory. Roodenrys S, Booth D, Bulzomi S, Phipps A, Micallef C, Smoker *J Neuropsychopharmacology.* 2002 Aug; 27(2):279-81.

[1927] Effects of a standardized Bacopa monnieri extract on cognitive performance, anxiety, and depression in the elderly: a randomized, double-blind, placebo-controlled trial. Calabrese C, Gregory WL, Leo M, Kraemer D, Bone K, Oken B *J Altern Complement Med.* 2008 Jul; 14(6):707-13.

[1928] Morgan A, Stevens J *J Altern Complement Med.* 2010 Jul; 16(7):753-9.

[1929] Liu RX, Song GH, Wu PG, Zhang XW, Hu HJ, et al. (2017). Distribution patterns of the contents of five biologically activate ingredients in the root of Scutellaria baicalensis. *Chin J Nat Med.* 15:152-160.

[1930] Tarragó T, Kichik N, Claasen B, Prades R, Teixidó M, et al. (2008). Baicalin, a prodrug able to reach the CNS, is a prolyl oligopeptidase inhibitor. *Bioorg Med Chem.* 2008;16(15):7516–7524.

[1931] Ouyang CH, Wu JL. (2006). Protective effect of baicalin on inflammatory injury following transient focal cerebral ischemia-reperfusion in rats. *Chin J Pharmacol Toxicol.* 2006;20(4):288-294.

[1932] Hui KM, Wang XH, Xue H. (2000). Interaction with Flavones from the Roots of Scutellaria baicalensis with the Benzodiazepine Site. *Planta Med.* 2000;66(1): 91-93

[1933] Wang F, Xu Z, Ren L, Tsang SY, Xue H. (2008). GABAA receptor subtype selectivity underlying selective anxiolytic effect of baicalin. *Neuropharmacology.* Dec;55(7):1231-7.

[1934] Liang W, Huang X, Chen W. (2017). The Effects of Baicalin and Baicalein on Cerebral Ischemia: A Review. *Aging Dis.* Dec;8(6): 850–867.

[1935] Letiembre M, Hao W, Liu Y, Walter S, Mihaljevic I, et al. (2007). Innate immune receptor expression in normal brain aging. *Neuroscience.* Apr 25;146(1):248-54.

[1936] Ridder DA, Schwaninger M. (2009). NF-κB signaling in cerebral ischemia. *Neuroscience.* 2009;158(3):995–1006.

[1937] Shieh DE, Liu LT, Lin CC. (2000). Antioxidant and free radical scavenging effects of baicalein, baicalin and wogonin. *Anticancer Res.* Sep-Oct;20(5A):2861-5.

[1938] Chen C, Li X, Gao P, Tu Y, Zhao M, et al. (2015). Baicalin attenuates alzheimer-like pathological changes and memory deficits induced by amyloid β1-42 protein. *Metab Brain Dis.* Apr;30(2):537-44.

[1939] Ding H, Wang H, Zhao Y, Sun D, Zhai X. (2015). Protective Effects of Baicalin on $A\beta_{1-42}$-Induced Learning and Memory Deficit, Oxidative Stress, and Apoptosis in Rat. *Cell Mol Neurobiol.* Jul;35(5):623-32.

[1940] Zhuang PW, Cui GZ, Zhang YJ, Zhang MX, Guo H, et al. (2013). Baicalin regulates neuronal fate decision in neural stem/progenitor cells and stimulates hippocampal neurogenesis in adult rats. *CNS Neurosci Ther.* Mar;19(3):154-62.

[1941] Gasiorowski K, Lamer-Zarawska E, Leszek J, Parvathaneni K, Yendluri BB, et al. (2011). Flavones from root of Scutellaria baicalensis Georgi: Drugs of the future in neurodegeneration? *CNS Neurol Disord Drug Targets.* Mar;10:184-191.

[1942] Chirumbolo S, Bjorklund G. (2016). Commentary: The Flavonoid Baicalein Rescues Synaptic Plasticity and Memory Deficits in a Mouse Model of Alzheimer's Disease. *Front Neurol.* Aug 29;7:141.

[1943] Chen M, Lai L, Li X, Zhang X, He X, et al. (2016). Baicalein attenuates neurological deficits and preserves blood-brain barrier integrity in a rat model of intracerebral hemorrhage. *Neurochem Res.* 41:3095-3102.

[1944] Wang CX, Xie GB, Zhou CH, Zhang XS, Li T, et al. (2015). Baicalein alleviates early brain injury after experimental subarachnoid hemorrhage in rats: Possible involvement of TLR4/NF-κB-mediated inflammatory pathway. *Brain Res.* 1594:245-255.

[1945] Ono K, Yoshiike Y, Takashima A, Hasegawa K, Naiki H, Yamada M. Potent anti-amyloidogenic and fibril-destabilizing effects of polyphenols in vitro: implications for the prevention and therapeutics of Alzheimer's disease. *J Neurochem.* 2003;87:172–181.

[1946] Subash S, Essa MM, Al-Adawi S, Memon MA, Manivasagam T, et al. (2014). Neuroprotective effects of berry fruits on neurodegenerative disease. *Neural Regen Res.* Aug 15;9(16):1557-1566.

f Alzheimer's disease. *J Neurochem.* 2003;87:172–181

[1947] Ibid. Pandey. (2009). *Oxid Med Cell Longev.*

[1948] Devore EE, Kangs JH, Breteler MM, Grodstein FA. (2012). Dietary intakes of berries and flavonoids in relation to cognitive decline. *Neurology.* Jul 12;72(1):135-43.

[1949] Joseph JA, Shukitt-Hale B, Willis LM. (2009). Review: Grape juice, berries, and walnuts affect brain aging and behavior. *J Med,* Sep;139(9):1813S-7S.

[1950] Krikorian R, Shidler MD, Nash TA, Kalt W, Vinqvist-Tymchuk MR, et al. (2010). Blueberry supplementation improves memory in older adults. *J Agric Food Chem.* Apr 14;58(7):3996-4000.

[1951] Small BJ, Rawson KS, Martin C, Eisel SL, Sanberg CD, et al. (2014). Nutraceutical intervention improves older adults' cognitive functioning. *Rejuvenation Res.* Feb;17(1):27-32.

[1952] Dai Q, Borenstein AR, Wu Y, Jackson JC, Larson EB. (2006). Fruit and vegetable juices and Alzheimers Disease: The kame project. *Am J Med.* Sep;1119(9):751-9.

[1953] Lau FC, Shukitt-Hale B, Joseph JA. (2007). Nutritional intervention in brain aging: Reducing the effects of inflammation in brain aging and oxidative stress. *Subcell Biochemistry.* 2007;42:299-318.

[1954] Joseph JA, Denisova NA, Arendash G, Gordon M, Diamond D, et al. (2003). Blueberry supplementation enhances signaling and prevents behavioral deficits in Alzheimer disease model. *Nutr Neurosci.* Jun;6(3):153-62.

[1955] Joseph JA, Carey A, Brewer GJ, Lau FC, Fisher DR. (2007). Dopamine and abera-induced stress signaling and decrements in Ca2+ buffering in primary neonatal hippocampal cells are antagonized by blueberry extract. *J Alz Dis.* Jul;11(4D):433-46 .

[1956] McGuire SO, Sortwell CE, Shukitt-Hale B, Joseph JA, Hejna MJ, et al. (2006). Dietary supplementation with blueberry extract improves survival of transplanted dopamine neurons. *Nutr Neurosc* Oct;9(5-6):251-8.

[1957] Suh N, Paul S, Hao X, Simi B, Xioa H, et al (2007). Pterostilene, an active constituent of blueberries, suppresses aberrant crypt foci formation in the azoxymethane-induces colon carcinogenesis model in rats. *Clin Can Res.* Jan 1;13(1):350-5.

[1958] Zafra-Stone S, Yasmin T, Bagchi M, et al. (2012). Berry anthocyanins as novel antioxidants in human health and disease prevention. *Int J Dev Neurosc.* Jun;30(4)303-313.

[1959] Sweeney MI, Kalt W, MacKinnon SL, Ashby J, Gottschall-Pass KT. (2002). Feeding rats diets enriched in lowbush blueberries for six weeks decreases ischemia-induced brain damage. *Nutr Neurosci.* Dec;5(6):427-31.

[1960] Joseph JA, Fisher DR, Bielinski D. (2006). Blueberry extract alters oxidative stress-mediated signaling in COS-7 cells transfected with selectively vulnerable muscarinic receptor subtypes. *J Alzheimers Dis.* Mar;9(1):35-42.

[1961] Galli RL, Shukitt-Hale B, Youdim KA, Joseph JA. (2002). Fruit polyphenolics and brain aging: nutritional interventions targeting age-related neuronal and behavioral deficits. *Ann N Y Acad Sci.* Apr;959:128-32.

[1962] Lazze MC, Pizzala R, Savio M, Stivala LA, Prosperi E, et al. (2003). Anthocyanins protect against DNA damage induced by tert-butyl-hydroperoxide in rat smooth muscle and hepatoma cells. *Mutat Res.* Feb 5;535(1):103-15.

[1963] Casadesus G, Shukitt-Hale B, Stellwagen HM, Zhu X, Lee HG, et al. (2004). Modulation of hippocampal plasticity and cognitive behavior by short-term blueberry supplementation in aged rats. *Nutr Neurosci.* 2004;7:309–316

[1964] Williams CM, El Mohsen MA, Vauzour D, Rendeiro C, Butler LT, et al. (2008). Blueberry-induced changes in spatial working memory correlate with changes in hippocampal CREB phosphorylation and brain-derived neurotrophic factor (BDNF) levels. *Free Radic Biol Med.* 2008;45:295–305.

[1965] Joseph JA, Shukitt-Hale B, Denisova NA, Bielinski D, Martin A, et al. (1999). Reversals of age-related declines in neuronal signal transduction, cognitive, and motor behavioral deficits with blueberry, spinach, or strawberry dietary supplementation. *J Neurosci.* Sep 15;19(18):8114-21.

[1966] Safayhi H, Mack T, Sabieraj J, Anazodo MI, Subramanian LR, et al. (1992). Boswellic acids: novel, specific, nonredox inhibitors of 5-lipoxygenase. *J Pharmacol Exp Ther.* Jun;261(3):1143-6.

[1967] Baram SM, Karima S, Shateri S, Tafakhori A, Fotouhi A, et al. (2019). Functional improvement and immune-inflammatory cytokines profile of ischaemic stroke patients after treatment with boswellic acids: a randomized, double-blind, placebo-controlled pilot trial. *Inflammopharmacology.* Aug 12.

[1968] Vasanthi HR, Mukherjee S, Das DK. (2009). Potential health benefits of broccoli-a chemico-biological overview. *Mini Rev Med Chem.* 2009 Jun;9(6):749-59.

[1969] Frantz B, Nordby EC, Bren G, Steffan N, Paya CV, et al. (1994). Calcineurin acts in synergy with PMA to inactivate I kappa B/MAD3, an inhibitor of NF-kappa B. *EMBO J.* Feb 15;13(4):861-70.

[1970] Sailer ER, Subramanian LR, Rall B, Hoernlein RF, Ammon HP, et al. (1996). Acetyl-11-keto-beta-boswellic acid (AKBA): structure requirements for binding and 5-lipoxygenase inhibitory activity. *Br J Pharmacol.* Feb;117(4):615-8.

[1971] Sandoval M, Charbonnet RM, Okuhama NN, Roberts J, Krenova Z, et al. (2000). Cat's claw inhibits TNFalpha production and scavenges free radicals: role in cytoprotection. Free Radic Biol Med. Jul 1; 29(1):71-8.

[1972] Gilmore TD. (2004). NF-kB Transcription Factors. Retrieved Nov 8 2019.

[1973] Chen SQ, Wang ZS, Ma YX, Zhang W, Lu JL, et al. (2018). Neuroprotective Effects and Mechanisms of Tea Bioactive Components in Neurodegenerative Diseases. *Molecules.* Feb 25; 23(3):512.

[1974] Da Rocha MD, Viegas FP, Campos HC, Nicastro PC, Fossaluzza PC, et al. (2011). The role of natural products in the discovery of new drug candidates for the treatment of neurodegenerative disorders II: Alzheimer's disease. *CNS Neurol Disord Drug Targets.* Mar;10(2):251-70.

[1975] Godkar PB, Gordon RK, Ravindran A, Doctor BP. (2006). Celastrus paniculatus seed oil and organic extracts attenuate hydrogen peroxide- and glutamate-induced injury in embryonic rat forebrain neuronal cells. *Phytomedicine.* Jan;13(1-2):29-36.

[1976] Katekhaye S, Duggal S, Pal A. (2011). An Inside Preview of Nutritional and Pharmacological Profile of Celastrus paniculatus. *Int J Rec Adv Pharm Res.* 1

[1977] Godkar P, Gordon RK, Ravindran A, Doctor BP. (2003). Celastrus paniculatus seed water soluble extracts protect cultured rat forebrain neuronal cells from hydrogen peroxide-induced oxidative injury. *Fitoterapia.* Dec;74(7-8):658-69.

[1978] Bhanumathy M, Harish MS, Shivaprasad HN, Sushma G. (2010). Nootropic activity of Celastrus paniculatus seed. *Pharm Biol.* Mar;48(3):324-7.

[1979] Kumar MH, Gupta YK. (2002). Antioxidant property of Celastrus paniculatus willd.: a possible mechanism in enhancing cognition. *Phytomedicine.* May;9(4):302-11.

[1980] Ibid. Bhanumathy. (2010).

[1981] Ibid. Kumar. (2002).

[1982] Godkar PB, Gordon RK, Ravindran A, Doctor BP. (2004). Celastrus paniculatus seed water soluble extracts protect against glutamate toxicity in neuronal cultures from rat forebrain. *J Ethnopharmacol.* 2004;93(2-3):213-219.

[1983] Ibid. Godkar. (2006).

[1984] Shinomol GK, Muralidhara, Bharath MM. (2011). Exploring the Role of "Brahmi" (Bacopa monnieri and Centella asiatica) in Brain Function and Therapy. *Recent Pat Endocr Metab Immune Drug Discov.* Jan; 5(1):33-49.

[1985] Cervenka F, Jahodár L. (2006). [Plant metabolites as nootropics and cognitives]. *Ceska Slov Farm.* Sep;55(5):219-29.

[1986] Dhanasekaran M, Holcomb LA, Hitt AR, Tharakan B, Porter JW, et al. (2009). Centella asiatica extract selectively decreases amyloid beta levels in hippocampus of Alzheimer's disease animal model. *Phytother Res.* Jan; 23(1):14-9.

[1987] Gray NE, Sampath H, Zweig JA, Quinn JF, Soumyanath A. (2015). Centella asiatica Attenuates amyloid-B-induced Oxidative Stress and Mitochondrial Dysfunction. *J Alzheimers Dis.* 2015; 45(3):933-46.

[1988] Soumyanath A, Zhong YP, Henson E, Wadsworth T, Bishop J, et al. (2012). Centella asiatica Extract Improves Behavioral Deficits in a Mouse Model of Alzheimer's Disease: Investigation of a Possible Mechanism of Action. *Int J Alzheimers Dis.* 2012:381974.

[1989] Prakash A, Kumar A. (2013). Mitoprotective effect of Centella asiatica against aluminum induced neurotoxicity in rats: possible relevance to its antioxidant and anti-apoptosis mechanism. *Neurol Sci.* 2013 Aug; 34(8):1403-9.

[1990] Shinomol GK, Muralidhara. (2008). Prophylactic neuroprotective property of Centella asiatica against 3-nitropropionic acid induced oxidative stress and mitochondrial dysfunctions in brain regions of prepubertal mice. *Neurotoxicology*. Nov; 29(6):948-57.

[1991] Gray NE, Zweig JA, Murchison C, Caruso M, Matthews DG, et al. (2017). Centella asiatica attenuates AB-induced neurodegenerative spine loss and denritic simplification. *Neurosci Lett*. Apr 12;646:24-29.

[1992] Ibid. Shinomol. (2008). *Neurotoxicology*.

[1993] Gray NE, Zweig JA, Caruso M, Zhu JY, Wright KM, et al. (2018). Centella asiatica attenuates hippocampal mitochondrial dysfunction and improves memory and executive function in B-amyloid overexpressing mice. *Mol Cell Neurosci*. Dec;93:1-9.

[1994] Dev R. D. O. (2009). Comparison on cognitive effects of Centella asiatica in healthy middle age female and male volunteers. 2009;55:709.

[1995] Wattanathorn J, Mator L, Muchimapura S, Tongun T, Pasuriwong O, et al. (2008). Positive modulation of cognition and mood in the healthy elderly volunteer following the administration of Centella asiatica. *J Ethnopharmacol*. Mar 5; 116(2):325-32.

[1996] Field DT, Williams CM, Butler LT. (2011). Consumption of cocoa flavanols results in acute improvement in visual and cognitive functions. *Physiol Behav*. Jun 1;103(3-4):255-60.

[1997] Li Z, Vance DE. (2008). Phosphatidylcholine and choline homeostasis. *J Lipid Res*. Jun; 49(6):1187-94.

[1998] Zeisel SH. Choline. In Ross AC, Caballero B, Cousins RJ, Tucker KL, Ziegler TR (Eds.), *Modern Nutrition in Health and Disease*. 11th ed. Baltimore, MD: Lippincott Williams & Wilkins; 2014:416-26.

[1999] Zeisel SH, Corbin KD. Choline. In: Erdman JW, Macdonald IA, Zeisel SH, (Eds.), *Present Knowledge in Nutrition*. 10th ed. Washington, DC: Wiley-Blackwell; 2012:405-18.

[2000] Institute of Medicine. Food and Nutrition Board. Dietary Reference Intakes: Thiamin, Riboflavin, Niacin, Vitamin B6, Folate, Vitamin B12, Pantothenic Acid, Biotin, and Choline. Washington, DC: National Academy Press; 1998. (p 390-422)

[2001] Zeisel SH. Choline. In: Coates PM, Betz JM, Blackman MR, et al., eds. *Encyclopedia of Dietary Supplements*. 2nd ed. London and New York: Informa Healthcare; 2010:136-43.

[2002] Ibid. Zeisel. (2012). Encyclopedia of Dietary Supplements.

[2003] Ibid. Institute of Medicine. (1998). Dietary Reference Intakes.

[2004] Fisher MC, Zeisel SH, Mar MH, Sadler TW. (2002). Perturbations on choline metabolism cause neural tube defects in mouse embryos in vitro. *FASEB J*. Apr;16(6):619-21.

[2005] Ibid. Institute of Medicine. (1998).

[2006] Poly C, Massaro JM, Seshadri S, Wolf PA, Cho E, et al. (2011). The relation of dietary choline to cognitive performance and white-matter hyperintensity in the Framingham Offspring Cohort. *Am J Clin Nutr*. Dec;94(6):1584-91.

[2007] Clinical Application: Acetylcholine and Alzheimer's Disease. Retrieved Nov 2 2019 from https://web.williams.edu/imput/synapse/pages/IA5.html.

[2008] Cao C, Cirrito JR, Lin X, Wang L, Verges DK, et al. (2009). Caffeine suppresses β-amyloid levels in plasma and brain of Alzheimer's transgenic mice. *J Alzheimer's Dis*. 2009;17:681-697.

[2009] Mancini RS, Wang Y, Weaver DF. (2018). Phenylindanes in Brewed Coffee Inhibit Amyloid-Beta and Tau Aggregation. *Front Neurosci*. Oct 12;12:735.

[2010] Sauer A. (2017). 4 Surprising Benefits of Coffee. Retrieved Mar 17 2020 from https://www.alzheimers.net/2014-04-09/benefits-of-coffee.

[2011] Fukuyama K, Kakio S, Nakazawa Y, Kobata K, Funakoshi-Tago M, et al. (2018). Roasted Coffee Reduces B-Amyloid Production by Increasing Proteasomal B-Secretase Degradation in Human Neuroblastoma SH-SY5Y Cells. *Mol Nutr Food Res*. Aug;62(21).

[2012] Liu QP, Wu YF, Cheng HY, et al. (2016). Habitual coffee consumption and risk of cognitive decline/dementia: A systematic review and meta-analysis of prospective cohort studies. *Nutrition*. 2016;32(6):628-36

[2013] Wu L, Sun D, He Y. (2017). Coffee intake and the incident risk of cognitive disorders: A dose-response meta-analysis of nine prospective cohort studies. *Clin Nutr*. Jun;36(3):730-6.

[2014] Arendash GW, Cao C. (2010). Caffeine and coffee as therapeutics against Alzheimer's disease. *J Alzheimers Dis*. 2010;20 Suppl 1:S117-26.

[2015] Eskelinene MH, Kivipelto M. (2010). Caffeine as a protective factor in dementia and Alzheimer's disease. *J Alzheimers Dis*. 2010;20, no. Suppl 1:S167-74.

[2016] Cao C, Loewenstein DA, Lin X, Zhang C, Wang L, et al. (2012). High blood caffeine levels in MCI linked to lack of progression to dementia. *J Alzheimers Dis*. 2012;30(3): 559-72.

[2017] Van Gelder BM, Buijsse B, Tijhuis M, et al. Coffee consumption is inversely associated with cognitive decline in elderly European men: the FINE Study. *Eur J Clin Nutr*. 2007;61(2):226-32.

[2018] Nehlig A. (2016). Effects of coffee/caffeine on brain health and disease: What should I tell my patients? *Pract Neurol*. Apr;16(2):89-95.

[2019] Ibid. Nehllg. (2016).

[2020] Basurto-Islas G, Blanchard J, Tung YC, Fernandez JR, Stock M, et al. (2014). Therapeutic Benefits of a Component of Coffee in a Rat Model of Alzheimer's Disease. *Neurobiol Aging.* 2014 Dec;35(12):2701-2712.

[2021] Lee KW, Im JY, Woo JM, Grosso H, Kim YS, et al. (2013). Neuroprotective and Anti-Inflammatory Properties of a Coffee Component in the MPTP Model of Parkinson's Disease. *Neurotherapeutics.* 2013 Jan;10(1):143-53.

[2022] Ibid. Mancini. (2018). *Front Neurosci.*

[2023] Trinh K, Andrews L, Krause J, Hanak T, Lee D, et al. (2010). Decaffeinated Coffee and Nicotine-Free Tobacco Provide Neuroprotection in Drosophila Models of Parkinson's Disease through an NRF2-Dependent Mechanism. *J Neurosco.* Apr 21;30(16):5525-5532.

[2024] Ibid. Mancini. (2018). *Front Neurosci.*

[2025] Daniels JW, Mole PA, Shaffrath JD, Stebbins CL. (1998). Effects of caffeine on blood pressure, heart rate, and forearm blood flow during dynamic leg exercise. *J Appl Physiol.* Jul;85(1):154-59.

[2026] Mathew RJ, Wilson M. (1985). Caffeine induced changes in cerebral circulation. *Stroke.* Sep-Oct;16(5): 814-17.

[2027] Lotfi K, Grunwald JE. (1991). The effect of caffeine on the human macular circulation. *Invest Ophthalmol Vis Sci.* Nov;32(12):3028-32.

[2028] Casiglia E, Bongiovi S, Paleari CD, Petucco S, Boni M, et al. (1991). Haemodynamic effects of coffee and caffeine in normal volunteer: a placebo-controlled clinical study," *J Intern Med.* Jun;229(6):501-4.

[2029] Ibid. Farooqui. (2018). In *Role of the Mediterranean Diet.*

[2030] Witter S, Witter R, Vilu R, Samoson A. (2018). Medical Plants and Nutraceuticals for Amyloid-B Fibrillation Inhibition. *J Alzheimers Dis Rep.* Dec 24:2(1):239-252.

[2031] Bihaqi SW, Singh AP, Tiwari M. (2011). In vivo investigation of the neuroprotective property of Convolvulus pluricaulis in scopolamine-induced cognitive impairments in Wistar rats. *Indian J Pharmacol.* Sep;43(5):520-5.

[2032] Nahata A, Patil UK, Dixit VK. (2008). Effect of Convulvulus pluricaulis Choisy. On learning behavior and memory enhancement activity in rodents. *Nat Prod Res.* 2008;22(16):1472-82.

[2033] Malik J, Karan M, Vasisht K. (2011). Nootropic, anxiolytic and CNS-depressant studies on different plant sources of shankhpushpi. *Pharm Biol.* Dec;49(12):1234-42.

[2034] Kaur M, Prakash A, Kalia AN. (2016). Neuroprotective potential of antioxidant potent fractions from Convolvulus pluricaulis Chois. In 3-nitropropionic acid challenged rats. *Nutr Neurosci.* 19(2):70-8.

[2035] Sharma K, Arora V, Rana AC, Bhatnagar M. (2009). Anxiolytic effect of Convolvulus pluricaulis Choisy petals on elevated plus maze model of anxiety in mice. *J Herb Med Tox.* 2009.

[2036] Dubey NK, Kumar R, Tripathi P. Global promotion of herbal medicine: India's opportunity. Curr Sci. 2007;86:37–41.

[2037] Scheiber IF, Mercer JF, Dringen R. (2014). Metabolism and functions of copper in brain. *Prog Neurobiol.* May;116:33-57.

[2038] Opazo CM, Greenough MA, Bush AI. (2014). Copper: from neurotransmission to neuroproteostasis. *Front Aging Neurosci.* Jul 3;6:143.

[2039] Noda Y, Asada M, Kubota M, Maesako M, Watanabe K, et al. (2013). Copper enhances APP dimerization and promotes Aβ production. *Neurosci Lett.* Jun 28; 547():10-5.

[2040] Eskici G, Axelsen PH. (2012). Copper and oxidative stress in the pathogenesis of Alzheimer's disease. *Biochemistry.* Aug 14; 51(32):6289-311.

[2041] Arnal N, Morel GR, de Alaniz MJ, Castillo O, Marra CA. (2013). Role of copper and cholesterol association in the neurodegenerative process. Int *J Alzheimers Dis.* 2013:414817.

[2042] Hordyjewska A, Popiolek L, Kocot J. (2014). The many "faces" of copper in medicine and treatment. *Biometals.* Aug;27(4): 611–621.

[2043] Ibid. Scheiber. (2014).

[2044] Rosenfeldt FL, Pepe S, Ou R, Mariani JA, Rowland MA, et al. (1999). Coenzyme Q10 improves the tolerance of the senescent myocardium to aerobic and ischemic stress: studies in rats and in human atrial tissue. *Biofactors.* 1999;9(2-4):291-9.

[2045] Littarru GP, Langsjoen P. (2007). Coenzyme Q10 and statins: biochemical and clinical implications. *Mitochondrion.* Jun;7 Suppl:S168-74.

[2046] Nawarskas JJ. (2005). HMG-CoA reductase inhiitors and coenzyme Q10. *Cardiol Rev.* Mar-Apr;13(2):76- 9.

[2047] Ghirlanda G, Oradei A, Manto A, Lippa S, Uccioli L, et al. (1993). Evidence of plasma CoQ10-lowering effect by HMG-CoA reductase inhibitors: a double-blind, placebo-controlled study. *J Clin Pharmacol.* Mar;33(3):226-9.

[2048] Shults CW, Haas R. (2005). Clinical trials of coenzyme Q10 in neurological disorders. *Biofactors.* 2005; 25(1-4):117-26.

[2049] Spindler M, Beal MF, Henchcliffe C. (2009). Coenzyme Q10 effects in neurodegenerative disease. *Neuropsychiatr Dis Treat.* 5:597-610.

[2050] Rosenfeldt F, Hilton D, Pepe S, Krum H. (2003). Systematic review of effect of coenzyme Q10 in physical exercise, hypertension and heart failure. *Biofactors.* 2003;18(1-4):91-100.

[2051] Saini R. (2011). Coenzyme Q10: The essential nutrient. *J Pharm Bioallied Sci.* Jul;3(3):466-7.

[2052] Chaturvedi RK, Beal MF. (2008). Mitochondrial approaches for neuroprotection. *Ann N Y Acad Sci.* Dec;1147():395 -412

[2053] Dumont M, Kipiani K, Yu F, Wille E, Katz M, et al. (2011). Coenzyme Q10 decreases amyloid pathology and improves behavior in a transgenic mouse model of Alzheimer's disease. *J Alzheimers Dis.* 2011;27(1):211-23.

[2054] Ibid. Chaturvedi. (2008).

[2055] Schmelzer C, Lindner I, Rimbach G, Niklowitz P, Menke T, et al. (2008). Functions of coenzyme Q10 in inflammation and gene expression. *Biofactors.* 2008;32(1-4):179-83.

[2056] Diaz-Casado ME, Quiles JL, Barriocanal-Casado E, Gonzalez-Garcia P, Battino M, et al. (2019). The Paradox of Coenzyme Q10 in Aging. *Nutrients.* Sep 14;11(9):2221.

[2057] Sharma SK, El Refaey H, Ebadi M. (2006). Complex-1 activity and 18F-DOPA uptake in genetically engineered mouse model of Parkinson's disease and the neuroprotective role of coenzyme Q10 via gene expression modification. *Brain Res Bull.* Jun 15;70(1):22-32.

[2058] Rathore P, Dohare P, Varma S, Ray A, Sharma U, et al. (2008). Curcuma oil: reduces early accumulation of oxidative product and is anti-apoptogenic in transient focal ischemia in rat brain. *Neurochem Res.* Sep;33(9):1672-82.

[2059] Shehzad A, Rehman G, Lee YS. (2013). Curcumin in inflammatory diseases. *Biofactors.* Jan-Feb; 39(1):69-77.

[2060] Menon VP, Sudheer AR. (2007). Antioxidant and anti-inflammatory properties of curcumin. *Adv Exp Med Biol.* 2007;595:105-25.

[2061] Dzamba D, Harantova L, Butenko O, Anderova M. (2016). Glial Cells – The Key Elements of Alzheimer's Disease. *Curr Alzheimer Res.* 2016;13(8):894-911.

[2062] Kim GY, Kim KH, Lee SH, Yoon MS, Lee HJ, et al. (2005). Curcumin inhibits immunostimulatory function of dendritic cells: MAPKs and translocation of NF-kappa B as potential targets. *J Immunol.* Jun 15;174(12):8116-24.

[2063] Mishra S, Palanivelu K. (2008). The effect of curcumin (turmeric) on Alzheimer's disease: An overview. *Ann Indian Acad Neurol.* Jan-Mar;11(1):13-19.

[2064] Tang M, Taghibiglou C. (2017). The Mechanisms of Action of Curcumin in Alzheimer's Disease. *J Alzheimers Dis.* 2017;58(4):1003-1016.

[2065] Goozee KG, Shah TM, Schrabi HR, Rainey-Smith SR, Brown B, et al. (2016). Examining the potential clinical value of curcumin in the prevention and diagnosis of Alzheimer's disease. *Br J Nutr.* Feb 14;115(3):449-65.

[2066] Reddy PH, Manczak M, Yin X, Grady MC, Mitchell A, et al. (2018). Protective Effects of Indian Spice Curcumin Against Amyloid-B in Alzheimer's Disease. *J Alzheimers Dis.* 2018;61(3):843-866.

[2067] Wang YL, Ju B, Zhang YZ, Yin HL, Liu YJ, et al. (2017). Protective Effect of Curcumin Against Oxidative Stress-Induced Injury in Rats with Parkinson's Disease Through the Wnt/ B-Catenin Signaling Pathway. *Cell Physiol Biochem.* 2017;43(6):2226-2241.

[2068] Cui Q, Li X, Zhu H. (2016). Curcumin ameliorates dopaminergic neuronal oxidative damage via activation of the Akt/Nrf2 pathway. *Mol Med Res.* Feb;13(2):1381-8.

[2069] Bigford GE, Del Rossi G. (2014). Supplemental substances derived from foods ad adjunctive therapeutic agents for treatment of neurodegenerative diseases and disorders. *Adv Nutr.* Jul 14; 5(4):394-403.

[2070] Siddique YH, Naz F, Jyoti S. (2014). Effect of Curcumin on Lifespan, Activity Pattern, Oxidative Stress, and Apoptosis in the Brains of Transgenic Drosophila Model of Parkinson's Disease. *Biomed Res Int.* 2014; 2014():606928.

[2071] Ng TP, Chiam PC, Lee T, Chua HC, Lim L, et al. (2006). Curry consumption and cognitive function in the elderly. *Am J Epidemiol.* Nov 1;164(9):898-906.

[2072] Kim, S.J., Son, T.G., Park, H.R., Park, M., Kimm, M.S., Kim, H.S., Chung, H.Y., Mattson, M.P., Lee, J. (23 May 2008), "Curcumin stimulations proliferation of embryonic neural progenitor cells and neurogenesis in the adult hippocampus." *Journal of Biological Chemistry.* 283(21):14497-505.

[2073] Dong S, Zeng Q, Mitchell ES, Xiu J, Duan Y, et al. (2012). Curcumin Enhances Neurogenesis and Cognition in Aged Rats: Implications for Transcriptional Interactions Related to Growth and Synaptic Plasticity. *PLOS One.* Feb 16.

[2074] Ibid. Ng. (2006). *Am J Epidemiol.*

[2075] Zhang L, Fiala M, Cashman J, Sayre J, Espinosa A, et al. (2006). Curcuminoids enhance amyloid-beta uptake by macrophages of Alzheimer's disease patients. *J Alzheimers Dis.* Sep; 10(1):1-7.

[2076] Ibid. Reddy. (2018). *J Alzheimers Dis.*

[2077] Mourtas S, Lazar AN, Markoutsa E, Duyckaerts C, Antimisiaris SG. (2014). Multifunctional nanoliposomes with curcumin-lipid derivative and brain targeting functionality with potential applications for Alzheimer disease. *Eur J Med Chem.* Jun 10; 80():175-83.

[2078] Ono K, Hasegawa K, Naiki H, Yamada M. (2004). Curcumin has potent anti-amyloiddogenic effects for Azheimer's disease beta-amyloid fibrils in vitro. *J Neurosci Res.* Mar 15;75(6):742-50.

[2079] Ringman JA, Frautschy SA, Cole GM, Masterman DL, Cummings JL. (2006). A potential role of the curry spice curcumin in Alzheimer's disease. *Curr Alzheimer Res.* Apr;2(2):131-136.

[2080] Yang F, Lim GP, Begum AN, Ubeda OJ, Simmons MR, et al. (2005). Curcumin inhibits formation of amyloid beta oligomers and fibrils, binds plaques, and reduces amyloid in vivo. *J Biol Chem.* Feb 18;280(7):5892-901.

[2081] Shoba G, Joy D, Joseph T, Majeed M, Rajendran R, et al. (1998). Influence of piperine on the pharmacokinetics of curcumin in animals and human volunteers. *Planta Med.* May;64(4):353-6.

[2082] Baum L, Lam CW, Cheung SK, Kwok T, Lui V, et al. (2008). Six-month randomized, placebo-controlled, double-blind, pilot clinical trial of curcumin in patients with Alzheimer disease. *J Clin Psychopharmacol.* 2008 Feb; 28(1):110-3.

[2083] Rasyid A, Lelo A. (1999). The effect of curcumin and placebo on human gall-bladder function: an ultrasound study. *Aliment Pharmacol Ther.* Feb; 13(2):245-9.

[2084] Rasyid A, Rahman AR, Jaalam K, Lelo A. (2002). Effect of different curcumin dosages on human gall bladder. *Asia Pac J Clin Nutr.* 2002;11(4):314-8.

[2085] Goncharov NP, Katsia GV. (2013). [Neurosteroid dehydroepiandrosterone and brain function]. *Fiziol Cheloveka.* Nov-Dec;39(6):120-8.

[2086] Perrini S, Laviola L, Natalicchio A, Giogino F. (2005). Associated hormonal declines in aging: DHEAS. *J Endocrinol Invest.* 2005;28(3 Suppl):85-93.

[2087] Jin RO, Mason S, Mellon SH, Epel ES, Reus VI, et al. (2016). Cortisol/DHEA ratio and hippocampal volume: A pilot study in major depression and healthy controls. *Psychoneuroendocrinology.* Oct;72:139-46.

[2088] Yamada S, Akishita M, Fukai S, Ogawa S, Yamaguchi K, et al. (2010). Effects of dehydroepiandrosterone supplementation on cognitive function and activities of daily living in older women with mild to moderate cognitive impairment. *Geriatr Gerontol Int.* Oct;10(4):280-7.

[2089] Moriguchi S, Shinoda Y, Yamamoto Y, Sasaki Y, Miyajima K. (2013). Stimulation of the sigma-1 receptor by DHEA enhances synaptic efficacy and neurogenesis in the hippocampal dentate gyrus of olfactory bulbectomized mice. *PLoS One.* Apr 8;8(4):e60863.

[2090] Van Niekerk JK, Huppert FA, Herbert J. (2001). Salivary cortisol and DHEA: association with measures of cognition and well-being in normal older men, and effects of three months of DHEA supplementation. *Psychoneuroendocrinology.* 2001;26(6):591-612.

[2091] Yang S, Gu YY, Jing F, Yu CX, Guan QB. (2019). The Effect of Statins on Levels of Dehydroepiandrosterone (DHEA) in Women with Polycystic Ovary Syndrome: A Systematic Review and Meta-Analysis. *Med Sci Monit.* Jan 20;25:590-597.

[2092] Malanga G, Agular MB, Martinez HD, Puntarulo S. (2012). New insights on dimethylaminoethanol (DMAE) features as a free radical scavenger. *Drug Metab Lett.* Mar;6(1):54-9.

[2093] Patel K. (2019). Centrophenoxine. Retrieved Nov 18 2019 from https://examine.com/supplements/centrophenoxine/.

[2094] Blin O, Audebert C, Pitel S, Kaladjian A, Casse-Perrot C, et al. (2009). Effects of dimethylaminoethanol pyroglutamate (DMAE p-Glu) against memory deficits induced by scopolamine: evidence from preclinical and clinical studies. *Psychopharmacology (Berl).* Dec;207(2):201-12.

[2095] Zs-Nagy I. (1989). On the role of intracellular physicochemistry in quantitative expression during aging and the effect of centrophenoxine. A review. *Arch Gerontol Geriatr.* Nov-Dec;9(3):215-29.

[2096] Zs-Nagy I. (2002). Pharmacological interventions against aging through the cell plasma membrane: a review of the experimental results obtained in animals and humans. *Ann N Y Acad Sci.* Apr;959:308-20.

[2097] Frank MJ. (2005). Dynamic dopamine modulation in the basal ganglia: a neurocomputational account of cognitive deficits in medicated and nonmedicated Parkinsonism. *J Cogn Neurosci.* Jan;17(1):51-72.

[2098] Bressan RA, Crippa JA. (2005). The role of dopamine in reward and pleasure behavior—review of data from preclinical research. *Acta Psychiatr Scand Suppl.* 2005;(427):14-21.

[2099] Chong TT, Husain M. (2016). The role of dopamine in the pathophysiology and treatment of apathy. *Prog Brain Res.* 2016;229:389-426.

[2100] Fernstrom JD, Fernstrom MH. (2007). Tyrosine, phenylalanine, and catecholamine synthesis and function in the brain. *J Nutr.* Jun;137(6 Suppl 1):1539S-1547S.

[2101] Colzato LS, de Haan AM, Hommel B. (2015). Food for creativity: tyrosine promotes deep thinking. *Psychol Res.* Sep;79(5):709-14.

[2102] Kuhn S, Duzel S, Colzato L, Norman K, Gallinat J, et al. (2019). Food for thought: association between dietary tyrosine and cognitive performance in younger and older adults. *Psychol Res.* Sep;83(6):1097-1106.

[2103] Fahn S. (2008). The history of dopamine and levodopa in the treatment of Parkinson's disease. *Mov Disord.* 2008;23 Suppl 3:S497-508.

[2104] Warren N, O'Gorman C, Lehn A, Siskind D. (2017). Dopamine dysregulation syndrome in Parkinson's disease: a systematic review of published cases. *J Neurol Neurosurg Psychiatry.* Dec;88(12):1060-1064.

[2105] Connolly BS, Lang AE. (2014). Pharmacological treatment of Parkinson disease: a review. *JAMA.* Apr 23-30;311(16):1670-83.

[2106] Zeisel SH, Corbin KD. Choline. In: Erdman JW, Macdonald IA, Zeisel SH, eds. Present Knowledge in Nutrition. 10th ed. Washington, DC: Wiley-Blackwell; 2012:405-18.

[2107] Fava M, Borus JS, Alpert JE, Nierenberg AA, Rosenbaum JF, et al. (1997). Folate, vitamin B12, and homocysteine in major depressive disorder. *Am J Psychiatry.* Mar; 154(3):426-8.

[2108] Durga J, van Boxtel MP, Schouten EG, Kok FJ, Jolles J, et al. (2007). Effect of 3-year folic acid supplementation on cognitive function in older adults in the FACIT trial: a randomized, double blind, controlled trial. *Lancet.* Jan 20; 369(9557):208-16.

[2109] Corrada MM, Kawas CH, Hallfrisch J, Muller D, Brookmeyer R. (2005). Reduced risk of Alzheimer's disease with high folate intake: the Baltimore Longitudinal Study of Aging. *Alzheimers Dement.* Jul; 1(1):11-8.

[2110] Fioravanti M, Ferrario E, Massaia M, Cappa G, Rivolta G, et al. (1998). Low folate levels in the cognitive decline of elderly patients and the efficacy of folate as a treatment for improving memory deficits. *Arch Gerontol Geriatr.* Jan-Feb; 26(1):1-13.

[2111] Ramos MI, Allen LH, Mungas DM, Jagust WJ, Haan MN, et al. (2005). Low folate status is associated with impaired cognitive function and dementia in the Sacramento Area Latino Study on Aging. *Am J Clin Nutr.* Dec; 82(6):1346-52. or in conjunction with other B vitamins

[2112] Nilsson K, Gustafson L, Hultberg B. (2001). Improvement of cognitive functions after cobalamin/folate supplementation in elderly patients with dementia and elevated plasma homocysteine. *Int J Geriatr Psychiatry.* Jun; 16(6):609-14.

[2113] Connelly PJ, Prentice NP, Cousland G, Bonham J. (2008). A randomised double-blind placebo-controlled trial of folic acid supplementation of cholinesterase inhibitors in Alzheimer's disease. *Int J Geriatr Psychiatry.* Feb;23(2):155-60.

[2114] Zingg JM, Jones PA. (1997). Genetic and epigenetic aspects of DNA methylation on genome expression, evolution, mutation and carcinogenesis. *Carcinogenesis.* May;18(5):869-82.

[2115] Duthie SJ. (2011). Folate and cancer: how DNA damage, repair and methylation impact on colon carcinogenesis. *J Inherit Metab Dis.* Feb; 34(1):101-9.

[2116] Lawson LD. (1998). Garlic: a review of its medicinal effects and indicated active compounds. *Phytomedicines of Europe. Chemistry and Biological activity.* 1998; series 691:176–209.

[2117] Rahman K, Lowe GM. (2006). Garlic and cardiovascular disease: a critical review. *J Nutr.* Mar; 136(3 Suppl):736S-740S.

[2118] Zeng T, Zhang CL, Zhao XL, Xie KQ. (2013). The roles of garlic on the lipid parameters: a systematic review of the literature. *Crit Rev Food Sci Nutr.* 53(3):215-30.

[2119] Raz L, Knoefel J, Bhaskar K. (2016). The neuropathology and cerebrovascular mechanisms of dementia. *J Cereb Blood Flow Metab.* Jan;36(1):172-86.

[2120] Durak I, Kavutcu M, Aytaç B, Avci A, Devrim E, et al. (2004). Effects of garlic extract consumption on blood lipid and oxidant/antioxidant parameters in humans with high blood cholesterol. *J Nutr Biochem.* Jun; 15(6):373-7.

[2121] Lau BH. (2001). Suppression of LDL oxidation by garlic. *J Nutr.* Mar; 131(3s):985S-8S.

[2122] Bordia AK, Sanadhya SK, Rathore AS, Bhu N. (1978). Essential oil of garlic on blood lipids and fibrinolytic activity in patients of coronary artery disease. *J Assoc Physicians India.* 1978 May; 26(5):327-31.

[2123] Chutani SK, Bordia A. (1981). The effect of fried versus raw garlic on fibrinolytic activity in man. *Atherosclerosis.* Feb-Mar; 38(3-4):417-21.

[2124] Hfaiedh N, Murat JC, Elfeki A. (2011). Compared ability of garlic (Allium sativum) extract or α-tocopherol + magnesium association to reduce metabolic disorders and oxidative stress in diabetic rats. *Phytother Res.* Jun;25(6):821-7.

[2125] Avci A, Atli T, Erguder IB, Varli M, Devrim E, et al. (2008). Effects of garlic consumption on plasma and erythrocyte antioxidant parameters in elderly subjects. *Gerontology.* 2008;54(3):173-6.

[2126] Bordia AK, Sanadhya SK, Rathore AS, Bhu N, Verma SK, Srivastava KC. (1998). Effect of garlic (Allium sativum) on blood lipids, blood sugar, fibrinogen and fibrinolytic activity in patients with coronary artery disease. *Prostaglandins Leukot Essent Fatty Acids.* Apr;58(4):257-63.

[2127] Chutani SK, Bordia A. The effect of fried versus raw garlic on fibrinolytic activity in man. *Atherosclerosis.* 1981 Feb-Mar; 38(3-4):417-21.

[2128] Ibid. Bordia. (1978).

[2129] Bordia A, Sharma KD, Parmar YK, Verma SK. (1982). Protective effect of garlic oil on the changes produced by 3 weeks of fatty diet on serum cholesterol, serum triglycerides, fibrinolytic activity and platelet adhesiveness in man. *Indian Heart J.* Mar-Apr; 34(2):86-8.

[2130] Ide N, Lau BH. (1997). Garlic compounds protect vascular endothelial cells from oxidized low-density lipoprotein-induced injury. *J Pharm Pharmacol.* ; 49(9):908-11.

[2131] Anoush M, Eghbal MA, Fathiazad F, Hamzeiy H, Kouzehkonani NS. (2009). The protective effects of garlic extract against acetaminophen-induced oxidative stress and glutathione depletion. *Pak J Biol Sci.* May 15;12(10):765-71.

[2132] Ho CY, Cheng YT, Chau CF, Yen GC. (2012). Effect of diallyl sulfide on in vitro and in vivo Nrf2-mediated pulmonic antioxidant enzyme expression via activation ERK/p38 signaling pathway. *J Agric Food Chem.* Jan 11;60(1):100-7.

[2133] Anoush M, Eghbal MA, Fathiazad F, Hamzely H, Kouzehkonani NS. (2009). The protective effects of garlic extract against acetaminophen-induced oxidative stress and glutathione depletion. *Pak J Biol Sci.* May 15;12(10):765-71.

[2134] Bruck R, Aeed H, Brazovsky E, Noor T, Hershkoviz R. (2005). Allicin, the active component of garlic, prevents immune-mediated, concanavalin A-induced hepatic injury in mice. *Liver Int.* Jun;25(3):613-21.

[2135] Butt MS, Sultan MT, Butt MS, Iqbal J. (2009). Garlic: nature's protection against physiological threats. *Crit Rev Food Sci Nutr.* Jun;49(6):538-51.

[2136] Hasan N, Siddiqui MU, Toossi Z, Khan S, Iqbal J. (2007). Allicin-induced suppression of Mycobacterium tuberculosis 85B mRNA in human monocytes. *Biochem Biophys Res Commun.* Apr 6;355(2):471-6.

[2137] Yeh YY, Liu L. (2001). Cholesterol-lowering effect of garlic extracts and organosulfur compounds: human and animal studies. *J Nutr.* Mar; 131(3s):989S-93S.

[2138] Amagase H. (2006). Clarifying the real bioactive constituents of garlic. *Amagase HJ Nutr.* Mar; 136(3 Suppl):716S-725S

[2139] Borek C. (2006). Garlic reduces dementia and heart-disease risk. *J Nutr.* Mar; 136(3 Suppl):810S-812S

[2140] Qu Z, Mossine VV, Cui J, Sun GY, Gu Z. (2016). Protective Effects of AGE and Its Components on Neuroinflammation and Neurodegeneration. *Neuromolecular Med.* Sep;18(3):474-82.

[2141] Rojas P, Serrano-Garcia N, Medina-Campos ON, Pedraza-Chaverri J, Maldonado PD, et al. (2011). S-Allylcysteine, a garlic compound, protects against oxidative stress in 1-methyl-4-phenylpyridinium-induced parkinsonism in mice. *J Nutr Biochem.* Oct:22(10):937-44.

[2142] Ibid. Rojas. (2011).

[2143] Jeong JH, Jeong HR, Jo YN, Kim HJ, Shin JH, et al. (2013). Ameliorating effects of aged garlic extracts against AB-induced neurotoxicity and cognitive impairment. *BMC Complement Altern Med.* Oct 18;13:268.

[2144] Ray B, Cauhan NB, Lahiri DK. (2011). The "aged garlic extract:" (AGE) and one of its active ingredients S-allyl-L-cysteine (SAC) as potential preventive and therapeutic agents for Alzheimer's disease (AD). *Curr Med Chem.* 2011;18(22):330-13.

[2145] Ibid. Jeong. (2013).

[2146] Li F, Kim MR. (2019). Effect of Aged Garlic Ethyl Acetate Extract on Oxidative Stress and Cholinergic Function of Scopolamine-Induced Cognitive Impairment in Mice. *Prev Nutr Food Sci.* Jun;24(2):165-170.

[2147] Ibid. Li. (2019).

[2148] Nillert N, Pannangrong W, Welbat JU, Chaijaroonkhanarak W, Sripanidkulchai K, et al. (2017). Neuroprotective Effects of Aged Garlic Extract on Cognitive Dysfunction and Neuroinflammation Induced by B-Amyloid in Rats. *Nutrients.* Jan 3;9(1):E24.

[2149] Jeong YY, Park HJ, Cho YW, Kim EJ, Kim GT, et al. (2012). Aged red garlic extract reduces cigarette smoke extract-induced cell death in human bronchial smooth muscle cells by increasing intracellular glutathione levels. *Phytother Res.* Jan;26(1):18-25.

[2150] Banerjee SK, Maulik SK. (2002). Effect of garlic on cardiovascular disorders: a review. *Nutr J.* 2002 Nov 19; 1():4.

[2151] Ried K, Frank OR, Stocks NP. (2013). Aged garlic extract reduces blood pressure in hypertensives: a dose-response trial. *Eur J Clin Nutr.* Jan;67(1):64-70.

[2152] Steiner M, Li W. (2001). Aged garlic extract, a modulator of cardiovascular risk factors: a dose-finding study on the effects of AGE on platelet functions. *J Nutr.* Mar; 131(3s):980S-4S.

[2153] Yeh YY, Lim HS, Yeh SM, Picciano MF. Garlic extract attenuate hyperhomocysteinemia caused by folic acid deficiency in the rat. *Nutr Res.* 2005;25:93–102.

[2154] Chandrashekar PM, Venkatesh YP. (2009). Identification of the protein components displaying immunomodulatory activity in aged garlic extract. *J Ethnopharmacol.* Jul 30;124(3):384-90.

[2155] Ishikawa H, Saeki T, Otani T, Suzuki T, Shimozuma K. (2006). Aged Garlic Extract Prevents a Decline of NK Cell Number and Actiity in Patients with Advanced Cancer. *J Nutr.* Mar;136(3 Suppl):816S-820S.

[2156] Morioka N, Sze LL, Morton DL, Irie RF. (1993). A protein fraction from aged garlic extract enchances cytotoxity and proliferation of human lymphocytes mediated by interleukin 2 and concanavalin A. *Cancer Immunol Immunother.* Oct;37(5):316-22.

[2157] Chandrashekar PM, Venkatesh YP. (2009). Identification of the protein components displaying immunobodulatory activity in aged garlic extract. *J Ethnopharmacol.* Jul 30;124(3):384-90.

[2158] Topic B, Tani E, Tsiakitzis K, Kourounakis PN, Dere E, et al. (2002). Enhanced maze performance and reduced oxidative stress by combined extracts of zingiber officinale and ginkgo biloba in the aged rat. *Neurobiol Aging.* 2002;23(1):135–43.

[2159] Halvorsen BL, Holte K, Myhrstad MC, Barikmo I, Hvattum E, et al. (2002). A systematic screening of total antioxidants in dietary plants. *J Nutr.* Mar;132(3):461–71

[2160] Ahmed RS, Suke SG, Seth V, Chakraborti A, Tripathi AK, et al. (2008). Protective effects of dietary ginger (Zingiber officinales Rosc.) on lindane-induced oxidative stress in rats. *Phytother Res.* 2008;22(7):902–6

[2161] El-Sharaky AS, Newairy AA, Kamel MA, Eweda SM. (2009). Protective effect of ginger extract against bromobenzene-induced hepatotoxicity in male rats. *Food Chem Toxicol.* 2009;47(7):1584–90.

[2162] Young H. Y, Luo Y. L, Cheng H. Y, Hsieh W. C, Liao J. C, Peng W. H. Analgesic and anti-inflammatory activities of [6]-gingerol. J *Ethnopharmacol.* 2005;96(1-2):207–10

[2163] Minghetti P, Sosa S, Cilurzo F, editors. et al. Evaluation of the topical anti-inflammatory activity of ginger dry extracts from solutions and plasters. *Planta Med.* 2007;73(15):1525–30

[2164] Marcus D. M, Suarez-Almazor M. E. Is there a role for ginger in the treatment of osteoarthritis? *Arthritis Rheum.* 2001;44(11):2461–2

[2165] Fernandes RCL, da Silva KS, Bonan C, Zahar SEV, Marinheiro LPF. Cognitive function in menopausal women evaluated with the mini-mental state examination and word-list memory test. *Cadernos de Saude Publica.* 2009;25(9):1883–1893.

[2166] Saenghong N, Wattanathorn J, Muchimapura S, Tongun T, Piyavhatkul N, et al. (2011). Zingiber officinale improves cognitive function in Middle-Aged Healthy Women. *Evid Based Complement Alternat Med.* 2012;2012: 383062.

[2167] Ibid. Saenghong. (2011).

[2168] Grzanna R, Phan P, Polotsky A, Lindmark L, Frondoza CG. (2004). Ginger extract inhibits beta-amyloid peptide-induced cytokine and chemokine expression in cultured THP-1 monocytes. *J Altern Complement Med.* Dec;10(6):1009-13.

[2169] Zeng GF, Zhang ZY, Lu L, Xiao DQ, Zong SH, et al. (2013). Protective effects of ginger root extract on Alzheimer disease-induced behavioral dysfunction in rats. *Rejuvenation Res.* Apr;16(2):124-33.

[2170] Lim S, Choi JG, Moon M, Kim HG, Lee W, et al. (2016). An Optimized Combination of Ginger and Peony Root Effectively Inhibits Amyloid-B Accumulation and Amyloid-B-Mediated Pathology in ABPP/PS1 Double-Transgenic Mice. *J Alzheimers Dis.* 2016;50(1):189-200.

[2171] Wu YZ, Li SQ, Zu WG, Du J, Wang FF. (2008). Ginkgo biloba extract improves coronary artery circulation in patients with coronary artery disease: contribution of plasma nitric oxide and endothelin-1. *Phytother Res.* Jun;22(6):734-9

[2172] Qiu Y, Rui YC, Li TJ, Zhang L, Yao PY. (2004). Inhibitory effect of extracts of Ginkgo biloba leaves on VEGF-induced hyperpermeability of bovine coronary endothelial cell in vitro. *Acta Pharmacol Sin.* 2004 Oct;25(10):1306-11.

[2173] Welt K, Weiss J, Martin R, Hermsdorf T, Drews S, et al. (2007). Ginkgo biloba extract protects rat kidney from diabetic and hypoxic damage. *Phytomedicine.* Feb;14(2-3):196-203.

[2174] Hong F, Wang L, Wu SL, Tang HC, Sha O, et al. (2017). A Review of Three Commonly Used Herbs Which Enhance Memory and New Evidences Which Show Their Combination Could Improve Memory in Young Animals. *Mini Rev Med Chem.* 2017;17(16):1537-1547.

[2175] Tchantchou F, Lacor PN, Cao Z, Lao L, Hou Y, et al. (2009). Stimulation of neurogenesis and synaptogenesis bilobalide and quercetin via common final pathway in hippocampal neurons. *J Alzheimer Dis.* 18(4):787-98.

[2176] Allain H, Raoul P, Lieury A, LeCoz F, Gandon JM, et al. (1993). Effect of two doses of ginkgo biloba extract (EGb 761) on the dual-coding test in elderly subjects. *Clin Ther.* May-Jun; 15(3):549-58.

[2177] Yoo DY, Nam Y, Kim W, Yoo KY, Park J, et al. (2011). Effects of Gingko Biloba extract on promotion of neurogenesis in the hippocampal dentate gyrus in C57BL/6 mice. *J Vet Med Sci.* Jan;73(1):71-6.

[2178] Hou Y, Aboukhatwa MA, Lei D, Manaye K, Khan I, et al. (2010). Antidepressant flavonols modulate BDNF and beta amyloid in neurons and hippocampus of double TgAD mice. *Neurophamarcology.* May;58(6): 911-920.

[2179] Wesnes K, Simmons D, Rook M, Simpson P. (1987). A double-blind placebo-controlled trial of Tanakan in the treatment of idiopathic cognitive impairment in the elderly. *Hum Psychopharmacol.* Sep;2(3).

[2180] Elsabagh S, Hartley DE, Ali O, Williamson EM. (2005). Differential cognitive effects of Ginkgo biloba after acute and chronic treatment in healthy young volunteers. *Psychopharmacology (Berl).* May; 179(2):437-46.

[2181] Kaschel R. (2009). Ginkgo biloba: specificity of neuropsychological improvement--a selective review in search of differential effects. *Hum Psychopharmacol.* 2009 Jul; 24(5):345-70

[2182] Li H, Sun X, Yu F, Xu L, Miu J, et al. (2018). In Silico Investigation of the Pharmacological Mechanisms of Beneficial Effects of Ginkgo biloba L. on Alzheimer's Disease. *Nutrients.* May 10;10(5);E589.

[2183] Wan W, Zhang C, Danielsen M, Li Q, Chen W, et al. (2016). Ebb761 improves cognitive function and regulates inflammatory responses in the APP/PS1 mouse. *Exp Gerontol.* Aug;81:92-100.

[2184] Zimmermann M, Colciaghi F, Cattabeni F, Di Luca M. (2002). Ginkgo biloba extract: from molecular mechanisms to the treatment of Alzhelmer's disease. *Cell Mol Biol (Noisy-le-grand).* Sep;48(6):613-23.

[2185] Weinmann S, Roll S, Schwarzbach C, Vauth C, Willich SN. (2010). Effects of Ginkgo biloba in dementia: systematic review and meta-analysis. *BMC Geriatr.* Mar 17; 10():14.

[2186] Mazza M, Capuano A, Bria P, Mazza S. (2006). Ginkgo biloba and donepezil: a comparison in the treatment of Alzheimer's dementia in a randomized placebo-controlled double-blind study. *Eur J Neurol.* Sep;13(9):981-5.

[2187] Andrieu S, Ousset PJ, Coley N, Ouzid M, Mathiex-Fortunet H, et al. (2008). GuidAge study: a 5-year double blind, randomised trial of EGb 761 for the prevention of Alzheimer's disease in elderly subjects with memory complaints. i. rationale, design and baseline data. *Curr Alzheimer Res.* Aug; 5(4):406-15.

[2188] IPSEN. Encouraging results of GuidAge, large scale European trial conducted in the prevention of Alzheimer's Dementia. 2010. 22 June. http://www.ipsen.com/en/encouraging-results-guidage-large-scale-european-trial-conducted-prevention-alzheimer-s-dementia.

[2189] Shi C, Xiao S, Liu J, Guo K, Wu F, et al. (2010). Ginkgo biloba extract Ebb761 protects against aging-associated mitochondrial dysfunction in platelets and hippocampi of SAMP8 mice. *Platelets.* 2010;21(5):373-9.

[2190] Soholm B. (1998). Clinical improvement of memory and other cognitive functions by Ginkgo biloba: a review of relevant literature. *Adv Ther.* Jan-Feb;15(1):54-65.

[2191] Biecharz-Klin K, Piechal A, Joniec I, Pyrzanowska J, Widy-Tyskiewicz E. (2009). Pharmacological and biochemical effects of Ginkgo biloba extract on learning, memory consolidation and motor activity in old rats. *Acta Neurobiol Exp* (Wars). 2009;69(2):217-31.

[2192] Ihl R, Tribanek M, Bachinskaya N. (2012). Efficacy and tolerability of a once daily formulation of Ginkgo biloba extract EGb 761® in Alzheimer's disease and vascular dementia: results from a randomised controlled trial., GOTADAY Study Group. *Pharmacopsychiatry.* Mar; 45(2):41-6.

[2193] McKenna DJ, Jones K, Hughes K. (2001). Efficacy, safety, and use of ginkgo biloba in clinical and preclinical applications. *Altern Ther Health Med.* Sep-Oct;7(5):70-86, 88-90.

[2194] Ramassamy C, Longpré F, Christen Y. (2007). Ginkgo biloba extract (EGb 761) in Alzheimer's disease: is there any evidence? *Curr Alzheimer Res.* 2007 Jul; 4(3):253-62.

[2195] DeFeudis FV, Drieu K. (2000). Ginkgo biloba extract (EGb 761) and CNS functions: basic studies and clinical applications. *Curr Drug Targets.* Jul; 1(1):25-58.

[2196] Ahlemeyer B, Krieglstein J. (2003). Neuroprotective effects of Ginkgo biloba extract. *Cell Mol Life Sci.* Sep; 60(9):1779-92.

[2197] Kennedy DO, Scholey AB, Wesnes KA. (2000). The dose-dependent cognitive effects of acute administration of Ginkgo biloba to healthy young volunteers. *Psychopharmacology (Berl).* Sep; 151(4):416-23.

[2198] Stough C, Clarke J, Lloyd J, Nathan P. (2001). Neuropsychological changes after 30-day Ginkgo biloba administration in healthy participants. *J Int J Neuropsychopharmacol.* Jun; 4(2):131-4.

[2199] Polich J, Gloria R. (2001). Cognitive effects of a Ginkgo biloba/vinpocetine compound in normal adults: systematic assessment of perception, attention and memory. Hum *Psychopharmacol.* Jul; 16(5):409-416.

[2200] Pizzorno J, Murray M. *Textbook of Natural Medicine.* Edinburg, NY: Churchill Livingstone, 1999, p. 752-3.

[2201] Yuan Q, Wang CW, Shi J, Lin ZX. (2017). Effects of Ginkgo biloba on dementia: An overview of systematic reviews. *J Ethnopharmacol.* Jan 4;195:1-9.

[2202] Wang Y, Liu J, Zhang Z, Bi P, Qi Z, et al. (2011). Anti-neuroinflammation effect of ginsenoside Rbl in a rat model of Alzheimer disease. *Neurosci Lett.* 2011;487:70–72.

[2203] Liao B, Newmark H, Zhou R. (2002). Neuroprotective effects of ginseng total saponin and ginsenosides Rb1 and Rg1 on spinal cord neurons in vitro. *Exp Neurol.* 2002;173:224–234.

[2204] Lee E, Kim S, Chung KC, Choo MK, Kim DH, et al. (2006). 20(S)-Ginsenoside Rh2, a newly identified active ingredient of ginseng, inhibits NMDA receptors in cultured rat hippocampal neurons. *Eur J Pharmacol.* 2006;536:69–77.

[2205] Ibid. Liao. (2002).

[2206] Ibid. Lee. (2006).

[2207] Qiao C, Den R, Kudo K, Yamada K, Takemoto K, et al. (2005). Ginseng enhances contextual fear conditioning and neurogenesis in rats. *Neurosci Res.* 2005;51:31–38.

[2208] Kim HJ, Jung SW, Kim SY, Cho IH, Kim HC, et al. (2018). Panax ginseng as an adjuvant treatment for Alzheimer's disease. *J Ginseng Res.* Oct; 42(4): 401–411.

[2209] Lee CH, Kim JM, Kim DH, Park SJ, Liu X, et al. (2013). Effects of sun ginseng on memory enhancement and hippocampus neurogenesis. *Phytother Res.* 27(9):1293-9.

[2210] Lin T, Liu Y, Shi M, Liu X, Li L, et al. (2012). Promotive effect of ginsenoside Rd on proliferation of neural stem cells in vivo and in vitro. *J Ethnopharmacol.* Aug;142(3):754-61.

[2211] Zheng GQ, Cheng W, Wang Y, Wang XM, Zhao SZ, et al. (2011). Ginseng total saponins enhance neurogenesis after focal cerebral ischemia. *J Ethnopharmacol.* Jan 27;133(2):724-8.

[2212] Wesnes KA, Ward T, McGinty A, Petrini O. (2000). The memory enhancing effects of a Ginkgo biloba/Panax ginseng combination in healthy middle-aged volunteers. *Psychopharmacology* (Berl). Nov; 152(4):353-61.

[2213] Schliebs R, Liebmann A, Bhattacharya SK, Kumar A, Ghosal S, et al. (1997). Systemic administration of defined extracts from Withania somnifera (Indian Ginseng) and Shilajit differentially affect cholinergic but not glutamatergic and GABAergic markers in rat brain. *Neurochem In.* Feb;30(2):181-90.

[2214] Li L, Liu J, Yan X, Qin K, Shi M, et al. (2011). Protective effects of ginsenoside Rd against okadaic acid-induced neurotoxicity in vivo and in vitro. *J Ethnopharmacol.* 2011;138:135–141.

[2215] Ibid. Kim. (2018).

[2216] Kuboyama T, Tohda C, Komatsu K. (2005). Neuritic regeneration and synaptic reconstruction induced by withanolide A. *Br J Pharmacol.* Apr;144(7):961-971.

[2217] Jayaprakasam B, Padmanabhan K, Nair MG. (2010). Withanamides in Withania somnifera fruit protect PC-12 cells from beta-amyloid responsible for Alzheimer's disease. *Phytother Res.* Jun;24(6):859-63.

2218 Jiang B, Xiong Z, Yang J, Wang W, Wang Y, et al. (2012). Antidepressant-like effects of ginsenoside Rg1 are due to activation of the BDNF signaling pathway and neurogenesis in the hippocampus. *Brit J Pharmacol*. Jul;166(6):1872-87.

2219 Xu C, Teng J, Chen W, Ge Q, Yang Z, et al. (2010). 20(S)-Protopanaxadiol, an active ginseng metabolite, exhibits strong antidepressant-like effects in animal tests. *Prog Neuropsychopharmacol Biol Psychiatry*. Dec;34:1402–1411.

2220 Al-Harbi KS. (2012). Treatment-resistant depression: therapeutic trends, challenges, and future directions. *Patient Prefer Adherence*. 2012;6:369–388

2221 Dong HS, Han C, Jeon SW, Yoon S, Jeong HG, et al. (2016). Characteristics of neurocognitive functions in mild cognitive impairment with depression. *Int Psychogeriatr*. Jul;28:1181–119.

2222 Van Kampen JM, Baranowski DB, Shaw CA, Kay DG. (2014). Panax ginseng is neuroprotective in a novel progressive model of Parkinson's disease. *Exp Gerontol*. 2014;50:95–105.

2223 Thatte U, Bagadey S, Dahanukar S. (2000). Modulation of programmed cell death by medicinal plants. *Cell Mol Biol*. 2000;46:199–214

2224 Xu C, Teng J, Chen W, Ge Q, Yang Z, et al. (2010). 20(S)-Protopanaxadiol, an active ginseng metabolite, exhibits strong antidepressant-like effects in animal tests. *Prog Neuropsychopharmacol Biol Psychiatry*. 2010;34:1402–1411.

2225 Rege NN, Thatte UM, Dahanukar SA. (1999). Adaptogenic properties of six rasayana herbs used in Ayurvedic medicine. *Phytother Res*. 1999;13:275–291.

2226 Churchill JD, Gerson JL, Hinton KA, Mifek JL, Walter MJ, et al. (2002). The nootropic properties of ginseng saponin Rb1 are linked to effects on anxiety. *Integr Physiol Behav Sci*. 2002;37:178–187.

2227 Radad K, Moldzio R, Rausch WD. (2011). Ginsenosides and their CNS targets. CNS *Neurosci Ther*. Dec;17(6):761-8.

2228 Nah SY, Kim DH, Rhim H. (2007). Ginsenosides: are any of them candidates for drugs acting on the central nervous system? *CNS Drug Rev*. 2007;13:381–404.

2229 Helms S. (2004). Cancer prevention and therapeutics: Panax ginseng. *Altern Med Rev*. 2004;9:259–274.

2230 Nguyen CT, Luong TT, Lee SY, Kim GL, Kwon H, et al. (2015). Panax ginseng aqueous extract prevents pneumococcal sepsis in vivo by potentiating cell survival and diminishing inflammation. *Phytomedicine*. 2015;22:1055–1061.

2231 Heo JH, Lee ST, Chu K, Oh MJ, Park HJ, et al. (2008). An open-label trial of Korean red ginseng as an adjuvant treatment for cognitive impairment in patients with Alzheimer's disease. *Eur J Neurol*. 2008;15:865–868.

2232 Heo JH, Lee ST, Oh MJ, Park HJ, Shim JY, et al. (2011). Improvement of cognitive deficit in Alzheimer's disease patients by long term treatment with Korean red ginseng. *J Ginseng Res*. 2011;35:457–461.

2233 Lee ST, Chu K, Sim JY, Heo JH, Kim M. (2008). Panax ginseng enhances cognitive performance in Alzheimer disease. *Alzheimer Dis Assoc Disord*. 2008;22:222–226.

2234 Kim JH. (2012). Cardiovascular diseases and Panax ginseng: a review on molecular mechanisms and medical applications. *J Ginseng Res*. 2012;36:16–26.

2235 Hong CE, Lyu SY. (2011). Anti-inflammatory and anti-oxidative effects of Korean Red Ginseng extract in human keratinocytes. *Immune Netw*. 2011;11:42–49.

2236 Huang T, Fang F, Chen L, Zhu Y, Zhang J, et al. (2012). Ginsenoside Rg1 attenuates oligomeric Aβ(1-42)-induced mitochondrial dysfunction. *Curr Alzheimer Res*. 2012;9:388–395.

2237 Shi C, Zheng D, Fang L, Wu F, Kwong WH, et al. (2012). Ginsenoside Rg1 promotes nonamyloidgenic cleavage of APP via estrogen receptor signaling to MAPK/ERK and PI3K/*Akt*. *Biochim Biophys Acta*. 2012;1820:453–460.

2238 Wu J, Yang H, Zhao Q, Zhang X, Lou Y. (2016). Ginsenoside Rg1 exerts a protective effect against Aβ25-35-induced toxicity in primary cultured rat cortical neurons through the NF-κB/NO pathway. *Int J Mol Med*. 2016;37:781–788.

2239 Nah SY, Kim DH, Rhim H. (2007). Ginsenosides: are any of them candidates for drugs acting on the central nervous system? *CNS Drug Rev*. 2007;13:381–404.

2240 Ibid. Helms. (2004).

2241 Ibid. Nguyen. (2015).

2242 Howarth C, Gleeson P, Attwell D. (2012). Updated energy budgets for neural computation in the neocortex and cerebellum. *J Cereb Blood Flow Metab*. Jul; 32(7):1222-32.

2243 Erbsloh F, Bernsmeier A, Hillesheim H. (1958). [The glucose consumption of the brain & its dependence on the liver] Arch Psychiatr Nervenkr Z Gesamte *Neurol Psychiatr*. 1958; 196(6):611-26.

2244 Dienel GA. (2012). Fueling and imaging brain activation. *ASN Neuro*. Jul 20; 4(5):e00093.

2245 Harris JJ, Jolivet R, Attwell D. (2012). Synaptic energy use and supply. *Neuron*. Sep 6; 75(5):762-77.

2246 Hertz L, Gibbs ME. (2009). What learning in day-old chickens can teach a neurochemist: focus on astrocyte metabolism. *J Neurochem*. May; 109 Suppl 1():10-6.

[2247] Suzuki A, Stern SA, Bozdagi O, Huntley GW, Walker RH, et al. (2011). Astrocyte-neuron lactate transport is required for long-term memory formation. *Cell.* Mar 4; 144(5):810-23.

[2248] Lubos E, Loscalzo J, Handy DE. (2011). Glutathione peroxidase-1 in health and disease: from molecular mechanisms to therapeutic opportunitites. *Antioxid Redox Signal.* Oct 1;15(7):1957-97.

[2249] Dringen R, Gutterer JM, Hirrlinger J (2000). Glutathione metabolism in brain metabolic interaction between astrocytes and neurons in the defense against reactive oxygen species. *Eur J Biochem.* Aug;267:4912-6.

[2250] Liu R, Choi J. (2000). Age-associated decline in gamma-glutamylcysteine synthetase gene expression in rats *Free Radic Biol Med.* Feb 15;28(4):566-574.

[2251] Mazzetti AP, Fiorile MC, Primavera A, Lo Bello M. (2015). Glutathione transferases and neurodegenerative diseases. *Neurochem Int.* Mar;82:10-8.

[2252] Saharan S, Mandal PK. (2014). The emerging role of glutathione in Alzheimer's disease. *J Alzheimers Dis.* 2014;40(3):519-29.

[2253] Ibid. Liu. (2000).

[2254] Rinaldi P, Polidori MC, Metastasio A, Mariani E, Mattioli P, et al. (2003). Plasma antioxidants are similarly depleted in mild cognitive impairment and in Alzheimer's disease. *Neurobiol Aging.* Nov;24(7):915-9.

[2255] Shukla D, Mandal PK, Ersland L, Gruner ER, Tripathi M, et al. (2018). Multi-Center Study on Human Brain Glutathione Conformation using Magnetic Resonance Spectroscopy. *J Alzheimers Dis.* 2018;66(2):517-532.

[2256] Ibid. Dringen. (2000).

[2257] Pocernich CB, Butterfield DA. (2012). Elevation of glutathione as a therapeutic strategy in Alzheimer disease. *Biochim Biophys Acta.* May;1822(5):525-30.

[2258] Chiang GC, Mao X, Kang G, Chang E, Pandya S, et al. (2017). Relationships among Cortical Glutathione Levels, Brain Amyloidosis, and Memory in Healthy Older Adults Investigated In Vivo with 1H-MRS and Pittsburgh Compound-B PET. *AJNR Am J Neuroradiol.* Jun;38(6):1130-1137.

[2259] Calabrese V, Sultana R, Scapagnini G, Guagliano E, Sapienza M, et al. (2006). Nitrosative stress, cellular stress response, and thiol home-ostasis in patients with Alzheimer's disease. *Antioxid Redox Signal.* Nov-Dec; 8(11-12):1975-86.

[2260] Lloret A, Badía MC, Mora NJ, Pallardó FV, Alonso MD, et al. (2009). Vitamin E paradox in Alzheimer's disease: it does not prevent loss of cognition and may even be detrimental. *J Alzheimers Dis.* 2009;17(1):143-9.

[2261] Lu SC. (2013). Glutathione synthesis. *Biochim Biophys Acta.* May;1830(5):3143–3153.

[2262] Xing X, Liu F, Xiao J, So KF. (2016). Neuro-protective Mechanisms of Lycium barbarum. *Neuromolecular Med.* Sep;18(3):253-63.

[2263] Cheng J, Zhou ZW, Sheng HP, He LJ, Fan XW, et al. (2014). An evidence-based update on the pharmacological activities as possible molecular targets of Lycium barbarum polysaccharides. *Drug Des Devl Ther.* Dec 17;9:33-78.

[2264] Long YC, Tan TM, Takao I, Tang BL. (2014). The biochemistry and cell biology of aging: metabolic regulation through mitochondrial signaling. *Am J Physiol Endocrinol Metab.* Mar;306(6):E581-91.

[2265] Dai DF, Chiao YA, Marcinek DJ, Szeto HH, Rabinovitch PS. (2014). Mitochondrial oxidative stress in aging and healthspan. *Longev Healthspan.* 2014; 3():6.

[2266] Amro MS, Teoh SL, Norzana AG, Srijit D. (2018). The potential role of herbal products in the treatment of Parkinson's disease. *Clin Ter.* Jan-Feb;169(1):e23-e33.

[2267] Ibid. Cheng. (2014). *Drug Des Devl Ther.*

[2268] Yu MS, Leung SK, Lai SW, Che CM, Zee SY, et al. (2005). Neuroprotective effects of anti-aging oriental medicine Lycium barbarum against beta-amyloid peptide neurotoxicity. *Exp Gerontol.* 2005;40:716–27.

[2269] Ibid. Cheng. (2014).

[2270] Amagase H, Nance DM. (2008). A randomized, double-blind, placebo-controlled, clinical study of the general effects of a standardized Lycium barbarum (Goji) Juice, GoChi. *Altern Complement Med.* May;14(4):403-12.

[2271] Bucheli P, Vidal K, Shen L, Gu Z, Zhang C, et al. (2011). Goji Berry Effects on Macular Characteristics and Plasma Antioxidant Levels. *Optom Vis Sci.* Feb;88(2):257-62.

[2272] Yu MS, Lai CS, Ho YS, Zee SY, So KF, et al. (2007). Characterization of the effects of anti-aging medicine Fructus lycii on beta-amyloid peptide neurotoxicity. *Int J Mol Med.* 2007;20:261–8.

[2273] Balu M, Sangeetha P, Murali G, Panneerselvam C. (2005). Age-related oxidative protein damages in central nervous system of rats: modulatory role of grape seed extract. *Int J Dev Neurosci.* Oct;23(6):501-7.

[2274] Zhen J, Qu Z, Fang H, Fu L, Wu Y, et al. (2014). Effects of grape seed proanthocyanidin extract on pentylenetetrazole-induced kindling and associated cognitive impairment in rats. *Int J Mol Med.* Aug;34(2):391-398.

[2275] Hwang IK, Yoo KY, Kim DS, Jeong YK, Kim JD, et al. (2004). Neuroprotective effects of grape seed extract on neuronal injury by inhibiting

DNA damage in the gerbil hippocampus after transient forebrain ischemia. *Life Sci.* Sep 3;75(16):1989-2001.

[2276] Solanki I, Parihar P, Mansuri ML, Parihar MS. (2015). Flavonoid-based therapies in the early management of neurodegenerative diseases. *Adv Nutr.* Jan; 6(1): 64–72.

[2277] Liu Y, Lukala TL, Musgrave IF, Williams DM, Dehle FC, et al. (2013). Gallic acid is the major component of grape seed extract that inhibits amyloid fibril formation. *Bioor Med Chem Lett.* Dec 1;23(23):6336-40.

[2278] Ono K, Condron MM, Ho L, Wang J, Zhao W, et al. (2008). Effects of grape seed-derived polyphenols on amyloid beta protein self-assembly and cytoxicity. *J Biol Chem.* Nov 21;283(47):32176-87.

[2279] Asha Devi S, Sagar Chandrasekar BK, Manjula KR, Ishii N. (2011). Grape seed proanthocyandin lowers brain oxidative stress in adult and middle-aged rats. *Exp Gerontol.* Nov;46(11):958-64.

[2280] Wang J, Ho L, Zhao W, Ono K, Rosensweig C, et al. (2008). Grape-derived polyphenolics prevent Abeta oligomerization and attenuate cognitive deterioration in a mouse model of Alzheimer's disease. *J Neurosci.* Jun 18;28(25):6388-92.

[2281] Ibid. Ono. (2008).

[2282] Sarkaki A, Rafiereirad M, Hossini SE, Farbood Y, Motamedi F, et al. (2013). Improvement in Memory and Brain Long-term Potentiation Deficits Due to Permanent Hypoperfusion/Ischemia by Grape Seed Extract in Rats. *Iran J Basic Med Sci.* 2013 Sep;16(9):1004-10.

[2283] Wang JY, Thomas P, Zhong JH, Bi FF, Kosaraju S, et al. (2009). Consumption of grape seed extract prevents amyloid-beta deposition and attenuates inflammation in brain of an Alzheimer's disease mouse. *Neurotox Res.* Jan;15(1):3-14.

[2284] Kang JH, Ascherio a, Grodstein F. (2005). Fruit and vegetable consumption and cognitive decline in aging women. *Ann Neurol.* May;57(5):713–720.

[2285] Morris MC, Evans DA, Tangney CC, Bienias JL, Wilson RS. (2006). Associations of vegetable and fruit consumption with age-related cognitive change. *Neurology.* 2006 Oct 24;67(8):1370–1376.

[2286] Morris MC, Wang Y, Barnes LL, Bennett DA, Dawson-Hughes B, et al. (2018). Nutrients and bioactives in green leafy vegetables and cognitive decline. *Neurology.* Jan 15;90(3):e214-e222.

[2287] Wu L, Sun D, Tan Y. (2017). Intake of Fruit and Vegetables and the Incident Risk of Cognitive Disorders: A Systematic Review and Meta-Analysis of Cohort Studies. *J Nutr Health Aging.* 2017;21(10):1284-1290.

[2288] Farooqui AA, Farooqui T, Madan A, Ong JH, Ong WY. (2018). Ayurvedic Medicine for the Treatment of Dementia: Mechanistic Aspects. *Evid Based Complement Alternat Med.* May 15;2018:2481076.

[2289] Ojha S, Bhatia J, Arora S, Golechha M, Kumari S, et al. (2011). Cardioprotective effects of Commiphora mukul against isoprenaline-induced cardiotoxicity: a biochemical and histopathological evaluation. *J Environ Biol.* Nov;32(6):731-8.

[2290] Chen Z, Huang C, Ding W. (2016). Z-Guggulsterone Improves the Scopolamine-Induced Memory Impairments Through Enhancement of the BDNF Signal in C57BL/6J Mice. *Neurochem Res.* Dec;41(12):3322-3332.

[2291] Liu FG, Hu WF, Wang JL, Wang P, Gong Y, et al. (2017). Z-Guggulsterone Produces Antidepressant-Like Effects in Mice through Activation of the BDNF Signaling Pathway. *Int J Neuropsychopharmacol.* Jun 1;20(6):485-497.

[2292] Saxena G, Singh SP, Pal R, Singh S, Pratap R, et al. (2007). Gugulipid, an extract of Commiphora whighitii with lipid-lowering properties, has protective effects against streptozotocin-induced memory deficits in mice. *Pharmacol Biochem Behav.* Apr;86(4):797-805.

[2293] Ibid. Chen. (2016).

[2294] Ibid. Saxena. (2007).

[2295] Nones J, E Spohr TC, Gomes FC. (2011). Hesperidin, a flavone glycoside, as mediator of neuronal survival. *Neurochem Res.* Oct; 36(10):1776-84.

[2296] Nones J, Spohr TC, Gomes FC. (2012). Effects of the flavonoid hesperidin in cerebral cortical progenitors in vitro: indirect action through astrocytes. *Int J Dev Neurosci.* Jun; 30(4):303-13.

[2297] Thenmozhi JA, Raja WTR, Manivasagam T, Janakiraman U, Essa MM. (2017). Hesperidin ameliorates cognitive dysfunction, oxidative stress, and apoptosis against aluminum chloride induced rat model of Alzheimer's disease. *Nutr Neurosci.* Jul;20(6):360-366.

[2298] Chakraborty S, Bandyopadhyay J, Chakraborty S, Basu S. (2016). Multi-target screening mines hesperidin as a multi-potent inhibitor: Implication in Alzheimer's disease therapeutics. *Eur J Med Chem.* Oct 4;121:810-822.

[2299] Howes MJ, Perry E. (2011). The role of phytochemicals in the treatment and prevention of dementia. *Drugs Aging.* Jun 1; 28(6):439-68.

[2300] Perlmutter, D. (2013). *Grain brain.* New York: Little, Brown and Company.

[2301] Li J, Wu HM, Zhou RL, Liu GJ, Dong BR. (2008). Huperzine A for Alzheimer's disease. Cochrane Database *Syst Rev.* 2008 Apr 16;(2):CD005592.

[2302] Desilets AR, Gickas JJ, Dunican KC. (2009). Role of huperzine a in the treatment of Alzheimer's disease. *Ann Pharmacother.* Mar;43(3):514-8.

2303 Bauer BA. Huperzine A: Can it treat Alzheimer's? Retrieved Oct 15 2019 from https://www.mayoclinic.org/diseases-conditions/alzheimers-disease/expert-answers/huperzine-a/faq-20058259

2304 Munoz P, Humeres A. (2012). Iron deficiency on neuronal function. *Biometals.* Aug;25(4):825-35.

2305 More MI, Freitas U, Rutenberg D. (2014). Positive effects of soy lecithin-derived phosphatidylserine plus phosphatidic acid on memory, cognitions, daily functioning, and mood in elderly patients with Alzheimer's disease and dementia. *Adv Ther.* Dec;31(12):1247-62.

2306 Jung HA, Karki S, Kim JH, Choi JS. (2015). BACE1 and cholinesterase inhibitory activities of Nelumbo nucifera embryos. *Arch Pharm Res.* Jun;38(6):1178-87.

2307 Motoi Y, Shimada K, Ishiguro K, Hattori N. (2014). Lithium and autophagy. *ACS Chem Neurosci. 2014 Jun 18;5(6):434-42.*

2308 Sofola O, Kerr F, Rogers I, Killick R, Augustin H, et al. (2010). Inhibition of GSK-3 ameliorates Abeta pathology in an adult onset Drosophila model of Alzheimer's disease. *PLoS Genet. 2010 Sep;6(9):e1001087.*

2309 Cohen P, Goedert M. (2004). GSK3 inhibitors: development and therapeutic potential. *Nat Rev Drug Discov.* Jun;3(6):479-87.

2310 Nunes MA, Schowe NM, Monteiro-Silva KC, Baraldi-Tomisielo T, Sousa SI, et al. (2015). Chronic Microdose Lithium Treatment Prevented Memory Loss and Neurohistopathological Changes in a Transgenic Mouse Model of Alzheimer's Disease. *PLoS One.* 2015;10(11):e0142267.

2311 Yang WM, Shim KJ, Choi MJ, Park SY, Choi BJ, et al. (2008). Novel effects of Nelumbo nucifera rhizome extract on memory and neurogenesis in the dentate gyrus of the rat hippocampus. *Neurosci Lett.* Oct 3;443(2):104-7.

2312 Kumaran A, Ho CC, Hwang LS. (2018). Protective effect of Nelumbo nucifera extracts on beta amyloid protein induced apoptosis in PC12 cells, in vitro model of Alzheimer's disease. *J Food Drug Anal.* Jan;26(1):172-181.

2313 Wong VK, Wu AG, Wang JR, Liu L, Law BY. (2015). Neferine attenuates the protein level and toxicity of mutant huntingtin in PC-12 cells via induction of autophagy. *Molecules.* Feb 18;20(3):3496-514.

2314 Widomska J, Subczynski WK. (2014). Why has Nature Chosen Lutein and Zeaxanthin to Protect the Retina? *J Clin Exp Ophthalmol.* Feb 21; 5(1):326.

2315 Johnson EJ, Vishwanathan R, Johnson MA, Hausman DB, Davey A, et al. (2013). Relationship between Serum and Brain Carotenoids, α-Tocopherol, and Retinol Concentrations and Cognitive Performance in the Oldest Old from the Georgia Centenarian Study. *J Aging Res.* 2013():951786.

2316 Vishwanathan R, Iannaccone A, Scott TM, Kritchevsky SB, Jennings BJ, et al. (2014). Macular pigment optical density is related to cognitive function in older people. *Age Ageing.* Mar; 43(2):271-5.

2317 Johnson EJ. (2014). Role of lutein and zeaxanthin in visual and cognitive function throughout the lifespan. *Nutr Rev.* Sep; 72(9):605-12.

2318 Ibid. Johnson. (2013).

2319 Ibid. Vishwanathan. (2014).

2320 Feeney J, Finucane C, Savva GM, Cronin H, Beatty S, et al. (2013). Low macular pigment optical density is associated with lower cognitive performance in a large, population-based sample of older adults. *Neurobiol Aging.* 2013 Nov; 34(11):2449-56.

2321 Renzi LM, Dengler MJ, Puente A, Miller LS, Hammond BR Jr. (2014). Relationships between macular pigment optical density and cognitive function in unimpaired and mildly cognitively impaired older adults *Neurobiol Aging.* Jul; 35(7):1695-9.

2322 Ibid. Vishwanathan. (2014).

2323 Ibid. Feeney. (2013).

2324 Ibid. Renzi. (2014).

2325 Renzi LM, Hammond BR Jr. (2010). The relation between the macular carotenoids, lutein and zeaxanthin, and temporal vision. *Ophthalmic Physiol Opt.* Jul; 30(4):351-7.

2326 Bovier ER, Renzi LM, Hammond BR. (2014). A double-blind, placebo-controlled study on the effects of lutein and zeaxanthin on neural processing speed and efficiency. *PLoS One.* 2014;9(9):e108178.

2327 Edman JW, Smith JW, Kuchan MJ, Mohn ES, Johnson EJ, et al. (2015). Lutein and Brain Function. *Foods.* Dec;4(4):547-564.

2328 Ibid. Vishwanathan. (2014).

2329 Johnson EJ, McDonald K, Caldarella SM, Chung HY, Troen AM, et al. (2008). Cognitive findings of an exploratory trial of docosahexaenoic acid and lutein supplementation in older women. *Nutr Neurosci.* Apr; 11(2):75-83.

2330 Johnson EJ. (2012). A possible role for zeaxanthin in cognitive function in the elderly. *Am J Clin Nutr.* Nov;96(5):1160S-5S.

2331 Min JY, Min KB. (2014). Serum lycopene, lutein and zeaxanthin, and the risk of Alzheimer's disease mortality in older adults. *Dement Geriatr Cogn Disord.* 2014;37(3-4).

2332 Nolan JM, Loskutova E, Howard A, Mulcahy R, Moran R, et al. (2015). The impact of supplemental macular carotenoids in Alzheimer's disease: a randomized clinical trial. *J Alzheimers Dis.* 2015;44(4):1157-69.

[2333] Chew EY, Clemons TE, Agron E, Launer LJ, Grodstein F, et al. (2015). Effect of Omega-3 Fatty Acids, Lutein/Zeaxanthin, or other Nutrient Supplementation on Cognitive Function: The AREDS2 Randomized Clinical Trial. *JAMA*. Aug 25;314(8):781-801.

[2334] Widomska J, Zareba M, Subczynski WK. (2016). Can Xanthophyll-Membrane Interactions Explain Their Selective Presence in the Retina and Brain? *Foods*. Jan 12;5(1):E7.

[2335] Gruszecki WI. Carotenoid orientation: Role in membrane stabilization. In: Krinsky N.I., Mayne S.T., Sies H., editors. *Carotenoids in Health and Disease*. Marcel Dekker, Inc.; New York, NY, USA: 2004. pp. 151–164

[2336] Ibid. Gruszecki. (2004).

[2337] Stahl W, Sies H. (2001). Effects of carotenoids and retinoids on gap junctional communication. *Biofactors*. 2001; 15(2-4):95-8.

[2338] Xiong J, Wang K, Yuan C, Xing R, Ni J, et al. (2017). Luteolin protects mice from severe acute pancreatitis by exerting HO-1-mediated anti-inflammatory and antioxidant effects. *Int J Mol Med*. Jan;39(1):113-125.

[2339] Yang SC, Chen PJ, Chang SH, Weng YT, Chang FR, et al. (2018). Luteolin attenuates neutrophilic oxidative stress and inflammatory arthritis by inhibiting Raf1 activity. *Biochem Pharmacol*. Aug;154:384-396.

[2340] Zhou WB, Miao ZN, Zhang B, Long W, Zheng FX, et al. (2019). Luteolin induces hippocampal neurogenesis in the Ts65Dn mouse model of Down syndrome. *Neural Regen Res*. Apr;14(4):613-620.

[2341] Jang RN, Johnson RW. (2010). Luteolin inhibits microglia and alters hippocampal-dependent spatial working memory in aged mice. *J Nutr*. Oct;140(10):1892-1898.

[2342] Crupi R, Paterniti, Ahmad A, Campolo M, Esposito E, et al. (2013). Effects of palmitoylethanolamide and luteolin in an animal model of anxiety/depression. *CNS Neurol Dis Drug Targets*. Nov;12(7):989-1001.

[2343] Xu SL, Bi CWC, Choi RCY, Zhu KY, Miernisha A, et al. (2013). Flavonoids induce the synthesis and secretion of neurotrophic factors in cultured rat astrocytes: A signaling response mediated by estrogen receptor. *Evid Based Complement Alternat Med*. 2013;127075.

[2344] Jang S, Kelley KW, Johnson RW. (2008). Luteolin reduces IL-6 production in microglia by inhibiting JNK phosphorylation and activation of AP-1. *Proc Natl Acad Sci U S A*. May 27; 105(21):7534-9.

[2345] Zhu LH, Bi W, Qi RB, Wang HD, Lu DX. (2011). Luteolin inhibits microglial inflammation and improves neuron survival against inflammation. *Int J Neurosci*. Jun; 121(6):329-36.

[2346] Chen HQ, Jin ZY, Wang XJ, Xu XM, Deng L, et al. (2008). Luteolin protects dopaminergic neurons from inflammation-induced injury through inhibition of microglial activation. *Neurosci Lett*. Dec 26; 448(2):175-9.

[2347] Dirscherl K, Karlstetter M, Ebert S, Kraus D, Hlawatsch J, et al. (2010). Luteolin triggers global changes in the microglial transcriptome leading to a unique anti-inflammatory and neuroprotective phenotype. *J Neuroinflammation*. Jan 14; 7:3.

[2348] Kao TK, Ou YC, Lin SY, Pan HC, Song PJ, et al. (2011). Luteolin inhibits cytokine expression in endotoxin/cytokine-stimulated microglia. *J Nutr Biochem*. Jul; 22(7):612-24.

[2349] Theoharides TC, Stewart JM, Hatziagelaki E, Kolaitis G. (2015). Brain "fog," inflammation and obesity: key aspects of neuropsychiatric disorders improved by luteolin. *Front Neurosci*. Jul; 9:225.

[2350] Ibid. Di Mascio. (1989). *Arch Biochem Biophys*.

[2351] Seo EJ, Fischer N, Efferth T. (2018) Phytochemicals as inhibitors of NF-kB for treatment of Alzheimer's disease. *Pharmacol Res*. Mar;129:262-273.

[2352] Ibid. Wang. (2018). *J Nutr Biochem*.

[2353] Liu CB, Wang R, Yi YF, Gao Z, Chen YZ. (2018). Lycopene mitigates B-amyloid induced inflammatory response and inhibits NF-kB signaling at the choroid plexus in early stages of Alzheimer's disease rats. *J Nutr Biochem*. Mar;53-66-71.

[2354] Sachdeva AK, Chopra K. (2015). Lycopene abrogates AB(1-42)-mediated neuroinflammatory cascade in an experimental model of Alzheimer's disease. *J Nutr Biochem*. Jul;26(7):736-44.

[2355] Ibid. Wang. (2019). *Int J Obes* (Lond).

[2356] Ibid. Chen. (2019). *Biomed Pharmacother*.

[2357] Serefko A, Szopa A, Wlaz P, Nowak G, Radziwon-Zaleska M, et al. (2013). Magnesium in depression. *Pharmacol Rep*. 2013;65(3):547-54.

[2358] Kieboom BCT, Licher S, Wolters FJ, Ikram MK, Hoorn, EJ, et al. (2017). Serum magnesium is associated with the risk of dementia. *Neurology*. Oct 17;89(16):1716-1722.

[2359] De Baaji JH, Hoenderop JG, Bindels RF (2015). Magnesium in man: implications for health and disease. *Physiol Rev*. 2015 Jan;95(1):1-46.

[2360] Grober U, Schmidt J, Kisters K. (2015). Magnesium in Prevention and Therapy. *Nutrients*. Sep;7(9):8199-8226.

[2361] Yu X, Guan PP, Guo JW, Wang Y, Cae LL, et al. (2015). By suppressing the expression of anterior pharynx-defective-1alpha and -1beta and inhibiting the aggregation of beta-amyloid protein, magnesium ions inhibit the cognitive decline of amyloid precursor protein/presenilin 1 transgenic mice. *FASEB J*. 2015;29(12):5044-58.

[2362] Slutsky I, Abumaria N, Wu LJ, Huang C, Zhang L, et al. (2010). Enhancement of learning and memory by elevating brain magnesium. *Neuron*. 2010;65(2):165-77.

[2363] Ibid. Yu. (2015).

[2364] Jin X, Liu MY, Zhang DF, Gao H. Wei MJ. (2018). Elevated circulating magnesium levels in patients with Parkinson's disease: a meta-analysis. *Neuropsychiatr Dis Treat*. Nov 19;14:3159-3168.

[2365] Grober U, Schmidt J, Kisters K. (2015). Magnesium in Prevention and Therapy. *Nutrients*. Sep;7(9):8199-8226.

[2366] Pandi-Perumal SR, BaHammam AS, Brown GM, Spence GM, Sharti VK, et al. (2013). Melatonin antioxidant defense: therapeutical ipications for aging and neurodegenerative processes. *Neurotox Res*. Apr;23(3):267-300.

[2367] Reiter JR. (1995). Oxygen radical detoxification processes during aging: the functional importance of melatonin. *Aging* (Milano). Oct1995;7(5):340-51.

[2368] Swiderska-Kolacz G, Klusek J, Kolataj A. (2006). The effect of melatonin on glutathione and glutathione transferase and glutathione peroxidase activities in the mouse liver and kidney in vivo. *Neuro Endocrinol Lett*. Jun;27(3):365-8.

[2369] Reiter RJ, Paredes SD, Korkmaz A, Jou MJ, Tan DX. (2008). Melatonin combats molecular terrorism at the mitochondrial level. *Interdiscip Toxicol*. Sep;1(2):137-49.

[2370] Chitsazi M, Faramarzie M, Sadighi M, Shirmohammadi A, Hashemzadeh A. (2017). Effects of adjective use of melatonin and vitamin C in the treatment of chronic periodontis: A randomized clinical trial. *J Dent Res Dent Clin Dent Prospects*. Autum;11(4):236-240.

[2371] Karaoz E, Gultekin F, Akdogan M, Oncu M, Gokcimen A. (2002). Protective role of melatonin and a combination of vitamin C and vitamin E on lung toxicity induced by chlorpyrifos-ethyl in rats. *Exp Toxicol Pathol*. Aug;54(2):97-108.

[2372] Rohr UD, Herold J. (2002). Melatonin deficiencies in women. *Maturitas*. 2002 Apr 15;41 Suppl 1:S85-104.

[2373] Mishima , Okawa M, Hozumi S, Hikikawa Y. (2000). Supplementary administration of artificial bright light and melatonin as potent treatment for disorganized circadin rhythm activity and dysfunctional autonomic and neuroendocrine systems in institutionalized demented elderly persons. *Chronobiol Int*. May;17(3):419-32.

[2374] Wang YY, Zheng W, Ng CH, Ungvari GS, Wei W, et al. (2017). Meta-analysis of randomized, double-blind, placebo-controlled trials of melatonin in Alzheimer's disease. *Int J Geriatr Psychiatry*. Jan;32(1):50-57.

[2375] Ibid. Pandi-Perumal. (2013).

[2376] Gupta YK, Gupta M, Kohli K. (2003). Neuroprotective role of melatonin in oxidative stress vulnerable brain. *Indian J Physiol Pharmacol*. Oct;47(4):373-86.

[2377] Bondy SC, Lahiri DK, Perreau VM, Sharman KZ, Campbell A, et al. (2004). Retardation of brain aging by chronic treatment with melatonin. *Ann N Y Acad Sci*. Dec;1035:197-215.

[2378] Ramirez-Rodriquez G, Vega-Rivera NM, Benetez-King G, Castro-Garcia M, Ortiz-Lopez L. (2012). Melatonin supplementation delays the decline if adult hippocampal neurogenesis during normal aging of mice. *Neurosci Lett*. Nov 14;530(1):53-8

[2379] Chern CM, Liao JF, Wang YH, Shen YC. (2012). Melatonin ameliorates through the MT2 melatonin receptor in ischemic -stroke mice. *Free Rad Biol Medi*. May 1;52(9):1634-47.

[2380] Sarlak G, Jenwitheesuk A, Chetsawang N, Govitrapong P. (2013). Effects of melatonin on nervous system aging: Neurogenesis and neurodegeneration. *J Pharm Sci*. Sep 20;123(1):9-24.

[2381] Ramirez-Rodriquez G, Klempin F, Babu H, Benitez-King G, Kempermann G. (2009). Melatonin modulates cell survival of new neurons in the hippocampus of adult mice. *Neuropsychopharmacology*. Aug;34(9):2180-91.

[2382] Lahiri DK, Chen DM, Lahiri P, Bondy S, Greig NH. (2005). Amyloid, cholinesterase, melatonin, and metals and their roles in aging and neurodegenerative diseases. *Ann N Y Acad Sci*. Nov;1056:430-49.

[2383] Lahiri DK, Chen D, Lahiri P, Rogers JT, Greig NH, Bondy S. (2004). Melatonin, metals, and gene expression: implications in aging and neurodegenerative disorders. *Ann N Y Acad Sci*. Dec;1035:216-30.

[2384] Fernandez-Tresquerres Hernandez JA. (2008). [Melatonina: old molecule, new medicament]. [Article in Spanish] *An R Acad Nac Med* (Madr). 2008;125(4):681-96.

[2385] West KE, Jablonski MR, Warfield B, Cecil KS, James M, et al. (2011). Blue light from light-emitting diodes elicits a dose-dependent suppression of melatonin in humans. *J Appl Physiol*. Mar;110(3):619-26.

[2386] Obulesu M, Rao DM. (2011). Effect of plant extracts on Alzheimer's disease: an insight into therapeutic avenues. *J Neurosci Rural Pract*. Jan;2(1):56-61.

[2387] Pakade V, Cukrowska E, Lindahl S, Turner , Chimuka L. (2013). Molecular imprinted polymer for solid-phase extraction of flavonols aglycones from Moringa oleifera extracts. *J Sep Sci*. Feb;36(3):548-55.

[2388] Zeng K, Li Y, Yang W, Ge Y, Xu L, Ren T, et al. (2019). Moringa oleifera seed extract protects against brain damage in both the acute and delayed stages of ischemic stroke. *Exp Gerontol*. Jul 15;122:99-108.

[2389] Sutalangka C, Wattanathorn J, Muchimapura S, Thukham-mee W. Moringa oleifera mitigates memory impairment and neurodegeneration in animal model of age-related dementia. *Oxid Med Cell Longev.* 2013;695936.

[2390] Omotoso GO, Gbadamosi IT, Afolabi TT, Abdulwahab AB, Akinlolu AA. (2018). Ameliorative effects of Moringa on cuprizone-induced memory decline in rat model of multiple sclerosis. *Anat Cell Biol.* Jun;51(2):119-127.

[2391] Ganguly R, Guha D. (2008). Alteration of brain monoamines and EEG wave pattern in rat model of Alzheimer's disease & protection by Moringa oleifera.

[2392] Mahaman YAR, Huang F, Wu M, Wang Y, Wiz Z, et al. (2018). Moringa Oleifera Alleviates Homocystein-Induced Alzheimer's Disease-Like Pathology and Cognitive Impairments. *J Alzheimers Dis.* 2018;63(3):1141-1159.

[2393] Giacoppo S, Rajan TS, De Nicola GR, Lori R, Rollin P, et al. (2017). The isothiocyanate isolated from Moringa oleifera shows potential anti-inflammatory activity: the Treatment of Murine Subacute Parkinson's Disease. *Rejuvenation Res.* Feb;20(1):50-63.

[2394] Kim HG, Oh MS. (2012). Memory enhancing effect of Mori Fructus via induction of nerve growth factor. *Brit J Nutr.* Jul 14;110(1):86-94.

[2395] Kim AJ, Park S. (2006). Mulberry extract supplements ameliorate the inflammation-related hematological parameters in carrageenan-induced arthritic rats. *J Med Food.* Fall;9(3):431-5.

[2396] Kim HG, Ju MS, Shim JS, Kim MC, Lee SH, et al. (2010). Mulberry fruit protects dopaminergic neurons in toxin-induced Parkinson's disease models. *Brit J Nutr.* Jul;104(1):8-16.

[2397] Shin WH, Park SJ, Kim EJ. (2006). Protective effect of anthocyanins in middle cerebral artery occlusion and reperfusion model of cerebral ischemia in rats. *Life Sci.* 79(2):130–137.

[2398] Kim HG, Ju MS, Park H, Seo Y, Jang YP, et al. (2010). Evaluation of Samjunghwan, a traditional medicine, for neuroprotection against damage by amyloid-beta in rat cortical neurons. *J Ethnopharmacol.* Aug 9;130(3):625-30.

[2399] Kuk EB, Jo AR, Oh SI, Sohn HS, Seong SH, et al. (2017). Anti-Alzheimer's disease activity of compounds from the root bark of Morus alba L. *Arch Pharm Res.* Mar;40(3):338-349.

[2400] Xia CL, Tang GH, Guo YQ, Xu YK, Huang ZS, et al. (2019). Mulberry Diels-Alder-type adducts from Morus alba as multi-targeted agents for Alzheimer's disease. *Phytochemistry.* Jan;157:82-91.

[2401] Manzi P, Gambelli L, Marconi S, Vivanti V, Pizzoferrato L. (1999). Nutrients in edible mushrooms: an inter-species comparative study. *Food Chem.* Jun;65(4):477-482.

[2402] Ferreira IC, Barros L, Abreu RM. (2009). Antioxidants in wild mushrooms. *Curr Med Chem.* 2009;16(12):1543-60.

[2403] Abdullah N, Ismail SM, Aminudin N, Shuib AS, Lau BF. (2012) Evaluation of Selected Culinary-Medicinal Mushrooms for Antioxidant and ACE Inhibitory Activities. *Evid Based Complement Alternat Med.* 2012:464238.

[2404] Sabaratnam V, Kah-Hui W, Naidu M, Rosie David P. (2013). Neuronal health – can culinary and medicinal mushrooms help? *J Tradit Complement Med.* Jan;3(1):62-8.

[2405] Elk LF, Naidu M, David P, Wong KH, Tan YS, et al. (2012). Lignosus rhinoceros (Cooke) Ryvarden: A Medicinal Mushroom That Stimulates Neurite Outgrowth in PC-12 Cells. *Evid Based Complement Alternat Med.* 2012:320308.

[2406] John PA, Wong KH, Naidu M, Sabaratnam V, David M. (2013). Combination effects of curcumin and aqueous extract of Lignosus rhinocerotis mycelium on neurite outgrowth stimulation activity in PC-12 cells. *Nat Prod Commun* 8:711–714

[2407] Seow SLS, Eik LF, Naidu M, David P, Wong KH, et al. (2015). Lignosus rhinocerotis (Cooke) Ryvarden mimics the neuritogenic activity of nerve growth factor via MEK/ERK1/2 signaling pathway in PC-12 cells. *Sci Rep.* Nov;5:15349.

[2408] Phan CW, Wong WL, David P, Naidu M, Sabaratnam V. (2012). Pleurotus giganteus (Berk). Karunrathna & K.D. Hyde: Nutritional value and in vitro neurite outgrowth activity in rat pheochromocytoma cells. *BMC Complement Altern Med.* Jul 19;12:102.

[2409] Lee B, Park J, Park J, Shin HJ, Kwon S, et al. (2011). Cordyceps Militaris improves neurite outgrowth in Neuro2A cells and reverses memory impairment in rats. *Food Sci Biotech.* Dec;20(6):1599-1608.

[2410] Gunawardena D, Shanmugam K, Low M, Bennett L, Govindaraghavan S, et al. (2014). Determination of anti-inflammatory activities of standardized preparations of plant- and mushroom-based foods. *Eur J Nutr.* Feb;53(1):335-43.

[2411] Lu MK, Cheng JJ, Lai WL, Lin YJ, Huang NK (2008). Fermented Antrodia cinnamomea extract protects rat PC12 cells from serum deprivation-induced apoptosis: the role of the MAPK family. *J Agric Food Chem.* 2008 Feb 13; 56(3):865-74.

[2412] Shi Y, Yang S, Lee DY, Lee C. (2016). Increasing anti-AB-induced neurotoxicity ability of Antrodia camphorate-fermented produce with deep ocean water supplementary. *J Sci Food Agric.* Nov;96(14):4690-4701.

[2413] Chang WH, Chen MC, Cheng IH. (2015). Antroquinonol Lowers Brain Amyloid-B Levels and Improves Spatial Learning and Memory in a Transgenic Mouse Model of Alzheimer's Disease. *Sci Rep.* Oct 15;5:15067.

[2414] Wang LC, Wang SE, Wang JJ, Tsai TY, Lin CH, et al. (2012). In vitro and in vivo comparisons of the effects of the fruiting body and mycelium of Antrodia camphorate against amyloid B-protein-induced neurotoxicity and memory impairment. *App Microbiol Biotechnol.* Jun;94(6):1505-19.

2415 Han C, Guo L, Yang Y, Li W, Sheng Y, et al. (2019). Study on antrodia camphorate polysaccharide in alleviating the neuroethology of PD mice by decreasing the expression of NLRP3 inflammasome. *Phytother Res.* Sep;33(9):2288-2297.

2416 Sabaratnam V, Kah-Hui W, Naidu M, David PR. (2013). Neuronal Health – Can Culinary and Medicinal Mushrooms Help? *J Tradit Complement Med.* Jan-Mar; 3(1): 62–68.

2417 Phan CW, David P, Naidu M, Wong KH, Sabaratnam V. (2015). Therapeutic potential of culinary-medicinal mushrooms for the management of neurodegenerative diseases: diversity, metabolite, and mechanism. *Crit Rev Biotechnol.* 2015;35(3):355-68.

2418 Seow SLS, Naidu M, David P, Wong KH, Sabaratnam V. (2013). Potentiation of neuritogenic activity of medinal mushrooms in rat pheochromocytoma cells. *BCM Complement Altern Med.* Jul 4;13:157.

2419 Vetvica V, Vetvickova J. (2014). Immune-enhancing effects of Maitake (Grifola frondosa) and Shiitake (Lentinula edodes) extracts. *Ann Transl Med.* Feb;2(2):14.

2420 Nagai K, Chiba A, Nishino T, Kubota T, Kawagishi HJ. (2006). Dilinoleoyl-phosphatidylethanolamine from Hericium erinaceum protects against ER stress-dependent Neuro2a cell death via protein kinase C pathway. *Nutr Biochem.* 2006 Aug; 17(8):525-30.

2421 Mori K, Inatomi S, Ouchi K, Azumi Y, Tuchida T. (2009). Improving effects of the mushroom Yamabushitake (Hericium erinaceus) on mild cognitive impairment: a double-blind placebo-controlled clinical trial. *Phytother Res.* 2009 Mar; 23(3):367-72.

2422 Mori K, Obara Y, Hirota M, Azumi Y, Kinugasa S, et al. (2008). Nerve growth factor-inducing activity of Hericium erinaceus in 1321N1 human astrocytoma cells. *Biol Pharm Bull.* 2008 Sep; 31(9):1727-32.

2423 Mori K, Obara Y, Hirota M, Azumi Y, Kinugasa S, et al. (2008). Lion's Mane stimulates nerve growth factors. *Biol Pharm Bull.* Sep; 31(9):1727-32.

2424 Wong K-H, Vikineswary S, Abdullah N, Naidu M, Keynes R. Activity of aqueous extracts of lion's mane mushroom Hericium erinaceus (Bull.: Fr.) Pers. (Aphyllophoromycetideae) on the neural cell line NG108-15. *International Journal of Medicinal Mushrooms.* 2007;9(1):57–65.

2425 Ibid. Mori. (2008).

2426 Li IC, Lee LY, Tzeng TT, Chen WP, Chen YP, et al. (2018). Neurohealth Properties of Hericium erinaceus Mycelia Enriched with Erinacines. *Behav Neurol.* May21;2018:5802634.

2427 Rossi P, Cesaroni V, Brandalise F, Occhinegro A, Ratto D, et al. (2018). Dietary Supplementation of Lion's Mane Medicinal Mushroom Hericium erinaceus (Agaricomycetes), and Spatial Memory in Wild-Type Mice. *Int J Med Mushrooms.* 2018;20(5):485-494.

2428 Lee LY, Li IC, Chen WP, Tsai TY, Chen CC, et al. (2019). Thirteen-Week Oral Toxicity Evaluation of Erinacine A Enriched Lion's Mane Medicinal Mushroom, Hericium erinaceus (Agaricomycetes), Mycelia in Spraque-Dawley Rats. *In J Med Mushrooms.* 2019;21(4):401-411.

2429 Hearst R, Nelson D, McCollum G, Millar BC, Maeda Y, et al. (2009). An examination of antibacterial and antifungal properties of Shiitake (Lentinula edodes) and oyster (Pleurotus ostreatus) mushrooms. *Complement Ther Clin Pract.* Feb; 15(1):5-7.

2430 Lee SS, Chang YS, Noraswati MN. (2009). Utilization of macrofungi by some indigenous communities for food and medicine in Peninsular Malaysia. For *Ecol Manage.* 2009;257:2062–5.

2431 Wong WL, Abdulla MA, Chua KH, Kuppusamy UR, Tan YS, et al. (2012). Hepatoprotective Effects of Panus giganteous (Berk.) Corner against Thioacetamide= (TAA-) Induced Liver Injury in Rats. *Evid Based Complement Alternat Med.* 2012():170303.

2432 Ibid. Phan. (2015).

2433 Phan CW, David P, Wong KH, Naidu M, Sabaratnam V. (2015). Uridine from Pleurotus giganteus and Its Neurite Outgrowth Stimulatory Effects with Underlying Mechanism. *PLoS One.* Nov 13;10(11):e0143004.

2434 Boh B, Berovic M, Zhang J, Zhi-Bin L. (2007). Ganoderma lucidum and its pharmaceutically active components. *Biotechnol Annu Rev.* 2007;13():265-301.

2435 Lee YH, Kim JH, Song CH, Jang KJ, Kim CH, et al. (2016). Ethanol Extract of Ganoderma lucidum Augments Cellular Anti-oxidant Defence through Activation of Nrf2/HO-1. *J Pharmacopuncture.* Mar;19(1):59-69.

2436 Rani P, Lal MR, Maheshwari U, Krishnan S. (2015). Antioxidant Potential of Lingzhi or Reishi Medicinal Mushroom, Ganoderma lucidum (Higher Basidiomycetes) Cultivated on Artocarpus heterophyllus Sawdust Substrate in India. *Int J Med Mushrooms*, 17: 1171-7.

2437 Wang J, Cao B, Zhao H, Feng J. (2017). Emerging Roles of Ganoderma Lucidum in Anti-Aging. *Aging Dis.* Dec 1; 8(6): 691–707.

2438 Lai CS, Yu MS, Yuen WH, So KF, Zee SY, et al. (2008). Antagonizing beta-amyloid peptide neurotoxicity of the anti-aging fungus Ganoderma lucidum. *Brain Res.* Jan 23;1190: 215-24

2439 Phan CW, David P, Naidu M, Wong KH, Sabaratnam V. (2015). Therapeutic potential of culinary-medicinal mushrooms for the management of neurodegenerative diseases: diversity, metabolite, and mechanism. *Crit Rev Biotechnol*, 35: 355-68.

2440 Ibid. Seow. (2013). BCM Complement Altern Med.

2441 Obara Y, Nakahata N, Kita T, Takaya Y, Kobayashi H, et al. (1999). Stimulation of neurotropic factor secretion from 1321N1 human astrocytoma cells by novel diterpenoids, scabronines A and G. *Eur J Pharmacol.* 1999 Apr 1; 370(1):79-84.

2442 Cheung WM, Hui WS, Chu PW, Chiu SW, Ip NY. (2000). Ganoderma extract activates MAP kinases and induces the neuronal differentiation of rat pheochromocytoma PC12 cells. *FEBS Lett.* Dec 15; 486(3):291-6.

2443 Vetvicka V, Vetvickova J. (2014). Immune-enhancing effects of Maitake (Grifola frondosa) and Shiitake (Lentinula edodes) extracts. *Ann Trans Med.* Feb;2(2):14.

2444 Nisar J, Mustafa I, Anwar H, Sohail MU, Hussain G, et al. (2017). Shiitake Culinary-Medicinal Mushroom, Lentinus edodes (Agaricomycetes): A Species with Antioxidants, Immunomodulatory, and Hepatoprotective Activities in Hypercholesterolemic Rats. *Int J Med Mushrooms.* 2017;19(11):981-990.

2445 Tan CS, Ng ST, Vikineswary S, Lo FP, Tee CS. Genetic markers for identification of a Malaysian medicinal mushroom, Lignosus rhinocerus (Cendawan Susu Rimau) *Acta Hortic.* 2010;859:161–8.

2446 John PA, Wong KH, David RP, Naidu M, Sabaratnam V. (2012). Combination effects on Lignosus rhinocerus (Cooke) Ryvarden mycelium and Gingko biloba aqueous extracts on PC-12 cells neurite outgrowth stimulation activity, in National Postgraduate Seminar (Kuala Lumpur:).

2447 Ibid. Mourtas. (2014). *Eur J Med Chem.*

2448 Ibid. Siddique. (2014). *Biomed Res Int.*

2449 Samberkar S, Gandhi S, Naidu M, Wong KH, Raman J, et al. (2015). Lion's Mane, Hericium erinaceus and Tiger Milk, Lignosus rhinocerotis (Higher Basiciomycetes) Medicinal Mushrooms Stimulate Neurite Outgrowth in Dissociated Cells of Brain, Spinal Cord, and Retina: An In Vitro Study. Int J *Med Mushrooms.* 2015; 17(11):1047-54.

2450 Ibid. John. (2012). *Nat Prod Comm.*

2451 Ibid. John. (2013). *Nat Prod Comm.*

2452 Nallathamby N, Phan CW, Seow SLS, Baskaran A, Lakshamanan H, et al. (2018). A Status Review of the Bioactive Activities of Tiger Milk Mushroom Lignosus rhinocerotis (Cooke) Ryvarden. *Front Pharmacol.* Jan 15;8:998.

2453 Sumi H, Hamada H, Tsushima H, Mihara H, Muraki H. (1987). A novel fibrinolytic enzyme (nattokinase) in the vegetable cheese Natto; a typical and popular soybean food in the Japanese diet. *Experientia.* Oct 15; 43(10):1110-1.

2454 Nagata C, Wada K, Tamura T, Konishi K, Goto Y, et al. (2017). Dietary soy and natto intake and cardiovascular disease mortality in Japanese adults: the Takayama study. *Am J Clin Nutr.* Feb; 105(2):426-431.

2455 Dabbagh F, Negahdaripour M, Berenjian A, Behfar A, Mohammadi F, et al. (2014). Nattokinase: production and application. *Appl Microbiol Biotechnol.* Nov; 98(22):9199-206.

2456 Huang Y, Ding S, Liu M, Gao C, Yang J, et al. (2013). Ultra-small and anionic starch nanospheres: formation and vitro thrombolytic behavior study. *Carbohydr Polym.* Jul 25; 96(2):426-34.

2457 Dogné JM, Hanson J, de Leval X, Pratico D, Pace-Asciak CR, et al. (2006). From the design to the clinical application of thromboxane modulators. *Curr Pharm Des.* 2006;12(8):903-23.

2458 Fujita M, Ohnishi K, Takaoka S, Ogasawara K, Fukuyama R, et al. (2011). Antihypertensive effects of continuous oral administration of nattokinase and its fragments in spontaneously hypertensive rats. *Biol Pharm Bull.* 2011; 34(11):1696-701.

2459 Jang JY, Kim TS, Cai J, Kim J, Kim Y, et al. (2013). Nattokinase improves blood flow by inhibiting platelet aggregation and thrombus formation. *Lab Anim Res.* Dec; 29(4):221-5.

2460 Suzuki Y, Kondo K, Matsumoto Y, Zhao BQ, Otsuguro K, et al. (2003). Dietary supplementation of fermented soybean, natto, suppresses intimal thickening and modulates the lysis of mural thrombi after endothelial injury in rat femoral artery. *Life Sci.* Jul 25; 73(10):1289-98.

2461 Ibid. Jang. (2013).

2462 Kurosawa Y, Nirengi S, Homma T, Esaki K, Ohta M, et al. (2015). A single-dose of oral nattokinase potentiates thrombolysis and anticoagulation profiles. *Sci Rep.* 2015 Jun 25; 5():11601.

2463 Shah AB, Rawat S, Mehta S. (2004). An open clinical pilot study to evaluate the safety and efficacy of natto kinaseas an add-on oral fibrinolytic agent tolow molecular weight heparin & anti-platelets in acute ischaemic stroke. *Japan Pharmacol Therap.* 2004;32:437–451

2464 Fujita M, Hong K, Ito Y, Misawa S, Takeuchi N, et al. (1995). Transport of nattokinase across the rat intestinal tract. *Nishimuro S Biol Pharm Bull.* Sep; 18(9):1194-6.

2465 Fadl NN, Ahmed HH, Booles HF, Sayed AH. (2013). Serrapeptase and nattokinase intervention for relieving Alzheimer's disease pathophysiology in rat model. *Hum Exp Toxicol.* Jul; 32(7):721-35.

2466 Hsu RL, Lee KT, Wang JH, Lee LY, Chen RP. (2009). Amyloid-degrading ability of nattokinase from Bacillus subtilis natto. *J Agric Food Chem.* Jan 28; 57(2):503-8.

2467 Bhatt PC, Verma A, Al-Abbasi FA, Anwar F, Kumar V, et al. (2017). Development of surface-engineered PLGA nanoparticulate-delivery system of Tet1-conjugated nattokinase enzyme for inhibition of AB40 plaques in Alzheimer's disease. *Int J Nanomedicine.* Dec 13;12:8749-8768.

359

[2468] Bhatt PC, Pathak S, Kumar V, Panda PB. (2018). Attenuation of neurobehavioral and neurochemical abnormalities in animal model of cognitive deficits of Alzheimer's disease by fermented soybean nanonutraceutical.

[2469] Kelly E, Vyas P, Weber JT. (2017). Biochemical Properties and Nueroprotective Effects of Compounds in Various Species of Berries. *Molecules.* Dec 22;23(1):E26.

[2470] Pribis P, Shukitt-Hale B. (2014). Cognition: the new frontier for nuts and berries. *Am J Clin Nutr.* Jul;100 Suppl 1:347S-52S.

[2471] Vinson JA, Cai Y. (2012). Nuts, especially walnuts have both antioxidant quantity and efficacy and exhibit significant potential health benefits. *Food Funct.* 2012 Feb;3(2):134-40.

[2472] O'Brien J, Okereke O, Devore E, Rosner B, Breteler M, et al. (2017). Long-term intake of nuts in relation to cognitive function in older women. *J Nutr Health Aging.* 2014 May; 18(5): 496–502.

[2473] Bazoti FN, Bergquist J, Markides KE, Tsarbopoulos A. (2006). Noncovalent interaction between amyloid-beta-peptide (1-40) and oleuropein studied by electrospray ionization mass spectrometry. *J Am Soc Mass Spectrom.* Apr; 17(4):568-75.

[2474] Farooqui AA, Tarooqui T. (2018). Effects of Mediterranean Diet Components on Neurodegenerative Diseases. In *Role of the Mediterranean Diet in the Brain and Neurodegenerative Diseases.*

[2475] Bazoti FN, Bergquist J, Markides K, Tsarbopoulos A. (2008). Localization of the noncovalent binding site between amyloid-beta-peptide and oleuropein using electrospray ionization FT-ICR mass spectrometry. *J Am Soc Mass Spectrom.* Aug; 19(8):1078-85.

[2476] Daccache A, Lion C, Sibille N, Gerard M, Slomianny C, et al. (2011). Oleuropein and derivatives from olives as Tau aggregation inhibitors. *Neurochem Int.* May;58(6):700-7.

[2477] Rigacci S, Guidotti V, Bucciantini M, et al. (2011). Abeta(1-42) aggregates into non-toxic amyloid assemblies in the presence of the natural polyphenol oleuropein aglycon. *Curr Alzheimer Res.* Dec;8(8):841-52.

[2478] Ibid. Daccache. (2011).

[2479] Giamarellos-Bourboulis EJ, Geladopoulos T, Chrisofos M, Koutoukas P, Vassiliadis J, et al. (2006). Oleuropein: a novel immunomodulator conferring prolonged survival in experimental sepsis by Pseudomonas aeruginosa. *Shock.* Oct; 26(4):410-6.

[2480] Omar SH. (2010). Cardioprotective and neuroprotective roles of oleuropein in olive. *Saudi Pharm J.* Jul; 18(3):111-21.

[2481] Bulotta S, Celano M, Lepore SM, Montalcini T, Pujia A, et al. (2014). Beneficial effects of the olive oil phenolic components oleuropein and hydroxytyrosol: focus on protection against cardiovascular and metabolic diseases. *J Transl Med.* Aug 3; 12():219.

[2482] Andreadou I, Iliodromitis EK, Mikros E, Constantinou M, Agalias A, et al. (2006). The olive constituent oleuropein exhibits anti-ischemic, antioxidative, and hypolipidemic effects in anesthetized rabbits. *J Nutr.* Aug; 136(8):2213-9.

[2483] Domitrović R, Jakovac H, Marchesi VV, Šain I, Romić Ž, et al. (2012). Preventive and therapeutic effects of oleuropein against carbon tetrachloride-induced liver damage in mice. *Pharmacol Res.* Apr; 65(4):451-64.

[2484] Park S, Choi Y, Um SJ, Yoon SK, Park T. (2011). Oleuropein attenuates hepatic steatosis induced by high-fat diet in mice. *J Hepatol.* May; 54(5):984-93.

[2485] Kim SW, Hur W, Li TZ, Lee YK, Choi JE, et al. (2014). Oleuropein prevents the progression of steatohepatitis to hepatic fibrosis induced by a high-fat diet in mice. M*ol Med.* Apr 25; 46():e92.

[2486] Mohagheghi F, Bigdeli MR, Rasoulian B, Hashemi P, et al. (2011). The neuroprotective effect of olive leaf extract is related to improved blood-brain barrier permeability and brain edema in rat with experimental focal cerebral ischemia. *Phytomedicine.* Jan 15;18(2-3):170-5.

[2487] Psaltopoulou T, Kosti RI, Haidopoulos D, Dimopoulos M, et al. (2011). Olive oil intake is inversely related to cancer prevalence: a systematic review and a meta-analysis of 13,800 patients and 23,340 controls in 19 observational studies. *Lipids Health Dis.* Jul 30; 10():127.

[2488] Nan JN, Ververis K, Bollu S, Rodd AL, Swarup O, et al. (2014). Biological effects of the olive polyphenol, hydroxytyrosol: An extra view from genome-wide transcriptome analysis. *J Nucl Med.* Jan-Apr; 17 Suppl 1():62-9.

[2489] Escrich E, Moral R, Grau L, Costa I, Solanas M. (2007).Molecular mechanisms of the effects of olive oil and other dietary lipids on cancer. *Mol Nutr Food Res.* 2007 Oct; 51(10):1279-92.

[2490] Scoditti E, Calabriso N, Massaro M, Pellegrino M, Storelli C, et al. (2012). Mediterranean diet polyphenols reduce inflammatory angiogenesis through MMP-9 and COX-2 inhibition in human vascular endothelial cells: a potentially protective mechanism in atherosclerotic vascular disease and cancer. *Arch Biochem Biophys.* Nov 15; 527(2):81-9.

[2491] Batarseh YS, Mohamed LA, Al Rihani SB, Mousa YM, Siddique AB, et al. (2017). Oleocanthal ameliorates amyloid-B oligomers' toxicity on astrocytes and neuronal cells: In vitro studies. *Neuroscience.* Jun 3;352:204-215.

[2492] Lauretti E, Juliano L, Pratico D. (2017). Extra-virgin olive oil ameliorates cognition and neuropathology of the 3xTg mice: role of autophagy. *Ann Clin Transl Neurol.* Jun 21;4(8):564-574.

[2493] Pang KL, Chin KY. (2018). The Biological Activities of Oleocanthal from a Molecular Perspective. *Nutrients.* May;10(5):570.

[2494] Canhada S, Castro K, Perry IS, Luft VC. (2018). Omega-3 fatty acids' supplementation in Alzheimer's disease: A systematic review. *Nutr Neurosci.* Oct;21(8):529-538.

[2495] Wysoczanski T, Sokola-Sysoczanska E, Pekala J, Lochynski S, Czyz K, et al. (2016). Omega-3 Fatty Acids and their Role in Central Nervous System: A Review. *Curr Med Chem.* 2016;23(8):816-31.

[2496] Ibid. Wysoczanski. (2016).

[2497] Ibid. Wysoczanski. (2016).

[2498] Rathod R, Kale A, Joshi S. (2016). Novel insights into the effect of vitamin B12 and omega-3 fatty acids on brain function. *J Biomed Sci.* Jan 25;23:17.

[2499] Thomas J, Thomas CJ, Radcliffe J, Itsiopoulos C. (2015). Omega-3 Fatty Acids in Early Prevention of Inflammatory Neurodegenerative Disease: A Focus on Alzheimer's Disease. *Biomed Res Int.* 2015:172801.

[2500] Avallone R, Vitale G, Bertolotti M. (2019). Omega-3 Fatty Acids and Neurodegenrative Diseases: New Evidence in Clinical Trials. *Int J Mol Sci.* Aug 30;20(17):E4256.

[2501] Fotuhi M, Mohassel P, Yaffe K. (2009). Fish consumption, long-chain omega-3 fatty acids and risk of cognitive decline or Alzheimer disease: a complex association. *Nat Clin Pract Neurol.* Mar; 5(3):140-52.

[2502] Chiu CC, Su KP, Cheng TC, Liu HC, Chang CJ, et al. (2008). The effects of omega-3 fatty acids monotherapy in Alzheimer's disease and mild cognitive impairment: a preliminary randomized double-blind placebo-controlled study. *Prog Neuropsychopharmacol Biol Psychiatry.* Aug 1; 32(6):1538-44.

[2503] Yurko-Mauro K, McCarthy D, Rom D, Nelson EB, Ryan AS,et al. (2010). Beneficial effects of docosahexaenoic acid on cognition in age-related cognitive decline. *Alzheimers Dement.* Nov; 6(6):456-64.

[2504] Morris MC, Evans DA, Tangney CC, Bienias JL, Wilson RS. (2005). Fish consumption and cognitive decline with age in a community study. *Arch Neurol.* Dec;62(12):1849-53.

[2505] Cole GM, Ma QL, Frautschy SA. (2019). Omega-3 fatty acids and dementia. *Prostaglandins Leukot Essent Fatty Acids.* Aug-Sep;81(2-3):213-21.

[2506] Devassy JG, Leng S, Gabbs M, Monirujjaman M, Aukema HM. (2016). Omega-3 Polyunsaturated Fatty Acids and Oxylipins in Neuroinflammation and Management of Alzheimer Disease. *Adv Nutr.* Sep 15;7(5):905-16.

[2507] McCann JC, Ames BN. (2005). Is docosahexaenoic acid, an n-3 long-chain polyunsaturated fatty acid, required for development of normal brain function? An overview of evidence from cognitive and behavioral tests in humans and animals. *Am J Clin Nutr.* Aug; 82(2):281-95.

[2508] Conklin SM, Gianaros PJ, Brown SM, Yao JK, Hariri AR, et al. (2007). Long-chain omega-3 fatty acid intake is associated positively with corticolimbic gray matter volume in healthy adults. *Neurosci Lett.* Jun 29;421(3):209-12.

[2509] Beltz BS, Tlusty MF, Benton JL, Sandeman DC. (2007). Omega-3 fatty acids upregulate adult neurogenesis. *Neurosci Lett.* Mar 25;415(2):154-8.

[2510] Zainuddin MSA, Thuret S. (2012). Nutrition, adult hippocampal neurogenesis and mental health. *Brit Med Bull.* 2012;103(1):89-114.

[2511] Ibid. Conklin. (2007).

[2512] Wurtman RJ, Cansev M, Sakamoto T, Ulus IH. (2009). Use of phosphate precursors to promote synaptogenesis. *An Rev Nutr.* 2009;29:59-87.

[2513] Wurtman RJ, Cansev M, Ulus IH. (Mar 2009). Synapse formation is enhanced by oral administration of uridine and DHA, the circulating precursors of brain phosphatides. *J Nutr Aging.* 13(3):189-97.

[2514] Heinrich SC. (2010). Dietary omega-3 fatty acid supplementation for optimizing neuronal structure and function. *Mol Nutr Food Res.* Apr;54(4):447-56.

[2515] Masterjohn C. (2014). Learning your memory, and cholesterol. Retrieved Oct 10 2019 from www.cholesterl-and-health.com.

[2516] Fotuli M, Mohassel P, Yaffe K. (2009). Fish consumption, long-chain omega-3 fatty acids and risk of cognitive decline or Alzheimer's disease: a complex association. *Nat Clin Pract Neurol.* Mar;5(3):140-52.

[2517] Barberger-Gateau P, Raffaitin C, Letenneur L, Berr C, Tzourio C, et al. (2007). Dietary patterns and risk of dementia: the Three City Cohort study. *Neurology.* Nov 13;69(20):1921-30.

[2518] Ibid. Morris. (2005). *Arch Neurol.*

[2519] Lin PY, Su KP. (2007). A meta-anlaytic review of double-blind, placebo-controlled trials of antidepressant efficacy of omega-3 fatty acids. *Clin Psychiatry.* Jul;68(7):1056-61.

[2520] Freeman MP, Hibbein JR, Wisner KL, Davis JM, Mischoulon D, et al. (2006). Omega-3 fatty acids: evidence basis for treatment and future research in psychiatry. *J Clin Psychiatry.* Dec;67:1954–1967.

[2521] Cameron-Smith D, Albert BB, et al. (2015). Fishing for answers: is oxidation of fish oil supplements a problem? *J Nutr Sci.* Nov 23;4:e36.

[2522] Kajla P, Sharma A, Sood DR. (2015). Flaxseed—a potential functional food source. *J Food Sci Technol.* Apr;52(4):1857-1871.

[2523] Kris-Etherton PM, Taylor DS, Yu-Poth S, Huth P, Moriaty K, et al. (2000). Polyunsaturated fatty acids in the food chain in the United States. *Am J Clin Nutr.* Jan;71(1 Suppl):179S-88S.

[2524] Sun GY, Simonyi A, Fritsche KL, Chuang DY, Hannink M, et al. (2018). Docosahexaenoic acid (DHA): An essential nutrient and a nutraceutical for brain health and diseases. *Prostaglandins Leukot Essent Fatty Acids.* Sep;136:3-13.

[2525] Walczewska A, Stephien T, Bewicz-Binkowska D, Zgorzynska E. (2011). [The role of docosahexaenoic acid in neuronal function]. [Article in Polish] *Postepy Hig Med Dosw (Online).* Jun 2;65:314-27.

[2526] Farooqui AA, Horrocks LA, Farooqui T. (2007). Modulation of inflammation in brain: a matter of fat. *J Neurochem.* May;101(3):577-99.

[2527] Litman BJ, Niu SL, Polozova A, Mitchell DC. (2001). The role of docosahexaenoic acid containing phospholipids in modulating G protein-coupled signaling pathways: visual transduction. *J Mol Neurosci.* Apr;16(2-3):237-42.

[2528] Turner N, Else PL, Hulbert AJ. (2003). Docosahexaenoic acid (DHA) content of membranes determines molecular activity of the sodium pump: implications for disease states and metabolism. *Naturwissenschaften.* Nov;90(11):521-3.

[2529] Cunnane SC, Chouinard-Watkins R, Castellano CA, Barberger-Gateau P. (2013). Docosahexaenoic acid homeostasis, brain aging and Alzheimer's disease: Can we reconcile the evidence? *Prostalandins Leukot Essent Fatty Acids.* Jan;88(1):61-70.

[2530] Sugasini D, Thomas R, Yalagala PCR, Tai LM, Subbaiah PV. (2017). Dietary docosahexaenoic acid (DHA) as lysophosphatidylcholine, but not as free acid, enriches brain DHA and improves memory in adult mice. *Sci Rep.* Sep;7:11263.

[2531] Sugasini D, Yalagala PCR, Googin A, Tai LM, Subbaiah PV. (2019). Enrichment of brain docosahexaenoic acid (DHA) is highly dependent upon the molecular carrier or dietary DHA: lysophosphatidylcholine is more efficient than either phosphatidycholine or triacylglycerol. *J Nutr. Biochem.* Aug 31;74:108231.

[2532] Rondanelli M, Opizzi A, Faliva M, Mozzoni M, Antoniello N, et al. Effects of a diet integration with an oily emulsion of DHA-phospholipids containing melatonin and tryptophan in elderly patients suffering from mild cognitive impairment. *Nutr Neurosci.* 2012 Mar;15(2):46-54.

[2533] Bradbury J. (2011). Docosahexaenoic acid (DHA): an ancient nutrient for the modern human brain. *Nutrients.* May;3(5):529-54.

[2534] Bazan NG, Musto AE, Knott EJ. (2011). Endogenous signaling by omega-3 docosahexaenoic acid-derived mediators sustains homeo-static synaptic and circuitry integrity. *Mol Neurobiol.* Oct;44(2):216-22.

[2535] Cao D, Kevala K, Kim J, et al. (2009). Docosahexaenoic acid promotes hippocampal neuronal development and synaptic function. *J Neurochem.* Oct;111(2):510-21.

[2536] Dyall SC, Michael GJ, Michael-Titus AT. (2010). Omega-3 fatty acids reverse age-related decreases in nuclear receptors and increase neurogenesis in old rats. *J Neurosci Res.* Aug 1;88(10):2091-102.

[2537] Hooijmans CR, Van der Zee CE, Dederen PJ, et al. (2009). DHA and cholesterol containing diets influence Alzheimer-like pathology, cognition and cerebral vasculature in APPswe/PS1dE9 mice. *Neurobiol Dis.* Mar;33(3):482-98.

[2538] Bradbury J. (2011). Docosahexaenoic acid (DHA): an ancient nutrient for the modern human brain. *Nutrients.* May;3(5):529-54.

[2539] Bazan NG. (2005). Neuroprotectin D1 (NPD1): a DHA-derived mediator that protects brain and retina against cell injury-induced oxidative stress. *Brain Pathol.* Apr;15(2):159-66.

[2540] Wu A, Ying Z, Gomez-Pinilla F. (2008). Docosahexaenoic acid dietary supplementation enhances the effects of exercise on synaptic plasticity and cognition. *Neuroscience.* Aug 26;155(3):751-9.

[2541] Chytrova G, Ying Z, Gomez-Pinilla F. (2010). Exercise contributes to the effects of DHA dietary supplementation by acting on membrane-related synaptic systems. *Brain Res.* Jun 23;1341:32-40.

[2542] Hashimoto M, Hossain S, Shimada T, Shido O. (2006). Docosahexaenoic acid-induced protective effect against impaired learning in amyloid beta-infused rats is associated with increased synaptosomal membrane fluidity. *Clin Exp Pharmacol Physiol.* Oct;33(10):934-9.

[2543] Hashimoto M, Hossain S, Agdul H, Shido O. (2005). Docosahexaenoic acid-induced amelioration on impairment of memory learning in amyloid beta-infused rats relates to the decreases of amyloid beta and cholesterol levels in detergent-insoluble membrane fractions. *Biochim Biophys Acta.* Dec 30;1738(1-3):91-8.

[2544] Cole GM, Frautschy SA. (2006). Docosahexaenoic acid protects from amyloid and dendritic pathology in an Alzheimer's disease mouse model. *Nutr Health.* 2006;18(3):249-59.

[2545] Oster T, Pillot T. (2010). Docosahexaenoic acid and synaptic protection in Alzheimer's disease mice. *Biochim Biophys Acta.* Aug;1801(8):791-8.

[2546] Pauwels EK, Volterrani D, Mariani G, Kairemo K. (2009). Fatty acid facts, Part IV: docosahexaenoic acid and Alzheimer's disease. A story of mice, men and fish. *Drug News Perspect.* May;22(4):205-13.

[2547] Xiao Y, Wang L, Xu RJ, Chen ZY. (2006). DHA depletion in rat brain is associated with impairment on spatial learning and memory. *Biomed Environ Sci.* Dec;19(6):474-80.

[2548] Geng X, Yang B, Li R, Teng T, Ladu MJ, et al. (2019). Effects of Docosahexaenoic Acid and Its Peroxidation on Amyloid-B Peptide-Stimulated Microglia. *Mol Neurobiol.* Nov 1. [Epub ahead of print]

[2549] Morris MC, Evans DA, Tangney CC, Bienias JL, Wilson RS. (2005). Fish consumption and cognitive decline with age in a large community study. *Arch Neurol.* Dec;62(12):1849-53.

[2550] Ibid. Cunnane. (2013). Prostalandins Leukot Essent Fatty Acids

[2551] Levi FY, Vedin I, Cederholm T, Basun H, Faxen Irving G, et al. (2014). Transfer of omega-3 fatty acids across the blood-brain barrier after dietary supplementation with a docosahexaenoic acid-rich omega-3 fatty preparation in patients with Alzheimer's disease: The OmegAD study. *J Intern Med.* Apr;275(4):428-36.

[2552] Balkouch M, Hachem M, Elgot A, Lo Van A, Picq M, et al. (2016). The pleiotropic effects of omega-3 docosahexaenoic acid on the hallmarks of Alzheimer's disease. *J Nutr Biochem.* Dec;38:1-11.

[2553] Lim GP, Calon F, Morihara T, Yang F, Teter B, et al. (2005). A diet enriched with the omega-3 fatty acid docosahexaenoic acid reduces amyloid burden in an aged Alzheimer mouse model. *J Neurosci.* Mar 23; 25(12):3032-40.

[2554] Calon F, Lim GP, Yang F, Morihara T, Teter B, et al. (2004). Docosahexaenoic acid protects from dendritic pathology in an Alzheimer's disease mouse model. *Neuron.* Sep 2; 43(5):633-45.

[2555] Kim HY, Akbar M, Lau A, Edsall L. (2000). Inhibition of neuronal apoptosis by docosahexaenoic acid (22:6omega-3). Role of phosphatidylserine in antiapoptotic effect. *J Biol Chem.* Nov 10;275(45):35215-23.

[2556] Schaefer EJ, Bongard V, Beiser AS, Lamon-Fava S, Robins SJ, et al. (2006). Plasma phosphatildylcholine docosahexaenoic acid content and risk of dementia and Alzheimer's disease: the Framingham Heart Study. *Arch Neurol.* 63 Nov;63(11):1545-50.

[2557] Morris MC, Evans DA, Bienias JL, Tangney CC, Bennett DA, et al. (2003). Consumption of fish and omega-3 fatty acids and risk of incident Alzheimer disease. *Arch Neurol.* Jul;60(7):940-6.

[2558] Kalmijn S, Launer LJ, Ott A, Witteman JC, Hofman A, et al. (1997). Dietary fat intake and the risk of incident dementia in the Rotterdam Study. *Ann Neurol.* Nov;42(5):776-82.

[2559] Chalon S, ion-Vancassel S, Belzung C, Guilloteau D, Leguisquet, AM, et al. (1998). Dietary fish oil affects monoaminergic neurotransmission and behavior in rats. *J Nutr.* Dec;128(12):2512.

[2560] Smedler E, Uhlen P. (2014). Frequency decoding of calcium oscillations. *Biochim Biophys Acta.* Mar;1840(3):964-9.

[2561] Sergeeva M, Strokin M, Reiser G. (2005). Regulation of intracellular calcium levels by polyunsaturated fatty acids, arachidonic acid and docosahexaenoic acid, in astrocytes: possible involvement of phospholipase A2. *Reprod Nutr Dev.* Sep;45(5):633-46.

[2562] Cao D, Kevala K, Kim J, Moon HS, Jun SB, et al. (2009). Docosahexaenoic acid promotes hippocampal neuronal development and synaptic function. *J Neurochem.* Oct;111(2):510-21.

[2563] Su HM. (2010). Mechanisms of n-3 fatty acid-mediated development and maintenance of learning memory performance. *J Nutr Biochem.* May;21(5):364-73.

[2564] Connor S, Tenorio G, Clandinin MT, Sauve Y. (2012). DHA supplementation enhances high-frequency, stimulation-induced synaptic transmission in mouse hippocampus. *Appl Physiol Nutr Metab.* Oct;37(5):880-7.

[2565] Hashimoto M, Katakura M, Hossain S, Rahman A, Shimada T, et al. (2011). Docosahexaenoic acid withstands the Abeta(25-35)-induced neurotoxicity in SH-SY5Y cells. *J Nutr Biochem.* Jan;22(1):22-9.

[2566] Kim HY, Moon HS, Cao D, Lee J, Kevala K, et al. (2011). N-Docosahexaenoylethanolamide promotes development of hippocampal neurons. *Biochem J.* Apr 15;435(2):327-36.

[2567] Tanaka K, Farooqui AA, Nikhat JS, Alhomida AS, Ong WY. (2012). Effects of Docosahexaenoic acid on Neurotransmission. *Biomol Ther (Seoul).* Mar;20(2):152-157.

[2568] Ibid. Walczewska. (2011). *Postepy Hig Med Dosw*

[2569] Ibid. Farooqui. (2007). *J Neurochem.*

[2570] Litman BJ, Niu SL, Polozova A, Mitchell DC. (2001). The role of docosahexaenoic acid containing phospholipids in modulating G protein-coupled signaling pathways: visual transduction. *J Mol Neurosci.* Apr;16(2-3):237-42.

[2571] Serhan CN, Arita M, Hong S, Gotlinger K. (2004). Resolvins, docosatrienes, and neuroprotectins, novel omega-3-derived mediators, and their endogenous aspirin-triggered epimers. *Lipids.* Nov;39(11):1125-32.

[2572] Pauwels EK, Volterrani D, Mariani G, Kairemo K. (2009). Fatty acid facts, Part IV: docosahexaenoic acid and Alzheimer's disease. A story of mice, men and fish. *Drug News Perspect.* May;22(4):205-13.

[2573] Xiao Y, Wang L, Xu RJ, Chen ZY. (2006). DHA depletion in rat brain is associated with impairment on spatial learning and memory. *Biomed Environ Sci*. Dec;19(6):474-80.

[2574] Turner N, Else PL, Hulbert AJ. Docosahexaenoic acid (DHA) content of membranes determines molecular activity of the sodium pump: implications for disease states and metabolism. *Naturwissenschaften*. 2003 Nov;90(11):521-3.

[2575] Begin ME, Plourde M, Pifferi F, Cunnane SC. (2010). What is the Link Between Docosahexaenoic Acid, Cognitive Impairment, and Alzheimer's Disease in the Elderly? In Montmayeur JP, le Coutre J. (eds). Fat Detection: Taste, Texture, and Post Ingestive Effects. *Frontiers in Neuroscience*. CRC Press. Taylor & Francis; 2010. Chapter 19.

[2576] Yalagala PCR, Sugasini D, Dasarathi S, Pahan K, Subbaiah PV. (2019). Dietary lysophosphatidylcholine-EPA enriches both EPA and DHA in the brain: potential treatment for depression. *J Lipid Res*. Mar;60(3):566-578.

[2577] Ibid. Yalagala. (2019).

[2578] Ibid. Yalagala. (2019).

[2579] Virtanen JK, Mursu J, Voutilainen S, Tuomainen TP. (2018). The associations of serum n-6 polyunsaturated fatty acids with serum C-reactive protein in men: the Kuopio Ischaemic Heart Disease Risk Factor Study. *Eur J Clin Nutr*. Mar;72(3):342-348.

[2580] Mercola.com. Borage Oil. Retrieved Nov 2 2019 from https://articles.mercola.com/herbal-oils/borage-oil.aspx.

[2581] Bolsoni-Lopes A, Festuccia WT, Chimin P, Farias TS, Torres-Leal FL. (2014). Palmitoleic acid (n-7) increases white adipocytes GLUT4 content and glucose uptake in association with AMPK activation. *Lipids Health Dis*. 2014;13:199.

[2582] Bernstein AM, Roizen MF, Martinez L. (2014). Purified palmitoleic acid for the reduction of high-sensitivity C-reactive protein and serum lipids: a double-blinded, randomized, placebo controlled study. *J Clin Lipidol*. 2014;8(6):612-7.

[2583] Yang ZH, Miyahara H, Hatanaka A. (2011). Chronic administration of palmitoleic acid reduces insulin resistance and hepatic lipid accumulation in KK-Ay Mice with genetic type 2 diabetes. *Lipids Health Dis*. 2011;10:120.

[2584] Stefan N, Kantartzis K, Celebi N, Staiger H, Machann J, et al. (2010). Circulating palmitoleate strongly and independently predicts insulin sensitivity in humans. *Diabetes Care*. 2010;33(2):405-7.

[2585] Bolsoni-Lopes A, Festuccia WT, Farias TS, Chimin P, Torres-Leal FL, et al. (2013). Palmitoleic acid (n-7) increases white adipocyte lipolysis and lipase content in a PPARalpha-dependent manner. *Am J Physiol Endocrinol Metab*. 2013;305(9):E1093-102.

[2586] Bernstein AM, Roizen MF, Martinez L. (2014). Purified palmitoleic acid for the reduction of high-sensitivity C-reactive protein and serum lipids: a double-blinded, randomized, placebo controlled study. *J Clin Lipidol*. 2014;8(6):612-7.

[2587] Kallio HP, Yang B. (2014). Health effects of sea buckthorn berries; research and strategies at the university of Turku, Finland. *Acta Hortic*. 2014;1017:343–349.

[2588] Sayegh M, Miglio C, Ray S. (2014). Potential cardiovascular implications of Sea Buckthorn berry consumption in humans. *Int J Food Sci Nutr*. Aug; 65(5):521-8.

[2589] Squire, LR; Schacter DL. *The Neuropsychology of Memory*. Guilford Press. 2002

[2590] Kim HY, Huang BX, Spector AA. (2014). Phosphatidylserine in the brain: metabolism and function. *Prog Lipid Res*. Oct;56:1-18.

[2591] Kidd PM. (2002). Phospholipids: Versatile Nutraceuticals for Functional Foods. *Func Foods Nutraceut*. 2002

[2592] Glade MJ, Smith K. (2015). Phosphatidylserine and the human brain. *Nutrition*. Jun;31(6):781-6.

[2593] Ibid. Kidd. (2002). *Func Foods Nutraceut*.

[2594] More MI. (2014). Positive Effects of Soy Lecithin-Derived Phosphatidylserine plus Phosphatidic Acid on Memory, Cognition, Daily Functioning, and Mood in Elderly Patients with Alzheimer's Disease and Dementia. *Adv Ther*. Dec;31(12):1247-1262.

[2595] *Acta Psychiatr Scand*. 1990 Mar;81(3):265-70 Effects of phosphatidylserine therapy in geriatric patients with depressive disorders. Maggioni M1, Picotti GB, Bondiolotti GP, Panerai A, Cenacchi T, Nobile P, Brambilla F.

[2596] Shen X, Liu Y, Luo X, Yang Z. (2019). Advances in Biosynthesis, Pharmacology, and Pharmacokinetics of Pinocembrin, a Promising Natural Small-Molecule Drug. *Molecules*. June 24;24(12):E2323.

[2597] Calatayud-Vernich P, Caltayud F, Simo E, Pico Y. (2018). Pesticide residues in honey bees, pollen and beeswax: Assessing beehive exposure. *Environ Pollut*. Oct:241:106-114.

[2598] Shoba G, Joy D, Joseph T, Majeed M, Rajendran R, et al. (1998). Influence of piperine on the pharmacokinetics of curcumin in animals and human volunteers. *Planta Med*. May;64(4):353-6.

[2599] Butt MS, Pasha I, Sultan MT, Randhawa MA, Saeed F, et al. (2013). Black pepper and health claims: a comprehensive treatise. *Crit Rev Food Sci Nutr*. 2013;53(9):875-86.

[2600] Guo S, Wang J, Xu H, Rong W, Gao C, et al. (2019). Classic Prescription, Kai-Xin-San, Ameliorates Alzheimer's Disease as an Effective Multitarget Treatment: From Neurotransmitter to Protein Signaling Pathway. *Oxid Med Cell Longev*. Jul 1;2019:9096409.

[2601] Hui S, Yang Y, Peng WJ, Sheng CX, Gong W, et al. (2017). Protective effects of Busen Tiansui decoction on hippocampal synapses in a rat model of Alzheimer's disease. *Neural Regen Res.* Oct;12(10):1680-1686.

[2602] Ibid. Castillo S. (2015). Pomegranate Health Benefits.

[2603] Hartman RE, Shah A, Fagan AM, Schwetye KE, Parsadanian M, et al. (2006) Pomegranate juice decreases amyloid load and improves behavior in a mouse model of Alzheimer's disease. *Neurobiol Dis* 24: 506-515.

[2604] Aviram M, Dornfeld L, Kaplan M, Coleman R, Gaitini D, et al. (2002). Pomegranate juice flavonoids inhibit low-density lipoprotein oxidation and cardiovascular diseases: studies in atherosclerotic mice and in humans. *Drugs Exp Clin Res.* 2002;28(2-3):49-62.

[2605] Ibid. Hartman. (2006).

[2606] Rojanathammanne L, Puig KL, Combs CK. (2013). Pomegranate polyphenols and extract inhibit nuclear factor of activated T-cell and microglial activation in vitr and in a transgenic mouse model of Alzheimer's disease. *J Nutr.* May;143(5):597-605.

[2607] Amri Z, Chorbel A, Turki M, Akrout FM, Ayadi F, et al. (2017). Effect of pomegranate extracts on brain antioxidant markers and cholinesterase activity in high fat-high fructose diet inducing obesity in rat model. *BMC Complement Altern Med.* Jun 27;17(1):339.

[2608] Yuan T, Ma H, Liu W, Niesen DB, Shah N, et al. (2016). Pomegranate's Neuroprotective Effects against Alzheimer Disease are Mediated by Urolithins, Its Ellagitannin-Gut Microbial Derived Metabolites. *ACS Chem Neurosci.* Jan 20;7(1):26-33.

[2609] Nawirska-Olszanska A, Kita A, Biesiada A, Sokol-Letowska A, Kucharska AZ. (2013). Characteristics of antioxidant activity and composition of pumpkin seed oils in 12 cultivars. *Food Chem.* Aug 15;139(1-4):155-61.

[2610] *Phytomedicine.* 2018 Nov 29;57:39-48. doi: 10.1016/j.phymed.2018.11.033. [Epub ahead of print] French maritime pine bark treatment decelerates plaque development and improves spatial memory in Alzheimer's disease mice. Paarmann K1, Prakash SR2, Krohn M2, Möhle L3, Brackhan M2, Brüning T2, Eiriz I2, Pahnke J4.

[2611] Cho KJ, Yun CH, Yoon DY, Cho YS, Rimbach G, et al. (2000). Effect of bioflavonoids extracted from the bark of Pinus maritima on proinflammatory cytokine interleukin-1 production in lipopolysaccharide-stimulated RAW 264.7. *Toxicol Appl Pharmacol.* Oct 1; 168(1):64-71.

[2612] Hu S, Belcaro G, Cornelli U, Luzzi R, Cesarone M, et al. (2015). Effects of Pycnogenol® on endothelial dysfunction in borderline hypertensive, hyperlipidemic, and hyperglycemic individuals: the borderline study. *Int Angiol.* Feb;34(1):43-52.

[2613] Gulati OP. (2014). Pycnogenol® in chronic venous insufficiency and related venous disorders. *Phytother Res.* Mar;28(3):348-62.

[2614] Rohdewald P. (2002). A review of the French maritime pine bark extract (Pycnogenol), a herbal medication with a diverse clinical pharmacology. *Int J Clin Pharmacol Ther.* Apr;40(4):158-68.

[2615] Liu X, Wei J, Tan F, Zhou S, Wurthwein G, et al. (2004). Antidiabetic effect of Pcynogenol French maritime pine bark extract in patients with diabetes type II. *Life Sci.* Oct 8;75(21):2505-13.

[2616] Grimm T, Chovanova Z, Muchova J, Sumegova K, Liptakova A, et al. (2006). Inhibition of NF-kappaB activation and MMP-9 secretion by plasma of human volunteers after ingestion of maritime pine bark extract (Pycnogenol). *J Inflamm* (Lond). Jan 27;3:1.

[2617] Jessberger S, Hogger P, Genest F, Salter DM, Seefried L. (2017). Cellular pharmacodynamic effects of Pyconogenol® in patients with severe osteoarthritis: a randomized controlled pilot study. *BMC Complement Altern Med.* Dec 16;17(1):537.

[2618] Nikpayam O, Rouhani MH, Pourmasoumi M, Roshanravan N, Ghaedi E, et al. (2018). The Effect of Pycnogenol Supplementation on Plasma C-Reactive Protein Concentration: a Systematic Review and Meta-Analysis. *Clin Nutr Res.* Apr;7(2):117-125.

[2619] Chovanova Z, Muchova J, Sivonova M, Dyorakova M, Zitnanova K, et al. (2006). Effect of polyphenolic extract, Pycnogenol, on the level of 8-oxoguanine in children suffering from attention deficit/hyperactivity disorder. *Free Radic Res.* Sep;40(9):1003-10.

[2620] Dvorakova M, Sivonova M, Trebaticka J, Skodacek I, Waczulikova I, et al. (2006). The effect of polyphenolic extract from pine bark, Pycnogenol on the level of glutathione in children suffering from attention deficit/hyperactivity disorder (ADHD). *Redox Rep.* 2006;11(4):163-72.

[2621] Ryan J, Croft K, Mori T, Wesnes K, Spong J, et al. (2008). An examination of the effects of the antioxidant Pycnogenol on cognitive performance, serum lipid profile, endocrinological and oxidative stress biomarkers in an elderly population. *J Psychopharmacol.* Jul;22(5):553-62.

[2622] Belcaro G, Luzzi R, Dugall M, Ippolito E, Saggino A. (2014). Pycnogenol® improves cognitive function, attention, mental performance and specific professionals aged 35-55. *J Neurosurg Sci.* Dec;58(4):239-48.

[2623] Ibid. Ryan. (2008).

[2624] Paarmann K, Prakash SR, Krohn M, Mohle L, Brackhan M, et al. (2019). French maritime pine bark treatment decelerates plaque development and improves spatial memory in Alzheimer's disease mice. *Phytomedicine.* Apr;57:39-48.

[2625] Ishrat T, Parveen K, Hoda MN, Khan MB, Yousuf S, et al. (2009). Effects of Pycnogenol and vitamin E on cognitive deficits and oxidative damage induced by intraverebroventricular streptozotocin in rats. *Behave Pharmacol.* Oct;20(7):567-75.

[2626] Ansari MA, Keller JN, Scheff SW. (2008). Protective effect of Pycnogenol in human neuroblastoma SH-SY5Y cells following acrolein-induced cytotoxicity. *Free Radic Biol Med.* Dec 1;45(11):1510-9.

[2627] Simpson T, Kure C, Stough C. (2019). Assessing the Efficacy and Mechanisms of Pycnogenol® on Cognitive Aging From In Vitro Animal and Human Studies. *Front Pharmacol.* Jul 3;10:694.

[2628] Khan MM, Kempuraj D, Thangavel R, Zaheer A. (2013). Protection of MPTP-induced neuroinflammation and neurodegeneration by Pycnogenol. *Neurochem Int.* Mar;62(4):379-88.

[2629] Itoh Y, Hine K, Miura H, Uetake T, Nakano M, et al. (2016). Effect of the Antioxidant Supplement Pyrroloquinoline Quinone Disodium Salt (BioPQQ™) on Cognitive Functions. *Adv Exp Med Biol.* 2016;876:319-325.

[2630] Akagaaw M, Nakano M, Ikemoto K. (2016). Recent progress in studies on the health benefits of pyrroloquinoline quinone. *Biosci Biotechnol Biochem.* 2016;80(1):13-22.

[2631] Zhang P, Xu Y, Sun J, Li X, Wang L, Jin L. (2009). Protection of pyrroloquinoline quinone against methylmercury-induced neurotoxicity via reducing oxidative stress. *Free Radic Res.* Mar;43(3):224-33.

[2632] Hara H, Hiramatsu H, Adachi T. (2007). Pyrroloquinoline quinone is a potent neuroprotective nutrients against 6-hydroxydopamine-induced neurotoxicity. *Neurochem Res.* Mar;32(3):489-95.

[2633] Kobayashi M, Kim J, Kobayashi N, Han S, Nakamura C, et al. (2006). Pyrroloquinoline quinone (PQQ) prevents fibril formation of alpha-synuclein. *Biochem Biophys Res Commun.* Oct 27;349(3):1139-44.

[2634] Zhang JJ, Zhang RF, Meng XK. (2009). Protective effect of pyrroloquinoline quinone against Abeta-induced neurotoxicity in human neuroblastoma SH-SY5Y cells. *Neurosci Lett.* Oct 30;464(3):165-9.

[2635] Itoh Y, Hine K, Miura H, Uetake T, Nakano M, et al. (2016). Effect of the Antioxidant Supplement Pyrroloquinoline Quinone Disodium Salt (BIOPQQ™) on Cognitive Functions. *Adv Exp Med Biol.* 2016;876:319-325.

[2636] Lu J, Chen S, Shen M, He Q, Zhang Y, et al. (2018). Mitochondrial regulation by pyrroloquinoline quinone prevents rotenone-induced neurotoxicity in Parkinson's disease. *Neurosci Lett.* Nov 20;687:104-110.

[2637] Ohwada K, Takeda H, Yamazaki M, Isogai H, Nakano M, et al. (2008). Pyrroloquinoline Quinone (PQQ) Prevents Cognitive Decline Caused by Oxidative Stress in Rats. *J Clin Biochem Nutr.* Jan; 42(1): 29–34.

[2638] Harris CB, Chowanadisai W, Mishchuk DO, Satre MA, Slupsky CM, et al. (2013). Dietary pyrroloquinoline quinone (PQQ) alters indicators of inflammation and mitochondrial-related metabolism in human subjects. *J Nutr Biochem.* Dec;24(12):2076-84.

[2639] Zhang P, Ye Y, Qian Y, Yin B, Zhao J, et al. (2017). The Effect of Pyrroloquinoline Quinone on Apoptosis and Autophagy in Traumatic Brain Injury. *CNS Neurol Disord Drug Targets.* 2017;16(6):724-736.

[2640] Ibid. Elumalai. (2016). *Adv Neurobiol.*

[2641] Lee M, McGeer EG, McGeer PL. (2016). Quercetin, not caffeine, is a major neuroprotective component in coffee. *Neurobiol Aging.* Oct;46:113-23.

[2642] Bournival J, Plouffe M, Renaud J, Provencher C, Martinoli MG. (2012). Quercetin and sesamin protect dopaminergic cells from MPP+-induced neuroinflammation in a microglial (N9)-neuronal (PC12) coculture system. *Oxid Med Cell Longev.* 2012;2012:921941.

[2643] Wenk GL, McGann-Gramling K, Hauss-Wegrzyniak B, et al. (2004). Attenuation of chronic neuroinflammation by a nitric oxide-releasing derivative of the antioxidant ferulic acid. *J Neurochem.* Apr;89(2):484-93.

[2644] Ibid. Bournival. (2012).

[2645] Wenk GL, McGann-Gramling K, Hauss-Wegrzyniak B, et al. (2004). Attenuation of chronic neuroinflammation by a nitric oxide-releasing derivative of the antioxidant ferulic acid. *J Neurochem.* Apr;89(2):484-93.

[2646] Hynd MR, Scott HL, Dodd PR. (2004). Glutamate-mediated excitotoxicity and neurodegeneration in Alzheimer's disease. *Neurochem Int.* 2004 Oct;45(5):583-95.

[2647] Silva B, Oliveira PJ, Dias A, Malva JO. (2008). Quercetin, kaempferol and biapigenin from Hypericum perforatum are neuroprotective against excitotoxic insults. *Neurotox Res.* May-Jun;13(3-4):265-79.

[2648] Yang EJ, Kim GS, Kim JA, Song KS. (2013). Protective effects of onion-derived quercetin on glutamate-mediated hippocampal neuronal cell death. *Pharmacogn Mag.* 2013 Oct;9(36):302-8.

[2649] Dong XX, Wang Y, Qin ZH. (2009). Molecular mechanisms of excitotoxicity and their relevance to pathogenesis of neurodegenerative diseases. *Acta Pharmacologica Sinica.* 2009;30(4):379-87.

[2650] Shi C, Zhao L, Zhu B, Li Q, Yew DT, et al. (2009). Protective effects of Ginkgo biloba extract (EGb761) and its constituents quercetin and ginkgolide B against beta-amyloid peptide-induced toxicity in SH-SY5Y cells. *Chem Biol Interact.* Sep 14;181(1):115-23.

[2651] Karuppagounder SS, Madathil SK, Pandey M, Haobam R, Rajamma U, et al. (2013). Quercetin up-regulates mitochondrial complex-I activity to protect against programmed cell death in rotenone model of Parkinson's disease in rats. *Neuroscience.* Apr 16;236:136-48.

[2652] Arredondo F, Echeverry C, Abin-Carriquiry JA, Blasina F, et al. (2010). After cellular internalization, quercetin causes Nrf2 nuclear translocation, increases glutathione levels, and prevents neuronal death against an oxidative insult. *Free Radic Biol Med.* Sep 1;49(5):738-47.

[2653] Pasinetti GM, Wang J, Ho L, Zhao W, Dubner L. (2015). Roles of resveratrol and other grape-derived polyphenols in Alzheimer's disease prevention and treatment. *Biochim Biophys Acta.* Jun; 1852(6):1202-8.

[2654] Costa LG, de Laat R, Dao K, Pellacani C, Cole TB, et al. (2014). Paraoxonase-2 (PON2) in brain and its potential role in neuro-protection. *Neurotoxicology.* Jul;43:3-9.

[2655] Costa LG, Tait L, de Laat R, Dao K, Giordano G, et al. (2013). Modulation of paraoxonase 2 (PON2) in mouse brain by the polyphenol quercetin: a mechanism of neuroprotection? *Neurochem Res.* 2013 Sep;38(9):1809-18.

[2656] Navarro A, Boveris A. (2007). The mitochondrial energy transduction system and the aging process. *Am J Physiol Cell Physiol.* 2007;292:C670–86.

[2657] Ibid. Costa. (2013). *Neurotoxicology.*

[2658] Ibid. Costa. (2013). *Neurochem.*

[2659] Navarro A, Boveris A. (2007). The mitochondrial energy transduction system and the aging process. *Am J Physiol Cell Physiol.* 2007;292:C670–86.

[2660] Karuppagounder SS, Madathil SK, Pandey M, Haobam R, Rajamma U, et al. (2013). Quercetin up-regulates mitochondrial complex-I activity to protect against programmed cell death in rotenone model of Parkinson's disease in rats. *Neuroscience.* Apr 16;236:136-48.

[2661] Hynd MR, Scott HL, Dodd PR. (2004). Glutamate-mediated excitotoxicity and neurodegeneration in Alzheimer's disease. *Neurochem Int.* 2004 Oct;45(5):583-95.

[2662] Silva B, Oliveira PJ, Dias A, Malva JO. (2008). Quercetin, kaempferol and biapigenin from Hypericum perforatum are neuroprotective against excitotoxic insults. *Neurotox Res.* May-Jun;13(3-4):265-79.

[2663] Ibid. Yang. (2013).

[2664] Dong XX, Wang Y, Qin ZH. (2009). Molecular mechanisms of excitotoxicity and their relevance to pathogenesis of neurodegenerative diseases. *Acta Pharmacologica Sinica.* 2009;30(4):379-87.

[2665] Xu XH, Zhao TQ. (2002). Effects of puerarin on D-galactose-induced memory deficits in mice. *Acta Pharmacol Sin.* Jul; 23(7):587-90.

[2666] Wu HQ, Chang MZ, Zhang GL, Chang MZ, Zhang GL, et al. (2009). The mechanism of protective effects of puerarin on learning-memory disorder after global cerebral ischemic reperfusion injury in rats. *J Apoplexy Nerv Dis.* Feb;15(1):54-9.

[2667] Yang D, Tang Y, Hu XM, Liu J, Chen Y, et al. (2005). Effects of puerarin on learning and memory of model mouse with beta amyloid peptide-induced dementia. *Chin J Tissue Eng Res.* 2005;9:169–71.

[2668] Sun X. (2005). Observation of 68 cases on effects of puerarin on the chronic alcoholism. *J Linyi Med Coll.* 2005;27:291–2.

[2669] Markus MA, Morris BJ. (2008). Resveratrol in prevention and treatment of common clinical conditions of aging. *Clin Interv Aging.* 2008;3(2): 331-9.

[2670] Szkudeiski T, Szkudeiska K. (2015). Resveratrol and diabetes: from animal to human studies. *Biochim Biophys Acta.* Jun;1852(6): 1145-54. Obes Rev. 2016 Dec; 17(12): 1329-1340.

[2671] Bitterman JL, Chung JH. (2015). Metabolic effects of resveratrol: addressing the controversies. *Cell Mol Life Sci.* Apr; 72(8): 1473-88.

[2672] Cho S, Namkoong K, Shin M, Park J, Yang E, et al. (2017). Cardiovascular Protective Effects and Clinical Applications of Resveratrol. *J Med Food.* Apr; 20(4):323-334.

[2673] Sawda C, Moussa C, Turner RS. (2017). Resveratrol for Alzheimer's disease. *Ann NY Acad Sci.* Sep;1403(1):142-119.

[2674] Ahmed T, Javed S, Javed S, Tariq A, Samec D, et al. (2017). Resveratrol and Alzheimer's Disease: Mechanistic Insights. *Mol Neurobiol.* May;54(4):2622-2635.

[2675] Kou X, Chen N. (2017). Resveratrol as a Natural Autophagy Regulator for Prevention and Treatment of Alzheimer's Disease. *Nutrients.* Aug 24;9(9):E927.

[2676] Pasinetti GM, Wang J, Ho L, Zhao W, Dubner L. (2015). Roles of resveratrol and other grape-derived polyphenols in Alzheimer's disease prevention and treatment. *Biochim Biophys Acta.* Jun; 1852(6):1202-8.

[2677] Moussa C, Hebron M, Huang X, Ahn J, Rissman, RA, et al. (2017). Resveratrol regulates neuro-inflammation and induces adaptive immunity in Alzheimer's disease. *J. Neuroinflammation.* Jan 3;14(1):1.

[2678] Turner RS, Thomas RG, Craft s, van Dyck CH, Mintzer J, et al. (2015). A randomized, double-blind, placebo-controlled trial of resveratrol for Alzheimer disease. *Neurology.* Oct 20;85(16):1383–1391.

[2679] Thordardottir S, Kinhult Ståhlbom A, Almkvist O, Thonberg H, Eriksdotter M, et al. (2017). The effects of different familial Alzheimer's disease mutations on APP processing in vivo. *Alzheimers Res Ther.* Feb 16; 9(1):9.

[2680] Song J, Cheon SY, Jung W, Lee WT, Lee JE. (2014). Resveratrol induces the expression of interleukin-10 and brain-derived neurotrophic factor in BV2 microglia under hypoxia. *Int J Mol Sci.* Sep 2; 15(9):15512-29.

[2681] Jardim FR, de Rossi FT, Nascimento MX, da Silva Barros RG, Borges PA, et al. (2018). Resveratrol and Brain Mitochondria: a Review. *Mol Neurobiol.* Mar;55(3):2085-2101.

[2682] Dasgupta B, Milbrandt J. (2007). Resveratrol stimulates AMP kinase activity in neurons. *Proc Natl Acad Sci U S A*. Apr 24; 104(17):7217-22.

[2683] Witte AV, Kerti L, Margulies DS, Flöel A. (2014). Effects of resveratrol on memory performance, hippocampal functional connectivity, and glucose metabolism in healthy older adults. *J Neurosci*. Jun 4; 34(23):7862-70.

[2684] Zhao L, Zhang Q, Ma W, Tian F, Shen H, et al. (2017). A combination of quercetin and resveratrol reduces obesity in high-fat diet-fed rats by modulation of gut microbiota. *Food Funct*. Dec 13;8(12):4644-4656.

[2685] Chen Q, Hu YE, Xia ZQ. (2000). Action of Sapogenin from Zhimu on learning and memory ability and free-radical metabolism in mouse D-galactose dementia model. *Pharmacol Clin Chin Mater Med*. 2000;16:14–16.

[2686] Ma YQ, Zhou XM, Wang LH, Cao YL. (2004). Anti-aging action of saponins from Anemarrhena asphodeloides Bge. on D-galactose model mice. *J Shenyang Pharma Univ*. 2004;21:450–3.

[2687] Deng Y, Ma BP, Xu QP, Xiong CQ. (2005). Effect and mechanism of effective component in Zhimu on ability of learning and memory in vascular dementia rats. *Chin Pharmacol Bull*. Jul;21:830–3.

[2688] Chen Q, Hu Y, Xia Z. (2001). [The effects of ZMS on learning and memory ability and brain choline acetyltransferase in scopolamine-induced mouse model]. *Zhong Yao Cai*. Jul; 24(7):496-8.

[2689] Hu M, Hu YE, Zhang W, Zongqin X. (2001). The effect of ZMS on brain M receptor in aged rats. *Chin J Nucl Med*. 2001;21:158–61.

[2690] Ibid. Chen. (2000).

[2691] Wang W, Wang W, Yao G, Ren Q, Wang D, et al. (2018). Novel sarsasapongenin-triazolyl hybrids as potential anti-Alzheimer's agents: Design, synthesis and biological evaluation. *Eur J Med Chem*. May 10;151:351-362.

[2692] Lee Y, Jung JC, Jang S, Kim J, Ali Z, Khan IA, et al. (2013). Anti-inflammatory and neuroprotective effects of constituents isolated from Rhodiola rosea. *Evid Based Complement Alt Med*. 2013:514049.

[2693] Nabavi SF, Braidy N, Orhan IE, Badiee A, Daglia M, et al. (2016). Rhodiola rosea L. and Alzheimer's disease: from farm to pharmacy. *Phyother Res*. Apr;30(4): 532-39.

[2694] Darbinyan V, Kteyan A, Panossian A, Gabrielian E, Wikman G, et al. (2000). Rhodiola rosea in stress induced fatique—a double blind cross over study of a standarized extract SHR-5 with a repeated low-dose regimen on the mental performance of healthy physicians during night duty. *Phytomedicine*. Oct;7:365-371.

[2695] Wu YQ, Yao WB, Gao XD, Wang H. (2004). Effects of the extracts of Rhodiola rosea L. on improving the ability of learning and memory in mice. *J China Pharm Univ*. Feb;35:69–72.

[2696] Qu ZQ, Zhou Y, Zeng YS, Li Y, Chung P. (2009). Pretreatment with *Rhodiola rosea* extract reduces cognitive impairment induced by intracerebroventrcular streptozotocin in rats: implication of anti-oxidative and neuroproteective effects. *Biomed Env Sci*. Aug;22(4):318-26.

[2697] Ma GP, Zheng Q, Xu MB, Zhou XL, Lu L, et al. (2018). Rhodiola rosea L. Improves Learning and Memory Function: Preclinical Evidence and Possible Mechanisms: Systematic Review Article. *Front Pharmacol*. Dec 4;9:1415.

[2698] Xie GQ, Sun XL, Tian SP, Chen, QS. (2004). Preventive effects of rhodosin and melatonin from damage induced by β-amyloid 1—40 in senile rats. *J Nanjing Med Univ*. 2004;18:203–6.

[2699] Jiang WH, Meng XT, Hao LM, Cui L, Dong Z, et al. (2001). Study of anti-aging and anti-dementia effects of Rhodosin on aging rats and experimental dementia rats. *J Jilin Univ*. 2001;27:127–9.

[2700] Van Dierman D, Marston A, Bravo J, Reist M. (2009). Monoamine oxidase inhibition by Rhodiola rosea L. roots. *J Ethnopharmacology*. Mar 18;122(2):397-401.

[2701] Hillhouse B, Ming DS, French CJ, Towers GHN.(2004). Acetylcholine esterase inhibitors in Rhodiola rosea. *Pharmaceu Biol*. 42;(1):68-72.

[2702] Palumbo DR, Occhiuto F, Spadaro F, Circosta C. (2012). Rhodiola rosea extract protects human cortical neurons against glutamate and hydrogen peroxide-induced cell death through reduction in the accumulation of intracellular calcium. *Phytother Res*. Jun;26(6): 878-83.

[2703] Kennedy DO, Scholey AB. (2006). The psychopharmacology of European herbs with cognition-enhancing properties. *Curr Pharm Des*. 12(35):4613-23.

[2704] Yesil-Celiktas O, Sevimli C, Bedir E, Vardar-Sukan F. (2010). Inhibitory effects of rosemary extracts, carnosic acid and rosmarinic acid on the growth of various human cancer cell lines. *Plant Foods Hum Nutr*. Jun; 65(2):158-63.

[2705] Bakirel T, Bakirel U, Keleş OU, Ulgen SG, Yardibi H. (2008). In vivo assessment of antidiabetic and antioxidant activities of rosemary (Rosmarinus officinalis) in alloxan-diabetic rabbits. *J Ethnopharmacol*. Feb 28; 116(1):64-73.

[2706] Pérez-Fons L, Garzón MT, Micol V. (2010). Relationship between the antioxidant capacity and effect of rosemary (Rosmarinus officinalis L.) polyphenols on membrane phospholipid order. *J Agric Food Chem*. Jan 13; 58(1):161-71.

[2707] Yamamoto J, Yamada K, Naemura A, Yamashita T, et al. (2005). Testing various herbs for antithrombotic effect. *Nutrit*. May;21(5):580-7.

[2708] Haloui M, Louedec L, Michel JB, Lyoussi B. (2000). Experimental diuretic effects of Rosmarinus officinalis and Centaurium erythraea. *J Ethnopharmacol*. Aug;71(3):465-72.

[2709] Gülçin I, Küfrevioglu OI, Oktay M, Büyükokuroglu ME. (2004). Antioxidant, antimicrobial, antiulcer and analgesic activities of nettle (Urtica dioica L.). *J Ethnopharmacol.* Feb;90(2-3):205-15.

[2710] Dias PC, Foglio MA, Possenti A, de Carvalho JE. (2000). Antiulcerogenic activity of crude hydroalcoholic extract of Rosmarinus officinalis *J Ethnopharmacol.* Jan;69(1):57-62.

[2711] Bozin B, Mimica-Dukic N, Samojlik I, Jovin E. (2007). Antimicrobial and antioxidant properties of rosemary and sage (Rosmarinus officinalis L. and Salvia officinalis L., Lamiaceae) essential oils. *J Agric Food Chem.* Sep 19; 55(19):7879-85.

[2712] Cheung S, Tai J. (2007). Anti-proliferative and antioxidant properties of rosemary Rosmarinus officinalis. *Oncol Rep.* Jun; 17(6):1525-31.

[2713] González-Trujano ME, Peña EI, Martínez AL, Moreno J, Guevara-Fefer P, et al. (2007). Evaluation of the antinociceptive effect of Rosmarinus officinalis L. using three different experimental models in rodents. *Ethnopharmacol.* May 22; 111(3):476-82.

[2714] Estévez M, Ramírez R, Ventanas S, Cava R. (2007). Sage and rosemary essential oils versus BHT for the inhibition of lipid oxidative reactions in liver pâté. *LWT Food Sci Technol.* Jan;40(1):58–65.

[2715] Sotelo-Félix JI, Martinez-Fong D, Muriel De la Torre P. (2002). Protective effect of carnosol on CCl(4)-induced acute liver damage in rats. *Eur J Gastroenterol Hepatol.* Sep;14(9):1001-6.

[2716] Al-Dhabi NA, Arasu MV, Park CH, Park SU. (2015). An up-to-date review of rutin and its biological and pharmacological activities. *EXCLI Journal.* Jan 9;14:59-63.

[2717] Perk AA, Shatynska-Mytsyk I, Gerçek YC, Boztas K, Yazgan M, et al. (2014). Rutin mediated targeting of signaling machinery in cancer cells. *Cancer Cell Int.* Nov 30;14(1):124.

[2718] Park SE, Sapkota K, Choi JH, Kim MK, Him YH, et al. (2014). Rutin from Dendropanax morbifera Leveille protects human dopaminergic cells against rotenone induced cell injury through inhibiting JNK and p38 MAPK signaling," *Neurochemical Res.* Apr;39(4):707-18.

[2719] Magalingam KB, Radhakrishnan A, Haleagrahara N. (2013). Rutin, a bioflavonoid antioxidant protects rat pheochromocytoma (PC-12) cells against 6-hydroxydopamine (6-OHDA)-induced neurotoxicity. *Int J Mol Med.* Jul;23(1):235-40.

[2720] Wang YB, Ge ZM, Kang WQ, Lian ZX, Yao J, Zhou CY. (2015). Rutin alleviates diabetic cardiomyopathy in a rat model of type 2 diabetes. *Exp Ther Med.* Feb;9(2):451-455.

[2721] Ibid. Park. (2014).

[2722] Yu XL, Li YN, Zhang H, Su YJ, Zhou WW, et al. (2015). Rutin inhibits amylin-induced neurocytotoxicity and oxidative stress. *Food Funct.* Oct;6(10):3296-306.

[2723] Enogieru AB, Haylett W, Hiss DC, Bardien S, Ekpo OE. (2018). Rutin as a Potent Antioxidant: Implications for Neurodegenerative Disorders. *Oxid Med Cell Longev.* Jun 27;2018:6241017.

[2724] Hablemariam S. (2016). Rutin as a Natural Therapy for Alzheimer's Disease: Insights into its Mechanisms of Action. *Curr Med Chem.* 2016;23(9):860-73.

[2725] LuY, Foo LY. (2002). Polyphenolics of Salvia—a review. *Phytochemistry.* Jan;59(2):117-40.

[2726] Huang. *The Pharmacology of Chinese Herbs*, 2nd ed. CRC Press, 1999, p. 94.

[2727] Lopresti AL. (2017). Salvia (Sage):A Review of its Potential Cognitive-Enhancing and Protective Effects. *Drgus R D.*, Mar;17(1):53-64.

[2728] Zhang XZ, Qian SS, Zhang YJ, Wang RQ. (2016). Salvia miltiorrhiza: A source for anti-Alzheimer's disease drugs. *Pharm Biol.* 2016;54(1):18-24.

[2729] Li LX, Dai JP, Ru LQ, Yin GF, Zhao B. (2004). Effects of tanshinone on neuropathological changes induced by amyloid beta-peptide(1-40) injection in rat hippocampus. Acta *Pharmacol Sin.* Jul; 25(7):861-8;

[2730] Ibid. Wightman. (2017).

[2731] Zhuang PY, Cui G, Bian Y, Zhang M, Zhang J, et al. (2012). Direct stimulation of adult neural stem/progenitor cells in vitro and neurogenesis in vivo by salviaolic acid B. *PLoS One.* Apr;7(4):e35636.

[2732] Chong CM, Su H, Lu JJ, Wang Y. (2019). The effects of bioactive components from the rhizome of Salvia miltiorrhiza (Danshen) on the characteristics of Alzheimer's disease. *Chin Med.* May 21;14:19.

[2733] Ibid. Chong. (2019).

[2734] Ibid. Chong. (2019).

[2735] Eidi M, Eidi A, Bahar M. (2006). Effects of Salvia officinalis L. (sage) leaves on memory retention and its interaction with the cholinergic system in rats. *Nutrition.* Mar;22(3):321-6.

[2736] Akhondzadeh S, Noroozian M, Mohammadi M, Ohadinia S, Jamshidi AH, et al. (2003). Salvia officinalis extract in the treatment of patients with mild to moderate Alzheimer's disease: a double blind, randomized and place-controlled trial. *J Clin Parm Ther.* Feb;28(1):53-9.

[2737] Kolac UK, Ustuner, MC, Tekin N, Ustuner D, Colak E, et al. (2017). The Anti-Inflammatory and Antioxidant Effects of Salvia officinalis on Lipopolysaccharide-induced Inflammation in Rats. *J Med Food.* Dec;20(12):1193-1200.

[2738] Smorgan C, Mari E, Atti AR, Dalla Nora E, Zamboni PF, et al. (2004). Trace elements and cognitive impairment.: an elderly cohort study. *Arch Gerontol Geriatr Suppl.* 2004;(9): 393-402.

[2739] Davis CD, Uthus EO. (2004). DNA methylation, cancer susceptibility, and nutrient interactions. *Exp Biol Med (Maywood).* Nov; 229(10):988-95.

[2740] Davis CD, Uthus EO. (2002). Dietary selenite and azadeoxycytidine treatments affect dimethylhydrazine-induced aberrant crypt formation in rat colon and DNA methylation in HT-29 cells. *J Nutr.* Feb; 132(2):292-7.

[2741] Davis CD, Uthus EO, Finley JW. (2000). Dietary selenium and arsenic affect DNA methylation in vitro in Caco-2 cells and in vivo in rat liver and colon. *J Nutr.* Dec; 130(12):2903-9.

[2742] Xiang N, Zhao R, Song G, Zhong W. (2008). Selenite reactivates silenced genes by modifying DNA methylation and histones in prostate cancer cells. *Carcinogenesis.* Nov; 29(11):2175-81.

[2743] Davis CD, Milner J. (2004). Frontiers in nutrigenomics, proteomics, metabolomics and cancer prevention. *Mutat Res.* Jul 13; 551(1-2):51-64.

[2744] Kryscio RJ, Abner EL, Caban-Holt A, Lovell M, Goodman P, et al. (2017). Association of Antioxidant Supplement Use and Dementia in the Prevention of Alzheimer's Disease by Vitamin E and Selenium Trial (PREADViSE). *JAMA Neurol.* May 1;74(5):567-573.

[2745] Aaseth J, Alexander J, Biorklund G, Hestad K, Dusek P, et al. (2016). Treatment strategies in Alzheimer's disease: a review with focus on selenium supplementation. *Biometals.* Oct;29(5):827-39.

[2746] Ellwanger JH, Franke SI, Bordin DL, Pra D, Henriques JA. (2016). Biological functions of selenium and its potential influence on Parkinson's disease. *An Acad Bras Cienc.* 2016;88(3 Suppl):1655-1674.

[2747] Zhang X, Liu RP, Cheng WH, Zhu JH. (2019). Prioritied brain selenium retention and selenoprotein expression: Nutritional insights into Parkinson's disease. *Mech Ageing Dev.* Jun;180:89-96.

[2748] van Driel LM, Eijkemans MJ, de Jonge R, de Vries JH, van Meurs JB, et al. (2009). Body mass index is an important determinant of methylation biomarkers in women of reproductive ages. *J Nutr.* Dec; 139(12):2315-21.

[2749] Sack JS, Thieffine S, Bandiera T, Fasolini M, Duke GJ, et al. (2011). Structural basis for CARM1 inhibition by indole and pyrazole inhibitors. *Biochem J.* Jun 1; 436(2):331-9.

[2750] Papakostas GI. (2009). Evidence for S-adenosyl-L-methionine (SAM-e) for the treatment of major depressive disorder. *J Clin Psychiatry.* 2009;70 Suppl 5:18-22.

[2751] Young SN, Shalchi M. (2005). The effect of methionine and S-adenosylmethionine on S-adenosylmethionine levels in the rat brain. *J Psychiatry Neurosci.* Jan;30(1):44-48.

[2752] Walder J, Popp S, Lange MD, Kem R, Kolter JF, et al. (2017). Genetically driven brain serotonin deficiency facilitates panic-like escape behavior in mice. *Transl Psychiatry.* Oct 3;7(10):e1246.

[2753] Southwick SM, Vythilingam M, Charney DS. (2005). The psychobiology of depression and resilience to stress: implications for prevention and treatment. *Annu Rev Clin Psychol.* 2005; 1():255-91.

[2754] Bhagat S, Agarwal M, Roy V. (2013). Serratiopeptidase: a systematic review of the existing evidence. *Int J Surg.* 2013;11(3):209-17.

[2755] Perry TL, Bratty PJ, Hansen S, Kennedy J, Urquhart N, et al. (1975). Hereditary mental depression and Parkinsonism with taurine deficiency. *Arch Neurol.* Feb;32(2):108-13.

[2756] Zhang L, Yuan Y, Tong Q, Jiang S, Xu Q, et al. (2015). Reduced plasma taurine level in Parkinson's disease: association with motor severity and levodopa treatment. *Int J Neurosci.* May 23:1-24

[2757] Ibid. Perry. (1975).

[2758] Ibid. Zhang. (2015).

[2759] Jang H, Lee S, Choi SL, Kim HY, Baek S, Kim Y. (2017). Taurine Directly Binds to Oligomeric Amyloid-B and Recovers Cognitive Deficits in Alzheimer Model Mice. *Adv Exp Med Biol.* 2017;975 Pt 1:233-241.

[2760] Chen C, Xia s, He J, Lu G, Xie Z, et al. (2019). Roles of taurine in cognitive function of physiology, pathology, and toxication. *Life Sci.* Aug 15;231:116584.

[2761] Gebara E, Udry F, Sultan S, Toni N. (2015). Taurine increases hippocampal neurogenesis in aging mice. *Stem Cell Res.* May;14(3):369-79.

[2762] Pasantes-Morales H, Ramos-Mandujano G, Hernandez-Benitez R. (2015). Taurine enhances proliferation and promotes neuronal specification of murine and human neural stem/progenitor cells. *Adv Exp Med Biol.* 2015;803:457-72.

[2763] Liu J, Wang HW, Liu F, Wang XF. (2015). Antenatal taurine improves neuronal regeneration in fetal rats with intrauterine growth restriction by inhibiting the Rho-ROCK signal pathway. *Metab Brain Dis.* Feb;30(1):67-73.

[2764] Ibid. Gebara. (2015).

[2765] Toyoda A, Koike H, Nishihata K, Iio W, Goto T. (2015). Effects of chronic taurine administration on gene expression, protein translation and phosphorylation in the rat hippocampus. *Adv Exp Med Biol.* 2015;803:473-80.

[2766] Wang Q, Huang H, Huang Z. (2015). Taurine inhibited the apoptosis of glial cells induced by hypoxia. *Wei Sheng Yan Jiu*. Mar;44(2):284-7.

[2767] Ward R, Dexter D, Crichton R. (2015). Ageing, neuroinflammation and neurodegeneration. *Front Biosci* (Schol Ed). 2015;7:189-204.

[2768] Xu S, He M, Zhong M, Li L, Lu Y, et al. (2015). The neuroprotective effects of taurine against nickel by reducing oxidative stress and maintaining mitochondrial function in cortical neurons. *Neurosci Lett*. Mar 17;590:52-7.

[2769] Wang Q, Zhu GH, Xie DH, Wu WJ, Hu P. (2015). Taurine enhances excitability of mouse cochlear neural stem cells by selectively promoting differentiation of glutamatergic neurons over GABAergic neurons. *Neurochem Res*. May;40(5):924-31.

[2770] Neuwirth LS, Volpe NP, Ng S, Marsillo A, Corwin C, et al. (2015). Taurine recovers mice emotional learning and memory disruptions associated with fragile x syndrome in context fear and auditory cued-conditioning. *Adv Exp Med Biol*. 2015;803:425-38.

[2771] Chang H, Lee DH. (2015). Analysis of Taurine as Modulator of Neurotransmitter in Caenorhabditis elegans. *Adv Exp Med Biol*. 2015;803:489-99.

[2772] Sun Q, Wang B, Li Y, Sun F, Li P. (2016). Taurine Supplementation Lowers Blood Pressure and Improves Vascular FUnciton in Prehypertension: Randomized, Double-Blind, Placebo-Controlled Study. *Hypertension*. Mar;67(3):541-9.

[2773] Moloney MA, Casey RG, O'Donnell DH, Fitzgerald P, Thompson C, et al. (2010). Two weeks taurine supplementation reverses endothelial dysfunction in young male type 1 diabetics. *Diab Vasc Dis Res*. Oct;7(4):300-10.

[2774] Ibid. Sun. (2016).

[2775] Ra SG, Choi Y, Akazawa N, Ohmori H, Maeda S. (2016). Taurine supplementation attenuates delayed increase in exercise-induced arterial stiffness. *Appl Physiol Nutr Metab*. Jun;41(6):618-23.

[2776] Wu JY, Schaffer SW, Azuma J. (2009). Taurine – a wonder molecule. Proceedings of the 17th International Taurine Conference. *J Biomed Sci*. 2010;17 Suppl 1:S2.

[2777] Hu J, Webster D, Cae J, Shao A. (2018). The safety of green tea and green tea extract consumption in adults – Results of a systematic review. *Regul Toxicol Pharmacol*. 2018 Jun;95:412-433.

[2778] Mandel SA, Amit T, Weinreb O, Youdim MB. (2011). Understanding the broad-spectrum neuroprotective action profile of green tea polyphenols in aging and neurodegenerative diseases. *J Alzheimers Dis*. 2011;25(2):187-208.

[2779] Rezai-Zadeh K, Arendash GW, Hou H, Fernandez F, Jensen M, et al. (2012). Green tea epigallocatechin-3-gallate (EGCG) reduces beta-amyloid mediated cognitive impairment and modulates tau pathology in Alzheimer transgenic mice. *Brain Res*. 1214 (2008): 177-87;

[2780] Williams RJ, Spencer JP. (2012). Flavonoids, cognition, and dementia: actions,, mechanisms, and potential therapeutic utility for Alzheimer disease. *Free Rad Bio Med*. 52 (2012): 35-45.

[2781] Kuriyama S, Hozawa A, Ohmori K, Shimazu T, Matsui T, et al. (2006). Green tea consumption and cognitive function: a cross-sectional study from the Tsurugaya Project 1. *Am J Clin Nutr*. 83 (2006): 355-61.

[2782] Ng TP, Feng L, Niti M, Kua EH, Yap KB. (2008). Tea consumption and cognitive impairment and decline in older Chinese adults. *Am J Clin Nutr*. 88 (2008):224-31.

[2783] Feng L, Gwee X, Kua EH, Ng TP. (2010). Cognitive function and tea consumption in community dwelling older Chinese in Singapore. *J Nutr Health Aging*. 14 (2010: 433-38.

[2784] Sueoka N, Suganuma M, Sueoka E, Okabe S, Matsuyama S. (2001). New function of green tea: prevention of lifestyle-related diseases. *Ann NY Acad Sci*. Apr; 928():274-80.

[2785] Raederstorff DG, Schlachter MF, Elste V, Weber P (2003). Effect of EGCG on lipid absorption and plasma lipid levels in rats. *J Nutr Biochem*. Jun; 14(6):326-32.

[2786] Yang YC, Lu FH, Wu JS, Wu CH, Chang CJ. (2004). The protective effect of habitual tea consumption on hypertension. *Arch Intern Med*. 2004;164:1534-40.

[2787] Hodgson JM, Puddey IB, Woodman RJ, Mulder TPJ, Fuch D, et al. (2012). Effects of black tea on blood pressure: a randomized controlled trial. *Arch Intern Med*. 2012;172:186-8.

[2788] Arab L, Liu W, Elashoff D. (2009). Green and black tea consumption and risk of stroke: a meta-analysis. *Stroke*. 2009;40:1786-92.

[2789] Kavanagh KT, Hafer LJ, Kim DW, Mann KK, Sherr DH, et al. (2001). Green tea extracts decrease carcinogen-induced mammary tumor burden in rats and rate of breast cancer cell proliferation in culture. *J Cell Biochem*. 2001; 82(3):387-98.

[2790] Lee AH, Su D, Pasalich M, Binns CW. (2013). Tea consumption reduces ovarian cancer risk. *Cancer Epidemiol*. 2013;37:54-9.

[2791] Nechuta S, Shu XO, Li HL, Yang G, Ji BT, et al. (2012). Prospective cohort study of tea consumption and risk of digestive system cancers: results from the Shanghai Women's Health Study. *Am J Clin Nutr*. 2012;96:1056-63.

[2792] Yan L, Wu S. (2001). Studies on the early prevention of tea polyphenol on senile dementia. *Zhejiang J Integ Trad Chin West Med*. 2001;11:538–40.

[2793] Li B, Wang BC, Yang WH. (2006). Effects of green tea polyphenols on learning behavior and AChE activity of mice with Alzheimer's disease. *J Beihua Univ (Nat Sci)* 2006;7:47–50.

2794 Osada K, Takahashi M, Hoshina S, Nakamura M, Nakamura S, et al. (2001). Tea catechins inhibit cholesterol oxidation accompanying oxidation of low density lipoprotein in vitro. *Comp Biochem Physiol C Toxicol Pharmacol.* Feb; 128(2):153-64.

2795 Slikker W, Youdim MB, Palmer GC, Hall E, Williams C, et al. (1999). The future of neuroprotection. *Ann NY Acad Sci.* 890:529-33.

2796 Salah N, Miller NJ, Paganga G, Tijburg L, Bolwell GP, et al. (1995). Polyphenolic flavanols as scavengers of aqueous phase radicals and as chain-breaking antioxidants. *Arch Biochem Biophys* 1995;322:339 –46.

2797 Nanjo F, Goto K, Seto R, Suzuki M, Sakai M, et al. (1996). Scavenging effects of tea catechins and their derivatives on 1,1-diphenyl-2picrylhydrazyl radical. *Free Radic Biol Med* 1996;21:895–902.

2798 Forester SC, Lambert JD. (2011). The role of antioxidant versus pro-oxidant effects of green tea polyphenols in cancer prevention. *Mol Nutr Food Res.* Jun;55(6):844-54.

2799 Donà M, Dell'Aica I, Calabrese F, Benelli R, Morini M, et al. (2003). Neutrophil restraint by green tea: inhibition of inflammation, associated angiogenesis, and pulmonary fibrosis. *Immunol.* Apr 15; 170(8):4335-41.

2800 Weinreb O, Mandel S, Amit T, Youdim MB. (2004). Neurological mechanisms of green tea polyphenols in Alzheimer's and Parkinson's diseases. *J Nutr Biochem.* Sep; 15(9):506-16.

2801 Khalabary AR, Khademi E. (2018). The green tea polyphenolic catechin epigallocatechin gallate and neuroprotection. *Nutr Neurosci.* 2018 Jul 25:1-14.

2802 Pervin M, Unno K, Ohishi T, Tanabe H, Miyoshi N, et al. (2018). Beneficial Effects of Green Tea Catechins on Neurodegenerative Diseases. *Molecules.* May 29;23(6).

2803 Machova Urdzikova L, Ruzicka J, Karova K, Kloudova A, Svobodova B, et al. (2017). A green tea polyphenol epigallocatechin-3-gallate enhances neuroregeneration after spinal cord injury by altering levels of inflammatory cytokines. *Neuropharmacology.* Nov;126:213-223.

2804 Schimidt HL, Garcia A, Martins A, Mello-Carpes PB, Carpes FP. (2017). Green tea supplementation produces better neuroprotection effects than red and black tea in Alzheimer-like rat model. *Food Res Int.* Oct;100(Pt 1):442-448.

2805 Ibid. Weinreb. (2004). *J Nutr Biochem.*

2806 Kim HS, Quon M, Jim JA. (2014). New insights into the mechanisms of polyphenols beyond antioxidant properties; lessons from the green tea polyphenol epigallocatechin 3-gallate. *Redox Biology.* Jan 10;2:187–195.

2807 Borgwardt S, Hammann F, Scheffler K, Kreuter M, Drewe J, et al. (2012). Neural effects of green tea extract on dorsolateral prefrontal cortex. *Eur J Clin Nutr.* Nov;66(11): 1187-92.

2808 Suzuki Y, Miyoshi N, Isemura M. (2012). Health-promoting effects of green tea. *Proc Jpn Acad Ser B Phys Biol Sci.* 2012;88(3):88-101.

2809 Hidese S, Ogawa S, Ota M, Ishida I, Yasukawa Z, et al. (2019). Effects of l-theanine administration on stress-related symptoms and cognitive functions in healthy adults: A randomized controlled trial. *Nutrients.* 2019;11(10):2362.

2810 Wakabayashi C, Numakawa T, Ninomiya M, Chiba S, Kunugi H. (2012). Behavioral and molecular evidence for psychotropic effects in L-theanine. *Psychopharmacology (Berl).* Feb; 219(4):1099-109.

2811 Tamano H, Fukura K, Suzuki M, Sakamoto K, Yokogoshi H, et al. (2014). Advantageous effect of theanine intake on cognition. *Nutr Neurosci.* Nov; 17(6):279-83.

2812 Ibid. Wakabayashi. (2012).

2813 Ibid. Tamano. (2014).

2814 Kakuda T, Nozawa A, Sugimoto A, Niino H. (2002). Inhibition by theanine of binding of [3H]AMPA, [3H]kainate, and [3H]MDL 105,519 to glutamate receptors. *Biosci Biotechnol Biochem.* Dec; 66(12):2683-6.

2815 Kakuda T. (2011). Neuroprotective effects of theanine and its preventive effects on cognitive dysfunction. *Pharmacol Res.* Aug; 64(2):162-8.

2816 Di X, Yan J, Zhao Y, Zhang J, Shi Z, et al. (2010). L-theanine protects the APP (Swedish mutation) transgenic SH-SY5Y cell against glutamate-induced excitotoxicity via inhibition of the NMDA receptor pathway. *Neurosc.* Jul 14; 168(3):778-86.

2817 Ibid. Hidese. (2019). *Nutrients.*

2818 Funakoshi H, Kanai M, Nakamura T. (2011). Modulation of tryptophan metabolism, promotion of neurogenesis and alteration of anxiety-related behavior in tryptophan 2,3-dioxygenase-deficient mice. *Int J Tryptophan Res.* 4:7-18.

2819 Olson CR, Mello CV. (2010). Significance of vitamin A to brain function, behavior and learning. *Mol Nutr Food Res.* Apr;54(4):489-95.

2820 Ono K, Yamada M. (2012). Vitamin A and Alzheimer's disease. *Geriatr Gerontol Int.* Apr;12(2):180-8.

2821 Sommer A. (2008). Vitamin A Deficiency and Clinical Disease: An Historical Overview. *J Nutr.* Oct;138(10):1835-1839.

2822 Troesch B, Weber P, Mohareri MH. (2016). Potential Links between Impaired One-Carbon Metabolism Due to Polymorphisms, Inadequate B-Vitamin Status, and the Development of Alzheimer's Disease. *Nutrients.* Dec 10;8(12):E803.

2823 De Jager CA, Oulhaj A, Jacoby R, Refsum H, Smith AD. (2012). Cognitive and clinical outcomes of homecysteine-lowering vitamin treatment in mild cognitive impairment: a randomized controlled trial. *Int J Geriatr Psychiatry.* Jun;27(6):592-600.

[2824] Smith AD, Smith SM, de Jager CA, Whitbread P, Johnston C, et al. (2010). Homocysteine-lowering by B vitamins slows the rate of accelerated brain atrophy in mild cognitive impairment: a randomized controlled trial. *PLoS One.* Sep 8;5(9):e12244.

[2825] Kinsella LJ, Riley DE. (1999). Nutritional deficiencies and syndromes associated with alcoholism. In: Goetz CG, Pappert EJ, (eds). *Textbook of Clinical Neurology.* Philadelphia: *W.B. Saunders Company.* (pp. 803–806).

[2826] Gibson GE, Hirsch JA, Fonzetti P, Jordan BD, Cirio RT, et al. (2016). Vitamin B1 (thiamine) and dementia. *Ann N Y Acad Sci.* Mar;1367(1):21-30.

[2827] Ibid. Kinsella. (1999).

[2828] Ba A. (2012). Effects of thiamine deficiency on food intake and body weight increment in adult female and growing rats. *Behav Pharmacol.* Sep;23(5-6):575-81.

[2829] Liu M, Alimov AP, Wang H, Frank JA, Katz W, et al. (2014). Thiamine deficiency induces anorexia by inhibiting hypothalamic AMPK.*Neuroscience.* May 16;267:102-13.

[2830] Singleton CK, Martin PR. (2001). Molecular mechanisms of thiamine utilization. *Curr Mol Med.* May; 1(2):197-207

[2831] Hegyi J, Schwartz RA, Hegyi V. (2004). Pellagra: dermatitis, dementia, and diarrhea. *Int J Dermatol.* 2004 Jan; 43(1):1-5.

[2832] Rajakumar K. (2000). Pellagra in the United States: a historical perspective. *South Med J.* Mar; 93(3):272-7.

[2833] Wu XY, Lu L. (2012). Vitamin b6 deficiency, genome instability and cancer. *Asian Pac J Cancer Prev.* 2012;13(11):5333-8.

[2834] Morris MS, Jacques PF, Rosenberg IH, Selhub J. (2002). Elevated serum methylmalonic acid concentrations are common among elderly Americans. *J Nutr.* Sep; 132(9):2799-803.

[2835] Carmel R. (1997). Cobalamin, the stomach, and aging. *Am J Clin Nutr.* 1997 Oct; 66(4):750-9.

[2836] E. Andres, Loukii NH, Noel E, Kaltenbach G, Abdelgheni MB, et al. (2004). Vitamin B12 (cobalamin) deficiency in elderly patients. *Can Med Ass J.* Aug 3;171(3).

[2837] Miller AL. (2008). The methylation, neurotransmitter, and antioxidant connections between folate and depression. *Alt Med Rev.* Sep;12(3): 216-26.

[2838] Clarke R, et al. (1998). Folate, Vitamin B12, Vitamin B12, and serum total homocysteine levels in confirmed Alzheimer's disease. *Arch Neurol.* 55(11): 1449-55.

[2839] Haan MN, Miller JW, Aiello AE, Whitmer RA, Jagust WJ, et al. (2007). Homocystein, B vitamins, and the incidence of dementia and cognitive impairment: results from the Sacramento Area Latino Study on Aging. *Am J Clin Nutr.* Feb;85(2): 511-17.

[2840] Quadri P, Fragiacomo C, Pezzati R, Zanda E, Forloni G, et al. (2007). Homocysteine, folate, and Vitamin B-12 in mild cognitive impairment, Alzheimer's disease, and vascular dementia. *Am J Clin Nutr.* Jul;80(1):114-22.

[2841] M. Ramos. (2005). Low folate status is associated with impaired cognitive function and dementia in the Sacramento Area Latino Study on Aging. *Am J Clin Nutr.* Dec;82(6): 1346-52.

[2842] Quinlivan EP, McPartlin J, McNulty H, Ward M, Strain JJ, et al. (2002). Importance of both folic acid and vitamin B12 in reduction of vascular disease. *Lancet.* Jan 19;359(9302):227-8.

[2843] Yajnik CS, Lubree HG, Thuse NV, Ramdas LV, Deshpande SS, et al. (2007). Oral vitamin B12 supplementation reduces plasma total homocysteine concentration in women in India. *Asia Pac J Clin Nutr.* 2007;16(1):103-9.

[2844] Cook S, Hess OM. (2005). Homocystein and B vitamins. *Handb Exp Pharmacol.* 2005;(170):325-38.

[2845] Miller AL. (2003). The methionine-homocystein cycle and its effects on cognitive diseases. *Altern Med Rev.* Feb;8(1):7-19.

[2846] Refsum H, Smith AD. (2003). Low vitamin B-12 status in confirmed Alzheimer's disease as revealed by serum holotranscobalamin. *J Neurol Neurosurg Psychiatry.* Jul;74(7):959-61.

[2847] Osimani A, Berger A, Friedman J, Porat-Katz BS, Abarbanel JM. (2005). Neuropsychology of vitamin B12 deficiency in elderly dementia patients and control subjects *J Geriatr Psychiatry Neurol.* Mar;18(1):33-8.

[2848] Vogiatzoglou A, Refsum H, Johnston C, Smith SM, Bradley KM, et al. (2008). Vitamin B12 status and rate of brain volume loss in community-dwelling elderly. *Neurology.* Sep 9;71(11):826-32.

[2849] Shen L, Ji HF. (2015). Associations between Homocysteine, Folic Acid, Vitamin B12 and Alzheimer's Disease: Insights from Meta-Analyses. *J Alzheimers Dis.* 46(3):777-90.

[2850] Wang HX, Wahlin A, Basun H, Fastbom J, Winblad B, et al. (2001). Vitamin B(12) and folate in relation to the development of Alzheimer's disease. *Neurology.* May 8;56(9):1188-94.

[2851] Kruman II, Kumaravel TS, Lohani A, Pedersen WA, Cutler RG, et al. (2002). Folic acid deficiency and homocysteine impair DNA repair in hippocampal neurons and sensitize them to amyloid toxicity in experimental modes of Alzheimer's disease. *J Neurosci.* Mar 1;22(5):1752-62.

[2852] Gagliano Taliun SA. (2019). Genetic determinants of low vitamin B12 levels in Alzheimer's disease risk. *Alzheimers Dement (Amst).* Jun 6;11:430-434.

[2853] Reynolds EH. (2002). Folic acid, ageing, depression, and dementia. *BMJ.* Jun 22; 324(7352):1512-5.

[2854] Goetz CG, Pappert EJ. *Textbook of Clinical Neurology*. Philadelphia: W.B. Saunders; 1999.

[2855] Savage DG, Lindenbaum J. (1995). Neurological complications of acquired cobalamin deficiency: clinical aspects. *Baillieres Clin Haematol*. Sep; 8(3):657-78.

[2856] Allen RH, Stabler SP, Savage DG, Lindenbaum J. (1990). Diagnosis of cobalamin deficiency I: usefulness of serum methylmalonic acid and total homocysteine concentrations. *Am J Hematol*. Jun; 34(2):90-8.

[2857] Kuzminski AM, Del Giacco EJ, Allen RH, Stabler SP, Lindenbaum J. (1998). Effective treatment of cobalamin deficiency with oral cobalamin. *Blood*. Aug 15; 92(4):1191-8.

[2858] Stover P. (2004). Physiology of folate and Vitamin B12 in health and disease. *Nut Rev*. Jun;62(6 Pt 2):S3-12.

[2859] Oh R, Brown DL. (2003). Vitamin 12 deficiency. *Am Fam Phys*. 67(5):979-86.

[2860] Tiemeier H, van Tuijl HR, Hofman A, Meijer J, Kiliaan AJ, et al. (2002). Vitamin B12, folate, and homocysteine in depression in the Rotterdam Study. *Am J Psychaitry*. Dec;159(12):2099-101.

[2861] Hong CH, Falvey C, Harris TB, Simonsick EM, Satterfield S, et al. (2013). Anemia and risk of dementia in older adults. *Neurology*. Aug 6;81(6): 528-33.

[2862] Andro M, Le Squere P, Estivin S, Gentric A. (2013). Anaemia and cognitive performances in the elderly: a systemic review. *Eur J Neurol*. Sep;20(9):1234-40.

[2863] McCarty MF, O'Keefe JH, DiNicolantonio JJ. (2019). A diet rich in taurine, cysteine, folate, B12 and betaine may lessen risk for Alzheimer's disease by boosting brain synthesis of hydrogen sulfide. *Med Hypotheses*. Aug 12;132:109356.

[2864] Walker JG, Batterham PJ, Mackinnon AJ, Jorm AF, Hickie I, et al. (2012). Oral folic acid and vitamin B-12 supplementation to prevent cognitive decline in community-dwelling older adults with depressive symptoms-the Beyond Aging Project: a randomized, controlled trial. *Am J Clin Nutr*. 2012 Jan;95(1):194-203.

[2865] Das UN. (2008). Folic acid and polyunsaturated fatty acids improve cognitive function and prevent depression, dementia, and Alzheimer's disease – But how and why? *Prostaglandins, Leukot Essent Fatty Acids*.Jan;78(1):11-9.

[2866] Borel P, Caillaud D, Cano NJ. (2015). Vitamin D bioavailability: state of the art. *Crit Rev Food Sci Nutr*. 2015;55(9):1193-205.

[2867] Goodwill AM, Szoeke C. (2017). A Systematic Review and Meta-Analysis of the Effect of Vitamin D on Cognition. *J Am Geriatr Soc*. Oct;65(10):2161-2168.

[2868] Pettersen JA. (2017). Does high dose vitamin D supplementation enhance cognition? A randomized trial in healthy adults. *Exp Gerontol*. Apr;90:90-97.

[2869] Van der Schaft J, Koek HL, Dijkstra E, Verhaar HJ, van der Schouw YT, et al. (2013). The association between vitamin D and cognition: a systematic review. *Ageing Res Rev*. Sep;12(4):1013-23.

[2870] Balion C, Griffith LE, Strifler L, Henderson M, Patterson C, et al. (2012). Vitamin D, cognition, and dementia: a systematic review and meta-analysis. *Neurology*. Sep 25;79(13):1397-405.

[2871] Michaelson K, Baron JA, Snellman G, Gedeborg R, Byberg L, et al. (2010). Plasma vitamin and mortality in older men: a community-based prospective cohort study. *Am J Clin Nutr*. Oct;92(4): 841-48.

[2872] Littlejohns TJ, Henley WE, Lang IA, Annweiler C, Beauchet O, et al. (2014). Vitamin D and the risk of dementia and Alzheimer disease. *Neurology*. Sep 2;83(10):920-8.

[2873] Toffanello ED, Coin A, Perissinotto E, Zambon S, Sarti S, et al. (2014). Vitamin D deficiency predicts cognitive decline in older men and women. *Neurology*. Dec 9;83(24):2292-98.

[2874] Yang K, Chen J, Li X, Zhou Y. (2019). Vitamin D concentration and risk of Alzheimer disease: A meta-analysis of prospective cohort studies. *Medicine (Baltimore)*. Aug;98(35):e16804.

[2875] Landel V, Annweiler C, Millet P, Morelio M, Feron F. (2016). Vitamin D, Cognition and Alzheimer's Disease: The Therapeutic Benefit is in the D-tails. *J Alzheimers Dis*. May 11;53(2):419-44.

[2876] Masoumi A, Goldenson B, Ghirmal S, Avagyan H, Zaghi J, et al. (2009). 1 alpha, 25-dihydroxyvitamin D3 interacts with curcuminoids to stimulate amyloid-beta clearance by macrophages of Alzheimer's disease patients. *J J Alzheimers Dis. 2009*;17(3):703-17.

[2877] Folstein MF, Folstein SE, McHugh PR. (1975). "Mini-mental state". A practical method for grading the cognitive state of patients for the clinician. *J Psychiatr Res*. Nov; 12(3):189-98.

[2878] Miller JW, Harvey DJ, Beckett LA, Green R, Farias ST, et al. (2015). Vitamin D Status and Rates of Cognitive Decline in a Multiethnic Cohort of Older Adults. *JAMA Neurol*. Nov;72(11):1295-1303.

[2879] Copp RP, Wisniewski T, Hentati F, Larnaout A, Ben Hamida M, et al. (1999). Localization of alpha-tocopherol transfer protein in the brains of patients with ataxia with vitamin E deficiency and other oxidative stress related neurodegenerative disorders. *Brain Res*. Mar 20; 822(1-2):80-7.

[2880] Vatassery GT, Nelson MJ, Maletta GJ, Kuskowski MA. (1991). Vitamin E (tocopherols) in human cerebrospinal fluid. *Am J Clin Nutr*. Jan; 53(1):95-9.

[2881] Burton GW, Traber MG. (1990). Vitamin E: antioxidant activity, biokinetics, and bioavailability. *Annu Rev Nutr*. 1990; 10():357-82.

[2882] Morris MC, Schneider JA, Li H, Tangney CC, et al. (2015). Brain tocopherols related to Alzheimer's disease neuropathology in humans. *Alzheimers Dement*. Jan;11(1):32-9.

[2883] Baldeiras I, Santana I, Proença MT, Garrucho MH, Pascoal R, et al. (2010). Oxidative damage and progression to Alzheimer's disease in patients with mild cognitive impairment. *J Alzheimers Dis*. 21(4):1165-77

[2884] Juliano L, Monticolo R, Straface G, Spoletini I, Gianni W, et al. (2010). Vitamin E and enzymatic/oxidative stress-driven oxysterols in amnestic mild cognitive impairment subtypes and Alzheimer's disease. *J Alzheimers Dis*. 21(4):1383-92.

[2885] Rinaldi P, Polidori MC, Metastasio A, Mariani E, Mattioli P, et al. (2003). Plasma antioxidants are similarly depleted in mild cognitive impairment and in Alzheimer's disease. *Neurobiol Aging*. Nov; 24(7):915-9.

[2886] Dysken MW, Sano M, Asthana s, Vertrees JE, Pallaki M, et al. (2014). Effect of vitamin E and memantine on functional decline in Alzheimer disease: the TEAM-AD VA cooperative randomized trial. *JAMA*. Jan 1;311(1):33-44.

[2887] Douaud G, Refsum H, de Jager CA, Jacoby R, Nichols TE, et al. (2013). Preventing Alzheimer's disease-related gray matter atrophy by B-vitamin treatment. Proc *Natl Acad Sci U S A*. 2013 Jun 4; 110(23):9523-8.

[2888] Ibid. Dysken. (2014).

[2889] Mangialasche F, Kivipelto M, Mecocci P, Rizzuto D, Palmer K, et al. (2010). High plasma levels of vitamin E forms and reduced Alzheimer's disease risk in advanced age. *J Alzheimers Dis*. 2010;20(4):1029-37.

[2890] Morris MC, Evans DA, Bienias JL, Tangney CC, Bennett DA, et al. Dietary intake of antioxidant nutrients and the risk of incident Alzheimer disease in a biracial community study. *JAMA*. Jun 26; 287(24):3230-7.

[2891] Morris MC, Evans DA, Tangney CC, Bienias JL, Wilson RS, et al. (2005). Relation of the tocopherol forms to incident Alzheimer disease and to cognitive change. *Am J Clin Nutr*. Feb; 81(2):508-14.

[2892] Mangialasche F, Xu W, Kivipelto M, Costanzi E, Ercolani S, et al. (2012).Tocopherols and tocotrienols plasma levels are associated with cognitive impairment. *Add Neuro Med Consortium. Neurobiol Aging*. Oct;33(10):2282-90.

[2893] Engelhart MJ, Geerlings MI, Ruitenberg A, van Swieten JC, Hofman A, et al. (2002). Dietary intake of antioxidants and risk of Alzheimer disease. *JAMA*. Jun 26; 287(24):3223-9.

[2894] Grodstein F, Chen J, Willett WC. (2003). High-dose antioxidant supplements and cognitive function in community-dwelling elderly women. *Am J Clin Nutr*. Apr; 77(4):975-84.

[2895] Hensley K, Barnes LL, Christov A, Tangney C, Honer WG, et al. (2011). Analysis of postmortem ventricular cerebrospinal fluid from patients with and without dementia indicates association of vitamin E with neuritic plaques and specific measures of cognitive performance. *J Alzheimers Dis*. 2011;24(4):767-74.

[2896] Sano M., Ernesto C., Thomas R.G., Klauber M.R., Schafer K, et al. (1997). A controlled trial of selegiline, alpha-tocopherol, or both as treatment for Alzheimer's disease. *N Engl J Med*. Apr 24;336(17):1216-22.

[2897] Mocchegiani E, Costarelli L, Giacconi R, Malavolta M, Basso A, et al. (2014). Vitamin E-gene interactions in aging and inflammatory age-related diseases: implications for treatment. A systematic review. *Ageing Res Rev*. 2014 Mar;14:81-101.

[2898] Dietary intake of antioxidants and risk of Alzheimer disease. Engelhart MJ, Geerlings MI, Ruitenberg A, van Swieten JC, Hofman A, Witteman JC, Breteler MM *JAMA*. 2002 Jun 26; 287(24):3223-9.

[2899] Morris MC, Evans DA, Bienias JL, Tangney CC, Wilson RS. (2002). Vitamin E and cognitive decline in older persons. *Arch Neurol*. Jul;59(7):1125-32.

[2900] Ibid. Morris. (2002).

[2901] Kang JH, Cook N, Manson J, Buring JE, Grodstein F. (2006). A randomized trial of vitamin E supplementation and cognitive function in women. *Arch Intern Med*. Dec 11-25; 166(22):2462-8.

[2902] Jiménez-Jiménez FJ, de Bustos F, Molina JA, Benito-León J, Tallón-Barranco A, et al. (1997). Cerebrospinal fluid levels of alpha-tocopherol (vitamin E) in Alzheimer's disease. *J Neural Transm (Vienna)*. 104(6-7):703-10.

[2903] M. Morris. (2004). Diet and Alzheimer's disease: what the evidence shows. *Med Gen Med*. 2004;6(1):48.

[2904] Fotuhi M, Zandi PP, Hayden KM, Khachaturian AS, Szekely CA, et al. (2008). Better cognitive performance in elderly taking antioxidant vitamins E and C supplements in combination with nonsteroidal anti-inflammatory drugs: The Cache County Study. *Alzheimers Dement*. May; 4(3):223-7.

[2905] Fulgoni VL 3rd, Keast DR, Bailey RL, Dwyer J. (2011). Foods, fortificants, and supplements: Where do Americans get their nutrients? *J Nutr*. Oct; 141(10):1847-54.

[2906] Ortega RM, Requejo AM, López-Sobaler AM, Andrés P, Navia B, et al. (2002). Cognitive function in elderly people is influenced by vitamin E status. *J Nutr.* Jul; 132(7):2065-8.

[2907] Grodstein F, Chen J, Willett WC. (2003). High-dose antioxidant supplements and cognitive function in community-dwelling elderly women. *Am J Clin Nutr.* Apr; 77(4):975-84.

[2908] Schrag M, Mueller C, Zabel M, Crofton A, Kirsch WM, et al. (2013). Review Oxidative stress in blood in Alzheimer's disease and mild cognitive impairment: a meta-analysis. *Neurobiol Dis.* Nov; 59():100-10.

[2909] Ibid. Jiménez-Jiménez. (1997). *J Neural Transm (Vienna).*

[2910] Schippling S, Kontush A, Arlt S, Buhmann C, Stürenburg HJ, et al. (2000). Increased lipoprotein oxidation in Alzheimer's disease. *Free Radic Biol Med.* Feb 1; 28(3):351-60.

[2911] Tohgi H, Abe T, Nakanishi M, Hamato F, Sasaki K, et al. (1994). Concentrations of alpha-tocopherol and its quinone derivative in cerebrospinal fluid from patients with vascular dementia of the Binswanger type and Alzheimer type dementia. *Neurosci Lett.* 1994 Jun 6; 174(1):73-6.

[2912] Cervantes B, Ulatowski LM. (2017). Vitamin E and Alzheimer's Disease – Is it Time for Personalized Medicine? *Antioxidants (Basel).* Sep;6(3):45.

[2913] Sano M., Ernesto C., Thomas R.G., Klauber M.R., Schafer K., Grundman M., Woodbury P., Growdon J., Cotman C.W., Pfeiffer E., et al. A controlled trial of selegiline, alpha-tocopherol, or both as treatment for Alzheimer's disease. *N. Engl. J. Med.* 1997;336:1216–1222

[2914] Ibid. Kryscio. (2017). *JAMA Neurol.*

[2915] Ibid. Morris. (2005). *Am J Clin Nutr.*

[2916] Instititute of Medicine. (2000). Dietary Reference Intake for Vitamin C, Vitamin E, Selenium, and Carotenoids. National Academy Press; Washington, D.C., USA.

[2917] NIH. Vitamin E (Fact Sheet). Retrieved Nov 1 2019 from https://ods.od.nih.gov/factsheets/VitaminE-HealthProfessional/.

[2918] Gulyas B, Halldin C, Sovago J, Sandell J, Cselenyi Z, et al. (2002). Drug distribution in man: a positron emission tomography study after oral administration of the labelled neuroprotective drug vinpocetine. *Eur J Nucl Med Mol Imaging.* 2002 Aug;29(8):1031-8.

[2919] Hindmarch, Fuchs HH, Erzigkeit H. (1991). Efficacy and tolerance of vinpocetine in ambulant patients suffering from mild to moderate organic psychosyndromes. *Int Clin Psychopharmacol.* Spring;6(1):31-43.

[2920] Pereira C, Agostinho P, Oliveira CR. (2000). Vinpocetine attenuates the metabolic dysfunction induced by amyloid beta-peptides in PC12 cells. *Free Radic Res.* Nov;33(5):497-506.

[2921] Kiss B, Cai NS, Erdo SL. (1991). Vinpocetine preferentially antagonizes quisqualate/AMPA receptor responses: evidence from release and ligand binding studies. *Eur J Pharmacol.* Dec 10;209(1-2):109-12.

[2922] Gaal L, Moinar P. (1990). Effect of vinpocetine on noradrenergic neurons in rat locus coeruleus. *Eur J Pharmacol.* Oct 23;187(3):537-9.

[2923] Hadjiev D. (2003). Asymptomatic ischemic cerebrovascular disorders and neuroprotection with vinpocetine. Ideggyogy Sz. May 20;56(5-6):166-72.

[2924] Horvath S. (2001). [The use of vinpocetine in chronic disorders caused by cerebral hypoperfusion]. [article in Hungarian]. Orv Hetil. Feb 25;142(8):383-9.

[2925] Balestreri R, Fontana L, Astengo F. (1987). A double-blind placebo controlled evaluation of the safety and efficacy of vinpocetine in the treatment of patients with chronic vascular senile dysfunction. *J Am Geriatr Soc.* 1987 May;35(5):425-30.

[2926] Bagoly E, Feher G, Szapary L. (2007). [The role of vinpocetine in the treatment of cerebrovascular diseases based in human studies]. *Orv Hetil.* Jul 22;148(29):1353-8.

[2927] Szilagyi G, Nagy Z, Balkay L, Boros I, Emri M, et al. (2005). Effects of vinpocetine on the redistribution of cerebral blood flow and glucose metabolism in chronic ischemic stroke patients: a PET study. *J Neurol Sci.* Mar 15;229-230:275-84.

[2928] Hadjiev D. (2003). Asymptomatic ischemic cerebrovascular disorders and neuroprotection with vinpocetine. *Ideggyogy Sz.* May 20;56(5-6):166-72.

[2929] Bagoly E, Feher G, Szapary L. (2007). [The role of vinpocetine in the treatment of cerebrovascular diseases based in human studies]. *Orv Hetil.* Jul 22;148(29):1353-8.

[2930] Protective activity of ethyl apovincaminate on ischaemic anoxia of the brain. Biró K, Kárpáti E, Szporny L *Arzneimittelforschung.* 1976; 26(10a):1918-20.

[2931] Szatmari SZ, Whitehouse PJ. (2003). Vinpocetine for cognitive impairment and dementia. *Cochrane Database Syst Rev.* 2003;(1):CD003119.

[2932] Nagy Z, Vargha P, Kovacs L, Bonoczk P. (1988). Meta-analysis of Cavinton. *Praxis.* Sep 15;7(9):63-8.

[2933] Ibid. Hadjiev. (2003).

[2934] Szakall S, Boros I, Balkay L, Emri M, Fekete I, et al. (1998). Cerebral effects of a single dose of intravenous vinpocetine in chronic stroke patients: a PET study. *J Neuroimaging.* Oct;8(4):197-204.

[2935] Ibid. Szakall. (1998).

[2936] Tamaki N, Matsumoto S. (19850. [Agents to improve cerebrovascular circulation and cerebral metabolism –vinpocetine]. [article in Japanese]. *Nippon Rinsho.* Feb;43(2):376-8.

[2937] Trejo F, Nekrassov V, Sitges M. (2001). Characterization of vinpocetine effects on DA and DOPAC release in striatal isolated nerve endings. *Brain Res.* Aug 3;909(1-2):59-67.

[2938] Sitges M, Nekrassov V. (1999). Vinpocetine selectively inhibits neurotransmitter release triggered by sodium channel activation. *Neurochem Res.* Dec;24(12):1585-91.

[2939] Bhatti JZ, Hindmarch I. (1987). Vinpocetine effects on cognitive impairments produced by flunitrazepam. *Int Clin Psychopharmacol.* Oct;2(4):325-31.

[2940] McDaniel MA, Maier SF, Einstein GO. (2003). "Brain-specific" nutrients: a memory cure? *Nutrition.* Nov-Dec;19(11-12):957-75.

[2941] DeNoble VJ. (1987). Vinpocetine enhances retrieval of a step-through passive avoidance response in rats. *Pharmacol Biochem Behav.* Jan;26(1):183-6.

[2942] Valikovics A, Csanyi A, Nemeth L. (2012). [Study of the effects of vinpocetine on cognitive functions]. *Ideggyogy Sz.* Mar 30;65(3-4):115-20.

[2943] Valikovics A. (2007). [Investigation of the effect of vinpocetine on cerebral blood flow and cognitive functions]. [article in Hungarian]. *Ideggyogy Sz.* Jul 30;60(7-8):301-10.

[2944] Subhan Z, Hindmarch I. (1985). Psychopharmacological effects of vinpocetine in normal healthy volunteers. *Eur J Clin Pharmacol.* 1985;28(5):567-71.

[2945] Jeon KI, Xu X, Aizawa T, Lim JH, Jono H, et al. (2010). Vinpocetine inhibits NF-kB-dependent inflammation via an IKK-dependent but PDE-indpendent mechanism. *Proc Natl Acad Sci U S A.* May 25; 107(21): 9795–9800.

[2946] Medina AE. (2010). Vinpocetine as a potent anti-inflammatory agent. *Proc Natl Acad Sci U S A.* June 1; 107(22): 9921–9922.

[2947] Truss MC, Stief CG, Uckert S, Becker AJ, Wefer J, et al. Phosphodiesterase 1 inhibition in the treatment of lower urinary tract dysfunction: from bench to bedside. *World J Urol.* 2001 Nov;19(5):344-50.

[2948] Truss MC, Stief CG, Uckert S, Becker AJ, Schultheiss D, et al. Initial clinical experience with the selective phosphodiesterase-I isoenzyme inhibitor vinpocetine in the treatment of urge incontinence and low compliance bladder. *World J Urol.* 2000 Dec;18(6):439-43.

[2949] Pilgramm M, Schumann K. (1986). Need for rheologically active, vasoactive and metabolically active substances in the initial treatment of acute acoustic trauma. *HNO.* Oct;34(10):424-8.

[2950] Bi D, Zhao Y, Jiang R, Wang Y, Tian Y, et al. (2016). Phytochemistry, Bioactivity and Potential Impact on Health of Juglans: the Original Plant of Walnut. *Nat Prod Commun.* Jun;11(6):869-80.

[2951] Yin TP, Cai L, Chen Y, Li Y, Wang YR, et al. (2015). Tannins and Antioxidants Activities of the Walnut (Juglans regia) Pellicle. *Nat Prod Commun.* Dec;10(12):2141-4.

[2952] Vinson JA, Cai Y. (2012). Nuts, especially walnuts, have both antioxidant quality and efficacy and exhibit significant potential health benefits. *Food Funct.* Feb;3(2):134-40.

[2953] Jahaban-Esfahlan A, Ostadrahimi A, Tabibiazar M, Amarowicz R. (2019). A Comparative Review on the Extraction, Antioxidant Content and Antioxidant Potential of Different Parts of Walnut (Juglans regia L.) Fruit and Tree. *Molecules.* Jun;24(11):2133.

[2954] Muthaiyah B, Essa MM, Chauhan V, Chauhan A. (2011). Protective effects of walnut extract against amyloid beta peptide-induced cell death and oxidative stress in PC12 cells. *Neurochem Res.* Nov; 36(11): 2096–2103.]

[2955] Poulose SM, Miller MG, Shukitt-Hale B. (2014). Role of walnuts in maintaining brain health with age. J Nutr. Apr;144(4 Suppl):561S-566S.

[2956] Chauhan N,Wang KC, Wegiel J, Malik MN. (2004). Walnut extracts inhibits the fibrillation of amyloid beta-protein, and also defibrillizes its preformed fibrils. *Curr Alzheimer Res.* Aug;1(3): 183-88.

[2957] Haddad EH, Gaban-Chong N, Oda K, Sabate J. (2014). Effect of a walnut meal on postprandial oxidative stress and antioxidants in healthy individuals. *Nutr J.* 10;13:4.

[2958] Guasch-Ferre M, Li J, Hu FB, Salas-Salvado J, Tobias DK. (2018). Effects of walnut consumption on blood lipids and other cardiovascular risk factors: an updated meta-analysis and systematic review of controlled trials. *Am J Clin Nutr.* Jul 1;108(1):174-187.

[2959] Widomska J, Zareba M, Subczynski WK. (2016). Can Xanthophyll-Membrane Interactions Explain Their Selective Presence in the Retina and Brain? *Foods.* 2016;5(1).

[2960] Feeney J, O'Leary N, Moran R, O'Halloran AM, Nolan JM, et al. (2017). Plasma Lutein and Zeaxanthin Are Associated With Better Cognitive Function Across Multiple Domains in a Large Population-Based Sample of Older Adults: Findings from The Irish Longitudinal Study on Aging. *J Gerontol A Biol Sci Med Sci.* Oct 1;72(10):1431-6

[2961] Lindbergh CA, Renzi-Hammond LM, Hammond BR, Terry DP, Mewborn CM, et al. (2018). Lutein and Zeaxanthin Influence Brain Function in Older Adults: A Randomized Controlled Trial. *J Int Neuropsychol Soc.* Jan;24(1):77-90

[2962] Ibid. Lindbergh. (2018).

[2963] Frederickson CJ, Koh JY, Bush A. (2005). The neurobiology of zinc in health and disease. *I Nat Rev Neurosci*. Jun; 6(6):449-62

[2964] Prakash A, Bharti K, Majeed AB. (2015). Zinc: indications in brain disorders. *Fundam Clin Pharmacol*. Apr;29(2):131-49.

[2965] Marger L, Schubert CR, Bertrand D. (2014). Zinc: an underappreciated modulatory factor of brain function. *Biochem Pharmacol*. Oct 15;91(4):426-35.

[2966] Yuan Y, Niu F, Liu Y, Lu N. (2014). Zinc and its effects on oxidative stress in Alzheimer's disease. *Neurol Sci*. Jun;35(6):923-8.

[2967] Brewer GJ. (2012). Copper excess, zinc deficiency, and cognition loss in Alzheimer's disease. *Biofactors*. Mar-Apr;38: 107-113.

[2968] Rasmussen HM, Johnson EJ. (2013). Nutrients for the aging eye. *Clin Interv Aging*. 2013;8:741-8.

[2969] Li Y, Hough CJ, Frederickson CJ, Sarvey JM. (2001). Induction of mossy fiber --> Ca3 long-term potentiation requires translocation of synaptically released Zn2+. *J Neurosci*. Oct 15; 21(20):8015-25.

[2970] Lu YM, Taverna FA, Tu R, Ackerley CA, Wang YT, et al. (2000). Endogenous Zn(2+) is required for the induction of long-term potentiation at rat hippocampal mossy fiber-CA3 synapses. *Synapse*. Nov; 38(2):187-97

[2971] Ibid. Li. (2001). *J Neurosci*.

[2972] Ibid. Lu. (2000). *Synapse*.

[2973] Ibid. Frederickson. (2005). *Nat Rev Neurosci*.

[2974] Haase H, Rink L. (2009). The immune system and the impact of zinc during aging. *Immun Ageing*. 2009 Jun 12;6:9.

[2975] Putics A, Vodros D, Malavolta M, Mocchegiani E, Csermely P, et al. (2008). Zinc supplementation boosts the stress response in the elderly: Hsp70 status is linked to zinc availability in peripheral lymphocytes. *Exp Gerontol*. May;43(5):452-61.

[2976] Barnett JB, Hamer DH, Meydani SN. (2010). Low zinc status: a new risk factor for pneumonia in the elderly. *Nutr Rev*. 2010 Jan;68(1):30-7.

[2977] Kahmann L, Uciechowski P, Warmuth S, Malavolta M, Mocchegiani E, et al. (2006). Effect of improved zinc status on T helper cell activation and TH1/TH2 ratio in healthy elderly individuals. Biogerontology. 2006 Oct-Dec;7(5-6):429-35.

[2978] Prasad AS. (2009). Impact of the discovery of human zinc deficiency on health. *J Am Coll Nutr*. Jun; 28(3):257-65.

[2979] Bhatnagar S, Taneja S. (2001). Zinc and cognitive development. *Br J Nutr*. May; 85 Suppl 2():S139-45.

[2980] Gao HL, Xu H, Xin N, Zheng W, Chi ZH, et al. (2011). Disruption of the CaMKII/CREB signaling is associated with zinc deficiency-induced learning and memory impairments. *Neurotox Res*. May; 19(4):584-91.

[2981] Halas ES, Hunt CD, Eberhardt M. (1986). Learning and memory disabilities in young adult rats from mildly zinc deficient dams. *J Physiol Behav*. 1986;37(3):451-8.

[2982] Ibid. Prakash. (2015). *Fundam Clin Pharmacol*.

[2983] Brewer GJ, Kanzer SH, Zimmerman EA, Molho ES, Celmins DF, et al. (2010). Subclinical zinc deficiency in Alzheimer's disease and Parkinson's disease. *Am J Alzheimers Dis Other Demen*. Nov; 25(7):572-5.

[2984] Avan A, Hoogenraad TU. (2015). Zinc and Copper in Alzheimer's Disease. *J Alzheimers Dis*. 46(1):89-92.

[2985] Adlard PA, Parncutt JM, Finkelstein DI, Bush AI. (2010). Cognitive loss in zinc transporter-3 knock-out mice: a phenocopy for the synaptic and memory deficits of Alzheimer's disease? *J Neurosci*. Feb 3; 30(5):1631-6.

[2986] Brewer GJ. (2014). Alzheimer's disease causation by copper toxicity and treatment with zinc. *Front Aging Neurosci*. May 16;6:92.

[2987] Ibid. Yuan. (2014). *Neurol Sci*.

[2988] Holtby S. Understanding Soft Gel Encapsulation. Retrieved Nov 25 2019 from https://www.naturalproductsinsider.com/supplement-delivery/understanding-soft-gel-encapsulation.

[2989] Medicare-Europe. Liquids vs Pills. Retrieved Nov 25 2019 from https://medicare-europe.co.uk/science-clinical-data/liquids-vs-pills.html.

[2990] Ibid. Medicare-Europe. Liquids vs Pills.

[2991] Ibid. Holtby S. Understanding Soft Gel Encapsulation.

[2992] Physician Desk Reference NPPDR #18.

[2993] Ibid. NPPDR #18.

[2994] Ibid. NPPDR #18.

[2995] Ibid. Medicare-Europe. Liquids vs Pills.

[2996] Ibid. NPPDR #18.

[2997] Ibid. NPPDR #18.

[2998] Ostro MJ. (1987) Liposomes. *Sci Am*. Jan;256(1):103-111.

[2999] Peuhkuri K, Vapaatalo H, Korpela R. (2010). Even low-grade inflammation impacts on small intestinal function. *World J Gastroenterol*. Mar 7;16(9):1057-1062.

3000 [no author or date]. When Diabetes Causes Stomach Problems. Retrieved Oct 20 2019 from https://www.webmd.com/diabetes/type-1-diabetes-guide/diabetes-and-gastroparesis#1.

3001 Ali B, Al-Wabel NA, Shams S, Ahamad A, Khan SA, et al. (2015). Essential oils used in aromatherapy: A systemic review. *Asian Pac. J. Trop.* Biomed. 2015;5:601–611.

3002 Kako H, Fukumoto S, Kobayashi Y, Yokogoshi H. (2008). Effects of direct exposure of green odour components on dopamine release from rat brain striatal slices and PC12 cells. *Brain Res Bull.* Mar 28; 75(5):706-12.

3003 Kiecolt-Glaser JK, Graham JE, Malarkey WB, Porter K, Lemeshow S, Glaser R. (2008). Olfactory influences on mood and autonomic, endocrine, and immune function. *Psychoneuroendocrinology.* Apr; 33(3):328-39.

3004 Angelucci FL, Silva VV, Dal Pizzol C, Spir LG, Praes CE, et al. (2014). Physiological effect of olfactory stimuli inhalation in humans: an overview. *Int J Cosmet Sci.* Apr; 36(2):117-23.

3005 Sell C.S. *The Chemistry of Fragrances—From Perfumer to Consumer.* 2nd ed. Quest International; Irvine, CA, USA: 2006.

3006 Milan-Calenti JC, Lorenzo-Lopez L, Alonso-Bua B, de Labra C, Gonzalez-Abraides I, et al. (2016). Optimal nonpharmacological management of agitation in Alzheimer's disease: challenges and solutions. *Clin Interv Aging.* Feb 22;11:175-84.

3007 Mantle F. (2002). The role of alternative medicine in treating postnatal depression. *Complement Ther Nurs Midwifery.* Nov; 8(4):197-203.

3008 Ballard CG, Gauthier S, Cummings JL, Brodaty H, Grossberg GT, et al. (2009). Management of agitation and aggression associated with Alzheimer disease. *Nat Rev Neurol.* May; 5(5):245-55.

3009 Pinweha S, Wanikiat P, Sanvarinda Y, Supavilai P (2008).The signaling cascades of Ganoderma Lucidum extracts in stimulating non-amyloidegenic protein secretion in human neuroblastoma SH-SY5Y cell lines. *Neurosci Lett*, 448: 62-6.

3010 Jimbo D, Kimura Y, Taniguchi M, Inoue M, Urakami K. (2009). Effect of aromatherapy on patients with Alzheimer's disease. *Psychogeriatrics.* Dec;9(4):173-9.

3011 Ibid. Ballard. (2009).

3012 Grace, U-M. (2015). Reducing anxiety and restlessness in institutionalised elderly care patients in Finland: A qualitative update on four years of treatment. *I J Clin Aromather.* 10(1):22-29.

3013 Ballard C, O'Brien J, Reichelt K, Perry E. (2002). Aromatherapy as a safe and effective treatment for the management of agitation in severe dementia: The results of a double-blind placebo-controlled trial with melissa. *J Clin Psychiatry*, 63(7): 553-558.

3014 Ibid. Jimbo. (2009). *Psychogeriatrics.*

3015 Forrester LT, Maayan N, Orrell M, Spector AE, Buchan LD, et al. (2014). . Aromatherapy for dementia. *Cochrane Database Syst Rev.* 2014 Feb 25;(2):CD003150.

3016 Yang YP, Wang CJ, Wang JJ. (2016). Effect of Aromatherapy Massage on Agitation and Depressive Mood in Individuals With Dementia. *J Gerontol Nurs.* Sep 1;42(9):38-46.

3017 Roh SY, Kim KH. (2013). [Effects of aroma massage on pruritis, skin pH, skin hydration and sleep in elders in long-term care hospitals]. [article in Korean]. *J Korean Acad Nurs.* Dec;43(6):726-35.

3018 Sanchez-Vidana DI, Ngai SP, He W, Chow JK, Lau BW, et al. (2017). The Effectiveness of Aromatherapy for Depressive Symptoms: A Systematic Review. *Evid Based Complement Alternat Med.* 2017;2017:5869315.

3019 Takeda A, Watanuki E, Koyama S. (2017). Effects of Inhalation Aromatherapy on Symptoms of Sleep Disturbance in the Elderly with Dementia. *Evid Based Complement Alternat Med.* 2017:1902807.

3020 Harris M, Richards KC, Grando VT. (2012). The effects of slow-stroke back massage on minutes of nighttime sleep in persons with dementia and sleep disturbance in the nursing home: a pilot study. *J Holist Nurs.* Dec;30(4):255-63.

3021 Hwang E, Shin S. (2015). The effects of aromatherapy on sleep improvement: a systematic literature review and meta-analysis. *J Altern Complement Med.* 2015 Feb;21(2):61-8.

3022 Snow LA, Hovanec L, Brandt J. (2004). A controlled trial of aromatherapy for agitation in nursing home patients with dementia. *J Altern Complement Med.* Jun;10(3):431-7.

3023 Chioca LR, Antunes VD, Ferro MM, Losso EM, Andreatini R. (2013). Anosmia does not impair the anxiolytic-like effect of lavender essential oil inhalation in mice. *Life Sci.* May 30;92(20-21):971-5.

3024 Smallwood J, Brown R, Coulter F, Irvine E, Copland. (2001). Aromatherapy and behavior disturbances in dementia: A randomized controlled trial. *Int J Geriatr Psychiatry.* Oct;15(10):1010-3.

3025 Ibid. Ballard. (2002). *Psychogeriatrics.*

3026 Holmes C, Hopkins V, Hensford C, MacLaughlin V, Wilkinson D, et al. (2002). Lavender oil as a treatment for agitated behaviour in severe dementia: a placebo controlled study. *Int J Geriatric Psychiatry.* 17(4):305–308.

3027 Burns A, Byrne J, Ballard C, and Holmes C. (2002). Sensory stimulation in dementia. *Brit Med J.* 325(7376):1312–1313, 2002.

3028 Han X, Gibson J, Eggett DL, Parker TL. (2017). Bergamot (Citrus bergamia) Essential Oil Inhalation Improves Positive Feelings in the Waiting Room of a Mental Health Treatment Center: A Pilot Study. *Phytother Res.* May;31(5):812-816.

3029 McDonnell B, Newcomb P. (2019). Trial of Essential Oils to Improve Sleep for Patients in Cardiac Rehabilitation. *J Altern Complement Med.* Sep 26.

3030 Halcón LL. (2002). Aromatherapy: therapeutic applications of plant essential oils. *Minn Med.* Nov; 85(11):42-6.

3031 Wilkinson SM, Love SB, Westcombe AM, Gambles MA, Burgess CC, et al. (2007). Effectiveness of aromatherapy massage in the management of anxiety and depression in patients with cancer: a multicenter randomized controlled trial. *J Clin Oncol.* Feb 10; 25(5):532-9.

3032 Rombola L, Amantea D, Russo R, Adornetto A, Berliocchi L, et al. (2016). Rational Basis for the Use of Bergamot Essential Oil in Complementary Medicine to Treat Chronic Pain. *Mini Rev Med Chem.* 2016;16(9):721-8.

3033 Lee YR, Shin HS. (2017). Effectiveness of Ginger Essential Oil on Postoperative Nausea and Vomiting in Abdominal Surgery Patients. *J Altern Complement Med.* Mar;23(3):196-200.

3034 Pehlivan S, Karadakovan A. (2019). Effects of aromatherapy massage on pain, functional state, and quality of life in an elderly individual with knee osteoarthritis. *Jpn J Nurs Sci.* Oct;16(4):450-458.

3035 Wattanathorn J, Jittiwat J, Tongun T, Muchimapura S, Ingkaninan K. (2011). Zingiber officinale Mitigates Brain Damage and Improves Memory Impairment in Focal Cerebral Ischemic Rat. *Evid Based Complement Alternat Med.* 2011;2011:429505.

3036 Oboh G, Ademiluyi AO, Akinyemi AJ. (2012). Inhibition of acetylcholinesterase activities and some pro-oxidant induced liper peroxidation in rat brain by two varieties of ginger (Zingiber officinale). *Exp Toxicol Pathol.* 2012 May;64(4):315-9.

3037 Zeng GF, Zhang ZY, Lu L, Xiao DQ, Zong SH, et al. (2013). Protective effects of ginger root extract on Alzheimer disease-induced behavioral dysfunction in rats. *Rejuvenation Res.* Apr;16(2):124-33.

3038 Saenghong N, Wattanathorn J, Muchimapura S, Tongun T, Piyavhatkul N, et al. (2012). Zingiber officinale Improves Cognitive Function of the Middle-Aged Healthy Women. *Evid Based Complement Alternat* Med. 2012; 2012:383062.

3039 Wu KL, Rayner CK, Chuah SK, Changchien CS, Lu SN, et al. (2008). Effects of ginger on gastric emptying and motility in healthy humans. *Eur J Gastroenterol Hepatol.* 2008 May;20(5):436-40.

3040 Khandouzi N, Shidfar F, Rajab A, Rahideh T, Hosseini P, et al. (2015). The effects of ginger on fasting blood sugar, hemoglobin a1c, apolipoprotein B, apolipoprotein a-I and malondialdehyde in type 2 diabetic patients. *Iran J Pharm Res.* Winter; 14(1): 131–140.

3041 Al-Yasiry AR, Kiczorowsha B. (2016). Frankincense—therapeutic properties. Postepy Hig Med Dosw (Online). Jan 4;70:380-91.

3042 Han X, Rodriguez D, Parker TL. (2017). Biological activities of frankincense essential oil in human dermal fibroblasts. *Biochem Open.* Feb 3;4:31-35.

3043 Ammon HP. (2002). [Boswellic acids (components of frankincense) as the active principle in treatment of chronic inflammatory diseases). [article in German.] Wien Med Wochenschr. 2002;152(15-16):373-8.

3044 Grover AK, Samson SE. (2016). Benefits of antioxidant supplements for knee osteoarthritis rationale and reality. *Nutr J.* Jan 5;15:1.

3045 Bannuru RR, Wang C. (2018). Efficacy of curcumin and Boswellia for knee osteoarthritis: Systematic review and meta-analysis. *Sci Direct.* Dec;48(3):416-429.

3046 Sharifabad MH, Esfandiari E, Alaei H. Effects of frankincense aqueous extract during gestational period on increasing power of learning and memory in adult offsprings. *J Isfahan Med Sch.* 2004;21:16–20.

3047 O'Connor DW, Eppingstall, Taffe T, Van Der Ploeg ES. (2013). A randomized, controlled cross-over trial of dermally-applied lavender (Lavandula angustifolia) oil as a treatment of agitated behaviour in dementia. *BMC Comp Alt Med.* 2013;13(315).

3048 Lee SY. (2005). [The effect of lavender aromatherapy on cognitive function, emotion, and aggressive behavior of elderly with dementia.] [article in Korean.] *Taehan Kanho Hakhoe Chi.* Apr;35(2):303-12.

3049 Moorman Li R, Gilbert B, Orman A, Aldridge P, Leger-Krall S, et al. (2017). Evaluating the effects of diffused lavender in an adult day care center for patients with dementia in an effort to decrease behavioral issues: a pilot study. *J Drug Assess.* Jan 23;6(1):1-5.

3050 Holmes C, Hopkins V, Hensford C, McLaughlin V, Wilkinson D, et al. (2002). Lavender oil as a treatment for agitated behavior in severe dementia: a placebo controlled study. *Int J Geriatr Psychiatry.* Apr;17(4):305-8.

3051 Woelk H, Schläfke S. (2010). A multi-center, double-blind, randomised study of the Lavender oil preparation Silexan in comparison to Lorazepam for generalized anxiety disorder. *Phytomedicine.* Feb; 17(2):94-9.

3052 Huang L, Abuhamdah S, Howes MJ, Dixon CL, Elliot MS, et al. (2008). Pharmacological profile of essential oils derived from Lavandula angustifolia and Melissa officinalis with anti-agitation properties: focus on ligand-gated channels. *J Pharm Pharmacol.* Nov;60(11):1515–1522.

3053 Umezu T. (2000). Behavioral effects of plant-derived essential oils in the geller type conflict test in mice. *Jap J Pharmacol.* Jun;83(2):150-3.

3054 Shiina Y, Funabashi N, Lee K, Toyoda T, Sekine T, et al. (2008). Relaxation effects of lavender aromatherapy improve coronary flow velocity reserve in healthy men evaluated by transthoracid doppler echocardiography. *Int J Cardiol.* Sep26;129(2);193-7.

[3055] Ibid. McDonnell. (2019). *J Clin Psychiatry.*

[3056] Ibid. Jimbo. (2009). *Psychogeriatrics.*

[3057] Cavanagh HM, Wilkinson JM. (2002). Biological activities of lavender essential oil. *Phytother Res.* Jun; 16(4):301-8.

[3058] Kasper S, Gastpar M, Müller WE, Volz HP, Möller HJ, et al. (2010). Efficacy and safety of silexan, a new, orally administered lavender oil preparation, in subthreshold anxiety disorder - evidence from clinical trials. *Wien Med Wochenschr.* Dec; 160(21-22):547-56.

[3059] Kasper S, Gastpar M, Müller WE, Volz HP, Möller HJ, et al. (2010). Silexan, an orally administered Lavandula oil preparation, is effective in the treatment of 'subsyndromal' anxiety disorder: a randomized, double-blind, placebo controlled trial. *Int Clin Psychopharmacol.* Sep; 25(5):277-87.

[3060] Elisabetsky E, Marschner J, Onofre Souza D. (1995). Effects of linalool on glutamatergic system in the rat cerebral cortex. *Neurochem Res.* 20(4):461–465.

[3061] Hartman D, Coetzee JC. (2002). Two US practitioners' experience of using essential oils for wound care. *J Wound Care.* Sep; 11(8):317-20.

[3062] Kashani MS, Tavirani MR, Talaei SA, Salami M. (2011). Aqueous extract of lavender (Lavandula angustifolia) improves the spatial performance of a rat model of Alzheimer's disease. *Neurosci Bull.* Apr; 27(2):99-106.

[3063] Ibid. Ballard. (2002). *J Clin Psychiatry.*

[3064] Akhondzadeh S, Noroozian M, Mohammadi M, Ohadinia S, Jamshida AH, et al. (2003). Melissa officinalis extract in the treatment of patients with mild to moderate Alzheimer's disease: a double blind, randomised, placebo controlled trial. *J Neurol Neurosurg Psych.* 2003;74(7):863–866.

[3065] Perry EK, Pickering AT, Wang WW, Houghton P, Perry NSL. (1998). Medicinal plants and Alzheimer's disease: integrating ethnobotanical and contemporary scientific evidence. *J Alt Compl Med.* 1998;4(4):419–428.

[3066] Moss M, Hewitt S, Moss L, Wesnes K. (2008). Modulation of cognitive performance and mood by aromas of peppermint and ylang-ylang. *Int J Neurosci.* Jan;118(1):59-77.

[3067] Raudenbush B, Garyhem R, Sears T, Wilson I. (2009). Effects of Peppermint and Cinnamon Odor Administration on Simulated Driving Alertness, Mood and Workload. *N Am J Psychol.* 2009;11(2):245-256.

[3068] Moss M, Cook J, Wesnes K, Duckett P. (2003). Aromas of rosemary and lavender essential oils differentially affect cognition and mood in healthy adults. *Int J Neurosci.* Jan;113(1):15-38.

[3069] Ibid. Jimbo. (2009). *Psychogeriatrics.*

[3070] Atsumi T, Tonosaki K. (2007). Smelling lavender and rosemary increases free radical scavenging activity and decreases cortisol level in saliva. *Psychiatry Res.* Feb 28;150(1):89-96.

[3071] Perry EK, Pickering AT, Wang WW, Houghton PJ, Perry NS. Medicinal plants and Alzheimer's disease: from ethnobotany to phytotherapy. *J Pharm Pharmacol.* 1999;51(5):527–534.

[3072] Hongratanaworakit T, Buchbauer G. (2006). Relaxing effect of ylang ylang oil on humans after transdermal absorption. *Phytother Res.* Sep;20(9):758-63.

[3073] Sauer A. (2015). Manage Dementia's Side Effects with These 7 Essential Oils. Retrieved Nov 20 2019 from https://www.alzheimers.net/10-10-14-essential-oils-dementia/.

[3074] Saedi N, Crawford GH. (2006). Botanical briefs: ylang-ylang oil--extracts from the tree Cananga odorata. *Cutis.* Mar; 77(3):149-50.

[3075] Sink KM, Holden KF, Yaffe K. (2005). Pharmacological treatment of neuropsychiatric symptoms of dementia: a review of the evidence. *JAMA.* Feb 2; 293(5):596-608.

[3076] Peisah C, Chan DK, McKay R, Kurrle SE, Reutens SG. (2011). Practical guidelines for the acute emergency sedation of the severely agitated older patient. *Intern Med J.* Sep; 41(9):651-7.

[3077] Wollen KA. (2010). Alzheimer's disease: the pros and cons of pharmaceutical, nutritional, botanical, and stimulatory therapies, with a discussion of treatment strategies from the perspective of patients and practitioners. *Altern Med Rev.* Sep; 15(3):223-44.

[3078] Manyam BV. (1999). Dementia in Ayurveda. *J Altern Complement Med.* Feb; 5(1):81-8.

[3079] Schlebusch L, Bosch BA, Polglase G, Kleinschmidt I, Pillay BJ, Cassimjee MH. (2000). A double-blind, placebo-controlled, double-centre study of the effects of an oral multivitamin-mineral combination on stress. *S Afr Med J.* Dec; 90(12):1216-23.

[3080] Govindarajan R, Vijayakumar M, Pushpangadan P. (2005). Antioxidant approach to disease management and the role of 'Rasayana' herbs of Ayurveda. *J Ethnopharmacol.* Jun 3; 99(2):165-78.

[3081] Howes MJ, Perry NS, Houghton PJ. (2003). Plants with traditional uses and activities, relevant to the management of Alzheimer's disease and other cognitive disorders. *Phytother Res.* Jan; 17(1):1-18.

[3082] Ibid. Manyam. (1999). *J Altern Complement Med.*

[3083] Wollen KA. (2010). Alzheimer's disease: the pros and cons of pharmaceutical, nutritional, botanical, and stimulatory therapies, with a discussion of treatment strategies from the perspective of patients and practitioners. *Altern Med Rev.* 2010 Sep; 15(3):223-44

3084 Ibid. Schlebusch. (2000). S *Afr Med J.*

3085 Rege NN, Thatte UM, Dahanukar SA. (1999). Adaptogenic properties of six rasayana herbs used in Ayurvedic medicine. *Phytother Res.* Jun; 13(4):275-91.

3086 Oh JH, Lee TJ, Park JW, Kwon TK. (2008). Withaferin A inhibits iNOS expression and nitric oxide production by Akt inactivation and down-regulating LPS-induced activity of NF-kappaB in RAW 264.7 cells. *Eur J Pharmacol.* Dec 3; 599(1-3):11-7

3087 Abbas S, Singh N. In: Delhi D. R. A. D. O., (ed). New Delhi, India: Institute of Nuclear Medicine and Allied; 2006

3088 Ven Murthy MR, Ranjekar PK, Ramassamy C, Deshpande M. (2010). Scientific basis for the use of Indian ayurvedic medicinal plants in the treatment of neurodegenerative disorders: ashwagandha. *Cent Nerv Syst Agents Med Chem.* Sep 1; 10(3):238-46.

3089 Mishra LC, Singh BB, Dagenais S. (2000). Scientific basis for the therapeutic use of Withania somnifera (ashwagandha): a review. *Altern Med Rev.* Aug; 5(4):334-46.

3090 Ibid. Ven Murthy. (2010). Cent Nerv Syst Agents Med Chem

3091 Chaudhari KS, Tiwari NR, Tiwari RR, Sharma RS. (2017). Neurocognitive Effect of Nootropic Drug Brahmi Bacopa monnieri) in Alzheimer's Disease. *Ann Neurosci.* May; 24(2):111-122.

3092 Farooqui AA. (2010). Neurochemical aspects of neurotraumatic and neurodegenerative diseases. 2010:1–401.

3093 Sudhakara G, Ramesh B, Mallajah P, Sreenivasulu N, Saralakumari D. (2012). Protective effect of ethanolic extract of Commiphora mukul gum resin against oxidative stress in the brain of streptozotocin induced diabetic Wistar male rats. *EXCLI J.* Aug;11:592.

3094 Vestergaard M, Hamada T, Morita M, Takagi M. (2010). Cholesterol, lipids, amyloid Beta, and Alzheimer's. *Curr Alzheimer Res.* May; 7(3):262-70.

3095 Eckert GP, Kirsch C, Leutz S, Wood WG, Müller WE. (2003). Cholesterol modulates amyloid beta-peptide's membrane interactions. *Pharmacopsychiatry.* Sep; 36 Suppl 2():S136-43.

3096 Ibid. Vestergaard. (2010).

3097 Morley JE, Banks WA. (2010). Lipids and cognition. *J Alzheimers Dis.* 2010 20(3):737-47.

3098 Bihaqi SW, Sharma M, Singh AP, Tiwari M. (2009). Neuroprotective role of Convolvulus pluricaulis on aluminium induced neurotoxicity in rat brain. J *Ethnopharmacol.* Jul 30; 124(3):409-15.

3099 Malik J, Karan M, Vasisht K. (2011). Nootropic, anxiolytic and CNS-depressant studies on different plant sources of shankhpushpi. *Pharm Biol.* Dec; 49(12):1234-42.

3100 Rai KS, Murthy KD, Karanth KS, Nalini K, Rao MS, et al. (2002). Clitoria ternatea root extract enhances acetylcholine content in rat hippocampus. *Fitoterapia.* Dec; 73(7-8):685-9.

3101 Ibid. Bihaqi. (2009).

3102 Ibid. Malik. (2011).

3103 Yang F, Lim GP, Begum AN, Ubeda OJ, Simmons MR, et al. (2005). Curcumin inhibits formation of amyloid beta oligomers and fibrils, binds plaques, and reduces amyloid in vivo. *J Biol Chem.* Feb 18; 280(7):5892-901.

3104 Hong HS, Rana S, Barrigan L, Shi A, Zhang Y, et al. (2009). Inhibition of Alzheimer's amyloid toxicity with a tricyclic pyrone molecule in vitro and in vivo. *J Neurochem.* Feb; 108(4):1097-1108.

3105 Ibid. Yang. (2005).

3106 Ma QL, Yang F, Rosario ER, Ubeda OJ, Beech W, et al. (2009). Beta-amyloid oligomers induce phosphorylation of tau and inactivation of insulin receptor substrate via c-Jun N-terminal kinase signaling: suppression by omega-3 fatty acids and curcumin. *J Neurosci.* Jul 15; 29(28):9078-89.

3107 Shoba G, Joy D, Joseph T, Majeed M, Rajendran R, et al. (1998). Influence of piperine on the pharmacokinetics of curcumin in animals and human volunteers. *Planta Med.* May; 64(4):353-6.

3108 Glymphatic System May Play Key Role in Removing Brain Waste. (2016). *Neurology Reviews.* Oct;24(10):13

3109 Iliff JJ, Wang M, Liao Y, Plogg BA, Peng W, et al. (2012). A paravascular Pathway Facilitates CSF Flow Through the Brain Parenchyma and the Clearance of Interstitial Solutes, Including Amyloid B. *Sci Transl Med.* Aug 15;4(147):147ra111.

3110 Jessen NA, Munk ASF, Lundgaard I, Nedergaard M. (2016). The Glymphatic System—A Beginner's Guide. *Neurochem Res.* Dec;40(12):2583-2599.

3111 Newman T. (2019). How does your brain take out the trash? *Med News Today.* Retrieved Dec 4 2019 from https://www.medicalnewstoday.com/articles/325493.php#1.

3112 De Oliveria M, Radanovic M, Cotting P, de Mello H, Buchain PC, et al. (2015). Nonpharmacological Interventions to Reduce Behavioral and Psychological Symptoms of Dementia: A Systematic Review. *Biomed Res Int.* 2015:218980.

3113 Huang Di's Canon of Internal Medicine.

3114 Stan J. (2015). Dietary & Nutritional Guidelines from a TCM Perspective. *Eastern Currents* website. Easterncurrents.ca.

3115 Knopman D, Parisi J, Boeve BF, Cha RH, Apaydin H, et al. (2003). Vascular dementia in a population-based autopsy study. *Arch Neurol.* Apr;60(4):569-75.

3116 Sreenivasmurthy SG, Liu JY, Song JX, Yang CB, Malampati S, et al. (2017). Neurogenic Traditional Chinese Medicine as a Promising Strategy for the Treatment of Alzheimer's Disease. *Int J Mol Sci.* Jan 28;18(2):E272.

3117 Liu Q, Wang SC, Ding K. (2017). Research advances in the treatment of Alzhemer's disease with polysaccharides from traditional Chinese medicine. *Chin J Nat Med.* Sep;15(9):641-652.

3118 Guo X, Ma T. (2019). Effects of Acupuncture on Neurological Disease in Clinical Animal-Based Research. *Front Integr Neurosci.* Aug 30; 13:47.

3119 Lai HC, Chang QY, Hsieh CL. (2019). Signal Transduction Pathways of Acupuncture for Treating Nervous System Diseases. *Evid Based Complement Alternat Med.* Jul 11;2019:2909632.

3120 Jiang Y, Gao H, Turdu G. (2017). Traditional Chinese medicinal herbs as potential AChE inhibitors for anti-Alzheimer's disease: a review. *Biorg Chem.* Dec;75:50-61.

3121 Li L, Zhang L, Yang CC. (2016). Multi-Target Strategy and Experimental Studies of Traditional Chinese Medicine for Alzheimer's Disease Therapy. *Curr Top Med Chem.* 2016;16(5):537-48.

3122 Klimova B, Kuca K. (2017). Alzheimer's Disease and Chinese Medicine as a Useful Alternative Intervention Tool: A Mini-Review. *Curr Alzheimer Res.* 2017;14(6):680-685.

3123 Cao Y, Zhang LW, Wang J, Du SQ, Xiao LY, et al. (2016). Mechanisms of Acupuncture Effect on Alzheimer's Disease in Animal-Based Researches. *Curr Top Med Chem.* 2016;15(5):574.8.

3124 Dong W, Yang W, Li F, Guo W, Qian C, et al. (2019). Electroacupuncture Improves Synaptic Function in SAMP8 Mice Probably via Inhibition of the AMPK/eEF2K/eEF2 Signaling Pathway. *Evid Based Complement Alternat Med.* Sep 18;2019:82608.

3125 Jia Y, Zhang X, Yu X, Han J, Yu T, et al. (2017). Acupuncture for patients with mild to moderate Alzheimer's disease: a randomized controlled trial. *BMC Complement Altern Med.* Dec 29;17(1);556.

3126 Zhou S, Dong L, He Y, Xiao H. (2017). Acupuncture plus Herbal Medicine for Alzheimer's Disease: Systematic Review and Meta-Analysis. *Am J Chin Med.* 2017;45(7):1327-1344.

3127 Zeng BY. (2017). Effect and Mechanism of Chinese Herbal Medicine on Parkinson's Disease. *Int Rev Neurobiol.* 2017;135:57-76.

3128 Han L, Xie YH, Wu R, Chen C, Zhang Y, et al. (2017). Traditional Chinese medicine for modern treatment of Parkinson's disease. *Chin J Integr Med.* Aug;23(8):635-640.

3129 Wei W, Chen HY, Fan W, Ye SF, et al. (2017). Chinese medicine for idiopathic Parkinson's disease: A meta analysis of randomized controlled trials. *Chin J Integr Med.* Jan;23(1):55-61.

3130 Ahn S, Liu QF, Jang JH, Park J, Jeony HJ, et al. (2019). Gami-Chunggan Formula Prevents Motor Dysfunction in MPTP/p-Induced and A53T a-Synuclein Overexpressed Parkinson's Disease Mouse Model Through DJ-1 and BDNF Expression. *Front Aging Neurosci.* Aug ;11:230.

3131 Ma J, Yuan L, Wang SJ, Lei J, Wang Y, et al. (2019). [Electroacupuncture improved locomotor function by regulating expression of tyrosine hydroxylas and a-synuclein protein transcription activating factor 6 and transcription factor X box binding protein 1 mRNAs in substantia nigra of rats with Parkinson's disease.] [article in Chinese]. *Zhen Ci Yan Jiu.* Nov 25;44(11):805-9.

3132 Yu SW, Lin SH, Tsai CC, Chaudhuri KR, Huang YC, et al. (Acupuncture Effect and Mechanism for Treating Pain in Patients with Parkinson's Disease. *Front Neurol.* Oct 22;10:1114.

3133 Kwon S, Seo BK, Kim S. (2016). Acupuncture points for treating Parkinson's disease based on animal studies. *Chin J Integr Med.* Oct;22(10):723-7.

3134 Cheng FK. (2017). The use of acupuncture in patients with Parkinson's disease. *Geriatr Nurs.* Jul-Aug;38(4):301-314.

3135 Noh H, Kwon S, Cho SY, Jung SW, Moon SK, et al. (2017). Effectiveness and safety of acupuncture in the treatment of Parkinson's disease: A systematic review and meta-analysis of randomized controlled trials. *Complement Ther Med.* Oct;34:86-103.

3136 Kong KH, Ng HL, Li W, Ng DW, Tan SI, et al. (2017). Acupuncture in the treatment of fatigue in Parkinson's disease: A pilot, randomized, controlled, study. *Brain Behav.* Dec 29;8(1):e00897.

3137 Lee SH, Lim S. (2017). Clinical effectiveness of acupuncture on Parkinson disease: A PRISMA-compliant systematic review and meta-analysis. *Medicine (Baltimore).* Jan;96(3):35836.

3138 Sinclair-Lian N, Hollifield M, Menache M, Warner T, Viscaya J, et al. (2006). Developing a traditional Chinese medicine diagnostic structure for post-traumatic stress disorder. *J Altern Complement Med.* Jan-Feb;12(1):45-57.

3139 Khusid MA. (2015). Clinical indications for acupuncture in chronic post-traumatic headache management. *Mil Med.* Feb;180(2):132-6.

3140 Oh JY, Kim YK, Kim SN, Lee B, Jang JH, et al. (2018). Acupuncture modulates stress response by the mTOR signaling pathway in a rat post-traumatic stress disorder model. *Sci Rep.* aug 8;8(1):11864.

3141 Liu L, Liu H, Hou Y, Shen J, Qu X, et al. (2019). Temporal effect of electroacupuncture on anxiety-like behavior and c-Fos expression in the anterior cingulate cortex in a rat model of post-traumatic stress disorder. *Neurosci Lett.* Oct 15;711:134432.

3142 Zhang Y, Han Y, Zhao Z, Yan X. (2016). [Exploration of acupoints selection law for post-traumatic disorder treated with acupuncture and moxibustion]. *Zhongguo Zhen Jiu.* Nov 12;36(11):1229-1232.

3143 Church D, Feinstein D. (2017). The Manual Stimulation of Acupuncture Points in the Treatment of Post-Traumatic Stress Disorder: A Review of Clinical Emotional Freedom Techniques. *Med Acupunct.* Aug 1;29(4):194-205.

3144 Kang SS, Erbes CR, Lamberty GJ, Thuras P, Sponheim SR, et al. (2018). Transcendental Meditation for veterans with post-traumatic stress disorder. *Psychol Trauma.* Nov;10(6):675-680.

3145 Barnes VA. (2018). Transcendental Meditation and treatment for post-traumatic stress disorder. *Lancet Psychiatry.* Dec;5(12):946-947.

3146 Barnes VA, Monto A, Williams JJ, Rigg JL. (2016). Impact of Transcendental Meditation on Psychotropic Use Among Active Duty Military Service Members With Anxiety and PTSD. *Mil Med.* Jan;181(1):56-63.

3147 Tan L, Zeng L, Wang N, Deng M, Chen Y, et al. (2019). Acupuncture to Promote Recovery of Disorder of Consciousness after Traumatic Brain Injury: A Systematic Review and Meta-Analysis. *Evid Based Complement Alternat Med.* Mar 19:5190515.

3148 Chan ES, Bautista DT, Zhu Y, You Y, Long JT, et al. (2018). Traditional Chinese herbal medicine for vascular dementia. *Cochrane Database Syst Rev.* Dec 6;12:CD010284.

3149 Lin SK, Tsai YT, Lo PC, Lai JN. (2016). Traditional Chinese medicine therapy decreases the pneumonia risk in patients with dementia. *Medicine (Baltimore).* Sep;95(37):e4917.

3150 Ye Y, Zhu W, Wang XR, Yang JW, Xiao LY, et al. (2017). Mechanisms of acupuncture on vascular dementia- A review of animal studies. *Neurochem Int.* Jul;107:204-210.

3151 Harris ML, Titler MG, Struble LM. (2019). Acupuncture and Acupressure for Demential Behavioral and Psychological Symptoms: A Scoping Review. *West J Nurs Res.* Dec 5:193945919890552.

3152 Gimson A, Schlosser M, Huntley JD, et al, Support for midlife anxiety diagnosis as an independent risk factor for dementia: a systematic review, BMJ Open 2018; 8:e019399.

3153 Manoj K. Bhasin, Jeffery A. Dusek, Bei-Hung Chang, Marie G. Joseph, John W. Denninger, Gregory L. Fricchione, Herbert Benson, Towia A. Libermann. Relaxation Response Induces Temporal Transcriptome Changes in Energy Metabolism, Insulin Secretion and Inflammatory Pathways. PLoS ONE, 2013; 8 (5): e62817 DOI: 10.1371/journal.pone.0062817

3154 McCall T. (2019). 117 Health Conditions Benefited by Yoga (as found in scientific studies as of June 2019), Retrieved Dec 4 2019 from http://www.drmccall.com/117-health-conditions-helped-by-yoga.html.

3155 Fox KCR, Nijeboer S, Dixon ML, Floman JL, Ellamil M, et al. (2014). Is meditation associated with altered brain structure? A systematic review and meta-analysis of morphometrict neuroimaging in meditation practitioners. *Neurosci Biobehav Rev.* Jun;43:48-73.

3156 Streeter CC, Gerbarg RB, Saper RB, Ciraulo DA, Brown RP. (2012). Effects of yoga on the autonomic nervous system, gamma-aminobutyric acid, and allostasis in epilepsy, depression, and post-traumatic stress disorder. *Med Hypotheses.* May;78(5):571-9.

3157 Streeter CC, Whitfield TH, Owen L, Rein T, Karri SK, et al. (2010). Effects of yoga versus walking on mood, anxiety, and brain GABA levels: a randomized controlled MRS study. *J Alt Compl Med.* Nov;16(11):1145-1152.

3158 Solas M, Puerta E, Ramirez MJ. (2015) Treatment Options in Alzheimer´s Disease: The GABA Story. *Curr Pharm Des.* 21: 4960.

3159 Kiecolt-Glaser JK, Christian L, Preston H, Houts CR, Malarkey WB, et al. (2010). Stress, inflammation, and yoga practice. *Psychosomatic Med.* 72(2), 113-21.

3160 Cahn BR, Goodman MS, Peterson CT, Maturi R, Mills PJ. (2017). Yoga, Meditation and Mind-Body Health: Increased BDNF, Cortisol Awakening Response, and Altered Inflammatory Marker Expression after a 3-Month Yoga and Meditation Retreat. *Front Hum Neurosci.* Jun 26;11:315.

3161 Lazar SW, Kerr CE, Wasserman RH, Gray JR, Greve DN, et al. (2005). Meditation experience is associated with increased cortical thickness. *Neuroreport.* 16(17), 1893-7.

3162 Innes KE, Selfe TK, Khalsa DS, Kandati S. (2017). Meditation and Music Improve Memory and Cognitive Function in Adults with Subjective Cognitive Decline: A Pilot Randomized Controlled Trial. *J Alzheimers Dis.* 2017;56(3):899-916.

3163 Khalsa DS. (2015). Stress, Meditation, & Alzheimer's Disease Prevention: Where the Evidence Stands. *J Alzheimer's Dis.* 2015;48(1):1-12.

3164 Eyre HA, Siddarth P, Acevedo B, Van Dyk K, Paholpak P, et al. (2017). A randomized controlled trial of Kundalini yoga in mild cognitive impairment. *Int Psychogeriactrics.* 29(4), 557-567.

3165 Wells RE, Yeh GY, Kerr CE, Wolkin J, Davis RB, Tan Y, et al. (2013). Meditation's impact on default mode network and hippocampus in mild cognitive impairment: a pilot study. *Neurosci Lett.* 556,15–19.

3166 Hölzel BK, Carmody J, Vangel M Congleton C, Yerramsetti SM, et al. (2010). Mindfulness practice leads to increases in regional brain gray matter density. *Psych Res.* 191(1):36-43.

[3167] Paller, K. A., Creery, J. D., Florczak, S. M., Weintraub, S., Mesulam, M. M., Reber, P. J., ... Maslar, M. (2014). Benefits of mindfulness training for patients with progressive cognitive decline and their caregivers. American journal of Alzheimer's disease and other dementias, 30(3), 257–267.

[3168] Wong WP, Hassed C, Chambers R, Coles J. (2016). The Effects of Mindfulness on Persons with Mild Cognitive Impairment: Protocol for a Mixed-Methods Longitudinal Study. Front Aging Neurosci. 8, 156.

[3169] Wong WP, Coles J, Chambers R, Wu DB, Hassed C. (2017). The Effects of Mindfulness on Older Adults with Mild Cognitive impairment. J Alzheimers Dis Rep. Dec 2;1(1):181-193.

[3170] Travis F, Parim N. (2017). Default mode network activation and Transcendental Meditation practice: Focused Attention or Automatic Self-transcending? Brain Cogn. Feb;111:86-94.

[3171] Orme-Johnson DW, Barnes VA. (2014). Effects of the transcendental meditation technique on anxiety: a meta-analysis of randomized controlled trials. J Altern Complement Med. May;20(5):330-41.

[3172] Tomljenovic H, Begic D, Mastrovic Z. (2016). Changes in trait brainwave power and coherence, state and trait anxiety after three-month transcendental meditation [TM] practice. Psychiatr Danub. Mar;28(1):63-72.

[3173] Elder C, Nidich S, Moriaty F, Nidich R. (2014). Effect of transcendental meditation on employee stress, depression, and burnout: a randomized controlled study. Perm J. Winter;18(1):19-23.

[3174] Mahone MC, Travis F, Gevirtz R, Hubbard D. (2018). fMRI during Transcendental Meditation practice. Brain Cogn. Jun;123:30-33.

[3175] Ooi SL, Giovino M, Pak SC. (2017). Transcendental meditation for lowering blood pressure: an overview of systematic reviews and meta analysis. Complement Ther Med. Oct;34:26-34.

[3176] Urushidani S, Kuriyama A. (2016). Transcendental meditation and blood pressure. J Hum Hypertens. May;30(5):354.

[3177] Infante JR, Peran F, Rayo JI, Serrano J, Dominguez ML, et al. (2014). Levels of immune cells in transcendental meditation practitioners. Int J Yoga. Jul;7(2):147-51.

[3178] Ibid. Barnes. (2016). Mil Med.

[3179] Bonamer JR, Aquino-Russell C. (2019). Self-Care Strategies for Professional Development: Transcendental Meditation Reduces Compassion Fatigue and Improves Resilience for Nurses. J Nurses Prof Dev. Mar/Apr;35(2):93:97.

[3180] Leach MJ, Francis A, Ziaian T. (2015). Transcendental Meditation for the improvement of health and wellbeing in community-dwelling dementia caregivers [TRANSCENDENT]; a randomized wait-list controlled trial. BMC Complement Altern Med. May 8;15:145.

[3181] Russell-Williams J, Jaroudi W, Perich T, Hoscheidt S, El Haj M, et al. (2018). Mindfulness and meditation: treating cognitive impairment and reducing stress in dementia. Rev Neurosci. Sep 25;29(7):791-804.

[3182] Donovan NJ, Okereke OI, Vannini P, Amariglio RE, Rentz DM, et al. (2016). Association of higher cortical amyloid burden with loneliness in cognitively normal older adults. JAMA Psychiatry. Dec 1;73(12): 1230-37.

[3183] Schlegel AA, Rudelson JJ, Tse PU. (2012). White matter structure changes as adults learn a second language. J Cogn Neurosci. Aug;24(8):1664-70.

[3184] Belleville S, Clement F, Mellah S, Gilbert B, Fontaine F, et al. (2011). Training-related brain plasticity in subjects at risk of developing Alzheimer's disease. Brain. Jun;134(Pt 5):1623-34.

[3185] Landau SM, Marks SM, Mormino EC, Rabinovici GD, Oh H, et al. (2012). Association of lifetime cognitive engagement and low B-amyloid deposition. Arch Neurol. May;69:623-29.

[3186] Ibid. Horowitz. (2020). Science.

[3187] Muller S, Preische O, Sohrabi HR, Graber S, Jucker M, et al. (2018). Relationship between physical activity, cognition, and pathology in autosomal dominant Alzheimer's disease. Alzheimers Dement. Nov;14(11):1427-1437.

[3188] Head D, Bugg JM, Goate AM, Fagan AM, Mintun MA, et al. (2012). Exercise engagement as a moderator of the effect of ApoE genotype on amyloid deposition. Arch Neurol. May;69(5):636-43.

[3189] Reynolds G. (2019). The Right Kind of Exercise May Boost Memory and Lower Dementia Risk. New York Times. Nov. 6, 2019.

[3190] Kovacevic A, Fenesi B, Paolucci E, Heisz JJ. (2019). The effects of aerobic exercise intensity on memory in older adults. Appl Physiol Nutr Metab. Oct 30.

[3191] Delwel S, Binnekade TT, Perez RSGM, Hertogh CMPM, Scherder EJA, et al. (2018). Oral hygiene and oral health in older people with dementia: A comprehensive review with focus on oral soft tissues. Clin Oral Investig. Jan;22(1): 93–108.

[3192] Levy BR, Slade MD, Kunkel SR, Kasl SV. (2002). Longevity increased by positive self-perceptions of aging. J Pers Soc Psychol. Aug;83(2): 261-70.

[3193] Richardson K, Fox C, Maidment I, Steel N, Loke YK, et al. (2018). Anticholinergic drugs and risk of dementia: case-control study. BMJ. Apr 25;361:k1315.

3194 Perry EK, Kilford L, Lees AJ, Burn DJ, Perry RH. (2003). Increased Alzheimer pathology in Parkinson's disease related to antimuscarinic drugs. *Ann Neurol.* Aug; 54(2):235-8.

3195 Ray PG, Meador KJ, Loring DW, Zamrini EW, Yang XH, et al. (1992). Central anticholinergic hypersensitivity in aging. *J Geriatr Psychiatry Neurol.* Apr-Jun; 5(2):72-7.

3196 Fox C, Richardson K, Maidment ID, Savva GM, Matthews FE, et al. Anticholinergic medication use and cognitive impairment in the older population: the medical research council cognitive function and ageing study. *J Am Geriatr Soc.* Aug; 59(8):1477-83.

3197 Ibid. Fox. (2011).

3198 Gray SL, Anderson ML, Dublin S, Hanlon JT, Hubbard R, et al. (2015). Cumulative use of strong anticholinergics and incident dementia: a prospective cohort study. *JAMA Intern Med.* Mar 1; 175(3): 401–407.

3199 Ibid. Gray. (2015). *JAMA Intern Med.*

3200 Ibid. Richardson. (2018). *BMJ.*

3201 Flicker C, Serby M, Ferris SH. (1990). Scopolamine effects on memory, language, visuospatial praxis and psychomotor speed. *Psychopharmacology (Berl).* 1990; 100(2):243-50.

3202 Merz B. (2015). Common anticholinergic drugs like Benadryl linked to increased dementia. Retrieved Dec 12 2019 from https://www.health.harvard.edu/blog/common-anticholinergic-drugs-like-benadryl-linked-increased-dementia-risk-201501287667.

3203 Ibid. Gray. (2015).

3204 Ibid. Merz (2015).

3205 Lucchetta RC, da Mata BPM, Mastroianni PC. (2018). Association between Development of Dementia and Use of Benzodiazepines: A Systematic Review and Meta-Analysis.

3206 Ballard C, Orrell M, YongZong S, Moniz-Cook E, Stafford J, et al. (2015). Impact of Antipsychotic Review and Nonpharmacological Intervention on Antipsychotic Use, Neuropsychiatric Symptoms and Mortality in People with Dementia Living in Nursing Homes: A Factorial Cluster-Randomized Control Trial by the Well-Being and Health for People with Dementia (WHELD) Program. *Am J Psychiatry.* Mar 1;173(3):252-62.

3207 Phillips LJ, Birtley NM, Petroski GF, Siem C, Rantz M. (2018). An observational study of antipsychotic medication use among long-stay nursing home residents without qualifying diagnoses. *J Psychiatr Ment Health Nurs.* Oct;25(8):463-474.

3208 Chaudhary, N. Soak Your Nuts Grains & Legumes. Retrieved Apr 18 2018 from http://myindianroots.blogspot.com/2015/03/soak-your-nuts-seeds-grains-legumes.html.

3209 Morgan R. (2017). At What Temperature Are Enzymes in Raw Food Destroyed? Retrieved Nov 2 2019 from https://caloriebee.com/diets/Food-Enzyme-Facts.

3210 (no author or date). How long does it take to digest different foods? Retrieved Nov 2 2019 from http://www.9tofine.net/en/diet/digestion-time-of-different-foods/.

3211 Watanabe E, Kuchta K, Kimura M, Rauwald HW, Kamei T, et al. (2015). Effects of bergamot (Citrus bergamia (Risso) Wright & Arn.) essential oil aromatherapy on mood states, parasympathetic nervous system activity, and salivary cortisol levels in 41 healthy females. *Forsch Komplementmed.* 2015;22(1):43-9.

3212 Seol GH, Lee YH, Kang P, You JH, Park M, et al. (2013). Randomized controlled trial for Salvia sclarea or Lavandula augustifolia: differential effects on blood pressure in female patients with urinary incontinence underdoing urodynamic examination. *J Altern Complement Med.* 2013 Jul;19(7):664-70.

3213 Sienkiewicz M, Głowacka A, Poznańska-Kurowska K, Kaszuba A, Urbaniak A, et al. (2015). The effect of clary sage oil on staphylococci responsible for wound infections. *Postepy Dermatol Alergol.* 2015 Feb; 32(1): 21–26.

3214 Seol G, Shim HS, Kim P Moon HK, Lee KH, et al. (2010). Antidepressant-like effect of Salvia sclarea is explained by modulation of dopamine activities in rats. *J Ethnopharmacol.* Jul 6;130(1):187-90.

3215 Al-Yasiry AR, Kiczorowsha B. (2016). Frankincense—therapeutic properties. *Postepy Hig Med Dosw (Online).* Jan 4;70:380-91.

3216 Haniadka R, Saldanha E, Sunita V, Palatty PL, Fayad R, et al. (2013). A review of the gastroprotective effects of ginger (Zingiber officinale Roscoe). *Food Funct.* Jun;4(6):845-55.

3217 Lee YR, Shin HS. (2017). Effectiveness of Ginger Essential Oil on Postoperative Nausea and Vomiting in Abdominal Surgery Patients. *J Altern Complement Med.* Mar;23(3):196-200.

3218 Lei H, Wei Q, Wang Q, Su A, Xue M, et al. (2017). Characterization of ginger essential oil/palygoskite composite (GEO-PGS) and its anti-bacteria activity. *Mater Sci Eng C Mater Biol Appl.* Apr 1;73:381-387.

3219 Karadag E, Samancioglu S, Ozden D, Bakir E. (2017). Effects of aromatherapy on sleep quality and anxiety of patients. *Nurs Crit Care.* Mar;22(2):105-112.

3220 Holmes C, Hopkins V, Hensford C, MacLaughlin V, Wilkinson D, et al. (2002). Lavender oil as a treatment for agitated behaviour in severe dementia: A placebo-controlled study. *Int J Geriatr Psychiatry*. Apr;17(4):305-8.

3221 Greenberg MJ, Slyer JT. (2018). Effectiveness of Silexan oral lavender essential oil compared to inhaled lavender essential oil aromatherapy on sleep in adults: a systemtic review. *JBI Database System Rev Implement Rep*. Nov;16(11):2109-2117.

3222 Nasiri A, Mahmodi MA, Nobakht Z. (2016). Effect of aromatherapy massage with lavender essential oil on pain in patients with osteoarthritis of the knee: A randomized controlled clinical trial. *Complement Ther Clin Pract*. Nov;25:75-80.

3223 Yazgan H, Ozogul Y, Kuley E. (2019). Antimicrobial influence of nanoemulsified lemon essential oil and pure lemon essential oil on foodborne pathogens and spoilage bacteria. *In J Food Microbiol*. Oct 2;306:108266.

3224 Ballard CG, O'Brien JT, Reichelt K, Perry EK. (2002). Aromatherapy as a safe and effective treatment for the management of agitation in severe dementia: *J Clin Psychiatry*. 2002 Jul;63(7):553-8.

3225 Salehi B, Valussi M, Morais-Braga MFB, Carneiro JNP, Leal ALAB, et al. (2018). Tagetes spp.Essential Oils and Other Extracts: Chemical Characterization and Biological Activity. *Molecules*. Nov 1;23(11):E2847.

3226 Kennedy D, Okelio E, Chazot P, Howes MJ, Ohiomokhare S, et al. (2018). Volatile Terpenes and Brain Function: Investigation of the Cognitive and Mood Effects of Menta x Piperita L. Essential Oil with In Vitro Properties Relevant to Central Nervous System Function. *Nutrients*. Aug 7;10(8):E1029.

3227 Raskovic A, Milanovic I, Paviovic N, Cebovic T, Vukmirovic S, et al. (2014). Antioxidant activity of rosemary (Rosmarinus officinalis L.) essential oil and itshepatoprotective potential. *BMC Complement Altern Med*. Jul 7;14:225.

3228 McCulloch M. (2018). 14 Benefits and Uses of Rosemary Essential Oil. Retrieved Dec 12 2019 from https://www.healthline.com/nutrition/rosemary-oil-benefits.

3229 Raman R. (2019). 11 Impressive Health Benefits of Saffron. Retrieved Dec 12 2019 from https://www.healthline.com/nutrition/saffron.

3230 Groves M. (2018). 11 Surprising Benefits of Spearmint Tea and Essential Oil. Retrieved Dec 12 2019 from https://www.healthline.com/nutrition/spearmint.

3231 (no author). Spike Lavender Essential Oil. Retrieved Dec 12 2019 from https://www.aromaweb.com/essential-oils/spike-lavender-oil.asp.

3232 (no author). Tangerine Oil Uses and Benefits. Retrieved Dec 12 2019 from https://www.doterra.com/US/en/blog/spotlight-tangerine-oil.

3233 Carson CF, Hammer KA, Riley TV. (2006). Melaleuca alternifolia (Tea Tree) oil: a review of antimicrobial and other medicinal properties. *Clin Microbiol Rev*. Jan;19(1):50-62.

3234 Dosoky NS, Setzer WN. (2018). Chemical composition and Biological Activites of Essential Oils of Curcuma Species. *Nutrients*. Sep 1;10(9):E1196.

3235 Moniri H. (2018). Evaluation of antioxidant properties of lemon verbena (Lippia citriodora) essential oil and its capacity in sunflower stabilization during storage time. *Food Sci Nutr*. Apr 2;6(4):983:990.

3236 (no author). Ylang Ylang: Benefits, Varieties & Uses. Retrieved Dec 12 2019 from https://www.newdirectionsaromatics.com/blog/products/all-about-ylang-ylang-oil.html.

3237 Liu SM, Wang SJ. Song SY, Zou Y, Wang JR, et al. (2017). Characteristic differences in essential oil composition of six Zanthoxylum bungeanum Maxim. (Rutaceae) cultivars and their biological significance. *J Zhejiang Univ Sci B*. Oct;18(10):917-920.

3238 Miller DH, Thompson AJ, Morrissey SP, MacManus DG, Moore SG, et al. (1992). High dose steroids in acute relapses of multiple sclerosis: MRI evidence for a possible mechanism of therapeutic effect. *J Neurol Neurosurg Psychiatry*. Jun; 55(6):450-3.

3239 Streeter CC, Whitfield TH, Owen L, Rein T, Karri SK, et al. (2010). Effects of yoga versus walking on mood, anxiety, and brain GABA levels: a randomized controlled MRS study. *J Alt Compl Med*. Nov;16(11):1145-1152.

3240 Morley JE. (2010). Nutrition and the brain. *Clin Geriatr Med*. 26, 89-98.

3241 Salerno-Kennedy R, Cashman KD. (2007). The relationship between nutrient intake and cognitive performance in people at risk of dementia. *Ir J Med Sci*. 176, 193-198.

3242 Mi W, van Wijk N, Cansev M, Sijben JW, Kamphuis PJ. (2013). Nutritional approaches in the risk reduction and management of Alzheimer's disease. *Nutrition*. 29, 1080-1089.

3243 Ibid. Nolan. (2015). *J Alzheimers Dis*.

3244 Nolan JM, Loughman J, Akkali MC, Stack J, Scanlon G, et al. (2011). The impact of macular pigment augmentation on visual performance in normal subjects: COMPASS. *Vision Res*. 51, 459-469.

3245 Beatty S, Chakravarthy U, Nolan JM, Muldrew KA, Woodside JV, et al. (2013). Secondary outcomes in a clinical trial of carotenoids with coantioxidants versus placebo in early age-related macular degeneration. *Ophthalmology*. 120, 600-606.

3246 Min JY, Min KB. (2014). Serum lycopene, lutein and zeaxanthin, and the risk of Alzheimer's disease mortality in older adults. *Dement Geriatr Cogn Disord*. 37, 246-256.

[3247] Rinaldi P, Polidori MC, Metastasio A, Mariani E, Mattioli P, et al. (2003). Plasma antioxidants are similarly depleted in mild cognitive impairment and in Alzheimer's disease. *Neurobiol Aging*. 24, 915-919.

[3248] Lee CS, Larson EB, Gibbons LE, Lee AY, McCurry SM, et al. (2019). Associations between recent and established ophthalmic conditions and risk of Alzheimer's disease. *Alzheimers Dement*. Jan;15(1)34-41.

[3249] Moon JY, Kim HJ, Park YH, Park TW, Park EC, et al. (2018). Association between Open-Angle Glaucoma and the Risks of Alzheimer's and Parkinson's Diseases in South Korea: a 10-year Nationwide Cohort Study. *Sci Rep*. Jul 24;(8)1:11161.

[3250] Chen YY, Lai YJ, Yen YF, Shen YC, Wang CY, et al. (2018). Association between normal tension glaucoma and the risk of Alzheimer's disease: a nationwide population-based cohort study in Taiwan. *BMJ Open*. Nov 5;8(11):e022987.

[3251] Giorgio A, Zhang J, Costantino F, De Stanfano N, Frezzotti P. (2018). Diffuse brain damage in normal tension glaucoma. *Hum Brain Mapp*. Jan;39(1):532-541.

[3252] Erasian M, Cerman E, Cekic O, Balci S, Dericioglu V, et al. (2015). Neurodegeneration in ocular and central nervouse systems: optical coherence tomography study in normal-tension glaucoma and Alzheimer disease. *Turk J Med Sci*. 2015;45(5):1106-14.

[3253] Ibid. Lee. (2019). *Alzheimers Dement*.

[3254] Ibid. Lee. (2019).

[3255] Ibid. Lee. (2019).

[3256] Cedars-Sinai. (2018). Cedars-Sinai Device May Provide Early Detection of Alzheimer's Disease. Retrieved Aug 24 2018 from https://www.cedars-sinai.edu/Research/Research-Areas/Neurosciences/Featured-Stories/Cedars-Sinai-Device-May-Provide-Early-Detection-of-Alzheimers-Disease.aspx.

[3257] Wikipedia. Sensitivity and specificity. Retrieved Aug 24 2018 from https://en.wikipedia.org/wiki/Sensitivity_and_specificity

[3258] (no author). Alzheimer's Association. Retrieved Jun 24 2020 from https://www.alz.org/alzheimers-dementia/research_progress/treatment-horizon.

[3259] Ibid. (no author). Alzheimer's Association. Treatment Horizon.

[3260] Vassar R. (2014). BACE1 inhibitor drugs in clinical trials for Alzheimer's disease. *Alzheimers Res Ther*. 2014;6:89.

[3261] Ibid. (no author). Alzheimer's Association. Treatment Horizon.

[3262] Sole-Domenech S, Rojas AV, Maisuradze GG, Scheraga HA, Lobel P, et al. (2018). Lysosomal enzyme tripeptidyl peptidase 1 destabilizes fibrillar AB by multiple endoproteolytic cleavages within the B-sheet domain. *PNAS*. Feb 13;115(7):1493-1498.

[3263] (no author). Alzheimer's Association. Retrieved Jun 24 2020 from https://www.alz.org/media/Documents/alzheimers-dementia-tau-ts.pdf

[3264] Zikova M, Nolle A, Kovacech B, Kontsekova E, Weisova P, et al. (2020). Humanized Tau Antibodies Promote Tau Uptake by Human Microglia Without Any Increase of Inflammation. *Act Neuropathol Commun*. May 29;8(1):74.

[3265] Ibid. (no author). Alzheimer's Association. Treatment Horizon.

[3266] Gutis P. (2020). FDA Gives Biogen Green Light to Relaunch Aducanumab Study of Trial Participants. Retrieved Jun 24 2020 from https://www.beingpatient.com/fda-approves-aducanumab-redosing-trial/.

[3267] Ibid. (no author). Alzheimer's Association. Treatment Horizon.

[3268] Ibid. (no author). Alzheimer's Association. Treatment Horizon.

[3269] Timmers M, Streffer JR, Russu A, Tominaga Y, Shimizu H, et al. (2018). Pharmacodynamics of Atabecestat (JNK-54861911), an Oral BACE1 Inihibitor in Patients with Early Alzheimer's Disease: Randomized, Double-Blind, Placebo-Controlled Study. *Alzheimers Res Ther*. Aug 23;10(1):85.

[3270] Novak G, Streffer JR, Timmers M, Henley D, Brashear HR, Bogert J, et al. (2020). Long-term Safety and Tolerabilty of Atabecestat (JNK-548861911), an Oral BACE1 Inhibitor, in Early Alzheimer's Disease Spectrum Patients: A Randomized,Double-Blind, Placebo-Controlled Study and a Two-Period Extension Study. *Alzheimers Res Ther*. May 14;12(1):58.

[3271] Ibid. (no author). Alzheimer's Association. Treatment Horizon.

[3272] Maquart FX, Siméon A, Pasco S, Monboisse C. (1993). Regulation of cell activity by the extracellular matrix: the concept of matrikines. *J Soc Biol*. 1999; 193: 423-428.

[3273] Pickart L, Margolina A. (2018). The Effect of the Human Plasma Molecule GHK-Cu on Stem Cell Actions and Expression of Relevant Genes. *OBM Geriatrics*. Aug 16;2(3).

[3274] Pickart L, Margolina A. (2018). Regenerative and Protective Actions of the GHK-Cu Peptide in the Light of New Gene Data. *Int J Mol Sci*. Jul;19(7):1987.

[3275] Pickart L. (2008). The human tri-peptide GHK and tissue remodeling. *J Biomater Sci Polym Ed*. 2008;19(8):969-988.

[3276] Chevalier G, Clark MD. (2019). Effect of LifeWave X39TM Patches on Brain as Seen with P3 Brain Mapping: Preliminary Results. Retrieved Oct 10 2020 from https://brainrenewal.nflalumni.org/wp-content/uploads/2020/10/EffectX39PatchBrain.pdf.

[3277] Muneta-Arrate I, Diez-Alarcia R, Horrillo I, Meana JJ. (2020). Pimavanserin Exhibits Serotonin 5_HT2A Receptor Inverse Agonism for Gai- and Neutral Antagonism for Gqa/11- proteins in Human Brain Cortex. *Eur Neuropsychopharmacol.* Jun 6;S0924-977X(20)30163-2.

[3278] Ibid. (no author). Alzheimer's Association. Treatment Horizon.

[3279] Sauer A. (2018). PET Scans Show Many Being Treated for Alzheimer's May Not Have Disease. Retrieved Jun 22 2020 from https://www.alzheimers.net/pet-scans-show-many-treated-for-alzheimers/.

[3280] Rapalino O, Weerasekera A, Moum SJ, Eikermann-Haerter K, Edlow BL, et al. (2020). Brain MR Spectroscopic Findings in 3 Consecutive Patients with COVID-19: Preliminary Observations. *ANJR Am J Neuroradiol.* Oct 29.

[3281] Mayo Clinic. (2020). COVID-19 (coronavirus): Long-term effects. Retrieved Jan 9 2021 from https://www.mayoclinic.org/diseases-conditions/coronavirus/in-depth/coronavirus-long-term-effects/art-20490351.

[3282] Lee Y, Min P, Lee S, Kim SW. (2020). Prevalence and Duration of Acute Loss of Smell or Taste in COVID-19 Patients. *J Korean Med Sci.* May 11;35(19:e174.

[3283] Passarelli PC, Lopez MA, Bonaviri GNM, Garcia-Godoy F, D'Addona A. (2020). Taste and smell as chemosensory dysfunctions in COVID-19 infection. *Am J Dent.* June;33(3):135-137.

[3284] Ibid. Mayo Clinic. (2020).

[3285] Ibid. Mayo Clinic. (2020).

[3286] Ellul MA, Benjamin L, Singh B, Lant S, Michael BD, et al. (2020). Neurological associations of COVID-19. *Lancet Neurol.* Sep;19(9):767-783.